A Barefoot Doctor's Manual

The American Translation of the
Official Chinese Paramedical Manual

Running Press
Philadelphia, Pennsylvania

*Canadian representatives: John Wiley & Sons Canada, Ltd.
22 Worcester Road, Rexdale, Ontario M9W 1L1*

*International representatives: Kaiman & Polon, Inc.
2175 Lemoine Avenue, Fort Lee, New Jersey 07024*

Printed in the United States of America

9   8   7   6   5
Digit on right indicates the number of this printing.

Library of Congress Cataloging in Publication Data

[Hu-nan Chung i yao yen chiu so. Ko wei hui]
 A Barefoot Doctor's Manual.

 Translation of Ch'ih chiao i sheng shou ts'e.
 Reprint of the 1974 ed. published by U. S. Dept. of Health, Educa-
tion, and Welfare, Public Health Service, National Institutes of Health,
Bethesda, Md., in series: DHEW publication no. (NIH) 75-695.
 1. Medicine, Popular. 2. Medicine, Chinese. I. Title. II. Series:
United States. Dept. of Health, Education, and Welfare. DHEW
publication; no. (NIH) 75-695.
RC82.H86 1977   610   77-364

ISBN 0-914294-91-1 lib. bdg.
ISBN 0-914294-92-X pbk.

Cover design by Jim Wilson

Text printed by Port City Press, Inc.

This book may be ordered directly from the publisher.
Please include 75 cents postage.
Try your bookstore first.

**Running Press
38 South Nineteenth Street
Philadelphia, Pennsylvania 19103**

Table of Contents

Preface to
A Barefoot Doctor's Manual

The "chijiao yisheng"—barefoot doctor—is the latest version of a venerable Chinese idea. Developed by the government of the People's Republic of China in the 1950's, the barefoot doctor program now includes some two million medical workers, stationed in the thousands of agricultural communes and hundreds of thousands of villages throughout the immense Chinese countryside. The term barefoot doctor may at first seem both confusing and inaccurate, for such workers are neither trained doctors, nor do they generally go about barefoot. The government defines them as being "peasants" who have had basic medical training and can handle medical emergencies, prescribe for simple injuries and illnesses, and apply treatments prescribed by a qualified doctor—and do all of this "without leaving productive work."

"Peasant" is the key word in the definition. Because it takes time to train sufficient doctors and nurses to serve a nation of almost a billion people, other supplementary measures were needed to bring at least primary health care to such a large, widely scattered population. It was the idea of the government to draw medical workers from among the people, especially from among the masses of farmers (or peasants), to teach them the basic medical skills, and to send them back to their homes to serve their neighbors and fellow villagers. In this way, any breach between the doctor and the patient, any acquisition of a false "status" by the "professional," could be avoided, while the people's primary medical needs could be met.

The word "barefoot" used in describing these medical workers further stresses their identification with the peasants, for it has long been the practice of farmers in some regions of China to work barefooted in their rice paddies. Thus the term "barefoot doctor," while it is not literally accurate, does communicate the essence of an idea.

Barefoot doctors compose the broad base of the health care pyramid in China. Practitioners of *preventive* medicine, they are responsible for recruiting all of the people to take an active role in health care and in sanitation, so that each individual may be responsible for fighting "against his own disease." Each commune or large village has a hospital staffed by one or more barefoot doctors. They are capable of responding to emergencies and of identifying and prescribing for such common illnesses as backaches, gastroenteritis, headaches, influenza, skin ailments, and sprains. Cases requiring more sophisticated treatments, or calling for an operation, are referred to the county hospitals, where fully trained doctors are available. Beyond the county level are yet larger hospitals, frequently allied to medical schools, where difficult cases may be sent for yet further tests, for diagnosis, and for complicated treatments. Often patients who have been sent on to a hospital are diagnosed and referred back to the local health care workes, who assume responsibility for monitoring the patient and providing the medication.

Barefoot doctors are selected by all the members of a village or commune, the basis of selection generally being an interest in medicine and an avowed desire to serve people. Their training at the county hospitals is conducted in periods lasting several months and is combined with closely supervised on-the-job work. The doctors are instructed both in Western medical technique and in the treatments and remedies developed in China over the span of a thousand years—including such unique practices as acupuncture, acupressure, and moxibustion. The use of a variety of herbs as medicines is also taught. For all their duties, the barefoot doctors are remunerated on the same scale as the other members of the commune.

An Explanation of the Manual

The *Barefoot Doctor's Manual* is not a textbook. The procedures discussed in the book are taught to the chijiao yishengs while they are attending classes at the county hospital. The *Manual* is a basic reference tool for the doctors, and it serves as a guide when they are uncertain of the techniques required for a certain procedure, or when the symptoms of an ailment have them perplexed. Although the *Manual* was originally prepared for the barefoot doctors of Hunan province, and published in 1970, the evidence now suggests that the book has been made available to barefoot doctors throughout the country. Some changes may be made in the manuals issued to a given province, for China embraces so many climatic regions that certain deseases and pests prevalent in one area are absent in another.

This translation, prepared by the Fogarty International Center, is of the original Hunan version. It lists one hundred and ninety-seven of the diseases occurring in the province, and a variety of traditional Chinese and Western treatments for the ailments. Descriptions are given for some five hundred herbs that are found in the province and considered helpful in the treatment of various problems, and their preparation and uses are explained. It should be noted that the inclusion of an illness in the *Manual* does not indicate that it is very prevalent. Rickets, for instance, was once a serious problem throughout China. Now, because of tremendous improvements in the diets of the Chinese, and because of the availability of Vitamin D, it has almost been eliminated—and when it does occur, it can be successfully treated.

The most arresting feature of the *Manual* for the Western reader is the inclusion of such treatments as acupuncture, massage, moxibustion, and herbal preparations. This is an important point, for the practice of such techniques makes Chinese medicine a hybrid science unlike any other medical system. When the new government of China began examining the health needs of the nation, there was a realization that traditional medical practices had been of great help to the people and, moreover, a large body of evidence suggesting that many of the treatments did, indeed, work. And, after 1949, there was neither enough manpower nor money to introduce Western medicine, with its drugs and elaborate machinery, to much of the country. Thus it was decided in 1950, and has been policy ever since, to integrate Western practices with traditional Chinese practices, using whatever worked, discarding what did not. This even-handed and pragmatic approach is evident throughout the *Manual*.

One further note: although this book was never intended to entertain or to provide a unique view of a distant and largely unknown culture, it does have an appeal besides its original purpose as a practical reference work for the use of barefoot doctors in the People's Republic of China. Not intended for presentation abroad, it remains free of doctrinaire messages and thus maintains a freshness and simplicity lacking in the official publications most countries prepare for distribution in other lands.

Publisher's Warning

The *Barefoot Doctor's Manual* has many potential applications. It is hoped that this re-issue will stimulate interest in the treatments discussed and present a model of what a *good*, simple medical text for the layperson should be. The book's discussion of symptoms is quite accurate, and its first aid techniques are comparable to those established by the Amerrican Red Cross. Its advocacy of a medical system based on prevention, a system in which all the people participate, is admirable.

However, there are certain ways in which this book should *not* be used. It is not the intention of the publisher to endorse for self-practice the treatments described in the text. Such treatments as acupuncture and moxibustion have only recently come under the study of Western medicine. While the techniques are beginning to receive validation, based on use in North America, some well intentioned laypeople and some medical charlatans have adapted the image, but not the substance, of acupuncture. The result has been some unusual, even bizarre, versions of the treatments used by the Chinese. Some qualified physicians are now practicing acupuncture in those cases where they judge it to be of help. Should the reader be interested in pursuing the possibility of such treatment, the best course would be to seek out a fully qualified physician who has incorporated such practices into his/her treatments. It is worth remembering that the only people in China allowed to prescribe and apply such treatments as acupuncture and moxibustion are personnel who have been trained intensively in the methods to be employed.

While the herbs and herbal. treatments recommended in *A Barefoot Doctor's Manual* may well be both harmless and effective, they require someone possessing both knowledge and experience in the identification and use of herbs as medicine to make proper use of them. Several people have obtained packets of herbs illegally imported from China, dosed themselves with the preparations, and obtained the most unfortunate results. The improper use of such herbs has evidently had at least some part in the death of one person on the West Coast.

There is an additional danger. Some Chinese herbs may have a close resemblance to varieties found growing in North America—but that does not mean that they can be assumed to act in the same way. There are qualified, very experienced, herbalists working in this country, and there exist a number of books dealing with American herbs and the uses to which they can be put. While the section of the *Manual* dealing with Chinese herbs is quite interesting as an indication of the extent to which the Chinese use herbs, and of the value of the different herbs, it should not be taken as a blueprint for self-treatment. Any reader interested in herbal remedies should consult the American texts available on the subject, or get in touch with an herbalist.

The treatments recommended in the *Barefoot Doctor's Manual* may well prove to be as effective, and less costly, than many of the traditional methods employed by Western physicians. However, the reader is advised to seek out competent medical advice before commencing any such treatments, and to seek out doctors qualified in such treatments. This re-issue of the *Manual* will hopefully contribute to an atmosphere in which such treatments can receive unbiased consideration.

It should be noted that this book is a reprint of the edition translated by the Fogarty International Center for Advanced Study in the Health Science, and was originally printed by the Superintendent of Documents for the U.S. Department of Health, Education and Welfare.

NOTES ON THE PREPARATION OF THIS MANUAL

1. All effort has been made to adapt the contents of this book -- the
signs and symptoms of diseases described, and their diagnosis and treatment
with the drugs listed -- to actual rural conditions in Hunan Province and to
the educational level of the rural barefoot doctors. For this reason, diagnosis
begins with a recognition of signs and symptoms, and descriptions of special
tests (such as X-rays, laboratory examinations) are largely omitted. In an
attempt to integrate traditional Chinese medicine and western medicine in
diagnosis, the names of disease and their type forms [according to traditional
Chinese medicine] are described together to facilitate treatment of cause and
use of discriminative therapy [treatment based on recognition of disease form/
type]. In the sections on treatment, the use of Chinese herbs and new therapeutic techniques are emphasized with the selective use of western medicines
appropriately mentioned (for the actual dosage and use of related western
medicines, and precautions connected with them, please consult section on
"Classification of Commonly Used Western Medicines" in the Appendix).

2. To cut down on the size of the manual and to simplify the use of
sub-divisions, descriptions of the various diseases in Chapter 6 follows a
general pattern. The first section of each description covers the name of
disease [and synonyms], etiology, pathology, signs and symptoms, important
diagnostic features, differential diagnosis and type/form classification of
the disease without any great detail. It is followed by subsequent sections
on "Prevention" and "Treatment" which go into greater detail.

3. In principle, the amounts of herbs given in the [cooked in water]
concoction-prescriptions listed for treating various diseases are for the
prescribed daily dosage, taken in two divided doses, the number of daily-
dosage prescriptions used based on the severity of illness. Where not spe-
cifically noted, the herbs called for are dried. If the fresh product is
used, the amounts are generally doubled, but an explanation is given.

4. This handbook records the prevention and treatment of illnesses we
are concerned with, and includes 338 illustrations describing common herbs seen
in Hunan Province. Another 184 drugs (including some Chinese herbs, other

own in Hunan Province, animal-origin drugs, minerals etc.)
illustrated only had their properties and action, the condi-
most used for, and preparation and usage mentioned briefly.

racteristic of Chinese-herb treatment of disease is the approach
of discriminative therapy [that treats according to the recognition of disease
condition]. Selection of tested single-and compound-ingredient prescriptions
used is based on the patient's actual condition such as his general physical
health, severity of illness, nature of the disease and its course of development [whether rapid or slow]. The amount of herbs used in each prescription
is also based on the severity of the patient's conditions, his age, and the
state of the herb [whether fresh or dried]. There is no need for blind adherence to the original amounts stated.

6. Because we are not thoroughly familiar with the conversion of complex characters [ideographs] into simpler forms, the listing in sequence of
"Common Chinese Medicinal Herbs" in Section 2 of Chapter 7 according to the
number of strokes in the first character may contain some errors. Please take
note when checking.

The units of weight and measure adopted in this manual are given
as follows:

Length:
meter (1 meter = 3 shih ch'ih [Chinese foot])
cm (1 cm = 3 shih-fen [0.03 Chinese inch])
mm (1 m = 3 shih-li [0.03 Chinese inch])
Volume:
liter (1 liter = 1 shih-sheng [Chinese liter])
ml (1 ml = 0.001 liter)

Drug-use weights:
chin (1 chin = 16 liang [Chinese ounce] = 500 gm)
liang (1 liang = 10 ch'ien = 31.2 gm)
ch'ien (1 ch'ien = 10 fen = 3.12 gm)
kg (1 kg = 2 chin = 1000 gm)

CHAPTER I. UNDERSTANDING THE HUMAN BODY

The human being is a complete unit formed by numerous cells undetected by the eye. Cells group to form tissues (such as muscle, skin etc.), and tissues group to form organs (such as the heart, liver, kidneys etc.) Certain organs assuming a similar function combine to form a system. An example is the digestive system formed by the alimentary canal, the stomach, large and small intestines, the liver, the gallbladder etc., which is responsible for the digestion of food in the human body. Other systems are the circulatory system, the respiratory system, the motor system, the urinary system, the nervous system, the sensory system, the endocrine system, the reproductive system etc. Though the various systems assume separate functions, they also interact. Controlled by the nervous and the endocrine systems, their activity is complimentary and synergistic.

Externally, the human body may be divided into the following parts: the head and neck, the trunk (including the thorax, abdomen, and back) and the extremities (including the upper and lower extremities) (Figure 1-1). The external layer covering the body is the skin (including the subcutis), under which is muscle tissue. The deeper layers of muscle tissue may wrap around the bony skeleton.

Within the body from top to bottom, are three cavities: the cranial cavity housing the brain; the thoracic cavity containing organs such as the heart, lungs, large blood vessels, etc.; and the abdominal cavity (which includes the pelvic cavity) containing the stomach, intestines, pancreas, liver, gallbladder, spleen, bladder, etc. In the female, the pelvis further contains organs such as the uterus, ovaries, fallopian tubes etc. (Figure 1-2).

The fact that living activity exists in the human body is due to the paradox of matter formation and breakdown. The human body continues to extract matter from its environment to convert it for use by the body through the digestive, respiratory, and absorption processes. At the same time, it continues to break down substances in the body producing waste matter such as carbon dioxide which is eliminated from the body through a process called metabolism. Only because the metabolic processes continue within the body can the body's viability be expressed. Once metabolic activity ceases, life also stops.

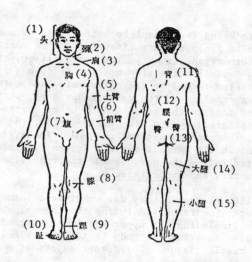

Figure 1-1. Parts of the human body.

Key:

(1)	Head	(6)	Forearm	(11)	Back
(2)	Neck	(7)	Abdomen	(12)	Waist
(3)	Shoulder	(8)	Knee	(13)	Buttock
(4)	Chest	(9)	Ankle	(14)	Thigh
(5)	Upper Arm	(10)	Toe	(15)	Leg

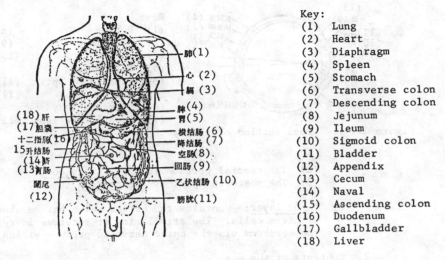

Key:
(1)   Lung
(2)   Heart
(3)   Diaphragm
(4)   Spleen
(5)   Stomach
(6)   Transverse colon
(7)   Descending colon
(8)   Jejunum
(9)   Ileum
(10) Sigmoid colon
(11) Bladder
(12) Appendix
(13) Cecum
(14) Naval
(15) Ascending colon
(16) Duodenum
(17) Gallbladder
(18) Liver

Figure 1-2. Organs of the thoracic and abdominal cavities.

The Eyes

The eyes primarily control vision. Each eye associated structure consists of the eyeball and accessories. The eyeball is formed by the eyeball surface layers and the contents they enclose (Figure 1-1-1).

1. <u>The surface layers</u>. Consists of the following:

    a. <u>External layer</u>

        (1) <u>Cornea</u>. A transparent membrane located anterior to the iris.

        (2) <u>Sclera</u>. A nontransparent covering over the whites of the eye.

    b. <u>Middle layer</u>. Contains a rich supply of blood vessels. It is also divided into anterior, middle, and posterior parts as follows:

        (1) The <u>iris</u>, located anteriorly, is commonly referred to as the "black eye-bead," in the center of which is the <u>pupil</u>. The muscles of the iris are very flexible and are able to control the size of the pupil. In strong light, the pupil contracts; in weak light, it dilates. This is called the <u>pupillar reflex.</u> In the presence of certain drugs used on it, or during a critical illness, or after death, the pupils are opened wide.

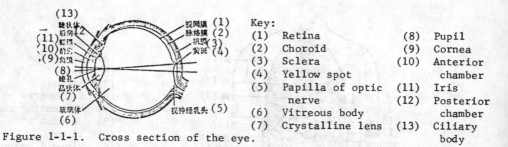

Key:

(1)	Retina	(8)	Pupil
(2)	Choroid	(9)	Cornea
(3)	Sclera	(10)	Anterior
(4)	Yellow spot		chamber
(5)	Papilla of optic	(11)	Iris
	nerve	(12)	Posterior
(6)	Vitreous body		chamber
(7)	Crystalline lens	(13)	Ciliary
			body

Figure 1-1-1. Cross section of the eye.

        (2) The central portion is the <u>ciliary body</u>.
        (3) The posterior part is the <u>choroid</u>.

    c. <u>Inner layer</u>: Contains the retina which has an abundant supply of nerve cells. The stimulation it receives is reflected to the cerebrum via the optic nerve to produce vision.

  2. <u>Contents of the eye</u>.

    a. <u>Aqueous humor</u>. Fills up the space between the anterior and posterior chambers.

    b. The <u>crystalline lens</u>. Located posterior to the iris as a double-convex elastic crystalline body. When the crystalline lens becomes cloudy, a cataract is formed, affecting vision to possibly cause blindness. Improper care of eyes may lead to <u>myopia</u>. When the crystalline lens become hardened, "old-age eyes" result in <u>hyperopia</u> or "far-sightedness."

    c. The <u>vitreous body</u>. The gelatinous and transparent humor filling the space posterior to the crystalline lens. When it becomes opaque, it may affect vision.

Associated structures of the eye (Figure 1-1-2) are listed as follows:

  1. The <u>orbit</u>. A bony cavity containing the eyeball, extrinsic muscle, blood vessels, nerves, lacrimal gland, fat and fasciae.

  2. The <u>extrinsic ocular muscles</u>. A total of six muscles that control eyeball movement in up, down, left and right directions.

  3. The <u>eyelid</u>. Bordered with eyelashes along the edges. Where the upper and lower eyelids meet at both ends are the <u>inner canthus</u> on the nasal aspect, and the <u>outer canthus</u> on the outer aspect near the T'ai-yang Yueh (acupuncture point). The sinal prominence on the inner canthus contains a tiny opening for the lacrimal point.

- 4 -

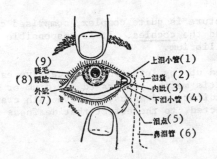

Key:
(1) Upper lacrimal duct
(2) Lacrimal sac
(3) Inner canthus
(4) Lower lacrimal duct
(5) Lacrimal point
(6) Nasolacrimal duct
(7) Outer canthus
(8) Eyelid
(9) Eyelashes

Figure 1-1-2. Anterior view of the eye and associated structures.

4. The conjunctiva. A transparent membrane layer over the eyes. The membrane lining the eyelid is the palpebral conjunctiva; that covering the eyeball in front is the bulbar conjunctiva. The connecting portion between these two membranes is called the fornical conjunctiva.

The Ear

The ear controls hearing and the body's sense of equilibrium. (Figure 1-1-3).

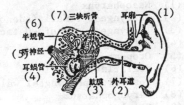

Key:
(1) Pinna of the ear
(2) External auditory meatus
(3) Eardrum
(4) Cochlea
(5) Auditory nerve
(6) Semilunar canals
(7) Auditory ossicles

Figure 1-1-3. Structure of the ear.

It consists of:

1. The external ear. Includes the pinna and the external auditory meatus. Several therapeutic acupuncture points are located on the pinna. The lobule of the pinna (the lower part) is a common site for pricking to obtain blood for laboratory examinations. The external auditory meatus is a passageway extending from the outer opening toward the middle ear.

2. The middle ear which is a tympanic chamber. The tympanic membrane (or ear drum) serves as the external wall, and the auditory ossicles are located just inside of it. When sound waves come through the external auditory meatus, the ear-drum caused vibrations in the ossicles are transmitted to the cochlea in the inner ear to produce the sensation of hearing.

3. The inner ear. Its structure is quite complex, comprised chiefly of a vestibule, semilunar canals, and the cochlea. It is responsible for hearing and maintenance of body equilibrium.

If the external ear is stopped up (by infection or excessive ear wax), or the middle ear is damaged (by otitis media, perforated ear drum or ossicle damage), or the inner ear and the auditory and acoustic nerve (8th cranial nerve) are diseased, hearing is affected, to the effect that deafness may result.

The Nose

The nose is primarily responsible for the sense of smell, though it also helps in the breathing function.

1. External nose. Cone-shaped. At the base are the anterior nares; laterally are the ala nasi or wings of the nose. Just inside the nares are some stiff hairs.

2. The nasal cavity. The left and right nasal fossae are separated by the nasal septum. Beyond the posterior nares, they merge into the nasopharynx, where the upper, middle and lower conchae form the lateral walls. As the uppermost part of the respiratory passage, the nasal cavity can warm, moisten, filter and disinfect the air (Figure 1-1-4).

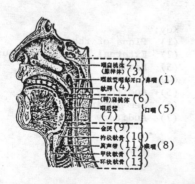

Key:
(1) Nasopharynx
(2) Pharyngeal tonsil (adenoid)
(3) Pharyngeal end of eustachian tube
(4) Soft palate
(5) Oropharynx
(6) (Palatine) tonsil
(7) Posterior pharyngeal wall
(8) Laryngopharynx
(9) Epiglottis
(10) Arytenoid cartilage
(11) True vocal cords
(12) Thyroid cartilage
(13) Cricoid cartilage

Figure 1-1-4. Anatomy of the nasopharynx and larynx.

3. Paranasal sinuses. As air spaces in the cranial bones opening into the nasal cavity, the parasanal sinuses are lined by one continuous membrane. The paranasal sinuses are the maxillary sinus, the ethmoidal air cells, and the paired frontal and sphenoidal sinuses. Inflammation of the upper respiratory tract can easily cause infection of these sinuses.

The Tongue

The tongue, a muscular tissue located inside the oral cavity, is responsible chiefly for the control of taste. On the surface of the tongue are many taste buds that can discern the various flavors of food and stimulate gastric juice secretion. Furthermore, the activity of the tongue is important for mastication, swallowing, and talking. On the under surface of the tongue is a fold, the frenum lingae. If it is too short, it can effect the clarity of speech.

Addendum

The Pharynx

The pharynx is the upper portion of the respiratory tract and the digestive tract at the same time. Superiorly, the pharynx joins the nasal cavity; inferiorly, the alimentary canal. Anteriorly, it opens into the nose, mouth, and larynx, to be designated as the nasopharynx, the oropharynx and the pharyngolarynx. Along both sides of the oropharynx are the tonsils, and between the tonsils is the uvula (commonly called the little tongue). The pharynx also plays a role in the tasting and swallowing function. Furthermore, the laryngopharynx also aids respiration, protects and aids the enunciation of speech. (See Figure 1-1-4).

The Larynx

The larynx, located at the anterior and upper part of the neck, is formed by several small cartilages. Superiorly, it connects with the pharyngolarynx, inferiorly, with the trachea. The vocal cords are a pair of membranous cords that produce the sound of the voice. Furthermore, the larynx is also a passageway for respiration.

Section 2. Skin Tissue

The skin is a soft and quite elastic tissue, with a coloring that varies with different individuals. Skin coloring of different parts of the body may also vary. Lines are found on the skin surface, such as those on the palms and fingers. These too, differ among different persons.

The skin is formed by three layers: the surface epithelium, the derma, and the tela subcutanea. Sweat glands, sebaceous glands, hair and nails are all accessories of the skin. Large sweat glands are found under the armpits, around the naval, genital and anal areas. Their secretions (especially that from under the arm) sometimes emit an unpleasant odor (called "B.O." when highly noticeable).

Sensory nerves and receptors are found throughout the skin, functioning chiefly to control the sense of touch, temperature and pain. Itchiness is a touch (tactile) sensation, a chief symptom of skin diseases.

Besides its tactile function, other functions of the skin are body protection, body temperature regulation, absorption, transpiration, metabolism and excretion. Furthermore, for certain ailments, acupuncture is applied through the skin at certain point locations to obtain dramatic results. Not only is the skin the first line of defense for the human body, it is also a tissue important for preserving life.

Section 3. The Nervous System

The nervous system controls the coordination and synergistic activity of all organs in the human body, provides appropriate reactions to environmental stimuli, in order to maintain the relative balance between man and the outside environment, and thus assure the normal course of life activities. The nervous system includes the central nervous system and the peripheral nervous systems (Figure 1-3-1). The <u>central nervous system</u> includes the brain and spinal cord, and it is the important component that controls various activities of the body. The <u>peripheral nervous system</u> refers to the cranial nerves

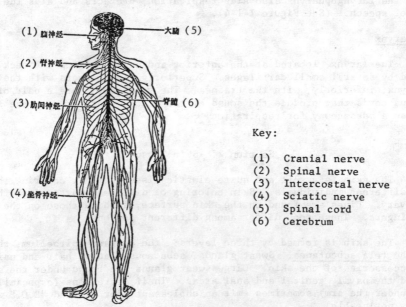

(1) 脑神经
(2) 脊神经
(3) 肋间神经
(4) 坐骨神经
大脑 (5)
脊髓 (6)

Key:

(1) Cranial nerve
(2) Spinal nerve
(3) Intercostal nerve
(4) Sciatic nerve
(5) Spinal cord
(6) Cerebrum

Figure 1-3-1. Cross section of the nervous system

that originate from the brain and the various spinal nerves that emit from the spinal cord. Afferent nerves in the peripheral system conduct sensations from inside and outside the body back to the brain, after which messages are sent out from the brain and spinal cord by the efferent nerves to coordinate various body activities, so that the appropriate organs can adapt to needs of the body at that time and produce a suitable reaction.

The Brain and the Cranial Nerves

1. <u>The brain</u>. Located inside the cranial cavity, it is divided into the cerebrum, the diencephalon, the midbrain, cerebellum, the pons and the oblongata (Figure 1-3-2).

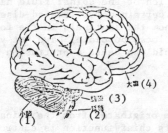

Key:

(1) Cerebellum
(2) Medulla oblongata
(3) Pons
(4) Cerebrum

Figure 1-3-2. The brain, external view.

a. The <u>cerebrum</u> which occupies most of the brain is divided into the left and right hemispheres. The hemispheres contain gray matter (the cerebral cortex), and white matter. Furthermore, such body activities and sensations as cold, heat, pain, vision, hearing and taste all depend on functional reflexes of the cerebrum. If one side of the cerebrum is damaged (as in a stroke), it can cause motor disturbance (paralysis) in extremities on the opposite side, and related sensations will be affected. When the brain encounters a severe vibration (concussion), or infection (encephalitis), coma will set in in severe cases.

b. The <u>cerebellum</u> is located under the cerebrum in the posterior part of the brain. Its chief function is maintaining balance in body position and coordination of body activity.

c. The <u>medulla oblongata</u>, also called the myelencephalon, is located under the cerebellum anteriorly, and connects superiorly with the pons. Its chief function is control of body activity such as respiration, cardiovascular activity, digestion etc.

2. <u>Cranial nerves</u>. Originating from the brain are 12 pairs of cranial nerves, some of them controlling receptor activity, facial expression, and cardiac action. The cranial nerves are peripheral nerves.

The Spinal Cord and Spinal Nerve

1. The <u>spinal cord</u> is located inside the spinal column, and classified as cervical, thoracic, lumbar and sacral parts. Except for the head and face, connections between the brain and all other body parts must go through the spinal cord. Therefore, spinal cord damage can disrupt connections between the brain, and related body parts and cause disturbance in motor activity and/ or tactile sensations.

2. The <u>spinal nerves</u>, a total of 31 pairs, originate from various points along both sides of the spinal cord. On the surface of the brain and spinal cord are three membranous layers. Between layers is a transparent fluid called <u>spinal fluid</u>. Examination of the spinal fluid has definite reference value in the diagnosis of certain nerve-related diseases. When encephalitis occurs in infants in whom the fontanels in the forebrain (called "ch'i-men" or gate of energy by the local populace) have not yet closed, the increased pressure of the spinal fluid can cause a protrusion or fullness in the forebrain.

The Vegetative Nervous System

The vegetative nervous system originates from the spinal cord, the medulla oblongata, and midbrain. Its chief function is control of visceral activity. The nerves are divided into sympathetic or parasympathetic nerves. Though both these types are found in the same organ, they generate different effects. If the sympathetic nerve is exerting a tonic action on the heart, and the parasympathetic nerve is exerting an opposite action, the two are complementing each other in a paradoxical sort of coordination.

Addendum: The Reflex

A reflex is a reaction of man to internal or external stimuli. Only through such reactions, can man adjust to internal and environmental changes. Reflexes may be classified as inborn and acquired.

During clinical examinations, certain reflex actions must be observed. For example, tapping the quadriceps just below the patella gently, a kicking motion results in what is called a <u>knee reflex</u>. In another example, using a wisp of cotton to touch the cornea of the eye will result quickly in closing the eye in what is called the <u>corneal reflex</u>. Again, using a light to shine directly on the pupils will result in a quick shrinking of pupil size, but quick removal of light source will see return of pupils to original size, in what is called the <u>light reflex.</u> These three examples are further referred to as physiological reflexes, which can disappear in presence of coma or certain infections. Furthermore, pathological reflexes such as <u>Babinski's reflex</u> oftentimes appear during course of diseases of the brain or meninges.

Section 4. The Endocrine System

The endocrine system includes the thyroid, the parathyroid glands, the adrenal glands, the pituitary gland, the pancreas, and the sex glands (Figure 1-4-1).

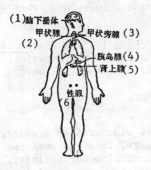

Key:

(1) Pituitary gland
(2) Thyroid
(3) Parathyroid gland
(4) Pancreas
(5) Adrenal gland
(6) Sex glands

Figure 1-4-1. Location of the endocrine glands.

Important hormones are manufactured by the endocrine glands and secreted directly into the blood strem by which they reach all parts of the body. Working together with the nervous system, the endocrine system and its hormones help control the coordination and synergism of all organ activity. These hormones can further affect body metabolism and growth development. When endocrine function is abnormal, certain abnormal changes leading to illness may occur.

The important endocrine glands are listed as follows:

1. The thyroid gland. Located in front of the neck and just below the trachea in front, the thyroid gland is divided into lobes. It secretes thyroxin which stimulates body metabolism and growth. Excessive thyroid secretion may result in thyroid gland enlargement, protruding eyeballs, increased appetite, weight loss and other signs of hyperthyroidism. When thyroid secretion is deficient, symptoms such as edema, mental retardation and dwarfism may be seen.

2. The adrenal glands. Paired, the adrenal glands are located one above each kidney. The cortical hormone secreted by these glands regulates body metabolism and increases body resistance to disease. Cortical hormone may increase the heart rate, blood vessel contraction, and blood pressure rise.

3. The island of Langerhans. Located within the pancreas, it secretes insulin. When insulin secretion is inadequate, diabetes may result. When secretion of insulin is excessive, the blood sugar may drop.

4. The pituitary body. Located at the base of the cerebrum, it is divided into posterior and anterior lobes. The pituitary secretes hormones that affect growth and development, urine volume, and other endocrine functions.

5. Sex glands. The testes in the male, and the ovaries in the female are both sex glands which determine individual characteristics that reflect certain differences in the anatomy and physiology of the two sexes.

Section 5. The Motor System

Work created the world, and work also created mankind. Since work is accomplished through various movements, this requires the complementary coordination between many tissues to control motor activity. These tissues are the body framework, joints, and muscles working under nervous system control.

The Bony Framework

The skeletal framework of the human body is made up of 206 bones of various sizes.

1. Bone structure and function. Bone tissue is comprised of three parts: the periosteum, osseous tissue, and bone marrow. On the basis of their shape, bones may be further classified as long, short, flat or irregular. Functions of bone are:

   a. Body support
   b. Protection of the brain and other internal organs.
   c. Completion of various body movements through lever action of muscles attached to bones.
   d. Manufacture of blood cells in the red marrow of bone.

2. Important bones (Figure 1-5-1).

   a. The cranium. Forms the cranial cavity and the bony framework of the face.
   b. The spinal column. Formed by seven cervical vertebrae, 12 thoracic vertebrae, five lumbar vertebrae, and the sacrum and coccyx. The prominence of the 7th vertebra is very noticeable when the head is lowered. It can be used as a land mark and originating point from which to count and locate the other vertebrae.
   c. The thoracic cage. Formed by the sternum, the thoracic vertebrae and 12 pairs of ribs.

d. The pelvis. Formed by the left and right hipbones, by the sacrum and coccyx posteriorly, and by the pubic bone anteriorly. In the female, the pelvis is more delicate and shallow, large at the entrance and broad at the exit, forming a circular shape to permit easy birth.

e. The extremities. The upper and lower extremities on the left and right are referred to as the four extremities. They are made up of several long bones. See (Figure 1-5-1) for further details.

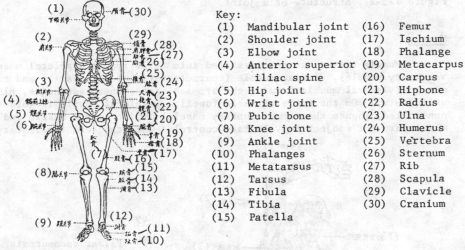

Key:
(1)	Mandibular joint	(16)	Femur
(2)	Shoulder joint	(17)	Ischium
(3)	Elbow joint	(18)	Phalange
(4)	Anterior superior iliac spine	(19)	Metacarpus
		(20)	Carpus
(5)	Hip joint	(21)	Hipbone
(6)	Wrist joint	(22)	Radius
(7)	Pubic bone	(23)	Ulna
(8)	Knee joint	(24)	Humerus
(9)	Ankle joint	(25)	Vertebra
(10)	Phalanges	(26)	Sternum
(11)	Metatarsus	(27)	Rib
(12)	Tarsus	(28)	Scapula
(13)	Fibula	(29)	Clavicle
(14)	Tibia	(30)	Cranium
(15)	Patella		

Figure 1-5-1. Bones of the skeleton and important joints.

The Joints

1. Structure and function. Individual bones meet at joints or junctures where movement is permitted. Depending on the range of joint movement, some are simple, some are more involved. A joint consists of an articular capsule, articulating surfaces and an articular cavity (Figure 1-5-2). A small amount of lubricating fluid is found inside the articular cavity that aids joint movement. When the joint is inflamed, this fluid may increase and become purulent. When this is serious, the articular surfaces become rough, to affect joint movement. When strong force is exerted on a joint, this may be serious enough to cause dislocation of the joint and affect its movement.

2. Important joints. These include the mandibular joint, the shoulder joint, the elbow joint, the wrist joint, the hip joint, the knee joint, the ankle joint etc.

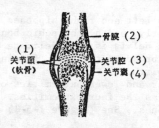

Key:

(1) Articular surface (cartilage)
(2) Periosteum
(3) Articular cavity
(4) Articular capsule

Figure 1-5-2. Structure of a joint.

Muscle

Muscle tissue may be classified into three types: skeletal muscle (or voluntary muscle), cardiac muscle (characteristic of the heart), and smooth muscle (visceral muscle forming the stomach, intestines, esophagus, bladder, uterus etc.) On the basis of their function, skeletal muscle is voluntarily controlled, (hence the term voluntary muscle), while smooth muscle and cardiac muscle are not subject to voluntary control (hence the term involuntary muscle).

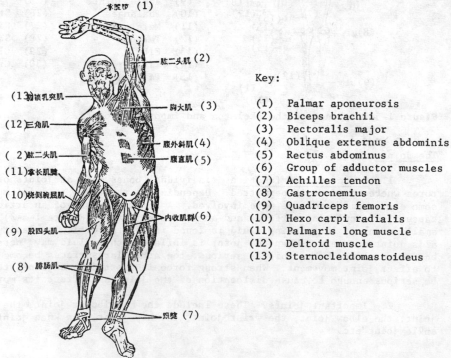

Key:

(1) Palmar aponeurosis
(2) Biceps brachii
(3) Pectoralis major
(4) Oblique externus abdominis
(5) Rectus abdominus
(6) Group of adductor muscles
(7) Achilles tendon
(8) Gastrocnemius
(9) Quadriceps femoris
(10) Hexo carpi radialis
(11) Palmaris long muscle
(12) Deltoid muscle
(13) Sternocleidomastoideus

Figure 1-5-3. Muscles of the body, anterior view.

The important superficial muscles of the human body are depicted in Figures 1-5-3 and 1-5-4. Muscle insertions at both ends of the muscle where they are attached to the bone undergo muscular contractions over the joints to permit joint extension, flexion, and rotation to accomplish such movements as raising the head, bending over at the waist, extending the hand, bending the knee, running etc. However, the completion of each movement is generally the result of synergistic muscular activity.

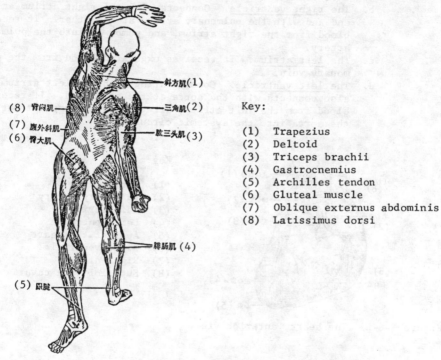

Key:

(1) Trapezius
(2) Deltoid
(3) Triceps brachii
(4) Gastrocnemius
(5) Archilles tendon
(6) Gluteal muscle
(7) Oblique externus abdominis
(8) Latissimus dorsi

Figure 1-5-4. Muscles of the body, posterior view.

Section 6. The Circulatory System

The circulatory system consists of the heart and blood vessels. It is also responsible for the lymphatic circulation.

1. The _heart_. Located in the thoracic cavity between the left and right lungs, it consists of four chambers (Figure 1-6-1): the right atrium, right ventricle, left atrium, and left ventricle. The heart is lined by the endocardium, and enveloped by the pericardium. The valves between the right atrium and right ventricle are called the tricupid valves; the valves between the left atrium and the left ventricle, the bicuspid valves. The valves between the left ventricle and the aorta is the aortic valve, and that between

the right ventricle and the pulmonary artery is the pulmonary valve. In certain disease conditions of the heart some of these valves may become narrowed or blocked incompletely.

a. The <u>right atrium</u>. Joined to the superior and inferior vena cava, it receives all the blood from the body returning to the heart.

b. The <u>right ventricle</u>. Connects with the right atrium at one end and with the pulmonary artery at the other. It receives blood from the right atrium, and pumps it into the pulmonary artery.

c. The <u>left atrium</u>. It receives oxgenated blood from the pulmonary vein.

d. The <u>left ventricle</u>. Communicating with the left atrium, it also connects with the aorta at the other end. It receives blood from the left atrium, after which it pumps it out through the aorta into the systemic circulation.

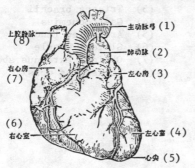

Key:

(1) Aortic arch
(2) Pulmonary artery
(3) Left atrium
(4) Left ventricle
(5) Apex of the heart
(6) Right ventricle
(7) Right atrium
(8) Superior vena cava

Figure 1-6-1. The heart, anterior view.

2. The <u>blood vessels</u>.

a. <u>Arteries</u>. The thick and elastic walls of the arteries help the heart transport the blood to all parts of the body.

b. <u>Veins</u>. Vessel walls of the veins are thinner and less elastic. Valves along the inner vessel lining assist blood from the rest of the body in its return to the heart.

c. <u>Capillaries</u>. Minute vessels that connect the arterioles (arteries) and the venules (veins). Their very thin walls allow exchange of certain substances through them. Through the capillaries, blood carries nutrients to various tissue cells, and carries out waste matter from the tissues.

3. Circulation of blood.

a. Body circulation. In this type of circulation, also called the systemic circulation, the blood is pumped from the left ventricle into the aorta where it is transported to all parts of the body via arteries and capillaries, and then returned via capillaries, veins, and the inferior and superior vena cava back into the right atrium and then the right ventricle.

b. Pulmonary circulation. Also called the lesser circulation. Blood from the right ventricle enters the pulmonary artery and then into the pulmonary capillary network where exchange of gases takes place. Fresh oxygen is absorbed and carbon dioxide is released. Finally, the blood is collected by the pulmonary vein for return to the left atrium and then the left ventricle.

The systemic circulation and the pulmonary circulation are inter-related in forming a complete and closed circulation passageway.

This circulation pattern is due chiefly to the regular contraction and relaxation of the heart. The heart beat of a normal person ranges from 60 to 100 times a minute. During ventricular contraction (systole), great pressure is generated to force the blood into the arteries and move the blood stream forward. In an adult, the normal pressure ranges between 90 to 100 mm of mercury. The reading is lower when the heart is relaxed -- about 60 to 90 mm of mercury (diastolic pressure). When the systolic and diastolic pressures are generally higher than normal values, hypertension is present. When the pressure readings are lower than normal values, hypertension is said to be present. With cardiac relaxation and contraction, the arterial walls show a regular beating action called the pulse. Feeling for the radial pulse (on the external aspect of the wrist which is the one used by traditional Chinese medical practitioners), the femoral pulse (on the medical aspect of the thigh), and the temporal pulse (at point posterior to the "T'ai-yang yueh" and about a finger's width anterior to the ear) during pulse-taking is often practiced to observe changes in the pulse pattern.

When the heart contracts and relaxes, certain heart sounds may be heard with a stethoscope placed over the chest. The sound heard during heart contraction is the first heart sound. When rales are detected in the first heart sound, that may reflect lesions in the tricuspid and bicuspid valves. The sound heard during diastole is the second heart sound. When rales are detected during diastole, that may indicate lesions in the aortic valve.

4. Tissue fluid. During the course of body circulation, part of the blood fluid content permeates the thin capillary walls and becomes tissue fluid.

Under normal circumstances, the production and return of tissue fluid maintains an equilibrium. However, during the course of certain diseases, because of excessive tissue fluid production or disrupted fluid return, excessive tissue fluid accumulation systematically or locally will cause edema. If tissue fluid or the fluid content of blood serum is greatly reduced during disease, dehydration will set in accompanied by a wrinkling of skin and reduced elasticity. In severe cases disturbances in circulation or acid-base balance may occur.

5. The lymphatic circulation.

 a. The lymphatics. Tissue fluid as lymph entering the lymphatic vessels is carried by the lymphatic network which reintroduces the fluid into the circulatory system via the veins.

 b. Lymph nodes. Before the lymphatic network joins with the veins, it converges on lymphatic nodes (located at various parts of the body) which filter out and destroy bacteria and other harmful matter in the lymph. Consequently, lymph nodes assume a protective function. When these nodes are inflamed, they became swollen and painful.

 c. The spleen. Located in the upper left part of the abdominal cavity. The spleen is rather soft, and hard to palpate under normal circumstances. However, when it is enlarged (as in malaria and schistosomiasis), it is readily palpable.

Addendum: The Blood Forming Organs and the Blood

Blood in the human body makes up 80 percent of the total body weight. When it is deficient (as in excessive hemorrhage or in cases where the blood formation process is deficient), anemia or other circulatory disturbance may be observed.

The important blood-making organs in the human body are listed as follows:

1. Bone morrow. The chief blood-making organ. It produces red cells (also called erythrocytes), white cells (also called leukocytes), and blood platelets.

2. The lymphatic system. Includes lymph nodes, the spleen, and lymphatic tissue in the bone marrow. It produces lymphocytes.

3. The reticuloendothelial system. Functioning chiefly through bone marrow, spleen, and lymphatic node tissue, reticular cells assume phagocytic properties in that certain foreign substances in the blood are swallowed up. Furthermore, this system also produces mononuclear leukocytes.

The blood is divided into two components: blood cells and blood serum.

1. Blood cells

    a. Red blood cells. In the normal adult, each millimeter of blood contains 4.5 to 5 million red blood cells. Red blood cells are important substances that carry oxygen and carbon dioxide. The hemoglobin of arterial blood contains more oxygen, which makes arterial blood a brighter red. On the other hand, hemoglobin of venous blood is a darker red.

    b. White blood cells. In the adult, each millimeter of blood contains 5000 to 10,000 white blood cells. In the presence of acute inflammatory disease or certain leukemias, the total number of white cells may increase. White blood cells exert a phagocytic action on bacteria and increase the body's immunity.

    c. Blood platelets. Exert coagulating action on the blood in bleeding. In the normal person, each millimeter of blood contains about 100,000 to 300,000 blood platelets.

2. Blood serum. Consisting chiefly of water, blood serum contains proteins, glucose, hormones and other nutrients which are transported to all parts of the body by the blood. At the same time, the waste products of metabolism are also carried to the kidneys for elimination outside the body.

Human blood is generally classed into four types: O, A, B, and AB. If blood used for transfusion is not compatible with that of the patient, serious consequences, even death, may result. Thus it is important to crossmatch and type blood for compatibility first before transfusion.

The important functions of blood are:

    (1) Supplying nutrients to body tissues.
    (2) Removing waste products of body metabolism.
    (3) Transporting hormones and participating in the immunization process.

Section 7. The Respiratory System

The important function of the respiratory system is inhalation of oxygen in the air and exhalation of carbon dioxide from the body. It consists of the nasopharynx, the larynx, the trachea, the bronchi and the lungs. The lungs are the sites of gaseous exchange, and the other parts are the air entrance and exit passageways.

    1. The nasopharynx and larynx. As the entrance and passageway for the respiratory tract, the nasopharynx and larynx prevent dust and foreign matter from entering the trachea.

    2. The trachea. Joined to the larynx above, the trachea subdivides at its lower junction into the left and right bronchi which further subdivides

into numerous <u>bronchioles</u> that connect with the <u>alveoli</u>. Walls of the trachea are formed by cartilage rings that maintain an open passageway. The mucous membrane lining the walls secrete a mucus that catches dust and bacteria from air coming through. When inflammation is present, this secretion is increased and becomes <u>sputum</u> that is usually coughed up.

3. The <u>lungs</u>. Divided into left and right. The lungs are made up of numerous alveoli that are lined with a rich vascular network. The gaseous exchange of oxygen and carbon dioxide takes place within these alveoli. Many adjacently connecting alveoli group to form small pulmonary <u>lobules</u>, and many lobules group to form a <u>lobe</u>. The left lung has two lobes, and the right lung three lobes (Figure 1-7-1).

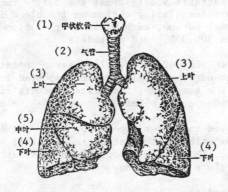

(1) 甲状软骨
(2) 气管
(3) 上叶
(3) 上叶
(5) 中叶
(4) 下叶
(4) 下叶

Key:

(1) Cricoid cartilage
(2) Trachea
(3) Upper lobe
(4) Lower lobe
(5) Middle lobe

Figure 1-7-1. The lungs, external view.

Because of movement by the chest wall and the diaphragm, the lungs will expand and contract to carry out gaseous exchange. In a normal person, the number of respirations ranges between 16 and 20 times. During physical exertion, nervous excitement or fever, the respirations are increased.

4. The <u>pleura</u>. Protects the lungs. The pleura consists of two thin membranes: one covering the surface of the lungs, and the other attached to the inner surface of the chest wall. The closed space between these two membranes is the <u>pleural cavity</u>.

Section 8. The Digestive System

The digestive system includes the oral cavity, the pharynx, esophagus, stomach, intestines, liver, gallbladder and pancrease (Figure 1-8-1). Through the synergistic action of these organs, the body partakes of food, digests it, absorbs its nutrients, and converts food residue into feces for removal outside the body.

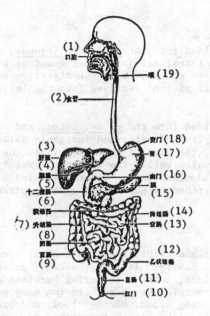

(1) 口腔
(19) 咽
(2) 食管
(3) 肝脏
(18) 贲门
(17) 胃
(4) 胆囊
(16) 幽门
(5) 十二指肠
(15) 胰
(6) 十二指肠
(14) 降结肠
(13) 空肠
(7) 升结肠
(8) 回肠
(9) 盲肠
(12)
乙状结肠
(11) 直肠
(10) 肛门

Key:

(1) Oral cavity
(2) Esophagus
(3) Liver
(4) Gallbladder
(5) Duodenum
(6) Transverse colon
(7) Ascending colon
(8) Ileum
(9) Cecum
(10) Anus
(11) Rectum
(12) Sigmoid colon
(13) Jejunum
(14) Descending colon
(15) Pancreas
(16) Pyloric orifice
(17) Stomach
(18) Cardiac orifice
(19) Pharynx

Figure 1-8-1. The digestive system.

The Oral Cavity, Pharynx and Esophagus

Inside the adult oral cavity are 32 teeth and three pairs of salivary glands that secrete saliva. One pair of salivary glands, the parotid glands, is located just below the ear toward the front. The pharynx connects with the esophagus, and the esophagus with the stomach. After food has been mixed around inside the mouth by the tongue and masticated by the teeth, it is swallowed via the pharynx, through the esophagus into the stomach. When the esophagus becomes narrowed as the result of tumor growth or other damage, it may become difficult for any swallowing to take place. Should veins along the esophageal wall become congested as the result of liver cirrhosis, venous rupture may occur and the patient vomits blood.

The Stomach

The largest and most expansive part of the digestive tract, the stomach, which is located in the upper abdominal cavity, receives and digests food. The upper opening of the stomach, called the cardiac orifice at its juncture with the esophagus, is usually tightly closed to prevent regurgitation of food back up the esophagus into the oral cavity. In the young infant, the cardiac orifice is not as strong, so regurgitation of milk is commonly seen. The exit of the stomach is the pyloric orifice which connects with the duodenum. The gastric mucosa secretes gastric juices containing hydrochloric acid. Gastric ulcers are usually found in the mucosa at the lesser stomach curvature and near the duodenum.

The Intestines

1. The <u>small intestine</u>: Divided into the <u>duodenum</u>, <u>jejunum</u>, and the <u>ileum</u>. The small intestine secretes intestinal juice that combines with bile and pancreatic juice in the duodenum to continue with the digestion of food, absorption of nutrients, and transport of food residues into the large intestine.

2. The <u>large intestine</u>: Divided into the <u>cecum</u>, <u>colon</u>, and <u>rectum</u>. Its function is continuing the absorption of water and inorganic salts and evacuation of feces through the <u>anus</u>, the exit of the rectum. At the terminal end of the cecum is a wormlike protrusion called the <u>appendix</u>. When the appendix is inflamed, it can cause abdominal pain. Sometimes veins along the rectal wall become congested and stretched because of stagnating circulation, to result in <u>hemorrhoids</u>.

The Liver

The liver is divided into left and right lobes, most of it located in the upper right part of the abdominal cavity. It is not usually palpable in adults. The liver has several functions, such as rendering harmless certain toxic byproducts of body metabolism, manufacturing and storing many nutrients (such as glucose, vitamins etc.), storing blood, making blood, and breaking down products of metabolism. Hence the liver is an important organ in the human body.

The Gallbladder and Bile Ducts

The gallbladder is located inferior to the liver. Bile produced by the liver is usually passed first into the gallbladder, via the hepatic and cystic ducts, for storage. Should stones be formed in the gallbladder, they could obstruct the bile ducts. Sometimes ascaris occur in the bile ducts and gallbladder and cause acute pain.

The Pancreas

Located posterior and inferior to the stomach, the pancreas secretes pancreatic juice which flows into the duodenum via the <u>pancreatic duct</u> to aid in the digestion of food.

The Peritoneum

The peritoneum is a smooth and white membraneous layer. The layer that adheres to the inner abdominal wall is the <u>parietal peritoneum</u>; that layer covering the visceral surfaces is the <u>visceral peritoneum</u>. The space between these two peritoneal layers is the <u>peritoneal cavity.</u> A small amount of synovial fluid is usually found in this cavity, but when the peritoneum is inflamed, this fluid increases and becomes purulent. In heart disease or kidney disease resulting in systemic edema or in liver cirrhosis, much of the vascular fluid is leaked into the peritoneal cavity to cause <u>ascites</u>.

Section 9. The Urinary System

The urinary system consists of the <u>kidneys</u>, the <u>ureters</u>, the <u>urinary bladder</u>, and the <u>urethra</u> (Figure 1-9-1).

1. The <u>kidneys</u>. Commonly called the "yao-tzu," the two kidneys are located on each side of the spine at the level of the waist or "yao" [hence "yao-tzu"]. Each kidney consists of several parts: the <u>cortex</u> and <u>medulla</u>, the <u>calyces</u> and the <u>renal pelvis</u>. Many glomerula and renal tubules wind through the cortical and medullary regions and join with other tubules as they enter the renal pelvis through the calyces.

The kidneys filter and excrete waste and toxic substances. When blood courses through the renal glomeruli and tubules, most of the water content and some useful substances it contains are reabsorbed into the circulation and leaves behind urine. The 24-hour volume of urine passed by an adult ranges between 1500 and 2000 ml. Normal urine should not contain any blood, albumin or sugar.

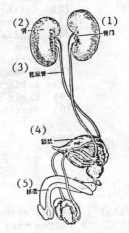

Key:

(1) Renal hilum
(2) Kidney
(3) Ureter
(4) Urinary bladder
(5) Urethra

Figure 1-9-1. Urinary system of the male.

2. The <u>ureters</u>. Located on each side of the spine inside the posterior abdominal wall. Superiorly it joins the renal pelvis, inferiorly, the urinary bladder.

3. The <u>urinary bladder</u>. Located in the center of the lower pelvis anterior to the rectum (in the female, anterior to the uterus), the urinary bladder is a highly elastic muscular sac used for the temporary storage of urine. Inferiorly, the bladder connects with the urethra.

4. The _urethra_. Superiorly, it connects with the bladder; inferiorly, it opens outside the body. The female urethra which is shorter is used only for passing urine. The longer male urethra is used for passage of urine and seminal fluid.

Section 10. The Reproductive System

The Female Reproductive System

The female genitals do not become mature until a girl has reached her teens. Generally, these organs do not undergo gradual degeneration until 30 some years after the female has attained maturity.

1. The _external genitals_. See Figure 1-10-1 for description of parts.

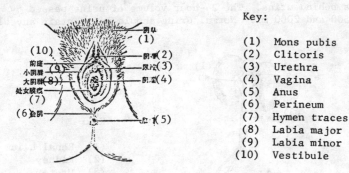

Key:

(1) Mons pubis
(2) Clitoris
(3) Urethra
(4) Vagina
(5) Anus
(6) Perineum
(7) Hymen traces
(8) Labia major
(9) Labia minor
(10) Vestibule

Figure 1-10-1. External genitals of the female

2. The _internal genitals_ (Figure 1-10-2).

    a. The _vagina_. The passage that joins the external and internal genitals. The upper part of the vagina that surrounds the cervix of the uterus is called the _fornix_. Inferiorly, the vagina opens out into the vulva. The anterior wall of the vagina is adjacent to the urinary bladder and the urethra; its posterior wall, to the rectum.

    b. The _uterus_. Located within the pelvis, the pear-shaped uterus is the site for fetal growth and development and for menses formation. The wall of the uterus is divided into three layers: the serous coat, the _muscular layer_, and the _membraneous lining_ (endometrium). The center of the uterus is a cavity that communicates with the vagina via the cervix. Uppermost is the _fundus_ of the uterus with two fallopian tubes opening laterally from each side. The central part is the _body_, and the

- 24 -

lower part is the cervix. The uterus is about 7.5 cm in length, tilted slightly anteriorly, and anchored inside the pelvic cavity by three pairs of ligaments. The bladder is located anterior to the uterus; the rectum, posterior to it.

c. Fallopian tubes. As the passageway for transporting the ovum, the fallopian tubes are located one on each side, leading laterally from the fundus of the uterus and opening into the peritoneal cavity through the upper part of the ovaries.

d. The ovaries. About the size of an almond, the ovaries are located one on each side of the uterus. Ova and female hormones are produced here.

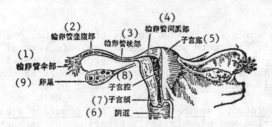

Key:

(1) Fimbriated end of fallopian tube
(2) Body section of fallopian tube
(3) Stem section of fallopian tube
(4) Interstitial part of fallopian tube
(5) Fundus of uterus
(6) Vagina
(7) Cervix of uterus

Figure 1-10-2. Internal genital organs of the female.

Ovalution generally occurs once a month, halfway between menstrual periods, when the ovum is discharged from the ovary. The period that the avum remains viable ranges from several hours to about 5 days. The female hormones can stimulate the sexual organs, the mammary glands and growth changes in the female figure. Furthermore, the ovaries and other endocrine organs also complement the action of each other.

The ovaries also affect the membranous lining of the uterus sufficiently for it to undergo cyclic changes. This cycle of proliferation, secretion, and denuding of the uterine mucosa, and bleeding from the uterus is menstruation. This cycle generally occurs every 28 days. The menstrual flow, lasting 3 to 5 days, generally measures 10-100 ml. The appearance [timing of puberty] of menstruation and the amount of menstrual flow sometimes are related to certain conditions such as the presence of tuberculosis or endocrine disturbances, or the nutritional state of the subject.

The Male Reproductive System

The male reproductive system consists of the testes, the epididymis, the seminal vesicles, the prostate gland, the penis, and the scrotum (Figure 1-10-3).

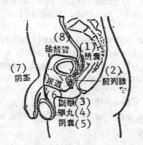

Key:

(1) Seminal vesicle
(2) Prostate gland
(3) Epididymis
(4) Testes
(5) Scrotum
(6) Urethra
(7) Penis
(8) Ductus deferens

Figure 1-10-3. The male reproductive system.

The testes. The testes, which are located inside the scrotum, one on each side, are glands responsible for sperm production and manufacture of the male sex hormone, testosterone. Testosterone stimulates growth and development of the male sexual organs and appearance of certain male physical characteristics (beard, muscular development, voice change to deeper pitch).

The epididymis, ductus deferens, seminal vesicle, and prostate gland all participate in semen production and ejaculation. Ligation of the ductus deferens which can prevent passage of sperm out from the testes is considered the simplest of birth control measures.

Section 11. Characteristics of Different Systems in Children

Description of the various systems before this generally refer to those in the adult. However, there are certain differences between the adult and the child in the anatomy and function of their various systems, though they share a common base. The fact that certain diagnostic characteristics are noted when a child is ill is due to peculiar characteristics in the structure and physiology of the young organ systems.

Now, what are some of the features that are characteristic of children under 10 years of age? They are seen chiefly as follows:

1. For the circulatory system:

    a. The presence of congenital heart disease if the special antrio-ventricular and the cardio-aortic passageways do not shut off in time.

    b. Location of the apex beat over the 4th rib slightly beyond the left nipple line. The younger the child, the higher this location.

c. A faster heart beat and pulse rate in children -- the younger the child, the more rapid the beat -- at a rate of 85 to 140 times a minute.

d. A lower blood pressure in children -- the younger the child, the lower the blood pressure -- ranging from 75-100/37-70 ml.

2. For the respiratory system: Small children are quite susceptible to colds, coughs, bronchitis, pneumonia etc., due chiefly to the following factors:

a. The narrow lumen of the nasal passages that easily become obstructed following infection, to cause great discomfort.

b. More rapid respirations in the child, generally 30 to 40 times a minute, because the small respiratory tract does not permit adequate gas exchange. In the presence of respiratory infections, this is aggravated as the wings of the nose quiver with each breath, and dyspnea and cyanosis set in.

c. The frequency of middle ear infections following throat infections. Furthermore, the incidence of pneumonia is also greater than that in adults.

3. For the digestive tract:

a. The greater susceptibility of the delicate oral mucosa in infants to injury. For this reason, cleaning of the mouth should be done gently. The fleshy protrusions on the buccal surfaces of the mouth (called "grasshoppers" by the people) and the hard yellowish-white splotches formed on the teeth (mistaken for "molars" usually) are normal, and should not be removed by force.

b. Drooling, a common physiological occurrence in milk-drinking infants, gradually diminishing after an infant is 7 months old.

c. Vomiting on the slightest excitation, as muscles around the cardiac orifice (of stomach) are more relaxed. The secretary and digestive functions of the stomach and intestines are also weak, so vomiting, diarrhea and poor digestion often appear during illness.

4. For the nervous system:

a. Immature development of the nervous system -- the younger the child, the greater the immaturity. Their reactions to external stimuli are sometimes slow, sometimes unclear. This is most obvious in nursing infants.

b. The presence of certain signs such as Kernig's sign (knee bend-
    ing) Babinski's sign (stimulating sole of foot), etc., as normal
    physiological reactions in young infants under 2 years of age.
    These are abnormal signs in sick adults being given neurologi-
    cal examinations.

c. Easy development of cramps in child during illness. Even healthy
    small children will jump and be frightened when a loud noise is
    heard in the midst of sound sleep.

5. For skin tissue:

a. The greater susceptibility of delicate baby skin to injury and
    subsequent infection.

b. The redder skin coloring in infants and their susceptibility
    to fever. The sweat glands of infants less than 6 months old
    are not developed and heat is dissipated less easily.

c. The greater amount of subcutaneous fat in infants less than
    1 year old which makes them look chubby and fat. Later on
    when the fat content gradually diminishes, growing children
    appear to be thinner (called "shooting up").

6. For the muscular system:

a. Development of muscles generally not noticeable, as infant
    muscle is very soft and delicate.

b. Rather tense muscles of the lower and upper extremities in in-
    fants less than 4 months old.

7. For the blood circulation system:

a. Varying normal values noted for the blood of infants. These
    values increase with age as they approximate those for adults.

b. A white blood count higher than that for adults, about 10,000
    to 11,000/ml, and a lower neutrophil white cell count of 40%.

c. The appearance of infantile physiologic anemia at 3 to 4 months
    of age. This generally corrects itself later on.

d. General instability in the function of blood-forming organs
    among infants, increasing susceptibility to illness.

8. For the urinary system:

a. A less efficient urinary system among infants and a greater
    suspectibility to uremia during dehydration.

b. A smaller urinary bladder that requires more emptying daily.

c. A shorter urethra in young girls, which increases susceptibility to cystitis or urinary tract infection.

From a very early time, traditional Chinese medicine has carefully observed the characteristics of infant physiology and pathology. For example, when it discusses changes taking place (with reference to the changes in growth and development continually going on), it indicates that the changes of growth and development occurring in children with respect to their cardio-pulmonary vitality, rib and bone structure, and the state of their visceral organs, mental awareness and emotions generally coincide with actual conditions. For example, the nonclosure of the anterior fontanels in small children indicates incomplete development. Certain traditional expressions show that some anatomical and physiologic characteristics in children provide specific inklings to their predisposition (hence the cause) to illness. Some of these are listed as follows:

Because of "delicate skin and muscle,"
    they "take chill easily";

Because of "flabby skin and muscle,"
    they "transmit changes [? infections] easily";

Because of "sensitive stomachs,"
    they "spit up milk and food easily";

Because of "weak organ vitality,"
    they "easily gain and lose weight";

Because of "listless spirit,"
    they "easily become emotional";

Because of "fetal poisons collected,"
    they are "more susceptible to measles and pox";

Because of "weak meridians,"
    they "easily become spastic";

Because of "weak [cardiopulmonary] vitality,"
    they "easily become chilled and feverish, hungry and full..."

For these reasons, measures taken for prevention, diagnosis, treatment and care of these conditions should be directed toward these specific signs and manifestations.

Section 12. Traditional Chinese Medicine
Understanding of the Human Body

The "chuang-fu" refers to the five viscera (chuang) and six "bowels" (fu) in the human body. The <u>five viscera</u> are the liver, heart (including the heart sac), spleen, lungs and kidneys. The <u>six bowels</u> are the gallbladder, stomach, large intestine, small intestine, urinary bladder and the "san-chiao". Functionally, the viscera and bowels share a coordinating division of labor. Between the viscera and bowels, their components also share a "paired-off" relationship that ties in the heart with the small intestine (the pericardium with the "san-chiao"), the liver with the gallbladder, the spleen with the stomach, the lungs with the large intestine, the kidneys with the bladder, etc. The different viscera and bowels stimulate, yet control each other. Moreover, these vital organs are also closely related to other tissues in the body. For example, the heart is joined to the blood vessels and involved with the tongue to illustrate how various components inter-relate to form an integral body organism.

Though the terms for "wu-chuang lu-fu" (five viscera and six bowels) in traditional Chinese medicine terminology generally resemble those used in modern medicine, there are some differences. The viscera or bowels that the traditional Chinese medicine practitioner refer to do not necessarily match those used by the western medicine practitioner from the standpoint of structure, location, and function. In our study and practice, we should not mechanically equate them.

A description of the five viscera and six bowels is now presented as follows:

The Heart

The heart is located in the chest, surrounded by the heart sac (pericardium). It is primarily concerned with the transport of blood, emotional feelings and mental activity, through connections with blood vessels and the tongue. It also shares a "paired relationship" with the small intestine.

During illness, the heart reflects unusual (disturbed) emotional and mental activity and blood transport disturbances. The sick patient may experience palpitation, forgetfulness, insomnia, involuntary ejaculation, madness, unconsciousness, asthma, hemetemesis, nosebleeds, ulcerated tongue or hematuria, etc.

However, these symptoms do not necessarily reflect the heart's pathological state. They must be considered with the other visceral and bowel organs. Symptoms affecting other vital organs to be discussed below should also be considered in this fashion.

The Small Intestine

The small intestine is connected to the stomach above and the large intestine below. It receives food from the stomach and retains the best [nutrients] of the digested food for nourishing the body. The residue is transported into the large intestine for evacuation via the anus, and the residue water content is transported to the bladder where it is excreted as urine.

In illness the small intestine reflects a muddled situation, and its transport function is disturbed, as evidenced by micturition difficulty or diarrhea. Because the heart and small intestine have a paired relationship, the heat from an overactive "heart fire" is transferred to the small intestine and is manifested as bloody stools or urine.

The Liver

The liver is located below the right flank, and serves to store and regulate the blood. The liver controls the sinews. Body sinews, bones, and joints all depend on the blood from the liver for sustenance. The liver is related to the eyes which also depend on blood from the liver for nourishment and the ability to see. The liver serves a great regulatory function which affects emotional and mental activity.

In presence of disease conditions the liver's blood storage and blood regulatory function is affected and signs such as hemetemesis, epistaxis, bleeding or clots are noted. When liver blood is deficient, nourishment to sinews and blood vessels is curtailed, and joints become stiff, muscles become spasmodic and numb. Because liver blood is difficult (or "hsu") the liver's yang element becomes dominant and symptoms such as stroke, dizziness, headache, tinnitus, deafness, fainting, or convulsions may appear. If the liver blood is so deficient that it cannot nourish the eyes, night blindness or blurring vision will result. When the liver is too heated, the eyes become red and inflamed. When the liver is affected by unhappy feelings, its vitality may become repressed, and the sides hurt, hiccups appear, the abdomen hurts, the bowels become constipated, hernia appears, or sleep is disturbed, accompanied by nightmares or insomnia.

The Gallbladder

The gallbladder is located underneath the liver. It stores bile, and with the liver, serves a laxative function. The bile that flows into the small intestine aids digestion.

When the gallbladder is diseased, it may be seen as yellow jaundice of the skin and whites of the eyes, dizziness, bad taste in mouth, painful flanks, vomiting of bile, aggravation and anger, insomnia and nightmares, or hot and cold flushes. Because the liver and gallbladder share a "paired" relationship, some symptoms of liver disease are seen the same as those for gallbladder disease.

The Spleen

The spleen is responsible for transport and conversion (hua), which includes digestion, absorption and transport of the best food nutrient. After food has been digested in the stomach, its nutrient component is transferred by the spleen to feed all tissues and vital organs. The spleen also regulates the fluid balance in the body, and exerts a great effect on the absorption, transport and removal of water content. The spleen moreover controls the muscle of the body extremities and is related to the mouth. Hence the body's muscular growth and the fresh coloring of the lips are supported by nourishment from the spleen. Besides this, the spleen also produces fresh blood, and affects blood circulation and ching-lo (meridian) transport.

In the presence of illness, the transport-conversion and regulatory function of the spleen may be disturbed, and such signs as a distended abdomen, watery stools, edema, weight loss, dry lips, no appetite, poor digestion, weakness, or hemorrhage may occur.

The Stomach

The stomach receives and digests incoming food and drink. It has a "paired" relationship with the spleen, so after the stomach has digested the food, the spleen converts and transfers the essence in a collateral role of digestion, absorption and transport of nutrients. The health (weak or strong) of the spleen and stomach directly affects the health of the body. Hence traditional Chinese medicine places great attention to spleen-stomach function. In disease, normal gastric function is affected, and mechanical (digestive) obstruction appear. Other symptoms such as post-meal abdominal distension, hiccups, sighing, vomiting and constipation may also appear.

The Lungs

The lungs direct air [function], control breathing and relate to the nose. When the lungs inhale fresh air (pure air), and exhale carbon dioxide (impure air), they carry out a renewal process to maintain normal life activity in the human body. The air protects the body and serves to regulate body temperature through perspiration. However, air [function] is controlled by the lungs, for the lungs also regulate the body's fluid channels and exert an important effect on elimination of fluid from the body.

When the lungs are affected by disease, signs such as fever, nasal catarrh, cough, congested nose associated with colds and influenza, and other symptoms such as hemoptysis, epistaxis, hoarseness, loss of voice, empyema, night sweats, edema of face, constipation etc. associated with lung abscess or tuberculosis, may appear.

The Large Intestine

The large intestine assumes a transport function by receiving food residue from the small intestine, further reduced by lung action. The large intestine then transforms it into fecal matter which is evacuated through the anus. Because the large intestine and lungs have a "paired" relationship, lung diseases usually affect the large intestine's transport function. For example, in tuberculosis patients in whom the lungs' regulatory role has been weakened, constipation is commonly seen. As the result, medication to "moisten" the lungs and "drop" vitality (or ch'i) should be used to relieve constipation.

When the large intestine is affected by disease, cramps, diarrhea, or constipation may be observed.

The Testes (shen)

The testes store the semen, hence they are capable of stimulating growth, development, and reproduction in the human body. The testes are responsible for bone (structure), and relate to the ears and hair. Therefore, skeletal growth, the healthy sheen of hair, and hearing sensitivity in the ears are all affected by the testes. The testes are also responsible for body fluid balance, urinary secretion and digestive function, so they play a role in the regulation of body fluid and the excretion of body wastes (urine and feces).

When the testes are affected by disease, disturbances to body growth and development, and reproduction or the regulation of body fluid may lead to the appearance of such symptoms as weakness of lower limbs, alopecia, tinnitus, deafness, listlessness, impotency, involuntary ejaculation, sterility, abdominal pain, difficult micturition, polyuria or edema.

The Urinary Bladder

The urinary bladder stores and eliminates urine. After distribution via the spleen and regulation by the lungs, body fluid is stored in the bladder. The kidneys and the bladder have a paired relationship -- after aeration by the kidneys, fluid stored in the bladder is eliminated outside the body.

When the bladder is affected by disease, the function of urine storage and elimination is disturbed and symptoms such as retention of urine, incontinence, polyuria, hematuria, and lack of micturition control may be seen.

CHAPTER II. HYGIENE

Section 1. The Patriotic Health Movement

To realize an effective Patriotic Health Movement, we must observe the following guidelines:

1. Carry out a policy emphasizing prevention.

2. Mobilize the masses on a large scale. Hygiene and disease prevention work must depend on the large masses of workers, peasants, and soldiers who fight unsanitary practices.

3. Popularize disease prevention knowledge.

Drinking Water Sanitation

Dirty drinking water can easily cause disease. Many gastrointestinal tract infections such as typhoid, acute gastroenteritis, dysentery etc., and many parasitical infections are due to contamination of the water supply. To assure that drinking water is sanitary and clean, the following measures must be observed.

1. **Protection of water supply source**

   (1) Place barns, latrines, manure pits, outhouses and waste water drains as far away as possible from the water supply source. They are located best below the source of water supply.

   (2) Wherever possible, line wells with bricks and cover the bottoms with gravel or coarse sand. It is best to build a platform for the well and to place a cover over it.

   (3) Do not pour garbage or excreta, nor wash night-waste buckets or diapers in ponds and rivers [that supply drinking water]. Drinking water ponds and other-usage ponds should be separate. If river water must be used for all purposes, delineate usage zones, with the upstream zone designated for drinking water supply, and the downstream zone designated for other uses. This way, the introduction of waste matter and disease parasites into the drinking water is kept to a minimum.

2. **Disinfection of drinking water**

- 35 -

The best method for disinfecting water is by boiling it. However, boiling must be maintained for 15 minutes to meet sterilization (disinfection) requirements. Advocate the drinking of boiled water, and not untreated water.

(1) <u>To purify water</u>: Place finely crushed alum, half an ounce to every 10 tans [man load of 2 buckets to each tan] in the water tank and stir well. After a while, the impurities will settle to the bottom, and the water become clear. If some impurities still remain, add a little lime to hasten the settling process.

(2) <u>To disinfect with bleaching powder</u>: The use of bleaching powder to disinfect drinking water is the most extensive and comparatively economical and effective method used at present. When the bleach breaks down in water, it has a germicidal effect. However, the tanks should still be tightly covered when water is stored. It is best to disinfect the water as it is being used up. If it is possible to disinfect the water twice a day, results will be even better.

(3) <u>To disinfect with traditional Chinese drugs</u>: Wrap in cloth and place in water tank the following:

Place 1 liang of "kuan-chung <u>(Cyrtomium fortunei</u> J. Sm.)
     3 ch'ien of "shih-chang-p'u" (<u>Acorus gramineus</u>, soland)
     3 ch'ien of realgar

After 1 hour, water is ready for use. Water so treated will prevent against gastrointestinal tract infections.

Excreta Management

Human and animal excreta are both used as agricultural fertilizers. To increase agricultural production, manure composting must be practiced, though certain infectious diseases and parasitical infections are transmitted because of improper excreta management. "Excreta management" is a measure designed to curtail multiplication/propagation of flies. It is also a measure that prevents disease transmission by curtailing the dispersal/loss of excreta (retained as fertilizers made effective for increasing production) and by eliminating/killing disease-causing bacteria and parasite ova.

1. <u>Principles of excreta management</u>.

(1) Determine definite collection points. Place excreta tanks in a suitable yet centralized location -- far enough from water supply sources and kitchens, but located close enough for the masses to conveniently transport the excreta away when tanks are full.

(2) Assign specific persons to this management responsibility. A certain number of persons from each production team should be assigned to excreta management and cleaning the outhouses and latrines.

(3) Schedule definite periods of chemical treatment. Health workers or specially appointed persons should be responsible for treating excreta with chemicals to prevent propagation of harmful insects (see section on "Destroying Pests To Eradicate Disease").

(4) Make definite plans for excreta use. Set up timetable for excreta to be used after proper fermentation and aging.

2. Excreta management

(1) Collect and store urine and feces. Place fresh feces in excreta crock (or pit) with lid, and date. Keep several crocks handy for use by rotation. Generally, store the excreta half a month during the summer and one month during the winter. This way, the stored excreta will gradually ferment and kill disease causing bacteria and parasite ova during the process. If the excreta fertilizer is urgently needed, add 1-2% ammonia, or lime 0.5 to 1%, to the crock, and note that the contents could be used after another 3 to 5 days. In schistosomiasis endemic areas, feces and urine may be mixed in proportions 1:7, whereby the ammonia produced by the urine may be used to kill the schistosoma ova. The excreta may be used as fertilizer after 3 to 5 days in the summer, and 7 to 10 days in the winter. When the excreta fertilizer is urgently needed, add the vermicide Ti-pai-ch'ung (Propanil) first, then stir and mix, 1 gram to a load. After a 24-hour wait, the excreta is ready for use.

(2) Compost manure. Human and animal feces, waste matter and various wild plants may be mixed together, covered tightly and "composted" for 10 to 20 days for the waste to become "hot," after which the composted material is ready for use.

Besides this, care of the animal stalls and pig stys must be heightened to eliminate breeding grounds for mosquitoes and flies.

Food Sanitation

Since disease enters by the mouth, attention should be given to cleanliness and hygiene in food handling, in order to maintain high on-the-job attendance and productivity. To accomplish this, the following points are raised:

(1) Do not eat raw and cold food. Food should only be eaten after being cooked, and cooked food kept overnight should be reheated or steamed again before eating. Fermented food should not be eaten.

(2) Select food stuffs including fish, meat, eggs, etc., for freshness. Any rotten or spoiled food should not be eaten.

(3) If possible, do not eat meat taken from animals who have died of disease. Do not eat wild plants and mushrooms that are not identifiable nor consume cultivated plants freshly sprayed with insecticide, to avoid food poisoning.

(4) Remember to wash hands -- after work, before, and after bathroom use.

Section 2. Industrial and Agricultural Occupational Health

Intoxication caused by chemical substances during industrial or agricultural production is called occupational intoxication.

1. Preventing occupational intoxication

During industrial and agricultural production certain chemical substances, in the form of dust, liquid, aerosol, gas or steam, may enter the respiratory tract or come in contact with the skin to produce a caustic effect, or become absorbed to cause poisoning. Sometimes, some toxic matter may adhere to the hands which introduce it into the body by the food handled, and cause intoxication. However, intoxication via this approach is rarely seen.

Because of the characteristics, amount and concentration of the toxic substance in the air, and differences in the state of health and body resistance among people, the severity of the intoxication reaction among different individuals also varies.

Now, what steps should be taken to prevent occupational intoxication?

First, eliminate the source of occupational intoxication. Depending on the situation, substitute nontoxic or mildly toxic substances for toxic ones used, after effecting reforms in certain industrial processes.

Second, arrange production shops according to a prepared plan and allow for proper ventilation. Wherever possible, mechanize, seal in a closed-in environment, and systemize operations in those shops where toxic gases and dusts gather. Use natural ventilation supported by ventilator fans to reduce the concentration of toxic substances in the air to the lowest level possible.

Third, strengthen personal hygiene and preventive measures as follows:

(1) Besides strict personal adherence to a reasonable program of exercise and calisthenics, make sure workers cultivate good health habits such as the following:

    (a) Do not smoke or eat on the job.
    (b) Do not use machine oil to clean greasy dirt from hands.
    (c) Do not inhale toxic substances through the mouth.
    (d) Remove working clothes after work. Wash hands and shower whenever necessary.
    (e) When necessary (and possible), wear protective clothing, face masks, protective gloves, shoes etc.

(2) Give pre-employment and periodic physical examinations to workers who are in contact with toxic materials and products on the job to assure prevention, early treatment, and change of work assignment when necessary.

(3) Pay attention to proper nutrition to increase body resistance.

Fourth, tear down the old to set up the new, by revising unreasonable regulations and systems, and observing strictly, various reasonable working procedures.

2. Agricultural occupational hygiene.

Agricultural occupational hygiene is an important aspect of rural health activity. It is an important front line activity supporting agricultural production.

Agricultural production presents itself in various forms, though certain characteristics listed below are common to all.

(1) Most agricultural activities are easily affected by high temperature, severe cold, baking sun, strong winds, rainfall amounts, etc.

(2) Production activity varies regularly with the seasons and climate changes, sometimes heavy, sometimes light.

(3) Infection and varying degrees of intoxication are likely to occur because of chemical and manure fertilizers, and insecticides being used.

(4) Participation of women in agricultural activity has become general practice now, so further attention to the health of women and children should be given.

For this reason, the following precautions should be observed during agricultural production.

(1) Adapt to climate changes. Guard against heat stroke in the summer. Schedule working hours wisely. Be sure to wear straw hats and light-colored clothing. Carry adequate salt and drinking water out to the fields to supplement fluid salt and water loss through perspiration. In the winter, guard against the cold and change wet clothing frequently. Intensify training to guard the skin against frostbites and cracking.

(2) Know how to use insecticides and chemical fertilizers properly. Train insecticide suppliers and users to observe necessary rules and procedures. Commune members who are in poor health and women who are menstruating, nursing, or pregnant, should not be given this task. During spraying, make sure that personal protective measures are observed -- by wearing long sleeves and trousers, face masks, and walking backwards while spraying with the wind (direction). Each contact with the insecticide should be as short as possible. Spraying is best done in early morning or evening. Take special care of insecticides, tools used, and fields sprayed after insecticide application to forestall accidental contact or oral consumption.

(3) Prevent accidental injury. When using agricultural implements, machines, or vehicles, be careful not to incur cuts, abrasions, tears and crush injuries. Watch out for bites by poisonous snakes, insects, centipedes etc., and electrical shock during thundershowers. Minor injuries must be cared for in time.

(4) Protect the working women. Suitable care should be given women commune members during menstrual periods, pregnancy, illness or nursing (babies), or their work load should be lightened. Strengthen health care of women, with particular attention to menstrual and childbirth hygiene.

Section 3. Eliminating Pests and Disease

"Prevention the chief objective" is an important item in Chairman Mao's proletarian revolution, one of the four guidelines. We must actively initiate a patriotic health movement for the masses centered around hygienic measures and elimination of the four pests, to reduce the incidence of disease and to strengthen the people's resistance, for the benefit of "grasping the revolution and production, and stimulating work and war preparedness."

Following are some simple methods that are effective for eliminating several common insect pests.

Elimination of Flies

Flies are the vectors of typhoid, dysentery, gastroenteritis, infectious hepatitis and other diseases of the gastrointestinal tract. Maturation of the fly is divided into four stages: larva, maggot, pupa, and adult fly. Development from larva to adult fly generally takes 1 to 2 weeks, so it propagates and multiplies rapidly. Coordination of patriotic health movement activities in the winter and spring by digging up pupae and eliminating flies, the annual density of the fly population is curtailed.

1. Eliminating the fly breeding grounds

Flies like to lay their larvae on odiferous matter such as feces, garbage, rot, feed, sugar mash etc., which are smelly, fragrant, sweet, or fishy. Sanitary management of places containing such matter is a must -- outhouses and cesspools must be kept clean at all times. It is best to keep lids on excreta crocks, fencing around stables and barns, and cages for chickens and ducks. People should not live under the same roof with domestic animals. Someone must be assigned the duties of sweeping and cleaning these areas regularly in connection with the goal of the Patriotic Health Movement to improve on compost-making and environmental sanitation.

2. To eliminate maggots

(1) Cover layers of compost piled over the maggots with dirt in sufficient amounts to seal them in and kill them.
(2) Pour cow manure into the latrine.
(3) Retrieve the maggots and feed them to ducks. Pouring boiling water and emptying hot ashes over the maggots is also an effective method.
(4) Use traditional Chinese medicinal herbs.

   (a) Crush whole plants of stargrass (Aletris spicata) or Clerodendron bungei (ch'ou mu-tan) and throw into excreta crock.
   (b) Mix and crush plants of groundsel chui-li-kuang (Senecio scandens), Japanese pepper, and plume poppy (Macleaya cordata), and pour into waste water or latrine.
   (c) Use a 5% extract of tea-seed bricks (compressed residue of tea seeds after oil has been extracted) or add 2-4 liang of the tea-seed brick into the latrine or cesspool and stir for maximum effectiveness in killing maggots and larvae.

   If possible, sprinkle 6% wettable 666 powder or 5% Ti-pai-ch'ung into the excreta crock.

3. To eliminate pupae

Pour concrete over area surrounding latrine and lavatories to seal off
cracks and prevent maggots from entering the soil to be transformed into pupae.
Avoid applying lime to areas around latrines since lime has a tendency to
hasten maggot penetration (into the soil) and pupae development. The best
method is mobilizing the masses during winter or spring to dig for the pupae,
seal off or flood areas around the latrines, to flush out and kill the pupae.

4. To eliminate adult flies

   (1) Swat: Use fly swat, or attract flies with fragrant odiferous
       substance first before swatting.

   (2) Bait-kill:

       (a) Crush tobacco leaves and add to rice gruel or congee
           which will bait and kill flies.
       (b) Cut up leaves of oleander, add as bait to food.
       (c) [not printed on xeroxed copy]
       (d) Prepare a 10% solution of Ti-pai-ch'ung or 0.1% DDT, add
           to gruel, soup stock, rotten fruits or vegetables and
           mix for use as bait.

   (3) Spray with insecticides:

       (a) Crush leaves of the castor plant, dilute the extracted
           juice and use as spray. Or make up a solution of pyrethrum
           for the same purpose.
       (b) To 10 ml of 80% DDT, add water to make 8000 ml of solu-
           tion, which is then sprayed over fly breeding areas.

   (4) Smoke-out: A good method for killing wintering-over flies.

       (a) Burn duckweed for smoke (food and clothes should be stored
           elsewhere during the smoking operation).
       (b) Burn crushed leaves of huang-ching [chenopodium?],
           artemesia, and red duckweed to which realgar (spirits
           of sulfur) is added.

Mosquito Elimination

Mosquitoes can transmit many diseases such as malaria, filariasis,
Japanese B encephalitis, etc. Reproducing rapidly, the mosquitoes go through
four stages of development: the ova, larva, pupa and imago stages. Because
of this rapid reproduction rate, they should be eliminated as early as possible.

1. __Eliminating the mosquito breeding areas__:

Development of the mosquito from the larva to pupa stages takes place
in winter. Hence any collections of water are potential mosquito breeding
grounds. Filling up swampy pits, turning over open-faced drums and crocks,
plugging up holes in tree trunks, draining off collections of water and cleaning out drainage ditches, removing weeds, and stocking fish in watery paddies
will prevent mosquitoes from breeding.

2. __Eliminating larvae and pupae__

Hygienic measures must be initiated early during summer and fall by
regular inspection of hidden places. The following Chinese medicinal herbs
may be used:

(1) Add half a chin of water to 1 chin of fresh marsh pepper
smartweed and let steep for 4 hours. Then pour over waste
water or latrine to kill larva and maggots.

(2) Crush the stems and leaves of Rhododendron sinese and steep
in water. The solution may be used as a spray to kill larvae.

(3) Cut up crowfoot plant __Ranunculus acris__, and throw the chopped-
up pieces into waste water collections and latrines to kill
larvae and maggots. Besides these agents a 0.1% of Ti-pai-
ch'ung solution may be used as a spray, about 40 ml of solution
to each square meter of area.

3. __Eliminating adult mosquitoes__

There must be no let-up in the winter and spring to kill over-winter
mosquitoes. During summer, the following measures may be used:

(1) Capture. In early morning or evening when mosquito activity
is at a peak, use a net to capture the mosquitoes, or use a
basin full of soapy water to attract the mosquitoes (which will
get stuck).

(2) Smoke-out.

(a) Burn a combination of camphor leaves, and rice husks to
smoke-kill the mosquitoes.
(b) Burn powdered pyrethrum (the dried plant crushed into
powder) for smoke-out.

(3) Spray. Boil tobacco stems and leaves and stalks from the
__Macleya cordata__, and spray indoor areas. Besides these agents,
a 0.1% solution of Ti-pai-ch'ung or a DDT suspension may be
used for spraying or sprinkling (Ti-pai-ch'ung solution at
the rate of 5-10 ml/cubic meter, DDT suspension at a rate of

- 43 -

2-4 ml/cubic meter). However, to prevent poisoning in animals and people, care must be taken during spraying or sprinkling, not to contaminate eating utensils.

Rat Elimination

Not only do rats transmit diseases such as plague, leptospirosis and hemorrhagic fever, they also steal food staples, chew on clothing, destroy dams and engage in other harmful activity. Great effort should be directed toward their elimination.

1. Protection against rats

Grain staples and other food should be properly stored to cut off the food source for rats. Rat holes must be sealed and frequently checked. Hygienic measures should be practiced with the following measures to flush out the rats.

2. Trapping.

(1) Traps, cages, rice polishings floated over water tank, latches, and other devices may be used to bait and capture rats. However, methods used must be varied and changed from time to time. The baits and trapping devices should be placed in places frequented by rats.

(2) Digging out rat holes and burrows. If suspicious burrows are found (The lower part of the burrow opening is smooth with fresh dirt, or a coat of frost in the winter is piled just outside the entrance.), dig along the burrow to capture the rats.

(3) Poisoning.

(a) Dry plants of plume poppy (Macleaya cordata), pulverize and mix with food for poison bait.

(b) Mix zinc phosphide and "An-to" with cooked sweet potatoes (or flour) to prepare bait. Used more often during winter and spring when food is more scarce for the rats. But make sure that it does not get mixed with food for human consumption to avoid poisoning.

(4) Smoke-out
Tobacco stems and pulverized parts from the pepper plant may be burned for smoking out the rat burrows.

Lice Elimination

Not only do lice bite and suck blood from humans they infest, they also transmit diseases such as scrub typhus. The most important measure in lice control is good personal hygiene, regular bathing and regular change of clothing.

According to the site of infestation on the human body, lice may be classified as head lice, body lice, and crab lice.

1. Eliminating head lice

(1) Soak hair in vinegar first, to make it easier for a fine comb to comb the nits out. Follow with a steamed concoction from the plant Stemona sessefolia (one liang of S. sessefolia boiled in two chin of water for half an hour, then strained) rubbed well onto the hair and scalp, and wrap a towel around the head. Leave overnight. All lice will be eliminated by the following morning.

(2) Sprinkle and rub one liang of 10% DDT powder or 0.5% 666 (hexachloro-cyclohexane) powder into the hair, wrap with a towel and keep on overnight. Wash hair in warm water the following day.

2. Eliminating body lice

(1) Bathe and change clothing frequently. Clothing and bed sheets should be boiled for 30 minutes to exterminate lice.

(2) Soak clothing in a 10% Stemona sessifolia solution for louse extermination and prevention.

(3) Boil flowers, leaves and roots from 2 chin of Rhododendron sinense, 4 liang of soap and 20 chin of water for 30 minutes, then strain. Use preparation with soap for washing clothes. Good for louse and flea extermination.

3. Eliminating crab lice

The stemona solution described before can also be used on crab lice. Also 10% DDT powder or 0.5% 666 can be sprinkled over the genital area after bathing, to be washed out by soapy water the following day.

Some lice contain pathogens. Do not squash after finding lice on body. Rather, throw them into a burning fire.

Flea Elimination

Besides biting, sucking blood, and disturbing sleep, fleas can also transmit plague. Hence it is important to have good environmental sanitation and to maintain clean and dry surroundings. At the same time, Chinese rhododendron (see "Lice Elimination"), slaked lime, lime water, gasoline, or wettable

666 powder may be used to sprinkle or spray the floor areas and eliminate fleas found on the bodies of domestic animals.

Bedbug Elimination

While bedbugs are blood suckers, they also disturb sleep and affect the working habits and health of the people. Development of the bedbug from ova to imago only take a little over a month's time, so its reproductive rate is quite high. However, if bedbugs are not thoroughly exterminated in time, they can multiply to sizeable numbers within a short time. Methods of bedbug elimination include the following:

(1) Maintain good indoor sanitation. Oil of horsetail pine may be dropped into wall cracks and bedboard cracks harboring the bedbugs. Or use 666, oil, and grouting to seal off crevices in tables, chairs, drawers and other household furniture.

(2) Flush cracks of furniture pieces with boiling water several times in a row.

(3) Sun the furniture. Bed mats, bedboards, straw cushions, bed clothing and other items that can easily harbor the bedbugs should be exposed to strong sunchine, turned frequently, and be beaten with a stick to shake down and crush the hiding bedbugs.

(4) Sandwich stalks, stems and leaves of Chinese rhododendron between bed mat and bedboard as a preventive measure.

(5) Prepare a mixture of gasoline (one chin) and pyrethrum (4 liang) for application over cracks and seams in furniture and walls.

(6) Prepare a solution from one-half chin of 6% wettable 666 and one chin of water for direct application on seams and cracks.

Grasshopper Elimination

The grasshopper is also called t'ou-yu-p'o (oil-stealing hag), and it likes to be active in areas of food storage. Not only does it like food, transmit diseases such as typhoid fever, tuberculosis, ascariasis etc., it also likes to chew on books and luggage. Hence it must be eliminated.

1. Eliminating breeding grounds.

The kitchen and food storage areas should be swept and cleaned regularly. Lime may be used to seal off (grasshopper-hiding cracks). Store food properly to cut off a means of grasshopper subsistence.

2. Capture-killing, by

    (1) Bottle snare: Place some strong-odored food inside a narrow-mouthed bottle, to attract grasshoppers. Once a grasshopper crawls in, he cannot get out.

    (2) Poison bait, with

        (a) A mixture of borax and flour in equal parts with a little sugar added.
        (b) Crushed leaves, with a little sugar mixed in.
        (c) Ti-pai-ch'ung in 1-2% solution added to food bait.

        Either one of the methods just described will be effective as an exterminating agent in places of high grasshopper activity.

    (3) Insecticide spray: Combined with mosquito and fly elimination, a 25% DDT or 2% 666 solution may be used for spray.

Snail Elimination

Snails of the species <u>Oncomelania sinensis</u> which transmits schistosomiasis are usually found in damp and warm areas with luxuriant reed and rush growth and abundant rainfall. Snail control work must be coordinated with production and the Patriotic Health Movement, well timed and suited to local needs, and repeated periodically. The program must be thorough -- kill [oncolemania snails] in a patch, clear a patch, and strengthen a patch.

    1. <u>Eliminating snail breeding grounds by remaking nature with the</u> following measures:

    (1) Reclaim-planting. Reclaim marshy areas with plantings. In a dry, no-grass environment, such snails will find living conditions unfavorable and gradually disappear.

    (2) Burning. In the spring before the reeds sprout, they should be cut, dried and piled up for burning in the right direction on a clear windy day toward the rushes and reeds. Areas not penetrated by the fire, such as ponds, ditches, etc., must be treated by other means.

    (3) Burying. This measure could be combined with water improvements made during the winter. When new ditches are dug and old ones are covered over, the snail growing areas, reeds and all, can be dug up -- to a depth of 4-5 inches -- for burying in old pits and old ditches being covered up, over which a layer of lime is applied and joined to the "snail-less" soil. Areas adjacent to snail growing areas can be sliced to a 4-cm depth, and the soil and reeds chopped off can be burned, added

to compost pile, (To 1 chin of lime or animal manure, add 1
tan of soil/rush grass slicings. Then cover over solid with
dirt uncontaminated by snails. When the manure pile of reeds
and ashes becomes sufficiently hot, it can be used to kill
oncomelania snails.)

2. Eliminating snails with Chinese herbs

   (1) Soak 1 part each of powdered tobacco and lime, or just 2 parts
       of tobacco in 160 parts warm water. Allow to soak for half
       a day, then strain. Add 0.4-0.5% soapy water, then spray over
       snail breeding areas.

   (2) To one chin of bark and roots (ground fine) from a vine, the
       "lei-kung-teng," add 5 chin of water and boil for 30 minutes.
       Strain, keep juice, add equal parts of clay and straw-wood
       ash. Stir thoroughly and spray over snail breeding areas.
       If this clay and straw-wood ash mixture is combined with
       powdered tobacco in equal parts, this measure becomes even
       more effective.

   (3) Apply tea-seed "bricks" (from residue remaining after seeds
       have been crushed for oil), at the rate of 30-50 chin per mou.

   (4) Apply Rhododendron sinensis at the rate of 10-20 chin per mou.

Elimination of Granary Beetles

Varieties of granary beetles that endanger storage and growing crops
are quite numerous. These highly adaptive beetles reproduce very rapidly.
They can damage up to 1% of stored staples. Not only is this a great economic
loss, it can also cause food quality to deteriorate and affect the people's
health. For this reason, "combined prevention-treatment" and "prevention-
over-treatment" measures must be realized.

   1. Preventing granary beetles

      (1) Inspect all food carefully before storage, and sift/separate
          beetles from the food.

      (2) Make sure moisture content of food before storage should be
          under 15%. Sun-dry and sterilize.

      (3) Store food in well ventilated and well lit room, preferably
          equipped with devices for protection against rats and birds.

      (4) Clean and disinfect the grain bins periodically, to cut off
          a supply source for insect pests.

2. <u>Eliminating granary beetles</u>

    (1) Use a 0.05-0.1% solution of 666 powder to spray empty bins, or mix in with rice husks lining the base of bins. Or a 0.3-0.5% suspension may be used for disinfecting empty bins.

    (2) Spray bins initially with 0.05-0.1% Ti-pai-ch'ung, and repeat every 7-10 days after.

    (3) Spray empty bins, and inside and outside the storage area with wettable or 25% suspension of DDT, one kg to 9 kg of water (do not spray directly on the stored grain).

Section 4. Personal Hygiene

1. <u>Oral hygiene</u>

Neglecting oral hygiene will easily damage the teeth and lead to gastrointestinal ailments. Sometimes it can lead to heart disease, arthritis, nephritis, etc. During the period of dentition, children must cultivate good hygiene habits so their teeth will erupt evenly, and not have dental caries, which in turn will lower disease incidence.

Generally, one must acquire the habit of brushing his teeth and rinsing his mouth daily, and not eat excessively cold or hot, sour or sweet, food. Nor chew on food that is too hard. Nor eat before retiring to avoid damage to teeth. Generally, salt water may be used for mouth rinsing to prevent infection. If dental caries or other oral diseases such as tonsillitis, pyorrhea, etc., are discovered, they should be taken care of early. Besides this, bad habits such as mouth breathing, thumb sucking, tongue sucking, lip biting and pencil chewing, or sleeping with hand supporting the chin, or chewing on one side of the mouth only, should be corrected.

2. <u>Skin hygiene and clothing care</u>

Since the skin has a secreting function, dust and dirt it comes in contact with often adheres to it. If the skin is not washed clean, some skin diseases may take hold, and affect the whole body. For this reason, habits must include regular bathing and change of clothes, frequent nail-trims, hand washing before meals and after use of toilet, to assure skin cleanliness. Regular cold water showers and sun baths can invigorate the skin and increase body resistance (to disease). Hair must be washed and cut regularly. Besides this, contact with skin irritants such as certain acids and alkalis should be avoided to prevent skin infections. During the winter, the skin must be kept warm to prevent chapping and cracking. Proper working clothes should be worn for specific jobs such as fire-prevention, flood prevention, heat prevention, poison prevention or dog-bite prevention.

CHAPTER III. INTRODUCTION TO DIAGNOSTIC TECHNIQUES

The physician's basic task is protection and improvement of the people's health and prevention, early diagnosis and proper treatment of disease, so that the sick can early regain their health.

Section 1. How To Understand Disease

Under certain conditions, the human body is affected internally and externally by disease-causing factors that cause the balance between the body and the environment or the balance between body components to be disturbed, and become sick.

To recognize and understand disease we must be in close contact with the patients and study them with care. Through case histories and thorough physical examinations, the physician is able to obtain significant data. On the basis of this data, he can apply medical theories of disease differentiation to carefully analyze and evaluate the etiology, pathology, diagnosis, treatment, and prognosis of disease in gradual steps.
Using such techniques as interviewing, observation, auscultation, (listening, "hearing,") touching, and percussion, the physician makes a correct diagnosis through comprehensive analysis and deduction of the data collected. Again, the treatment carried out on the basis of the diagnosis obtained must not be isolated, restricted, or based on a static metaphysical approach to disease analysis and recognition. Under most conditions, the physician must repeat and follow up his studies, and accumulate some practical experience before he can better understand disease and its management.

Some of these methods used to understand disease will now be described.

Interviewing

The interview takes the form of a highly responsible and concerned question-and-answer dialogue, in which the history of illness is taken. It is a direct approach to understanding the patient's illness and its development. In the case of infants, and deaf and dumb or unconsious patients who cannot personally describe their illness, the physician should ask the patient's relatives or companion who brought him, for a history. When the questions are asked, the important points must not be lost sight of, the characteristics of the important disease symptoms must be clarified. The interview must have a purpose and a focus. It must also be systematic, well-organized, and objective. The general content of an interview includes the following:

1. <u>Chief complaint</u>: This describes the most important signs or obvious symptoms giving the patient most trouble since he became ill, including the nature and duration of their onset. Examples are "fever for two days," "chest pain, hemoptysis for a week," etc.

2. <u>History of onset</u>: This covers the whole course of illness from the time the patient became ill to the time he presented himself for treatment. For example, this includes details on the appearance of the important signs and symptoms, their development and subsequent changes, and finally their diagnosis and prescribed treatment, etc. Some pre-planning should be used in asking patients about symptoms. For example, if the patient is asked about "pain," the physician should ask about its location, duration, and nature, as well as possible causes, possible means of pain alleviation, and other signs and symptoms that accompany the pain, etc. He should pay attention to the following:

    a. <u>Chills and fever</u>: New cases of chill and fever are usually the consequences of skin exposure. Perspiration, when present, indicates a superficial or external (piao) deficiency, while absence of perspiration indicates a superficial "solidness" (clogging). Intermittent fever and chills indicate an ailment affecting both external (piao) and internal (li) organs. Fever and thirst with no chills indicates an internal (li) ailment, but chills without fever generally indicate a deficiency of the yang, and fever without chills, usually an overabundance of the yang. Afternoon fevers accompanied by a flushed face, heat and restlessness around the five centers (hearts), and excessive perspiration indicate a yin deficiency and "hot" inner organs. Chills without fever, accompanied by cold hands and feet, and loose stools and diarrhea generally indicate an abundance of the yin and "cold" inner organs.

    b. <u>Perspiration</u>: Perspiration noted when the patient is awake (self-perspiration) indicates a deficiency in the yang. An

excessive and somewhat oily perspiration indicates a deficiency
and detachment of the yang energy, but perspiration noted only
around the region of the head generally means an external deficiency and an overly "hot" stomach. Perspiration along the
arms and legs is usually seen in anemic patients, or those who
have stomach and digestive problems.

c. Stools and urine: Constipation accompanied by a hard stool or
diarrhea generally indicates a disease of heat and "solidness"
(congestion). If the stool is loose or contains undigested
food, a "cold" and deficiency disease is present. A yin-deficient constipation is usually seen in weak, restless, warm,
perspiring (excessively), and dry-mouthed patients. A yang-
deficient constipation is usually seen in thin and short-breathed
patients who are aversive to cold. Those who pass yellowish
brown and watery stools following abdominal cramps, and those
who feel a burning sensation in the anus generally present a
"hot" disease. Fresh blood in the stool may indicate hemorrhoids. Red and white mucus in the stool generally indicate
dysentery.

A scanty and yellowish-red urine is generally seen in heat and
congestion type diseases. Large amounts of clear urine passed
at one time generally are seen in "cold" and deficient types
of diseases. A cloudy urine generally indicates moist heat,
and frequent and scanty amounts of urine, an energy deficiency.
Polyuria accompanied by excessive thirst (sugar in the urine)
or polyuria with little fluid intake may possibly indicate
diabetes.

d. Food, drink, and taste: A flat taste in the mouth with absence
of thirst, and an inclination for hot drinks generally indicate
a "cold" disease. An inclination for cold drinks and food
usually indicate a "hot" disease. A bitter taste in the mouth,
accompanied by thirst, restlessness, and an inclination for
cold drinks generally indicate a "hot" disease affecting the
inner organs. A flat taste in the mouth accompanied by a feeling of greasiness (resulting from too much rich food) and a
disinclination for [drinking] water generally indicate a "moist"
disease. Hiccups and abdominal distension with appetite loss
and a feeling of fullness and nausea on eating generally indicate indigestion. A liking for spicy, dried or fried, and
strange materials (such as tea leaves, dirt, candles, etc.)
generally indicate the presence of parasites.

e. Sleep: An inclination towards sleep is seen in those with yang
deficiency and "moist" obstruction. Insomnia is usually present
in patients with poor circulation, excessive worries, and heart
and spleen deficiencies. Fitful sleep generally indicates

overeating or emotional disturbances. Wakefulness and early
awakening usually point to an active heart fire, a deficient
gallbladder energy (ch'i), or weak energy in the aged.

    f. <u>Menstruation and pregnancy</u>: The most important questions to
be asked here concern the age of menstrual onset, length of
menstrual cycles, duration of each menstrual period, amount
of flow, the presence of clots, dysmenorrhea, if any, the age
of menopause, if applicable, and the date of last menstruation.
A general report of each pregnancy and delivery, and any history of abortion or difficult childbirth, etc. should also be
included. If the patient's menstrual period is always early,
and the menstrual flow excessive and red, this generally indicates a "hot" disease. If the period is prolonged, and the
menses are scanty and dark purple, this generally indicates a
"cold" disease. When the period is delayed, and the menses
are light and scanty, this generally indicates anemia. Scanty
amounts of dull purple menses containing clots, when preceded
by pre-menstrual abdominal pains, generally indicate the presence of blood clots. Besides these, the nature of any leukorrhea, if present, should be questioned.

        Other questions should relate to any discomfort felt in the
head, chest and abdomen, the general treatment given after
onset of disease, its effectiveness, etc.

    3. <u>Past history</u>: To learn about the patient's general health and his
past illness, a medical history should be taken. This information is helpful
in diagnosing and treating the disease encountered at the moment.

    Furthermore, a clear and detailed record should be made of the patient's
environment and living conditions, personal habits, previous surgery, if any,
vaccinations and inoculations, and allergic episodes. In the case of sick
infants, their feeding routine, and any history of chicken pox, measles, and
other infectious diseases should be included. The general health history of
the family should be taken also.

Observation

    A methodical visual observation of related parts of the patient's body
and its secretions, excretions, etc., is employed by the physician to understand changes in the human body's skin coloring and form, tongue picture, etc.,
which may reflect disease states in related organs of the human body. Hence
the visual examination is an important technique used in the diagnosis of
disease.

    1. <u>Patient's mental makeup</u>: The patient's mood, good or bad, must be
noted first. If he is only excited -- his eyes are shining, his coloring
normal, movements quick, conversation spirited, and his breathing regular,

the illness is not serious and the prognosis is good. If he is depressed or moody -- his eyes are listless, his body thin, face sunken, mind unclear, and speech confused and/or breathing irregular, the illness is more serious, prognosis is poor, and the patient needs special attention.

2. Patient's complexion: When the skin coloring or complexion of healthy individuals is a vital-looking rosy tan, and the face is open and bright, this indicates a balance between energy and circulation. If the skin coloring is dull, dry, and lusterless, this may be due to a breakdown in stomach energy or visceral energy, and the prognosis is poor. If the patient's face is flushed and red, then a deficient (heat) fever is present; if it is not, a "solid" heat is present. Generally, a pale, wrinkled and lusterless complexion indicates a blood deficiency; a pale complexion accompanied by an aversion to cold, a yang deficiency; a wilted yellow complexion, deficiency and weakness in the stomach, a dull dark complexion, kidney damage; and a tangerine-colored complexion, yellow jaundice due mostly to "moist" heat.

3. Patient's physical condition: The patient's general physical condition and body stamina (strong or weak) are observed through his body movements -- walking, sitting, lying down, standing up, and through his body build (obese or thin). For example, hemiplegia is seen mostly in stroke cases, tremors in the extremities in tetanus, of infantile convulsions, and muscular spasms in malaria or rabies. Mental confusion and a picking of the bedclothes often indicate the critical nature of an illness. Patients who do not like to be turned or be bent over usually have back or spinal trouble. Wheezing, breathlessness, or respiratory difficulty on lying down flat may indicate respiratory and/or heart trouble.

4. Visual examination of the tongue (noting its general appearance and checking for a coated tongue): The tongue structure generally means its muscular makeup and meridian characteristics. The tongue fur is the coated layer found on the surface of the tongue. Tongue examination will be used as a diagnostic aid to help determine the deficient-solid nature of the disease, as well as its severity.

      a. Tongue structure:
         (1) Morphology (form): A normal tongue is neither thick nor thin, but soft and moist. If the tongue appears tight and shriveled, no matter how the tongue fur looks, the disease is the "solid" type. If the tongue appears thick, porous and tender, or the sides and tip of the tongue look jagged, then regardless of how the tongue fur and color look, the disease is most likely deficient. If the tongue papillae appear rough and prickly, this indicates heat inside the body. If the tongue is fat and swollen, this indicates "moist" heat in the body. If the tongue is cracked, body heat is over active or the yin circulation is inadequate. If the tongue is dark red and hard, speech is muffled, this usually indicates heat damage to the salivation mechanism, or the penetration of heat into the

heart. Tongue wagging and tongue swallowing usually indicate heat in the heart and spleen.

(2) Coloring: The normal tongue is pink, fresh and moist looking. Generally, a light-colored tongue without any fur on it indicates an energy and blood deficiency; a bright red tongue, a hot, "solid" disease; and a red and dry unfurred tongue, salivation damage. The stiff and bright red papillae signal, an overactive "heating" in the blood, but a dark red tongue often means heat penetration into the blood, and a purplish one, the presence of contusions or bruises.

b. Tongue fur: On the normal tongue a thin, white and clear fur coating that is not too dry nor too moist is present. However, it usually becomes thick when disease sets in. Observation of the moistness or dryness of the tongue may provide an inkling of body fluid loss. Generally, a washed-out looking fur on the tongue indicates moisture and cloudiness in the digestive tract; and a yellow fur, a worsening of a "hot" ailment. A raw-looking white fur indicates "cold" and moistness; a raw-looking yellow fur, dominance of a "moist" heat. A smooth black fur mostly indicates a yang-deficient "cold" disease; but a dry black one, the presence of a saliva-damaging "hot" disease.

Besides this, attention should also be paid to false impressions often created on the tongue coating by dyes from food and drink.

Whenever possible, the patient's urine and stools, the menses, and leukorrhea discharge, if present, should be noted to assist in the diagnosis of "cold," "heat," "deficiency," and "solidness" in disease.

Listening

This technique includes examination by hearing and smelling. When the physician examines the patient with this technique, he uses his own sense organ (such as the ear) or depends on some simple examination instrument (such as the stethoscope) to listen to the patient's speech, respiration, coughing and visceral organ sounds (such as those for the heart, lungs, etc.) and changes in them. The physician can also use his nose to check on the smell of the patient and of his excretions. Combined use of the four examination techniques to note changes in sound and smell may help determine the location of the disease and its nature.

1. Listening to the patient's sounds: Though the speech sounds made by the patients vary according to their size, and differences in pitch and quality, the normal speech sounds are generally emitted naturally, harmoniously and smoothly. If the patient's speech sounds low and weak, it generally indicates a deficiency ailment. Restlessness and confused speech generally indicates a "solid" illness.

Breathing of a normal person is even and regular, at the rate of 15 times a minute. Generally, shallow breathing accompanied by weak sounds indicates a disease of deficiency. Rapid stertorous respirations generally indicate a disease of "solidness."

A weak, low-pitched cough indicates an ailment of deficiency; a heavy and loud cough, generally an ailment of "solidness."

2. Auscultation: Examination of the heart and abdomen by auscultation is described here briefly.

    a. Auscultation of the heart: This is an important technique used in examining for heart ailments. It is generally performed over four areas:

        (1) Over the bicuspid valve: located at the apex of the heart.
        (2) Over the aortic valve: located along the right border of the sternum between the second intercostal space.
        (3) Over the pulmonary aortic valve: located along the left border of the sternum between the second intercostal space.
        (4) Over the bicuspid valve: located slightly to the right of the lower sternum.

    The sounds provided by the pumping of the heart are called the heart sounds.

The first heart sound is caused by contraction of the heart chamber where the tricuspid and bicuspid valves suddenly close and muscles of the left and right ventricle contract. At the apex of the heart, one can hear a "tung-tung" sound.

The second heart sound is produced by vibration resulting from ventricular diastole and sudden closure of the pulmonary and aortic valves. At the base of the heart, that is, over the pulmonary aortic valve and the aortic valve, one can hear a "ta-ta" sound.

The interval between the first and second heart sounds is comparatively short. From the second heart sound to the appearance of the first heart sound the interval is longer.

Heart sounds of a normal person are regular, heard at the rate of 60-80 times per minute in an adult. In illness, murmurs may be heard during diastole or systole.

Systolic murmurs are heard during the interval between the first heart sound and the second heart sound. In illness, such murmurs rattle like wind, particularly noisy and long. Systolic murmurs heard at the apex usually imply

- 57 -

incomplete closure of the bicuspid valve. If the duration of the murmur is comparatively short and it sounds like a gentle wind, then it is not considered pathological.

Diastolic murmurs are those appearing during the interval after the second heart sound but before the first heart sound. These murmurs usually sound like thunder going "lung-lung," or "thump-thump," like wind. Such murmurs heard over the bicuspid valve area generally indicate mitral stenosis. However, heart murmurs heard do not necessarily prove that heart disease exists. Nor do heart murmurs not heard indicate the absence of heart disease.

      b. Auscultation of the lungs: When the patient is examined by auscultation, he should usually sit or lie down. The examination sequence starts from top to bottom, from left to right, the physician comparing his findings simultaneously. The patient should unbutton his upper garments to suitably expose the back and chest, and continue breathing regularly and perhaps deeply. During the examination, the patient should not talk or swallow. The stethescope must be placed firmly on the chest, and not rub back and forth.

The sounds heard over the lungs during normal breathing include the following:

(1) Vesicular respiratory sounds: These are the soft "foo-foo" sounds produced by air entering and leaving the lung alveoli during respiration that sound like blowing wind. Inspiration of air is deep and long, while expiration is short and weak. In the normal person, except for the areas over the trachea, the clavicle, and the interscapular space between the third and fourth thoracic vertebrae, such breathing sounds may be heard over all other areas.

(2) Bronchial breathing sounds: These are coarse "ha-ha" sounds produced by air coming through the trachea and bronchi. The sounds are stronger and longer on exhalation, but shorter and weaker on inhalation. In the normal person, such sounds may be heard in the areas over the trachea and the clavicles, and the interscapular space between the third and fourth thoracic vertebrae. These sounds heard over other locations indicate some pathologic condition.

(3) Broncho-vesicular respiratory sounds: These sounds are a mixture of vesicular breathing sounds and bronchial breathing sounds, manifested as vesicular during inspiration of air, and bronchial during expiration of air. In the normal person, they are generally heard over the right lung apex, the upper sternum and the interscapular space. Heard over other locations, these breathing sounds indicate a disease condition seen most commonly in bronchopneumonia, pulmonary tuberculosis, and empyema.

Pathologic breathing sounds are due chiefly to lesions in the chest or pleura. Other characteristics, besides an increase, decrease, or dissipation in breathing sounds, are the following:

(1) Rales: This is a type of attached murmur heard during respiration. They may be divided further as:

(a) Dry rales: A whistle or snoring sound emitted through the narrowed respiratory passages as the result of bronchitis, pulmonary edema or bronchial spasms. Heard mostly in cases of bronchial asthma or bronchitis.

(b) Moist rales (bubbling sounds): A crackling bubbling sound produced by air passing through bronchioles or lung cavities containing some secretions. According to the loudness of the bubble sound, moist rales may be classified as large, medium and fine. Bubbling rales generally indicate the presence of inflammation or fluid collection in the bronchi or lungs.

(2) Bronchial speech sounds: As the patient counts "one, two, three" quietly, the physician uses a stethoscope to examine symmetrically the force of the respiratory sounds in both lungs. Under normal conditions, except over part of the large bronchial tube, speech sounds generally are not detected. However, when there are "solid" changes in the lung, or cavities appear in the lungs, these speech sounds become stronger and clearer, because the broncho-tube speech sounds are intensified. Such sounds are not heard over the healthy side. In the presence of bronchial obstruction, pleural effusion, or emphysema, when the pleurae undergo proliferation, the speech sounds are weakened or dissipated.

c. Auscultation of the abdomen: Under normal conditions, the purring peristaltic sounds of the intestines are heard at the rate of two to three times each minute. If such sounds are not heard within a 10-minute period, peristalsis is lost, a sign seen frequently in intestinal paralysis. In the presence of acute enteritis or intestinal obstruction, peristalsis becomes stronger and more frequent.

Tactile Examination

This is a technique in which the physician employs pulse diagnosis to check the patient's pulse and uses other manual methods such as touch, palpation and percussion to examine the patient's skin, extremities, and abdomen.

1. _Pulse diagnosis_: The pulse is generally felt at the "ts'un-k'ou" (over the radial artery at the wrist). Different pulse findings supplementing data obtained by other diagnostic techniques, may uncover the nature of pathologic change in the human body, and help make a proper diagnosis.

a. _Technique_: Before the patient's pulse is checked, the patient should be resting, and the physician should be relaxed. During the pulse taking, the patient's wrist is placed resting on its side, while the physician places his index, middle and ring fingers over the "ts'un-k'ou," feeling first the "kuan-mai" site on the inner aspect of the bony prominence (the ulnar prominence) with his middle finger. Then he places the other two fingers over the "tsun" and "chih" sites, anterior and posterior to the middle finger. If the patient's arms are short, placement of the three fingers should be adjusted, but the same amount of pressure (light, medium, heavy) is used to detect pulse conditions over the ts'un, kuan, and ch'ih sites (Figure 3-1-1).

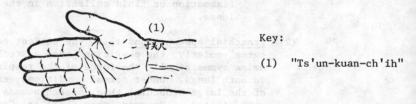

Key:

(1) "Ts'un-kuan-ch'ih"

Figure 3-1-1. "Ts'un-kuan-ch'ih" sites for pulse diagnosis.

b. _Pulse pictures_. The pulse of a normal person is not floating nor sunken, not rapid nor slow, but firm and regular, beating at the rate of 4 times between each respiration.

The commonly seen clinical pulse pictures are described below:

(1) _Floating pulse_: Felt lightly just under the skin, this pulse generally indicates superficial or external illness. Floating and forceful, the pulse indicates an external "solidness"; floating without force, an external deficiency.

(2) _Sunken pulse_: Felt only under heavy pressure (hardly felt on light pressure), a sunken pulse usually indicates internal disease involvement. Sunken and forceful, the pulse indicates internal "solidness"; sunken and weak, an internal deficiency.

(3) Slow pulse: A slow pulse, less than 4 beats during one respiration, generally indicates a "cold" disease. A slow but forceful pulse implies a cold accumulation into a "solid" disease, but a slow and weak pulse, a deficient "cold."

(4) Rapid pulse: A rapid pulse, in the excess of 5 times per respiration, generally indicates a "hot" disease; a frequent and forceful pulse, a solid "heat"; and a frequent and weak pulse, a deficient "heat."

(5) Deficient pulse: Such a pulse is weak under gentle pressure, hollow and deficient under heavier pressure. A patient deficient in energy and blood generally shows such a pulse picture.

(6) Solid pulse: Shows a forceful beat, whether felt under light or heavy pressure, this pulse is seen usually in "solid" type diseases.

(7) Slippery pulse: Felt to be smooth and easy, like pearls rolling around a smooth plate, this pulse is generally seen in patients producing a lot of mucus, or showing a "solid heat." In married women who have not menstruated for 2 or 3 months, such a slippery pulse (when considered with other signs), may indicate pregnancy.

(8) Full pulse: Full and long, hard and forceful, this pulse is felt like the tight cords of a musical instrument. Seen mostly in liver disease, pain, or malaria.

Other pulse nuances like a timid, hidden, fine pulse, weak pulse, and faint pulse, etc., are variations of a deficient pulse, differing only in the extent of their energy and blood deficiency.

2. Light massage examination

     a. Massaging the skin and muscles: A body in which disease is active is generally felt to be very hot, indicating a "solid" disease. A body cold to the feel indicates a weakening of the proper energy and a deficient disease.

     b. Massaging the arms and legs: The purpose of this examination is to check the temperature of the extremities. Generally, cold extremities indicate a deficient "yang"; but hot hands and legs imply a deficient "yin." Hot dorsal surfaces of the hands and feet generally indicate external exposure, wind and chills.

c. <u>Massaging the abdomen</u>: Abdominal pain that is heightened by gentle massage is usually a "solid" disease. Abdominal pain that is eased by such massage generally indicates a "deficient" disease.

3. <u>Palpation</u>: By applying pressure with the fingers to the body surface, this technique determines the consistency of organs underneath.

a. <u>Palpation of the thorax</u>: When the physician uses both hands to palpate symmetrical areas of the thorax and asks the patient to phonate by repeating sounds such as "one, two, three," he feels a slight tremor or vibration through the palms of his hands. The sound-produced fremitus felt by the hands is called the <u>vocal resonance</u>. This technique used for determining the amount of fremitus present is one of the important methods used for detecting respiratory disease.

Under normal conditions, vocal resonance in the male is stronger than that in the female, just as that in the adult is deeper than the voice in the child. People with thinner chest walls also display a deeper vocal resonance than those with thicker chest walls. Vocal resonance originating from the upper thorax is also stronger than that from the lower thorax, and resonance from the right chest is stronger than that from the left.

Under pathological conditions, the vocal resonance in patients with lobar pneumonia and serious tuberculosis is deeper, but that in patients with pleural effusion (or pneumothorax), bronchial obstruction, emphysema, thickening of the pleura, hydrothorax, or an excess of subcutaneous fat, is weaker.

b. <u>Palpation of the heart</u>: When the physician places his palms in the precordial area, if he feels a vibration similar to that felt when the hand is placed over the back of a cat ("feline wheeze"), this generally indicates some valvular stenosis, or incomplete blockage. "Feline wheeze" is generally felt at the base of the heart, apex, or left rib margins.

c. <u>Palpation of the abdomen</u>: When this examination is performed, the physician should stand on the right side of the patient, and let the patient lie with both knees flexed and the abdomen relaxed, for breathing deeply and naturally. The examination should be made from top to bottom with a light pressure of the hands, to determine the presence of pain on contact, the location and extent of the pain, and the relaxed or tensed-up state of the abdominal muscles. After this, deep palpation is performed to determine the presence of any enlargements in the deeper organs. When an inflammation of any abdominal organs is suspected during deep palpation, the physician should suddenly lift his fingers, and if the patient feels a "rebound pain," this generally indicates an inflammation of the peritoneum.

(1) Palpation of the stomach and duodenum: Pressure pain points in duodenal ulcers are found along the upper right part of the abdominal midline, about two fingers length from the navel. Pressure pain points for ulcers along the

lesser curvature of the stomach are found on the left
side of the midline. Pressure pain points in pyloric
ulcers are generally located on the right side of the
midline.

(2) Palpation of the appendix: Under normal conditions the
appendix cannot be felt. In acute appendicitis, the lower
right abdomen reacts obviously to pressure pain, the local
abdominal muscles show resistance and rebound tenderness
is present. In chronic appendicitis, because the inflamed
adhesions are fixed in one position, a belt or rope-like
mass is felt and pressure pain is present.

(3) Palpation of the liver: During this examination, the palm
of the right hand is placed flat on the patient's abdominal
wall, moving from the lower abdomen gradually up to the
right coastal margin. When the patient is exhaling and
the abdominal wall moves upward, the physician may use
the tip of his finger to exert pressure on the abdominal
wall so that when the patient inhales, the lower margin
of the liver slides downward along the abdominal wall and
is clearly felt if the liver is enlarged. If the liver
enlargement is not obvious, or the abdominal fat is thick
and the liver is not easily palpable, the patient should
be examined in the sitting position. If the patient has
a great amount of ascites, percussion should be used. When
the liver is palpated, its size (in cm below the ribs),
hardness, superficial features and margins, and pressure
pain etc., should be noted.

Under normal conditions, the liver cannot be felt. It is
soft, superficially smoth, and not painful to palpation.
In disease, such as hepatitis, cirrhosis, liver tumors,
liver cancer, late schistosomiasis or chronic right heart
failure etc., the liver is enlarged. In liver cirrhosis,
the liver first becomes enlarged after which it shrinks
and hardens. In liver carcinoma, hard nodes may be felt
on its surface.

When the liver is palpated, attention should be paid to
differentiating it from the right rib margin or other
internal organs.

(4) Palpation of the spleen: In this examination, the patient
lies down on his back or on his right side, both legs flexed,
to allow abdominal wall relaxation. The physician places
his left hand on the left lower thorax of the patient to
stabilize the patient's abdomen, moving it gradually upward toward the left rib margin. While he asks the patient
to breathe deeply from the abdomen, he watches the breathing motions and presses his slightly curved fingertips

lightly on the abdomen. When the patient inhales deeply
and the diaphragm pushes the spleen downward, the spleen
moves up towards the finger, and its size is measured by
noting its extension from under the rib (in cm). Besides
this, attention should be paid to surface features and the
presence of pressure pain, etc.

Under normal conditions, the spleen is not palpable. In
disease, such as typhoid, blood diseases, malaria, schistosomiasis, chronic and congestive heart failure, or splenic
abscess, etc., an enlarged spleen may be felt.

4. Percussion

During percussion the physician uses the middle finger of his right
hand to hit on the second interphalangeal joint of the left middle finger
placed over the patient's body, and determines any changes in the organ based
on the resonance produced by this percussion.

a. Percussion of the heart: The chief purpose of this examination
is determining the size of the heart, its shape, and location inside the thorax.
During percussion, the patient lies down and breathes in a relaxed manner. The
position of the physician's left middle finger should be parallel to the edge
of the heart. The left and right heart boundaries are percussed from the bottom up, and laterally toward the midline. That is, starting from the lungs
toward the heart, in a planned sequence over the intercostal spaces: on the
right, beginning from the first intercostal space over the liver-dullness border and left, beginning from the intercostal space over the apex impulse and
going upwards toward the second intercostal space. In a normal person, the
relative dullness boundaries generally do not go beyond the mid-clavicle on
the left, and not beyond the right margin of the thoracic cage on the right.
An increase in the boundaries of cardiac dullness indicates the possibility
of pericardial effusion or myocardial hypertrophy. If hydrothorax, pneumothorax, or emphysema exists, then the scope of cardiac dullness may be diminished
or dissipated.

b. Percussion of the lungs: It is best for the patient to be in
a sitting (or recumbent) position, his head tilted slightly forward, both
hands placed over the knees. Percussion begins from the apex of the lungs
over symmetrical parts, first anteriorly, then laterally, finally posteriorly,
from the top down. Under normal conditions, besides dullness noted over the
heart and liver, and a tympanic sound over the base of the stomach (the lower
part of a line drawn from the left armpit), clear lung sounds are noted on
percussion over the posterior part of the thorax from the 10th or 11th thoracic
vertebrae up.

Under pathological conditions, such as lung collapse or atelectasis,
pulmonary fibrosis, tuberculosis or pneumonia, etc., percussion reveals a dull
or solid sound. Pneumothorax or shallow but large cavities in the lung emit
a tympanic sound on percussion; pneumothorax emits an empty boxy sound (a high
clear sound).

c. **Percussion of the abdomen**: Under normal conditions, percussion of the abdomen generally presents a tympanic sound. If percussion presents movable dull sounds, it generally indicates the presence of ascites.

Characteristics of a movable dullness are generally presented as follows: when the patient is lying on his back, a tympanic sound noted over the central abdomen is accompanied by dull sounds over both sides; when the patient is lying on his side, this dull sound is noted over the lower abdomen, and the tympanic sound on the upper abdomen.

Appendix: Examination of Several Reflexes

1. <u>Pupillar reflex</u>: See section 3, "The Nervous System," in Chapter I.

2. <u>Corneal reflex</u>: When normal, a wisp of cotton applied lightly to the cornea will cause the eye to shut immediately. In coma, this reflex is lost.

3. <u>Knee-jerk reflex</u>: This reflex is checked with the patient either sitting up or lying down, so that the knee may be bent. The physician checks for the reflex by striking the quadriceps muscle at its fixation point (between the patella and the tibia), the reflex being a retraction of the muscle and extension of the leg. In disease, this reflex may be heightened or lost.

4. <u>Plantar reflex</u> (formerly called Babinski's sign): This is checked along the outer sole of the patient's foot, with a small pin scratching the skin from the ankle toward the toes of the foot. When normal, the toes flex toward the plantar surface of the foot. However, if the big toe shows dorsiflexion, and the other toes spread out like a fan, this is a positive sign.

5. <u>Knee-bend reflex</u> (Kernig's sign): This reflex is checked for with the patient lying down, both thighs and legs flexed to form two straight angles. After this, the physician extends the extremity by pulling the leg at the knee. If the extension is limited or the patient feels pain, this is a positive sign.

6. <u>Neck-flexion reflex</u> (formerly called Brezinski's sign): This reflex is checked for with the patient lying down, legs extended. When the physician raises the patient's head and flexes his neck, if the lower extremities immediately straighten out, this is a positive sign.

In case of meningitis where there is irritation of the meninges, both Kernig's sign and Brezinski's sign are usually positive.

Section 2. How To Analyze Causes of Disease

To find the cause of disease, on the basis of the patient's signs and symptoms and the physical examination results, is an important step in the diagnosis of disease. After a physician has gained a certain recognition of disease by using the examination techniques just described, he must, to further understand and make a correct diagnosis, make an overall study of the patient's attitudes and mental activity, and his illness to correctly differentiate between the etiology and the present course of the disease. The human body is an integral mechanism in which inconsistencies contradict each other. It also has a very close relationship with society and its natural environment. The onset and development of disease frequently are related to the body's makeup, its resistance, and the virulence and number of pathogens present, in a complex relationship.

The following sections list some causes of disease in the human body.

Body Factors

The important ones refer to mental activity and the physical makeup of the human being.

1. Nervous and emotional makeup

Mental and emotional activity among different individuals vary under the different influences of society and the natural environment. Examples are joy, excitement, happiness, anger, fright and sorrow. Under most conditions, emotional activity will not cause disease, but under certain conditions it can damage normal body function and cause disease or hasten its development, e.g., certain neuroses or functional digestive disturbances. However, we must feel the dynamic effect of the proletarian world view and its revolutionary optimism on preventing or overcoming disease. For example, for some of our comrades who have incurred large serious burns, because they can hold on to a fearless revolutionary determination to fight against disease, they ultimately overcome it. This fully explains how dynamic the patient's subjective, yet dynamic, outlook can have on overcoming a serious illness.

2. Body makeup or physical conditions

This includes the body build, and body reactions and differences such as age, sex, resistance to disease, etc. which are closely related to the incurrence and development of disease. After 1950, the large working masses were given regular training so their bodies become healthy and strong, and less susceptible to disease. Furthermore, the aged or the young, because of a weak body makeup, may, because of weak resistance, be easily affected by disease-causing factors to become ill.

The human body's reaction to external environmental and internal body factors may vary because of regional, age, sex, and sensitivity differences. For example, children can easily be affected by infantile paralysis, while older adults are more susceptible to cancer. Some people are allergic to pollen, shrimp and crab, and develop wheezing or urticaria. Certain other ailments are commonly seen in men, and others more commonly seen in females. These are all closely related to the human body's reaction.

- 66 -

External Factors

These include various social and natural environmental factors. Sometimes etiologic factors are quite complex.

1. Social factors

Differences in the social system often have a great effect on the incidence and elimination of certain diseases. China has early eliminated cholera, smallpox, venereal disease, plague, etc. With respect to certain diseases with more serious consequences, such as malaria, schistosomiasis, etc., better prevention and treatment measures have greatly reduced the disease incidence. Therefore, when causes of disease are analyzed, great emphasis must be given to the social system.

2. Natural factors

Often the frequently seen natural etiologic factors are:

a. **Physical factors:** Radiation, mechanical injuries, war injuries, high altitude, high temperature, and outer space activity, etc.

b. **Chemical factors:** Strong acids and alkalis, pharmaceuticals, cyanide products, organic phosphorous in agriculture insecticides, and snake venom. Though the liver exerts a detoxifying action, if the poison in the chemical is very strong, or the dose is sizeable, or the detoxifying capability is lowered, poisoning or intoxication will result.

c. **Biological factors:** Pathogenic viruses, bacteria, fungi, spirochetes, protozoa, tapeworms, etc. Biological pathogens attacking the human body are quite selective in their site of attack. For example, the dysentery bacillus acts chiefly on the colon, the encephalitis B virus acts chiefly on the cerebrum. Diseases caused by biologic pathogens are also specific in most cases, and have a definite incubation period, an orderly course of progression, specific pathologic changes, clinical manifestations and immunity mechanisms, etc. This is due chiefly to the different specificity of different pathogenic factors and the human body forming unusual contradictions.

d. **Climatic factors:** Under normal conditions, natural climatic factors, such as wind, cold, heat, humidity, aridity, etc., do not cause disease. However, when the climate changes suddenly and the body's resistance is lowered and cannot adapt immediately, disease may occur. At present, the traditional Chinese medicine approach to climatic factors as causes of disease will be described in the following discussion on excesses of the six elements of wind, cold, heat, humidity, aridity and fire, and their associated ailments.

(1) <u>Wind frequently causing disease</u>. Wind changes rapidly, and
its symptoms are usually uncertain. However, wind as a disease-causing factor is often combined with the excess of
other elements. For example, in a wind-heat combination,
its symptoms are headache or tension, perspiration and
fever, or slight perspiration, red sore throat, thin white
or slightly yellow coating on the tongue, and/or a floating
and rapid pulse. In a wind-moisture combination, the symptoms may be headache and depression, an aversion to cold,
feverishness, body aches and joint pains, and a thin white
coating of fur on the tongue.

(2) <u>Cold or chill:</u> Chills damaging to people are manifested
as headache, no sweat, fever, aversion to chills, aches and
pains over the body and joints, a thin white fur on the
tongue, a floating and bounding, or tight, pulse.

(3) <u>Heat or fever</u>: Divided into two types: summer and "fire"
heat. Summer heat or fever is the hot vapor [excess] abound-
ing in the heat of summer; usually accompanied by moisture.
Its symptoms are heavy-headedness, respiratory heaviness,
malaise, perspiration, a dirty-looking face, or a thirst
accompanying high fever, burning urination, deficient pulse,
red tongue, and a thin yellow film on the tongue. This may
be seen in various symptoms surrounding heat stroke.

"Fire" heat is a disease caused by overheating or trans-
ference of other disease vapors [excesses]. Its symptoms
are high fever with restlessness, thirst and sore throat,
flushed face and bloodshot eyes, rapid pulse, dry yellow
fur or rough papillae on the tongue, and a red or purplish
tongue base.

(4) <u>Moisture</u>: Oftentimes the damage from moisture affects the
lower parts of the body first, because of exposure to dew
and fog, or living in damp areas, or wading in water, or
getting soaked in the rain. Its symptoms are usually heaviness of the body, sore and tender joints which may limit
extension or bending of the joint, a slightly oily white
fur on the tongue, and a slow pulse.

(5) <u>Dryness</u>: Dryness becomes an ailment in the fall. Besides
fever, it is manifested by cracked lips, dry throat and
mouth, thirst, a dry non-productive cough, scanty urine,
slightly constipated stool, dry rough skin, etc. Such diseases are further classified as illnesses of warm dryness
and illnesses of cool dryness. Furthermore a "dryness"
disease may also be caused by an illness that affects saliva
secretion.

Other factors, such as unhygienic eating habits that lack discipline
and control, can also be indirect pathological factors.

Section 3: How To Make A Differential Diagnosis

The physician analyzes the clinical data collected by these four examination methods and makes some deductions to arrive at some conclusion about
the severity, location and nature of the disease, before he prescribes treatment. This is the course of diagnosis and treatment called disease differentiation and therapy in traditional Chinese medicine.

The differentiation of disease may be grouped by the name of the disease,
such as typhoid, dysentery, malaria, etc. Other diseases are named by the
symptoms, such as edema, coughing, hemoptysis, etc. In traditional Chinese
medicine, there are the eight principles of discriminative or disease-differen-
tiating classification (yin, yang, piao, li, han, jeh, hsu, and shih) and the
six meridians (t'ai-yang, yang-ming, shao-yang, t'ai-yin, hsueh-yin, and shao-
yin).

The important content of a symptom based on the eight principles will
be described as follows:

Yin-yang comprise the basis of disease differentiation by the eight
principles. On the basis of clinical manifestations, the diagnosis of all
diseases may be divided into two great categories: yin illnesses and yang
illnesses.

Yin Illnesses

Most deficient (hsu), cold (han) and internal (li) ailments are yin-
illnesses. Symptoms are a pale or light complexion, fatigue and drowsiness,
general malaise, soft and low voice, inclination for quiet and few words (of
speech), shallow respiration, shortness of breath, loose scanty stools containing undigested food, poor appetite, flat taste in the mouth, low fluid
intake (never thirsty), an inclination for hot drinks and pressure applied to
abdomen to alleviate cramps, cold hands and feet, urine clear (and passed in
large quantity), tongue pale and lightly coated (white), or the pulse may be
sunken, delayed (slow), deficient, or weak.

Yang Illnesses

Most "solid" (shih), hot (jeh) and external (piao) ailments are yang
illnesses. Symptoms are a flushed face, overly warm body and preference for
coolness; restlessness, loud mouthed talkativeness, coarse, loud, rapid breathing, use of coarse, loud language, aversion to applied pressure for relieving
abdominal cramps, hard stools or constipation, dry mouth and cracked lips,
great thirst and desire for fluids, scanty burning urine, a purplish red tongue
-- coated yellow, sometimes cracked or black and raw.

Changes for the yin and yang illnesses described above are quite complex
and sometimes they overlap. All the symptoms described do not necessarily
appear in any one patient, because the external, internal cold, heat, deficient or solid manifestations for the illnesses vary.

External (piao) Illnesses

"Piao" and "li" are indications differentiating the site (inside or outside) and the extent and seriousness of the illness. External illnesses generally are the beginning stages of exposure (chills) and may be classified as external cold or external heat.

1. **External cold**: Symptoms generally are fever and chills, no perspiration, painful joints, a floating and tight pulse, and a thin white coated tongue.

2. **External heat**: Symptoms are headache, fever, and aversion to wind, perspiration (may or may not be present), thirst (or no thirst), floating and rapid pulse, and a white or slightly yellow coated tongue.

Internal (li) Illnesses

Before recovery from its external manifestations, the illnesses may develop inward. When the illness has left the confines of external illness but before it reaches the level of an internal illness, it is a half-external half-internal illness. When the condition progresses internally, it is divided further into internal heat and internal cold.

1. **Half-external half-internal illness**: The symptoms are generally intermittent fever and chills, a heaviness in the chest, restlessness, nausea and vomiting, no appetite, dry throat and irritation in the mouth, dizziness, and a bounding pulse.

2. **Internal heat**: Symptoms are fever, an aversion to heat but not cold, perspiration, great thirst, bloodshot eyes and red lips, rapid pulse, red and coated (yellow) tongue, constipation and abdominal distension in many cases. Because of fever and increased blood flow in some cases, red spots, bleeding, vomiting of blood, nosebleeds, and a reddish purple tongue may be seen.

3. **Internal cold**: Symptoms are generally an aversion to cold, cold extremities, night sweats, loose stools, and a sunken and slow pulse.

Cold (han) Illnesses

Cold and heat are used to differentiate the nature of disease. Cold illnesses usually stem from a cold air (vapor) or a degeneration in body function. The illness is characterized by a pale or white complexion, an aversion to cold, cold hands and feet, drowsiness, loose stools, clear urine (of low specific gravity). The patient is not thirsty, but likes hot fluids. Tongue covered with a white and smooth coating, and the pulse is slow.

Heat (jeh) Illnesses

Heat illnesses are due mostly to heat or changes transferred from other etiological factors, or overactive reaction of the human body. Symptoms are generally a flushed face, fever, restlessness or even flaying of the arms and legs, delirium, constipation, a coarse yellow coating on the tongue, rapid bounding pulse, etc.

Deficient (hsu) Illnesses

Deficiency and "solidness" are indicators used to differentiate the extent or seriousness of the illness, and the resistance of the human body. Symptoms are a decrease in body function, a lowered resistance, and in more severe cases, a listless spirit, weakness, shortness of breath, aversion to talk, poor appetite, emaciation (weight loss) and a thick and tender tongue.

"Solid" (shih) Illnesses

In such illnesses, body functions are overactive (in healthy individuals) and symptoms such as abdominal distension that is sensitive to touch, difficulty in urination, constipation, loud speech and coarse breath, a hard tongue, and bounding pulse may be noticed.

Solid diseases may be due to:

1. Food accumulation. Symptoms are generally seen as no appetite, an aversion to the smell of grease, abdominal distension, hiccups and regurgitation of hydrochloric acid, and in severe cases vomiting of food consumed the night before, a thick-coated tongue, and sliding and forceful pulse.

2. Mucus. Symptoms are an abundant expectoration of a thin white sputum, dizziness, palpitation, and an aversion to fluids (water).

3. Moistness (shih). Symptoms are seen mostly as nausea, no appetite, a sweet and greasy taste in the mouth, watery stools, a white-coated and greasy-feeling tongue.

4. Energy stagnation. Congestion in the chest and abdomen. Symptoms are usually manifested as abdominal distension and pain, nausea, belching of air, and a tensed-up pulse.

5. Blood clots. When the blood circulation is poor, symptoms are usually manifested as sharp pains, localization of pain, and in some cases, hard masses felt in the abdomen, black stools, dry mouth and lips, aversion to drinking water, cyanosis, and petechia on the tongue.

This shows how yin and yang, piao (external) and li (internal), cold (chills) and heat, deficiency and "solidness" cover the general range of disease symptoms. During the course of an illness, these factors, under certain conditions, are variable and interchangeable. Therefore, in the diagnosis through recognition of symptoms, it is important to distinguish the true from the false. To grasp the important point, the physician must interrelate or tie things together and develop an understanding of the disease, and be flexible in his application of the eight principles for diagnosis. Only in this way can he continue to raise the level of diagnosis and treament through practical medical experience.

Appendix: Glossary of Common Terms

Triple warmer (san-chiao): The overall term for the upper warmer
(Shang-chiao), central warmer (chung-chiao), and the lower warmer (hsia-
chiao). On the basis of their locations, the upper warmer refers to those
parts above the diaphragm including the lungs and the heart; the central
warmer refers to those parts under the diaphragm but above the navel, including the stomach and spleen; the lower warmer refers to the abdomen below the
navel, including the liver and kidneys. When used to describe the stage of
disease development, the upper warmer refers to the early stages of the disease, the central warmer refers to the height (crisis) of the disease, and
the lower warmer refers to the latter or final stage of the disease.

Nutritents (or nutrition) reinforcing energy and blood (ying wei-ch'i-
hsueh). Has two meanings: one refers to the nourishment and protection of
the human body, and the circulation of energy and blood within the traditional
Chinese medicine concept of physiology; the second refers to the four stages
of high fever development in fevers, and is used as the basis for disease
diagnosis and treatment, within the traditional Chinese medicine concept of
pathology.

Pericardium (hsin-pao). The outer covering of the heart, whose function and pathological changes reflect the same within the heart. (Note: As
a traditional Chinese medical term, this has an interpretation different from
the "pericardium" in Western medicine.)

Upper orifices (shang-ch'iao) also called (ch'ih-ch'iao). The ears,
eyes, mouth, and nose.

Primordial energy (yuan-ch'i). The prime energy in the human body.

"Tan-t'ien". The site about two inches (ts'un) below the navel.

Parts controlled by the five viscera (wu-chuang-so-chu). Blood vessels
controlled by the heart, skin by the lungs, sinews by the liver, flesh by the
spleen, and bone by the kidney.

Saliva (tsun-I). All normal fluids in the human body are called "tsun-
I." Examples are perspiration, blood, semen, saliva, tears, urine, etc. The
production and excretion of "tsun-I" is an important factor for maintaining
the yin-yang balance in the body. If "tsun-I" consumption or loss is excessive, the deficiency will cause a shortage and lack in energy and blood, that
will require some drug to restore it to its normal state. This is called
"sheng-tsun" (fluid or saliva stimulation).

Correct or restore (cheng). The proper mechanism of body resistance to
disease or the reaction of body resistance to disease, like in "cheng-ch'i"
(to restore prime energy).

Deflection or improper (hsieh). On a wide scale, it is used to describe all pathological factors, such as wind, chill, heat, dampness, fire, and their improper aspects; now interpreted to include bacteria, viruses, protozoa, and other pathogenic factors in modern medicine.

Seven emotions (ch'ih-ch'ing). Emotional changes such as joy, anger, worry, pensiveness, sadness, sorrow, and fear, which generally fall within the scope of normal feelings. Illnesses resulting from an excess of these emotions is called "hurt by the seven emotions" (ch'ih-ch'ing-so-shang).

Deficient or empty activity (hsu-lao). A comprehensive term for several types of chronic diseases caused by injury or damage to the viscera and by a weakening of the prime energy.

Nosebleeds (niu). Bleeding not due to trauma, such as bleeding from the nose, the gums, the ears, the tongue and the skin. Examples are epistaxis and bleeding gums, etc.

Night sweats. A symptom commonly associated with yin-deficient illnesses. This is perspiration that appears after a person is asleep.

Sputum (t'an-yin). The thick sputum is called "t-an," the clear mucoid sputum is called "yin." Generally the term includes both of these characters: "t'an-yin," which is an illness as well as a cause of illness.

Tympanic distension (ku-chang). Drum-like abdominal distension as the result of body ascites or stagnant circulation of the energy (ch'i).

Recurring fever (ch'ao-jeh). Fever that recurs at regular intervals.

Insufficient central energy (chung-ch'i fu-chu). Insufficient energy in the spleen and stomach, termed so because the spleen and stomach are located in the central part of the body.

Very chilled hands and feet (shou-chu chueh-I). Excessive chills experienced by the patient whereby the chill in the hands and feet extend all the way up to the knee cap.

Alternating chills and fever (han-jeh wang-lai). An important symptom seen in shao-yang disease.

Accumulation or congestion? (chi-chu). Manifestation of energy-related illness. Its occurrence and subsequent pain became localized as a growth. When pin-pointed and a mass is felt upon palpation, it is called "chi" (accumulation). When its occurrence, pain and timing cannot be pin-pointed, it is called "chu" (settling). This symptom indicates some accumulation of energy in the viscera.

Numbness (pi). A numb feeling resulting from obstruction of the meridian that leads to painful joints, numbness and motor disturbance. Because of differences in the cause, its clinical manifestation may be classified into two types: wind-chill rheumatoid numbness and fever numbness.

Warm (low-grade fever) illness (wen-cheng). A term covering all feverish illnesses. Commonly seen are spring fever, dampness fever, summer fever, winter fever, etc. Illness occurring in the spring as a result of the malevolent feverishness (though the "malevolent" influences abound during winter and the yin-fluid is low) is called spring fever. Illness occurring in late summer and early fall as the result of dampness deflections invading the body is called dampness fever (shih-jeh); illness due to attack by summer heat, disposed toward fever with no dampness is called summer fever; disease occurring in early winter when the climate is normal and the body is affected by heat and hot and dry deflections is called winter fever.

Six-meridian disease (lu-ching-ping). The six meridians are the "t'ai-yang," "yang-ming," "shao-yang," "ta'i-yin," "shao-yin," and "hsueh-yin." In six-meridian disease, the changes and development of illness extend from the shallow to the deep, and from the superficial to the internal. It is also a method of classifying illnesses resulting from external exposure.

Yin depletion (mang-yin). A condition characterized by feverish skin, restlessness and aversion to heat, great thirst and a desire for cold fluids, noisy or coarse breathing, and a rapid and hollow pulse as the result of excessive perspiration, vomiting and diarrhea, or hemorrhage when the yin fluids are depleted.

Yang depletion (mang-yang). A condition characterized by cold skin, pallor, no thirst, shallow respiration, cold hands and feet, a weak, small pulse. These symptoms are the result of excessive perspiration that does not stop, as yin damage affects the yang to deplete it of its energy.

Fever (shang-han, literally chill injury). Characterized by a floating tight pulse, aversion to cold, body pains and aches, vomiting, etc. as the result of chill deflections received by the human body. The meaning of this term is distinctly different from that for "shang-han-ping" (typhoid fever) of modern medicine.

Summer injury (shang-shu). Characterized by a dirty complexion, a dry mouth, "hot" teeth, restlessness, etc. as the result of summer heat deflection received.

Tuberculosis (lao-ping). Broadly speaking, the deficient tuberculosis ("hsu-lao-ping" or the deficient work illness) caused by tuberculosis. Characterized by coughing, hemoptysis, recurrent fever, night sweats, wet dreams, insomnia, etc.

Sputum dampness (t'an-shih). According to traditional Chinese medicine, dampness is controlled by the spleen, and sputum is caused by dampness. When used together, the term "t'an-shih" refers to an impairment in transport function between the spleen and liver, or because of dampness attack by dampness deflections. The symptoms of dampness deflections are continuous coughing with a thin white mucus coughed up, tight feeling in the chest, constipation, dizziness, vomiting, etc.

Yang deficiency (yang-hsu). A symptom group describing functional impairment. Symptoms are pallor, pale lips, loose stools, cold and clammy skin of hands and feet, a large but weak pulse.

Deficient yin (yin-hsu). A group of symptoms describing inadequate body fluid. Symptoms are dark complexion, dry mouth and lips, afternoon fevers, restlessness around the five centers, contipation, dark urine, a weak rapid pulse, etc.

Deficient spleen (p'i-hsu). A group of symptoms describing impaired digestive function. Symptoms are indigestion, diarrhea, emaciation, cold hands and feet, yellow wrinkled complexion, etc. The spleen here is different from the one described by modern anatomy.

Deficient testes (shen-k'uei). Same as "shen-hsu." A group of symptoms describing impaired testicular function, which leads to dizziness, tinnitus, weakness of back and legs, impotency, wet dreams, etc. (Not to be confused with the "shen" used to describe the kidneys in modern medicine.)

Depressed liver (kan-yu). Indicates some depression and apprehension. Clinical signs are nausea, pain in the sides, poor appetite, listlessness, etc. Treatment by "loosening" (so) the liver and "rectifying" (li) the energy.

Liver-yang dominance (kan-yang shang-hang). A group of symptoms describing overactive liver energy on the ascendance. Seen as headache (top of head), dizziness, tinnitus, restlessness and apprehension, insomnia, bad temper, etc. Drug therapy relieving these symptoms is called "p'ing-kan t'i-yang" (quieting the liver and watering down the yang).

Wind and water (feng shui). A type of edema. Because vapor (shui-ch'i) and wind deflections are contained and felt within the body, the illness presents first with edematous eyelids, after which the edema spreads over the body rapidly, accompanied by chills, fever, scanty urine, etc. Medicinal preparations that suppress the wind and stimulate body fluid circulation may be used for treatment.

The Herbal (Pen-ts'ao). A book that records Chinese medicinal plants.

Prescription or **prescribed concoction** (fang-chi). Compounding several drugs (or just selecting one) for a purpose, and with accuracy and selectiveness in mind, into a specific mode for prevention or treatment.

Single concoction (I-chi). Taking one dose of one concoction. "Erh-fu," and "san-fu," etc., means two or three doses.

Fight poison with poison (I-tu kung-tu). Employing toxic substances to treat poison-deflected conditions. This method is used to treat many resistant boils, infected sores, leprosy, etc.

Muscle (tissue) building (sheng-chi). Regenerative growth of tissue eroded by sores. Medications are applied to stimulate the healing process called muscle (tissue) building.

Diuretic (li-shui). One of the principles of diuresis therapy. Drugs used to promote diuresis are called diuretics.

Energy-regulation (t'iao-ch'i). Drugs used to restore blocked or stagnating energy to normal in doses less strong than that given to stimulate energy circulation (hsing-ch'i).

Bruise-resorption (hsieh-yen). Use of drugs to resolve bruises and clots which cause fever and pain (inflammation).

Rectifying the center (li chung). Use of drugs to correct and regulate the stomach and spleen in the center (middle) warmer.

Measles breakout (t'ou-chen). Use of an antipyretic to hasten appearance of the measles.

Convulsions calming (chen-ching). Use of drugs to quiet infants and adults having convulsive fits.

T'i-ch'a (retract-insert). A needling technique used in acupuncture. After the needle has been introduced, a slight retraction made with the needle between the thumb and index fingers is "t'i;" deeper needle penetration is "ch'a."

Nien-ch'uan (hold and turn). A needle-manipulating technique used in acupuncture. Twirling movement made by the needle held between the thumb and index finger.

CHAPTER IV. THERAPEUTIC TECHNIQUES

Section 1. Treatment with Chinese Herbs

Traditional Chinese medicine is the sum total of the Chinese working people's experience in their struggle against disease over the last several thousand years. It contains the rich experiences and theoretical knowledge of their fight against disease over a long period of time.

Great numbers of barefoot doctors, workers, peasants, soldier, and workers have promoted, on a large scale, the use of Chinese herbs to treat disease. Not only have they obtained very good results toward the control of commonly seen rural ailments, they have also obtained valuable experience in treating difficult-to-treat diseases. From this, they have strengthened the development of cooperative medical therapeutics and contributed immensely to creating a new medicine and a new pharmacology for China based on a combination of the traditional Chinese and western medicine approaches. Chinese herb resources in Hunan Province are plentiful. For daily emergencies, they are valuable for treating disease; for wartime emergencies, good for treating wounds. Simple and easy to use, they are well received by the large masses of people.

Precautionary measures that should be taken in the use of Chinese herbs to treat disease are discussed in Chapter VII. For detailed information on medicinal plant recognition and identification, collection, processing, storage and use, please consult Chapter VII.

The use of Chinese herbs to treat disease generally takes eight approaches:

1. The perspiration method (chieh-piao fa). Literally meaning "to release externally," this method is suited for "superficial" or external exposure ailments. Chinese medicines used for this purpose are externally

releasing drugs (chia-piao yao), which are perspiration inducers. Divided into warm (hsin-wen) and cool (hsin-liang) perspiration inducers, the warm inducers are suited for wind-cold illnesses; the cool inducers, for wind-heat illnesses.

2. The vomit-inducing or emetic method. Suited for acute and "solid" illnesses affecting the upper parts. Any drug that can induce vomiting is an emetic. By causing the patient to vomit, pathogenic matter in the stomach and intestines are removed. To make vomiting more effective, using a finger or a goose feather [to press on the back of the tongue a few times] will induce retching and vomiting. If vomiting does not stop once it gets started, giving the patient some cold congre by mouth will stop it.

3. The purgative method. Also called "kung-hsia fa." The purgative lubricates the large intestine and induces loose, "hot" stools which also bring out "solid" heat already collected in the body. Drugs used are classified as purgatives and laxatives: the purgatives, exerting strong action, may be used for internally solid illnesses in patients still in good health; the laxatives, exerting milder lubricant action, are more suited for older, weaker and/or chronically ill patients.

4. The neutralizer method. Also called "ho-chieh fa" or "ho fa," this method uses drugs with neutralizing and "smoothing out" action to accomplish its purpose. Generally suited for combination half-internal and half-external illnesses as well as liver energy stagnation which causes irregular menstruation, and for liver disease affecting painful purge of the stomach-spleen.

5. The stimulation (warm center) method. Also called "wen fa." It warms the center to dispel cold, invigorates the yang and stimulates circulation with "warm" and "hot" drugs to stimulate body function and eliminate cold vapors (han-ch'i). Suited for chill-deficient illnesses.

6. Heat (fever) clearing method (ch'ing-jeh fa). Also called "ch'ing fa," it uses cooling medicines to clear the fever, lower the temperature, sustain saliva flow, and detoxity. Fever-clearing drugs are classified into four types: fever-clearing fire-purging drugs, fever-clearing blood-cooling drugs, fever-clearing moisture-drying (ts'ao-shih) drugs, and fever-clearing detoxifying drugs. Their use ranges over a broad scale. The fire-purging drugs are suited for "solid" heat fevers and associated thirst, stupor, delirium, parched throat, coated tongue, etc. The blood-cooling variety is suited for measles (that involve the blood) and all kinds of bleeding. The detoxifying variety is suited for cases of abscesses, boils, carbuncles, etc., in which the fever toxins are dominant. The moisture-drying variety is suited for cases of dysentery and jaundice caused by a dominance of "moist" fever in the internal organs.

7. The deflection method (hsiao-tao fa). Also called "hsiao fa," this method uses drugs to dispel, to channel stagnation, to correct energy-blood circulation, and to loosen sputum "moisture," etc. This group of drugs, suited for treating stagnation, accumulation, congestion, etc., is further divided into five types: energy-correcting, blood-correcting, digestion-promoting, sputum-liquifying, and moisture-converting. The energy-correcting drugs that stimulate energy circulation, improve appetite and stop pain are suited for cases of abdominal distension, hiccups, nausea, regurgitation or irregular menstruation. The blood-correcting drugs may be used in cases of irregular menstruation, post-natal abdominal pain, tumors, bruises, rheumatoid arthritis and abscesses. The digestion promoters are suited for indigestion and stomach ache, regurgitation of hydrochloric acid, nausea and vomiting, diarrhea, etc., resulting from indiscriminate eating and weak stomach-spleen. The sputum-liquifiers loosen up the mucus and "transform moisture" (hua-shih), suited best for productive coughs, asthma, epilepsy, convulsions, scrofulas, etc. The moisture-converters are also diuretic, suited for cases of edema, difficult and/or painful micturition, polyuria, etc., that are caused by water/moisture retention in the body.

8. The tonic method (pu-I fa). Also called "pu fa." Drugs that can supplement the yin-yang imbalance of energy (ch'i) and blood (hsueh) in the body and treat certain diseases of deficiency (hsu), are called supplementary tonics. These tonics are divided into four kinds: yang-supplementing, yin-supplementing, energy-supplementing, and blood-supplementing. The yang-supplements are suited for cases of yang-energy degeneration and cold deficient (hsu-han) type illnesses. The yin-supplements are suited for cases of fever-caused yin damage or convalescent yin-deficiency. The energy supplements are suited for convalescent weakness, fatigue exhausting the spleen. Blood tonics supplement and nourish blood deficiencies -- anemia, excessive post-partum loss of blood, etc.

Section 2. Folk Treatments

Many simple and effective treatments that meet the criteria of quantity, speed, quality, and economy are found in Hunan Province.

Skin Scrape (Kua-sha)

1. Conditions suited for treatment: heat stroke, catarrhal headaches, indigestion, painful joints, colic, etc.

2. Technique: First dip an old copper coin in wine or water. Then scrape the coin over patient's skin surface in a back and forth movement called "kua-sha." The folk practice often employs the fingers in a pinch-pull movement called "t'i-sha," "chih-sha," "nieh-sha" or "niu-sha."

Sites chosen for kua-sha may be in the occipital depression over the neck, both sides of the thoracic vertebrae, both sides of the Adam's apple, the bridge of the nose, the t'ai-yang depression, the "inter-eyebrow" space, the anterior chest, the elbow and knee spaces, etc. Scraping action generally goes from top to bottom, first from the back, then to the front along the intercostal spaces. When pinch-pulling is used, the index and middle fingers are used to pluck on the skin until reddish stripes begin to appear.

3. Precautions: During the kuo-sha treatment, be sure to observe the patient's expression. Do not use too much force in case the skin breaks open. If unfavorable changes are noticed, stop the procedure immediately and treat accordingly. The "kuo-sha" instrument must be blunt and smooth, otherwise the skin can easily be cut.

Blood Letting

Blood letting is a method of treatment employing a triangular needle or small magnetic disk to cut open the site of injury or an acupuncture point and allow a small amount of blood to flow out.

1. Conditions suited for treatment. Heat stroke, colic, vomiting and diarrhea, abscesses and swellings, stroke, traumatic injuries, etc.

2. Technique: Select site for blood letting. After routine sterilization of skin area, prick open the skin with the sterilized triangular needle and allow a small amount of blood to flow out.

3. Usual blood-letting sites: For summer stroke and colic, select the "shih-hsuan" and "ch'u-tse" points. For vomiting and diarrhea, select the "wei-chung." For traumatic injuries, abscesses and swellings, blood letting may be followed by cupping treatment for even better results, with pus drained, swelling reduced, and poisons neutralized.

Cupping (Pa-huo-kuan)

1. Conditions suited for treatment: Wind-chill moisture-based numbness (arthritis), stomach ache, abdominal pain, wind-chill catarrh, traumatic falls, bruises, abscesses, stroke paralysis, etc.

2. Sites and conditions to be avoided: All skin conditions, bony prominences (in thin patients), and sites prone to cramps, areas showing many superficial blood vessels and much hair growth. Also the abdomen, chest and breasts of pregnant women; and the precordium, tumor and lymphatic node sites.

3. Technique: Hold a flaming alcohol sponge with a pair of forceps and quickly flame the inside of the cup, then take out. At this time, the air inside the cup has become less dense, and the cup placed instantly over the selected spot will attach itself firmly to the skin, because of the atmospheric pressure outside. This method is quite safe.

4. Precautions:

   a. Generally, use large cups over muscular or fleshy areas, and small ones over less fleshy spots. Also use large cups on healthy young people or new patients still in good physical shape, but use small cups for the old and the weak, women and children and the chronically ill.

   b. Select cupping sites over the localized lesion or a swollen spot.

   c. Have patient in the recumbent position during the cupping procedure, in case he faints while standing. If the patient feels unwell during treatment, discontinue the cupping procedure immediately.

   d. Set duration of the procedure for 10-15 minutes, but make sure it is sufficient to induce reddish stripes in the cupping area.

   e. When the cup is removed, do not use strong pressure on the cup in case it cuts the skin. To remove, press skin around edges of cup. When outside air enters the cup, the cup will fall off by itself.

Massage (t'ui-na)

Massage by t'ui-na (pushing and grasping) and an-mo (palpate and massage) techniques is simple and effective. It is used to treat a wide range of illnesses. Massage can clear the meridian vessels, stimulate circulation of energy and blood, loosen up stiff joints, and increase body resistance to disease.

1. Conditions suited for treatment: Acute back strain/sprain, chronic backache, rheumatism, rheumatoid arthritis, facial nerve paralysis, post-encephalitis complications, prolapse of internal organs, digestive disturbances, etc.

2. Technique: T'ui-na has many techniques, such as

   a. Rolling method: suitable for shoulders and back, waist, and buttocks, and the four extremities (Figure 4-2-1).

   b. Rubbing method: suitable for all parts of the body (Figure 4-2-2).

   c. Kneading method (jou fa): suitable for the face, abdomen, and area around a swelling or tumor (Figure 4-2-3).

   d. Press-rotate method (mo fa): suitable for use on the abdomen (Figure 4-2-4).

e. Grasping method (na-fa): suitable for use on the neck,
    shoulders, underarms and the extremities (Figure 4-2-5).

f. Pressing method (an-fa): suitable for use on all body parts
    (Figure 4-2-6).

g. Wiping method (mo-fa): suitable for use on the head, face,
    and neck area (Figure 4-2-7).

h. Rotating method (yao-fa): suitable for use on all body joints
    (Figure 4-2-8).

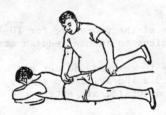

Figure 4-2-1.   Rolling method

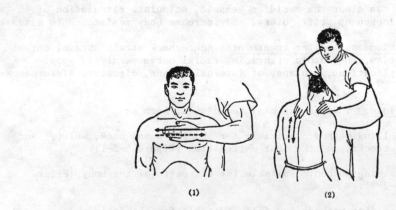

(1)   (2)

Figure 4-2-2.   Push-rub method

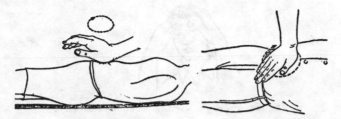

Figure 4-2-3. Kneading method   Figure 4-2-4. Press-rotate (mo-fa)
                                                        method

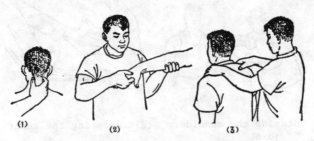

(1) Grasping the   (2) Grasping the   (3) Grasping the
    "feng-ch'ih" point   "ho-ku"   shoulders

Figure 4-2-5. Grasping method.

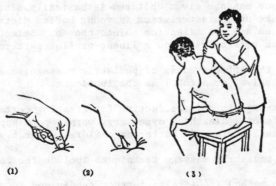

(1) Pressing with   (2) Pressing with   (3) Elbow-pressing-on-the-
    ball of thumb   knuckle of index   back technique
                              finger.

Figure 4-2-6. Pressing method (an-fa).

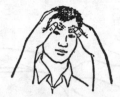

Figure 4-2-7. Wiping method (mo-fa).

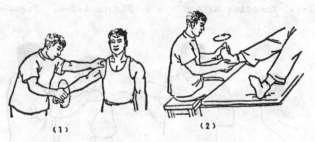

(1) Rotating the shoulder   (2) Rotating the ankle joint.
     joint

Figure 4-2-8. Rotating method (yao-fa).

4. T'ui-na massage of children.

Though t'ui-na massage given children is basically similar to that given adults, physical make-up characteristics in young bodies dictate differences in the technique used and the selection points chosen. Selection points in infants and children generally follow a linear or flat pattern.

To increase the effectiveness of pediatric massage, use fresh ginger juice, mentholated salve, or alcohol as the lubricant.

Pediatric massage is quite effective for treating certain childhood illnesses such as fevers, diarrhea, dysentery, worms, poor appetite, convulsions, etc. The results are even better in children under 5 years old.

Common used pediatric massage techniques include the following:

a. Push method (t'ui-fa): further subdivided into the direct push method and the partial push method. See figure 4-2-9.

b. Kneeding or inunction method (jou-fa) (Fig. 4-2-10).

c. Spine-pinch-pull method (nieh-chi-fa). Details will be described later on.

The sites and points most commonly selected for t'ui-na massage in small children and the techniques most often used are described in Table 4-2-1.

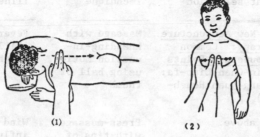

(1)   (2)

(1) Direct push method   (2) Simultaneous separate push method
                                          (with both hands)

Figure 4-2-9. Push method (t'ui-fa).

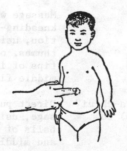

Figure 4-2-10. Kneading-inunction method.

To treat a small child burning from an "exposure" fever resulting from exposure to wind and cold, rub cold water onto [the vertebral process of the axis] the "ta-ch'ui hsueh" (1129 2785 4494) 100 times, over the "fei-yu" (5151 0358) [thoracic vertebra] 50 times, and push-massage the spinal column 300 times. If coughing is present, use both hands to push-massage simultaneously from the "t'an-chung" (5238 0022) point [over the sternum].

To treat infantile vomiting resulting from overeating, from exposure to cold or cold foods, push-massage the "t'an-chung" (5238 0022) over the sternum 50 to 100 times, press-rotate the "chung-wan" (0022 5184) point [located in mid-egigastrium, possibly over the cardiac orifice of stomach] for 5 minutes, and press massage the "tsu-san-li" (6398 0005 6849) [on lateral aspect of leg under kneecap] 20 times.

Table 4-2-1. Body Points and Techniques Commonly Used in Pediatric T'ui-na
Massage

Body sites and points	Point selection	Technique	Illnesses treated
Shoulder and back Ta-ch'ui (1129 2785)	See <u>New Acupuncture Therapy: Common Acupuncture Points</u> (Hsin-Chen Liao-fa: Ch'ang-yuan Hsueh-wei)	Massage with kneading-inunction motion, using ball of thumb	Fevers, convulsions, chills, and colds, coughing.
Chien-ching (5144 0064)	See above.	Press-massage with tips of both index fingers or middle fingers. Or grasp-massage with thumbs and index fingers.	Wind-chill caused influenza-like illnesses, and stomachache.
Fei-yu (5151 0358)	See above.	Massage with kneading-inunction, using both thumbs, or the tips of index and middle fingers.	Fevers, coughing, asthma, excessive mucus [formation], and recurring fevers.
Chi-chu (5182 2691)	From the "ta-ch'ui" hsueh [axis] to the sacrum.	Direct push-massage, using the balls of index and middle fingers in a pushing motion up and down the spinal column.	Fever, diarrhea, after-effects of poliomyelitis.
Ch'i-chieh (0003 4634)	From the 4th lumbar vertebra to the sacrum and coccyx in a straight line	Employ the push technique, using the balls of index and middle fingers or the thumb, in massaging motion up and down the spinal column.	Diarrhea treated with massage in upward direction; constipation with massage in downward direction.
Kuei-wei (7898 1442)	Tip [end] of spinal column	Massage, using the thumb in kneading-inunction motion.	Diarrhea, dysentery, prolapse of rectum, constipation.

Table 4-2-1 (Continued)

Body sites and points	Point selection	Technique	Illnesses treated
T h o r a x T'an-chung (5238 0022)	See New Acupuncture Therapy: Common Acupuncture Points (Hsin-chen Liao-fa: Ch'ang-yuan Hsueh-wei)	Push-massage simultaneously, using both thumbs, toward the nipples.	Vomiting, hiccups, excessive mucus in throat and respiratory tract, nausea, coughing.
a n d a b d o m e n Chung-wan (0022 5184)	See above	Massage with kneading-inunction motion, using the tip of middle finger. The base of the palm can also be used to press-massage in rotating motion.	Vomiting, diarrhea, abdominal distension, overeating, ulcers, indigestion.
Ch'i-hai (3051 3189)	See above	Massage with kneading-inunction motion, using the ball of the thumb or the middle finger.	Slight abdominal distension, passing of scanty and bloody urine, anuria, hernia, or weak physical condition.
Ch'i-chung (5247 0022)	See above	Massage with kneading-inunction motion, using the tip of the middle finger or the base of the palm.	Diarrhea, abdominal distension, abdominal cramps, indigestion, anuria, constipation, etc.
L o w e r e x t r e m i t y Tsu-san-li (6398 0005 6849)	See above	Massage with kneading or pressing motion, using the tip of the thumb.	Indigestion, abdominal distension, diarrhea, and vomiting.

To treat childhood spleen-stomach disturbances and malnutrition resulting from illness or ascariasis, press-rotate the "chung-wan" point 5 minutes, and the abdomen 3 minutes; inunction-rub the navel 3 minutes, push-massage the seven vertebral joints 200 times, and pinch-pluck the spine five times from top to bottom.

To treat indigestion in children, the result of overeating, inunction-rub the "chung-wan" point for 5 minutes, and push-massage the seven vertebral joints (in a downward motion) 200 times.

<u>Appendix</u>: Spinal Pinch-Pull

Physician use of fingers to pinch-pull the skin over the patient's spine (the passageway of the tu-mo (4206 9115) meridian clears the passageway of this meridian and allows regulation of blood and energy. For this reason, this technique is effective for certain illnesses.

1. <u>Conditions suited for treatment</u>: Neurasthenia, peptic and duodenal ulcers, functional intestinal disturbances, hypertension, etc. The technique may be used both on adults and children.

2. <u>Technique</u> (Figure 4-2-11). The physician uses his thumbs and index fingers to apply a pinch-pull action on the skin over the spine, going up the spine from the sacrum to the 7th cervical vertebra for three times in what is called the supplementary or additive method (pu-fa). When the pinch-pull sequence goes from the top of the spine downward, as used to treat hypertension, the technique is called the purging method (hsieh-fa). If additional points are massaged, according to differences in the patient's condition, (mostly by pressing or press-rotating massage of points on the back with the thumb) effectiveness of the technique will be even more pronounced.

For example, for neurathenia and deficiency (or hypofunction) in the heart and spleen, after spinal pinch-pull, the thumb may be used in pressing massage with or without circular motion over the following points: the "nei-kuan" (0355 7070) [on anterior aspect of forearm above the wrist], "tsu-san-li,"   the "shen-men" (4377 7024) [over the anterior ulnar aspect of wrist], the "yin-ling-ch'uan" (7122 7117 3123) [on inner aspect of lower limb just below the kneecap], the "p'i-yu" (5196 0358), "hsin-yu" (1800 0358), and "wei-yu" (5152 0358) [all vertebral prominances for the spleen, heart and stomach]. In cases with hyperactive liver and gallbladder fire, massage after spinal pinch-pull, using the thumb, may be done over the following points: the "san-yin-chiao" (0005 7113 0074) point [on the medical aspect of the leg], the "kan-yu" (5139 0358) "tan-yu" (9054 0358), "san-chiao-yu" (0005 3542 0358), "shen-yu" (5200 9358), [vertebral prominences for the liver, gallbladder, triple-warmer, and kidneys).

For ulcers, the thumb may be used to massage the "wei-yu," "p'i-yu" "tsu-san-li" and "san-yin-chiao" [see preceding paragraph for description of points].

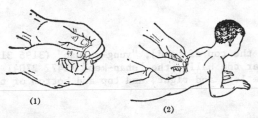

(1)　Position of hands　　　　　　(2)　Spinal pinch-pull in practice

Figure 4-2-11.　Spine pinch-pull method (nieh-chi-fa)

For chronic hepatitis, early recurring hepatitis or early liver cirrhosis, after spinal pinch-pull, the thumb may be used to massage with press-
rotating action over the following points:　the "kan-yu," "p'i-yu," "shen-
yu" [alongside vertebral prominences for the liver, spleen and kidneys],
"chih-shih" (1807 1358), the "tsu-san-li (6398 0005 6849), the "san-yin-chiao"
(0005 7113 0074), and the "feng-ch'ih" (7364 3069).　When pain is present
over the liver, the thumb should massage with heavy pressure the "kan-yu" and
other pain points found alongside the spinal column.

The spinal pinch-pull technique is used daily, for five to six times
in each treatment on the spine from the bottom up, 20 treatments making up
one course of therapy.　Tried before bedtime on patients who suffer from insomnia and headaches, this method has also been found effective.

Moxibustion (shao-teng-huo)

Moxibustion is a therapeutic technique that employs a flaming moxa
wick placed directly on the skin to burn it.

1.　Conditions suited for treatment:　For epidemic mumps, moxibustion
is often applied to the "chiao-sun" (6037 1327) [located on the upper part
of the pinna of the ear]; for convulsions in small children, to the "t'ai-
yang" (1132 7122) point [located in the depression of the temples]; for nosebleeds that do not stop, at the "shao-shang" (1421 0794) point [located on
anterior aspect of ball of thumb]; and for continuous vaginal bleeding, at
the "ta-tun" (1129 2415), [located on the outer aspect of big toe], 3-hairs
width from base of toe nail.　For rheumatism and numbness, the affected part
may be treated by a small bundle of burning moxa enveloped in dogskin.

2.　Technique:　For mild cases, a single moxa is used.　After it is
lit, the moxa is applied to the skin over the affected part and selected
points.　For more serious cases, several moxas are bundled and burned together,
producing quicker results.

3.　Commonly used points:　The "jen-chung" (0086 0022) [located in
groove over middle upper lip]; "ch'eng-chiang" (2110 3364) [located in dimple
over chin just below middle lower lip]; "pai-hui" (4102 2585) [located on

dorsal midline near the top of head]; "yung-ch'uan" (3196 3123 [located on midsole of foot, near the ball]; the "shan-ken" (1472 2704) point and points about an inch to the left and right, and top and bottom of the knee.

Section 3. New Therapeutic Techniques

The great masses of workers, peasants, soldiers and health workers have shown a daring and courageous spirit. They have, after much practice, discovered many new therapeutic techniques, such as, new acupuncture techniques, alkali treatments, "suture-buried-in-acupuncture point" technique, needle plucking, etc. The appearance of these new methods which are well received by the masses has greatly increased the effectiveness of treatments given. Not only are they important contributions to the people's health, they also represent a merger of western medicine and traditional Chinese medicine, and thus open new opportunities for the new medicine and pharmacology that China is inherently favorably disposed to.

New Acupuncture Therapy Techniques

Development of the acupuncture therapy techniques is based on the traditional practice of acupuncture-moxibustion. All-out efforts were channeled to "focus all medical and health care on the rural areas in service to the people." Development of these new techniques is one fruitful outocme, which contributed further to the precious heritage of traditional Chinese medicine.

The new acupuncture therapy techniques are simple to use, economical, and quickly effective. Moreover, the techniques are easy to learn and promote, and their range of use is extensive. Well received by the masses, acupuncture therapy is a treatment technique that embraces quantity, speed, quality and economy.

1. Characteristics of new acupuncture therapy.

   a. Grasping the important contradiction of disease.

   Though signs and symptoms of any one illness oftentimes are numerous, there are important and less important symptoms. By focussing

attention on the important symptoms and the basic cause, when selecting
the proper acupuncture point for treatment, we are able to obtain fairly
good results. For example, symptoms of hypertention include headache,
dizziness, insomnia, etc., but once its chief antagonist, high blood
pressure, is resolved, the other symptoms will follow suit.

b. Selection of fewer sites and points.

The new techniques does not use as many points as more conventional
treatments do. It is based on the principle of few points with better quality
of treatment. Generally, only two to three points are selected for a treatment; at the most, four to five needling sessions.

c. Quick needle insertion.

By doing so, the pain felt by patient is lessened.

d. Deep penetration possible.

Except for the chest, back and abdomen, which house important organs,
points on other sites may, depending on the situation, receive needles at
deeper penetration.

e. Penetration linkage of more points possible at one insertion.

Many points are suitable for such linkage, such as the "wai-kuan"
(1120 7070) with the "nei-kuan" (0355 7070) [one on posterior aspect, the
other on anterior aspect of forearm]; the "ch'u-ch'ih" (2575 3069) with the
"shao-hai" (1421 3189), [both located in the elbow space], and the "chia-che"
(7335 6508) with the "ti-tsang" (0966 0221) [one on side of cheek, other at
corner of mouth]. This way, fewer points need to be used, while effectiveness is increased.

f. Stronger stimulation.

The new acupuncture therapy also practices three kinds of stimulation: strong, medium, and weak. However, except for old, young, and weak
patients, strong stimulation through broad range needle twirling and needle
retraction and insertion is generally used. Experience has shown good results.

g. No needle retention.

Because needle penetration is deep, and stimulation is strong, the
needle is removed in most patients after it has evoked a tingling numbing

pain, sensation, and the time required for treatment is greatly reduced. However, in patients experiencing great pain and spasms, the needle should be retained.

2. Basics of the new acupuncture therapy.

a. Selection, inspection and care of acupuncture instruments.

(1) Commonly used needles.

(a) "Hao" needles (Hao-chen, 3032 6859). Comes in various gauges and lengths: in gauges No 26, No 28, No 30 and No 32; and in lengths of 0.5 ts'un, 1.0, 1.5, 2.0, 2.5, 3.0 and 3.05 ts'un. The selection of needle length is based on the amount of penetration needed. No 26 is the largest gauged needle, suitable only for use on epileptics. No 28 is used more often.

(b) Triple-edged needles. Used generally for blood-letting. Wedge-shaped, the point is extremely sharp. When used for blood-letting, be sure to place finger at a section of needle marking extent of penetration, to prevent excessive or inadequate needle insertion.

(c) Skin needles. This type consists of several needles inserted around a pipe stem -- called "seven-star" needles (ch'i-hsing chen) when seven are used, and "plum-blossom needles (mei-hua chen) when five are used. Exposed points of these needles are generally 0.3 ts'un long. These needles are commonly used for treating infants and skin conditions. During treatment, use the right hand to hold the body of the needle and gently hit the skin with the needle trip.

(d) Intradermal needles. Used chiefly to treat chronic organic (visceral) disease, and illnesses characterized by resistant and recurring pain. Intradermal needles come in two types: the circular model and the wheat grain model. The former is suited for buried treatment on the pinna of the ear; the latter, for treatment over various body acupuncture points or pain pressure points. In practice with these needles, first sterilize the local part with alcohol, then insert directly (vertically) if the circular needles are used, but inserting only horizontally if the wheat-grain model is used, and leave the stems of needles outside on the skin, anchored down by adhesive tape.

(2) <u>Inspection and repair</u>: Before each use, inspect needles for blunt tips, hooked ends, rust, bending and breaking. Also check to see if the stem (handle) is loose (detached) from the point. If the tip is no longer sharp, use fine sandpaper to sand off some of the bluntness. If the needle should break because of rust, it should be discarded.

(3) <u>Care</u>: After use, the needle must be cleaned and adjusted, then placed in a storage tube, the tip inserted first. Make sure some cotton provides cushioning at both ends of tube.

b. <u>Positions of the patient</u>.

The position assumed by the patient during acupuncture therapy must be comfortable for the patient, but also convenient for the acupuncturist to carry out the procedure. Common positions are the leaning-back, and leaning-forward sitting positions the lateral recumbent, recumbent, and prone positions (Figure 4-3-1). Before inserting the needle, make sure the patient is assuming the correct position. Also instruct the patient not to move after needle insertion, to guard against any bending or breakage of the needle and accidental burns by the moxa.

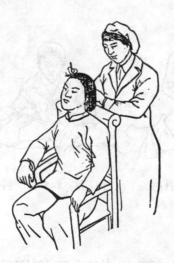

Figure 4-3-1. Acupuncture positions.
Sitting position, leaning back.

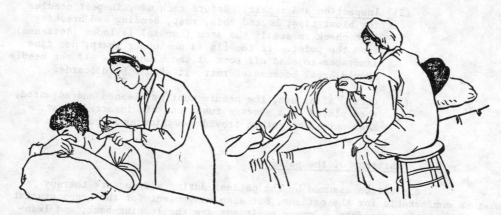

Figure 4-3-1. Sitting position,   Figure 4-3-1. Lateral recumbent
              leaning forward.   position.

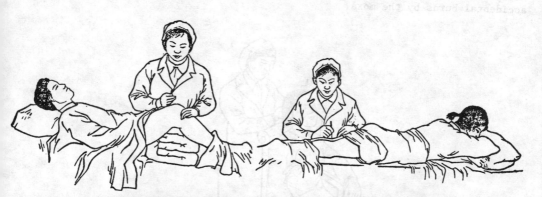

Figure 4-3-1. Recumbent position   Figure 4-3-1. Prone position.

c. <u>Sterlization</u>

All articles that come in direct or indirect contact with the acupuncture sites must be sterilized.

    (1) <u>Physician's fingers</u>. Nails must be closely trimmed, after
which hands are washed with soap and warm boiled (sterile)
water, and finally wiped with a 75% alcohol sponge.

- 94 -

(2) <u>Needle puncture site</u>. Sterilize the acupuncture point with a 75% alcohol sponge, wiping from the center out.

(3) <u>Needles and other utensils</u>. Sterilize needles and forceps by boiling. Or immerse in 75% alcohol for 5-10 minutes before use.

d. <u>Acupuncture technique</u>

(1) <u>Needle insertion technique</u> (Figure 4-3-2).

    (a) Quick method. Most commonly used. Hold needle by the lower stem section between the thumb and index finger of right hand, exposing about 0.2 ts'un of the point, and quickly but accurately insert needle into the acupuncture site (point). Rapid insertion reduces the patient's sensation of pain.

    (b) Pressure-cut method. Apply pressure to the acupuncture point with fingernail of the left index finger, after which the needle is quickly inserted into the skin with the right hand.

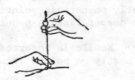

Figure 4-3-2. Methods of needle insertion
Quick method   Pressure cut method

(2) <u>Post-insertion technique</u>. After the needle has reached the desired depth, the patient will experience sensations of achiness, weight, swelling, numbness, etc., and the physician may feel that the needle has sunk and is anchored (called "energy-obtained" or "te ch'i"). At this time, the physician may twirl the needle or withdraw it slightly and reinsert to intensify this "energy-flooding-in" feeling. According to the amount of twirling or needle-pushing in and out, the stimulation may be classified as weak, moderate or strong. However, the amount of stimulation given must be according to the patient's tolerance.

(3) Needle withdrawal technique. Press a cotton ball alongside needle with the left hand, and grasp the needle
lightly with the right and quickly withdraw the needle.
Massage puncture site with left hand to prevent bleeding.
Should there be some slight bleeding, place cotton ball
over puncture site and apply pressure for 2 to 3 minutes.
If necessary, instruct the patient to apply hot compresses
to hasten absorption.

(4) Blood-letting technique. Also called "point-puncture"
(tien-tzu). After the skin has been sterilized, introduce a triple-edged needle (or No 5 injection, needle),
held between the thumb and index finger, quickly into
the acupuncture point, to a depth of about 0.1 inch (ts'un),
withdraw immediately, and squeeze out some blood (as will
happen in puncturing the "szu-feng" (0934 4911) and "shih-
hsuan" (0577 1357) points).

(5) Direction of acupuncture.

Vertical acupuncture: Used most frequently, the direction
of needle insertion here is perpendicular (at 90°) to the
skin. Used mostly on the waist, back, and the extremities.

Slanted acupuncture: Needle is inserted into the skin at
a 45° angle. Used mostly on certain points to bypass important organs, or for deeper linkage penetration.

Horizontal acupuncture: Needle is inserted into the skin
at a 15° angle. Used mostly on points located on the head
and face.

e. Handling of unusual situations.

(1) Acupuncture dizziness and shock (yun-chen). Seen mostly
in patients receiving acupuncture the first time due possibly to emotional tension, weak constitution, fatigue,
hunger, excessive perspiration, or an overly strong technique practiced on an older patient. Before the spell
sets in, the patient experiences apprehension, dizziness,
facial pallor, sweating, nausea and vomiting. In severe
cases, the patient may become unconscious, hands and feet
clammy and cold. At this point, the acupuncture should
be stopped, needle withdrawn, and the patient made to lie
flat, the head slightly lower than the legs. In mild cases,
give patient drink of hot sugar water. Severely affected
patients should receive acupuncture at the "jen-chung"
(0086 0022) and "pai-hui" (4102 2585) points to regain
consciousness.

(2) **Acupuncture slow-down** (chi-chen): Occurs after needle insertion when manipulating techniques, such as needle twirling and retraction, are difficult to execute. Due mostly to local muscular tension. To treat, leave needle in and ask the patient to relax. For severe cases, acupuncture may be applied to a nearby site to facilitate needle twirling and retraction before needle withdrawal.

(3) **Bent needles:** Due mostly to uneven digital pressure or too much force used during needle insertion, or to shifts in patient's position, or to needle holder being accidentally bumped into by outside object. In such a situation, withdraw needle gently in direction of the curve. Where the situation is caused by change in patient's position, see that the patient's position is first corrected before needle is withdrawn.

(4) **Broken needles:** Due mostly to some damage such as rust causing needle to crack and erode. Sometimes it is due to muscular tension in the patient (following energy obtained) and needle insertion is overly strong. When a needle is broken, maintain a calm composure, for needle to be taken out in time. Once a section of needle is exposed, use a hemostat to remove the broken needle. When broken-off end has penetrated deeper tissues, remove by surgical means. Broken needles can be avoided if the needles are checked beforehand and the acupuncture technique is practiced with care.

f. **Contraindications for acupuncture therapy.**

(1) Not recommended when patient is hungry, full, drunk, perspiring excessively, or tired. Acupuncture may be done after a period of rest or after an improvement in the conditions described above.

(2) Acupuncture contraindicated for the five organs [lungs, heart, liver, spleen, kidneys]. Deep acupuncture not to be done on surfaces corresponding to the five organs.

(3) Contraindicated for women less than 5 months pregnant at points located on the lower abdomen and lower back; for women over 5 months pregnant, additional points located on the upper abdomen. Other points that can provoke a strong response (such as the "ho-ku" (0678 6253), "san-yin-chiao" (0005 7115 0074) and the "yin-pai" (7148 4101)) should not be punctured, and only lightly, if done at all. Postpartum acupuncture (before a month has gone by) should be applied lightly.

(4) Other precuations and contraindications.

    (a) Extra care taken in acupuncture used on patients with heart disease.

    (b) Contraindicated for surface over anterior fontanels of infants before closure.

    (c) Contraindicated for eyeballs and testicles.

    (d) Contraindicated at points which may hit the aorta or vena cavae.

    (e) Contraindicated in certain diseases such as leukemia, thrombopenia.

3. Acupuncture points

    Acupuncture points (hsueh-wei) are locations where energy (ch'i) and blood converge. Those located on the meridians are called meridian points (ching-hsueh), and those located outside the meridians are called special points (ch'i-hsueh). Some experimental points found to be effective are new points. Those points located over a site of pain are the a-shih-hsueh (7093 2508 4494).

    a. Point location technique: Most commonly used are the following three methods.

    (1) Inch (ts'un) conversion from bone measurements (Table 4-3-1). This method assigns arbitrary inch measurements to specific anatomical parts regardless of sex or age differences, for use as a frame of reference. For example, the distance from the wrist flexor fold to the elbow flexure is "measured" as 12 inches (ts'un), meaning that this distance is divided into 12 equal parts (Figure 4-3-3). Locating an acupuncture point is based on this set of standards.

    (2) Body-inch conversion from middle finger measurements. This measurement standard is obtained by flexing the middle finger over to the thumb to form a circle, and taking the distance between folds formed by the 1st and 2nd interphalangeal joints as the standard inch (Figure 4-3-4). This method can be used for vertical measurements of the extremities and horizontal measurements of the back.

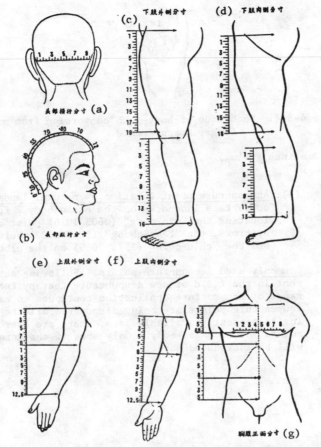

Figure 4-3-3. Inch (ts'un) conversion from bone measurements.

Key: (a) Assigned transverse measurements of the head.
       (b) Assigned measurements of the head (longitudinal section).
       (c) Assigned measurements of the lower extremity (lateral aspect).
       (d) Assigned measurements of the lower extremity (medial aspect).
       (e) Assigned measurements of the upper extremity (lateral aspect).
       (f) Assigned measurements of the upper extremity (medial aspect).
       (g) Assigned measurements of the chest and abdomen (anterior view).

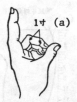

Figure 4-3-4. Technique of body-inch conversion from middle-finger measurements.

Key: (a)   One inch (ts'un)

> (3) <u>Acupuncture point location by natural landmarks</u>. Based on surface landmarks on the human body. For example, locating the "yin-tang" (0603 1016) point between the eyebrows, the "t'an-chung" (5238 0022) between the breasts, and the "ch'u-chih" (2575 3069) on the elbow flexure.

b. <u>Commonly used acupuncture points</u>. Following active development in the field of new acupuncture therapy techniques, the range of acupuncture application continues to expand, and new acupuncture points are being discovered all the time. According to presently available data, there are over 900 acupuncture points in the human body. Only some of the more common ones will be introduced here.

Table 4-3-1. Table of Inch (ts'un) Conversions from Bone Measurements.

Body part	Beginning and end points of part	Commonly used bone measurement	Measurement method	Explanation
Head	Longitudinal measurement -- Front hairline to back hairline	12 inches (ts'un)	Vertical measurement	If the hairlines are not well defined, measure the distance from point between eyebrows to the "ta-ch'iu-hsueh" [over the axis] as 18 inches, the distance from between the eyebrows to frontal hairline as 3 inches, that from the axis to the posterior hairline as 3 inches.
	Transverse measurement -- From one mastoid prominence ("wan-ku") behind one ear to mastoid prominence behind ear to other side of head	9 inches	Horizontal measurement	(1) Used to take horizontal measurements of the head (2) "Wan-ku" refers to the mastoid prominence.
Upper arm	Arm -- Transverse fold at anterior armpit to transverse fold at elbow flexure	9 inches	Vertical measurement	Used for measurements to locate the "shou-san-yin" (2087 0005 7113) and "shou-san-yang" (2087 0005 7122) points
Forearm	Forearm -- from transverse fold at elbow flexure to transverse fold at wrist	12 inches	Vertical measurement	

Table 4-3-1 (Continued)

Body part	Beginning and end points of part	Commonly used bone measurement	Measurement method	Explanation
Chest	From "t-ien-t'u" (1131 4499) to "ch'i-ku" (2978 7539)	9 inches	Vertical measurement	(1) Vertical measurements are taken to locate points on the chest and sides, based on spacing between ribs, generally calculated as 1.6 inches (ts'un).
	From the "ch'i-ku" to the navel	8 inches	Vertical measurement	(2) "T'ien-tu" is an acupuncture point. The "ch'i-ku" refers to the junction of the sternum with the xiphoid. The "heng-ku shang-lien" (2897 7539 0006 1670) refers to the upper margin of the pubic symphysis.
	From the navel to the "heng-ku shang-lien."	5 inches	Vertical measurement	
Abdomen	Between the two breast nipples	8 inches	Transverse horizontal measurement	Point location on the chest and abdomen using transverse measurements is based on the distance between the two breast nipples. For female patients, the distance between the left and right "ch-ueh-p'en-hsueh" (4972 4133 4494) points may be used to represent this spacing between the two nipples.
Back waist and	From the "ta-ch'ui" vertebra (axis) to the coccyx	21 vertebrae	Vertical measurement	Location of acupuncture points on the back is referred from the spine. Generally, points are selected on the basis of symptoms. The lower corner of the shoulder is located at level of the 7th thoracic vertebra; the haunch, at level of the 16th vertebra (the 4th lumbar prominence). Transverse measurements of the back are based on inch conversion from the patient's middle finger measurements.

Table 4-3-1. (Continued)

Body part	Beginning and end points of part	Commonly used bone measurement	Measurement method	Explanation
Lower Extremities	From the "heng-ku shang-lien" (upper margin pubic symphysis) to the "nei-fu ku shang-lien" (0355 7539 0006 1670)	18 inches	Vertical Measurement	(1) Used for location points on the "tsu-san-yin" meridian; (2) The "nei-fu-ku shang-lien" refers to the upper edge of the medial condyle of the femur
	From the "nei-fu-ku hsia-lien (lower edge of the femoral medial condyle) to the point of the inner malleolus	13 inches	Vertical measurement	
	Head of femur to the middle of knee ("hsi-chung" (5230 0022)	19 inches	Vertical measurement	(1) Used for locating points on the "tsu-yang"; (2) The "hsi-chung" refers to the center of the patella. (3) The transverse buttock fold to the center of the knee is calculated at 14 inches.
	Lateral knee prominence (the lateral condyle of femur?) to the lateral malleolus	16 inches	Vertical measurement	
	From lateral malleolus to sole of foot	3 inches	Vertical measurement	

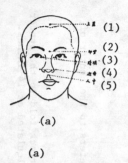

(a)

(a)

Key:
1. Shang-hsing (0006 2502)
2. Yin-t'ang (0603 1016)
3. Ching-ming (4200 2494)
4. Ying-hsiang (6601 7449)
5. Jen-chung (0086 0022)

Key:
6. Pai-hui (4102 2585)
7. Chiao-sun (6037 1327)
8. Lu-ku (3764 6253)
9. T'ai-yang (1132 7122)
10. Erh-men (5101 7024)
11. Lung-hsueh (5122 4494)
12. T'ing-kung (5121 1362)
13. T'ing-hui (5121 2585)
14. I-ming (6829 2494)
15. I-lung (6829 5122)
16. I-feng (6829 7364)
17. Chia-che (7335 6508)
18. Hsia-kuan (0007 7070)
19. Ti-ts'ang (0966 0221)
20. Shang-lien-ch'uan (0006 1670 3123)

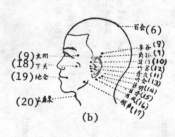

(b)

(b)

Key:
21. Feng-ch'ih (7364 3069)
22. T'ien-ch'u (1131 2691)
23. Ya-men (0800 7024)

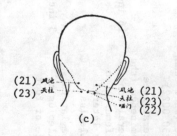

(c)

Figure 4-3-5. Commonly used acupuncture points of the head.
(a) Points on anterior aspect of face and head.
(b) Points on the lateral aspect.
(c) Points on the back of head.

Table 4-3-2. Common Acupuncture Points of the Head and Neck.

Acupuncture point	Meridian	Conditions treated	Location	Locating technique
Shang-hsing	The governing tu-mo (4202 9115) meridian	Headache, stuffi-ness of nose, epistaxis	On forehead, one inch into the hairline	Patient sitting down, facing acupuncturist.
Yin-t'ang	Special point (ch'i-hsueh, 1142 4494)	Frontal headache, infantile convul-sions, post-partum bleeding	Between the two eyebrows	Patient sitting down, with face tilted.
Ching-ming	Foot bladder meridian (tsu t'ai-yang p'ang-kuang ching)	Swollen and pain-ful eyes, styes, tearing	Alongside inner canthus of eye	Patient in recumbent position, with eyes closed. Locate acupuncture point medially, about 0.1 inch from the inner canthus.
Ying-hsiang	Hand large in-testine meridian (shou yang-ming ta-ch'ang ching)	Stopped-up nose, epistaxis	Alongside outer edge of nostril	Locate points about 0.5 inch alongside each nostril
Jen-chung	The governing "tu-mo" meridian	Facial edema, epi-lepsy, infantile convulsion, back-ache, sudden black-outs and fainting	On groove be-tween upper lip and nose	Locate point on groove between upper lip and nose, at one-third distance from the nose.
Pai-hui	The governing "tu-mo" meridian	Stroke, headache and dizziness, anal prolapse in infants, epilepsy	Center at top of head	Patient in sitting position, head bowed. Pin auricles of both ears forward, and draw imaginary lines upwards from pointed edges of both ears to top of head where they meet. Locate acupuncture point here at convergence.

Table 4-3-2. (Continued)

Acupuncture point	Meridian	Conditions treated	Location	Locating techniques
Chiao-sun	Hand triple-warmer meridian (shou shao-yang san-chiao ching)	Pterygium, tooth-ache, inflamed auricles; alveolar abscess	Over middle of auricle	Fold pinna of ear forward, and locate the acupuncture point where the pointed edge of ear intrudes into the hairline.
Lu-ku	Leg gallbladder meridian (tsu shao-yang tan ching)	Temporal headaches, conjunctivitis	Above the ear, about 1.5 inch into the hair-line	Locate point above the upper point of ear, about two fingers width into the hair-line. Perform technique with patient in sitting or recum-bent positions.
T'ai-yang	Special point (ch'i-hsueh)	Temporal headaches, eye ailments	In temporal depression about one inch behind the space between end of eyebrow and outer canthus	Patient in sitting position facing acupuncturist.
Erh-men	Hand triple-warmer meridian (shou t'ai-yang san-chiao ching)	Deafness, tinnitis, draining ears, dental caries, jaw pain	In depression anterior to external ear	Patient in sitting position with mouth wide open, facing the acupuncturist. Locate point in depression anterior to the anterior fold of the ear lobe.
Lung-hsueh	New acupuncture point	Deafness	Anterior to ear, in depres-sion that pre-sents itself when mouth is opened	Locate point between the two points, the "t'ing-kung" and the "t'ing-hui."

- 106 -

Table 4-3-2. (Continued)

Acupuncture Point	Meridian	Conditions treated	Location	Locating techniques
T'ing-kung	Hand small intestine meridian (shou yang-ming hsiao-ch'ang ching)	Deafness, tinnitus	In depression anterior to pinna of ear [over meatus]	Locate point in depression anterior to ear lobe. When digital pressure on point is suddenly released, ear rings.
T'ing-hui	Leg gallbladder meridian (tsu shao-yang tan ching)	Deafness, tinnitus	In lower part of depression anterior to ear	Locate point in lower part of ear that opens into a gap when the mouth is opened.
I-ming	New point	Myopia, night blindness, green and white cataract, retinal hemorrhage, optical neuritis, insomnia, headache, dizziness, parotitis	On upper part of base of the sternocleido-mastoid muscle, at juncture of the inferiorly directed mastoid prominence and the posteriorly directed ear lobe	Locate point at midway of line connecting the "I-feng" and "feng-ch'ih" points.
I-lung	New point	Deafness	In depression be-tween the mas-toid prominence and the pinna	Point located 0.5 inch above the I-feng point.
I-feng	Hand triple warmer meridian (shou shao-yang san-chiao ching)	Swollen jaws, toothache, deaf-ness, tinnitis, distorted oris	In depression behind pinna	Patient in sitting position facing acupuncturist. While holding ear lobe, locate point along edge of lobe.

Table 4-3-2. (Continued)

Acupuncture point	Meridian	Conditions treated	Location	Locating techniques
Chia-che	Foot stomach meridian (tsu yang-ming wei ching)	Distorted oris, toothache, lockjaw	In depression over the mandibular notch, just below the ear	Apply digital pressure to depression below ear on upper part of mandible. Locate point in area under finger that rises when teeth are grit.
Hsia-kuan	Foot stomach meridian (tsu yang-ming wei ching)	Toothache, distorted oris	In depression anterior to ear just under the cheekbone	Ask patient to close mouth in order to locate point.
Ti-ts'ang	Foot stomach meridian (tsu yang-ming wei ching)	Distorted oris, drooling	Outside corner of mouth	Locate site about 0.4 inch outside corner of mouth.
Shang-lien-ch'uan	New point	Aphasia	One inch above Adam's apple, above the hyoid bone	Locate site by having patient tilt head upwards slightly.
Feng-ch'ih	Foot gallbladder meridian (tsu shao-yang tan-ching)	Tearing, headache on top of head	In occipital depression behind the ear	Locate points in depressions along lateral sides of the ridges for the occipital groove in the hairline.
Ya-men	The governing "tu-mo"	Headache, deafness and aphasia backache, listlessness	In back of neck in occipital groove	Look for point with patient sitting and facing the acupuncturist, his head lowered. Be careful during acupuncture and not needle too deep, as the medulla oblongata is located in the deeper parts.

Table 4-3-2. (Continued)

Acupuncture point	Meridian	Conditions treated	Location	Locating techniques
T'ien-ch'u	Foot bladder meridian (chu t'ai-yang pang-kuang ching)	Violent pain in neck	Along ridges of occipital groove	Locate points on hairline 1.5 inch from ridges of occipital groove.

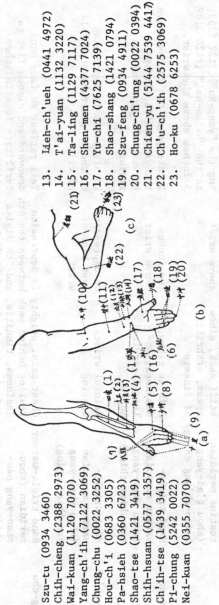

Figure 4.3.6. Commonly used acupuncture points of the upper extremity.

(a) Acupuncture points on lateral aspect of upper extremity.
(b) Acupuncture points on medial aspect of upper extremity.
(c) Acupuncture points on flexures of upper extremity.

Key:
1. Szu-tu (0934 3460)
2. Chih-cheng (2388 2973)
3. Wai-kuan (1120 7070)
4. Yang-ch'ih (7122 3069)
5. Chung-chu (0022 3252)
6. Hou-ch'i (0683 3305)
7. Pa-hsieh (0360 6723)
8. Shao-tse (1421 3419)
9. Shih-hsuan (0577 1357)
10. Ch'ih-tse (1439 3419)
11. Pi-chung (5242 0022)
12. Nei-kuan (0355 7070)
13. Lieh-ch'ueh (0441 4972)
14. T'ai-yuan (1132 3220)
15. Ta-ling (1129 7117)
16. Shen-men (4377 7024)
17. Yu-chi (7625 7139)
18. Shao-shang (1421 0794)
19. Szu-feng (0934 4911)
20. Chung-ch'ung (0022 0394)
21. Chien-yu (5144 7539 4417)
22. Ch'u-ch'ih (2575 3069)
23. Ho-ku (0678 6253)

Table 4-3-3. Common Acupuncture Points of the Upper Extremity

Acupuncture point	Meridian	Conditions treated	Location	Locating techniques
Szu-tu	Hand triple-warmer meridian (shou shao-yang san-chiao ching)	Paralysis of upper extremity, deafness	About 5 inches from the elbow, in the "wai-lien" depression	Locate the point between the radius and ulna, 5 inches from the angle of elbow.
Chih-cheng	Hand small intestine meridian (shou t'ai-yang hsiao-ch'ang ching)	Headache, vertigo, stiff neck, elbow spasm, arthritis of fingers	Five inches above wrist	Locate point along line joining the "yang-ku" (7122 6253) to the "hsiao-hai" (1420 3189) 5 inches above the wrist.
Wai-kuan	Hand triple-warmer meridian (shou shao-yang san-chiao ching)	Pain in elbow, deafness, enlarged cervical nodes	Two inches above wrist	Locate point two inches above the yangpch'ih, in space between the ulna and the radius.
Yang-ch'ih	Hand triple-warmer meridian (shou shao-yang san-chiao ching)	Painful wrists, wasting	On depression over back of wrist	Locate point in depression on the upper transverse fold of wrist.
Chung-chu	Hand triple-warmer meridian (shou shao-yang san-chiao ching)	Chest pain, weighty feeling behind neck deafness, tinnitis, pain in the shoulder and the 4th and 5th digits	In depression between the 4th and 5th digits of hand, 1 inch behind the "yi-men" (3210 7024) point	Tell patient to face hand downward and clench fist to facilitate locating the point.
Hou-ch'i	Hand small intestine meridian (shou t'i-yang hsiao-ch'ang ching)	Epilepsy, painful digits, malaria	Alongside the little finger at first phalan-phalangeal joint	Ask patient to clench fist. Locate point in fold of first phalan- phalangeal joint.

Table 4-3-3. (Continued)

Acupuncture point	Meridian	Conditions treated	Location	Locating techniques
Pa-hsieh	Special point	Swollen back of hand, exposure headache, tooth-ache	Three points on upper margins of the inter-digital webs.	Ask patient to clench fist.
Shao-tse	Hand small intestine meridian (shou t'ai-yang hsiao-ch'ang ching)	Apoplexy and fainting, malaria, inadequate milk (nursing mother) supply	On lateral aspect of little finger at base of finger nail	Locate point 0.1 inch from base of finger nail on lateral aspect of little finger.
Shih-hsuan	Special point	Tonsillitis, fever, heat stroke and general symptoms of acute unconsciousness	On all fingertips, 0.1 inch from fingernails	Locate points on fingertips.
Ch'ih-tse	Hand lung meridian (shou ta'i-yin fei ching)	Cough and hemoptysis, pain in arms	On thumb side of the elbow flexure	Have patient bend arm slightly (about 35°) palm upwards, and locate point along lateral edge of elbow flexure.
Pi-chung	New point	Upper extremity paralysis	Medial aspect of upper extremity	Locate point on imaginary line drawn between the "ta-ling" and "ch'u-ch'ih" points
Nei-kuan	Hand heart controller meridian (shou ch'ueh-yin Hsin-pao ching)	Stomach ache, nausea, hiccups, vomiting	Two inches above the wrist flexure	Locate point between two sinews beyond the wrist [anterior aspect].
Lieh-ch'ueh	Hand lung meridian (shou t'ai-yin fei ching)	Headache, cough	Above wrist on thumb (lateral) side	Lock hands across thumbs. Locate wrist just under finger-tips on index fingers.

Table 4-3-3. (Continued)

Acupuncture point	Meridian	Conditions treated	Location	Locating techniques
T'ai-yuan	Hand lung meridian (shou t'ai-yin fei ching)	Cough, hematemesis toothache	On radial side of wrist lines above the palm	Locate point in depression at the "head" of wrist flexure; on thumb side, over radial pulse.
Ta-ling	Hand heart controller meridian (shou ch'ueh-yin Hsin-pao ching)	Fever, gastric pain, pain in chest and sides, vomiting, hematemsis	Center of wrist joint (anterior aspect)	Locate point in depression at center of wrist flexure lines, between two sinews.
Shen-men	Hand heart meridian (shou shao-yin hsin ching)	Palpation, epilepsy insomnia	In wrist flexure depression, on little finger side	Have patient position hand with palm upward, and locate point in depression in front of styloid process of ulna.
Yu-chi	Hand lung meridian (shou t'ai-yin fei ching)	Numbness of throat, cough, hematemesis voice loss, vertigo headache, chest (heart) pain, mental disturbances, fever, abdominal pain	In fleshy part of palm under the thumb	Locate point on side of palm over the 1st metacarpal bone, in the fleshy part.
Shao-shang	Hand lung meridian (shou t'ai-yin fei ching)	Apoplexy, sore throat	On inner aspect of thumb about 0.1 inch from the inner corner of nail	Locate point 0.1 inch from base of nail, along medial aspect.

Table 4-3-3. (Continued)

Acupuncture point	Meridian	Conditions treated	Location	Locating techniques
Szu-feng	Special point	Ascariasis in small children, delicate constitution	In middle of transverse fold over the proximal interphalangeal joint of all four fingers on the palmer surface	Have patient extend palm and fingers to facilitate locating the point.
Chung-ch'ung	Hand heart controller meridian (shou ch'ueh-yin hsin-pao ching)	Stroke, fever, infantile convulsions	At tip of middle finger	Locate point on tip of middle finger, 0.1 inch from the nail
Chien-yu	Hand large intestine meridian (shou yang-ming ta-ch'ang ching)	Aches and pain in the shoulders and arm, upper extremity paralysis	In middle of space between arm and shoulder	Have patient extend arms outward to front, and locate point on fossa over the shoulder joint.
Ch'u-ch'ih	Hand large intestine meridian (shou yang-ming ta-ch'ang ching)	Fever, urticaria, painful arms and joint, paraplegia	In middle of elbow joint, on same aspect (proximal)	Ask patient to bend elbow joint, and locate point in middle of transverse fold.
Ho-ku	Hand large intestine meridian (shou yang-ming ta-ch'ang ching)	Toothache, fever, headache, pain in the eyes	In the interdigital space between the thumb and index finger	Have patient open up hand extending the thumb and index finger. Locate point on the interdigital space.

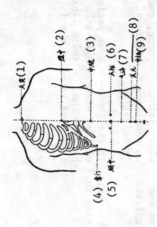

Key:
1. T'ien-tu (1131 4499)
2. T'an-chung (5238 0022)
3. Chung-wan (0022 5184)
4. Chang-men (4545 7024)
5. Ch'i-chung (5247 0022)
6. T'ien-shu (1131 2873)
7. Ch'i-hai (3051 3189)
8. Kuan-yuan (7070 0337)
9. Chung-chi (0022 2817)

Figure 4-3-7. Commonly used acupuncture points on the chest and abdomen.

Table 4-3-4. Acupuncture Points of the Chest and Abdomen

Acupuncture point	Meridian	Conditions treated	Location	Locating techniques
T'ien-tu	The special "jen-mo" meridian	Coughing, asthma, mucus in throat	In middle of fossa over manubrium of sternum	Ask patient to raise head, so point can be easily located. Be sure that needle is inserted obliquely in downward direction.
T'an-chung	The special "jen-mo" meridian	Chest pains, coughing, asthma, inadequate lactation	On midline of sternum, at level of the 4th intercostal space	Have patient lie in recumbent position, locate the point between the breasts.

- 114 -

Table 4-3-4. (Continued)

Acupuncture point	Meridian	Conditions treated	Location	Locating techniques
Chung-wan	The special "jen-mo" meridian	Stomach ache, abdominal distension, diarrhea, vomiting, weak stomach and spleen	Four inches above the navel	Have patient lie down in recumbent position, and locate point between the ch'i-ku (sternum) and the ch'i-chung (navel).
Chang-men	Foot liver meridian (tsu ch'ueh-yin kan ching)	Vomiting, diarrhea, weak and deficient spleen and stomach pain in chest and abdomen	At tip of 11th rib located on side of body between chest and abdomen	Have patient lie on side, arm at rest and elbow bent. The corner of the bent elbow indicates location of acupuncture point.
Ch'i-chung (shen ch'ueh)	The special "jen-mo" meridian	Vomiting, diarrhea abdominal cramps	In middle of navel	Have patient lie in recumbent position to locate point
T'ien-shu	Foot stomach meridian (tsu yang-ming wei ching)	Diarrhea, dysentery abdominal pain and distension, constipation, edema	Alongside the navel, 2 inches away	Have patient lie in recumbent position, and locate point 2 inches away from the navel.
Ch'i-hai	The special "jen-mo" meridian	Abdominal pain, leukorrhea, metrorrhagia, dysmenorrhea, hernia	Below the navel 1 1/2 inches	Have patient lie on back, to locate point.
Kuan-yuan	The special "jen-mo" meridian	Abdominal pain, diarrhea, impotency preliminary ejaculation, hernia, menstrual irregularity, leukorrhea, metrorrhagia	3 inches below the navel	Have patient in recumbent position. Locate point 1/2 inch below the "ch'i-hai" point

Table 4-3-4. (Continued)

Acupuncture point	Meridian	Conditions treated	Location	Locating techniques
Chung-chi	The special "jen-mo" meridian	Preliminary ejaculation, anuria, metorrhagia, leukorrhea. dysmenorrhea	On upper part of pubic bone 4 inches below the navel	Locate point by having patient lie in recumbent position.

Key:
1. Ta-ch'ui (1129 2785)
2. Ting-ch'uan (1353 0820)
3. Chien-ching (5144 0064)
4. Fei-yu (5151 0358)
5. Kao-mang-yu (5221 4159 0358)
6. Ling-t'ai (7227 0669)
7. Chih-yang (5267 7122)
8. Kan-yu (5139 0358)
9. Tan-yu (9054 0358)
10. P'i-yu (5196 0358)
11. Shen-yu (5200 0358)
12. Chih-shih (1807 1358)
13. Yao-ch'i (5212 1142)
14. Ch'ang-ch'iang (7022 1730)

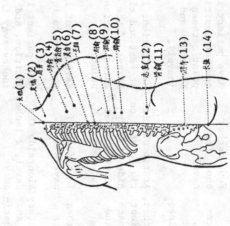

大椎(1)
天宗 肩井 (3)
膏肓俞(5)
天柱(6)
天阳(7)
肝俞(8)
胆俞(9)
脾俞(10)
志室(12)
肾俞(11)
腰奇(13)
长强 (14)

Figure 4-3-8. Commonly used acupuncture points for the back.

- 116 -

Table 4-3-5. Acupuncture Points of the Back

Acupuncture point	Meridian	Conditions treated	Location	Locating techniques
Ta-ch'ui	The governing "tu-mo" meridian	Influenza fever, malaria, intense pain in neck	Between prominences of the 7th cervical and 1st thoracic vertebrae	Have patient bow head. Locate point at level of shoulders.
Ting-chu'an (chu'an-hsi)	Special point	Labored breathing, hives	One inch to side of 7th cervical vertebra	Locate point with patient in prone position
Chien-ching	Foot gallbladder meridian (tsu shao-yang tan ching)	Shoulder pain, intense pain in neck, early mastites	In middle of shoulder	Draw imaginary line between the points "ta-ch'ui" and "chien-yu." Locate point at mid-point.
Fei-yu	Foot bladder meridian (tsu t'ai-yang pang-kuang ching)	Tuberculosis, cough, hemoptysis	About 1.5 inch (to the side) from the lower edge of the 3rd [thoracic] vertebra	Have patient sitting straight up to locate the acupuncture point.
Kao-mang-yu	Foot bladder meridian (tsu t'ai-yang pang-kuang ching)	Tuberculosis and all chronic ailments	3 inches away from lower part of the 4th [thoracic] vertebra	Have patient in prone position, arms locked with hands holding elbows. Locate point by following the medial margins of the shoulder blades down to where they face the 4th vertebra.
Ling-t'ai	The governing "tu-mo" meridian	Boils and abscesses	In fossa below prominence of 6th [thoracic] vertebra	Locate point with patient in prone position

Table 4-3-5. (Continued)

Acupuncture point	Meridian	Conditions treated	Location	Locating techniques
Chih-yang	The governing "tu-mo" meridian	Malaria, yellow jaundice	In fossa below prominence of 7th [thoracic] vertebra	Have patient in prone position. Locate point below 9th vertebra at level of lower margin of scapulae.
Kan-yu	Foot bladder meridian (tsu t'ai-yang pang-kuang ching)	Yellow jaundice, pain in the sides (thorax and flank)	About 1.5 inch [to the side] from point below the 9th [thoracic] vertebra	Locate point with patient in sitting or in prone position.
Tan-yu	See above	Jaundice, aching bones	About 1.5 inch [to the side] from point below the 10th vertebra.	See above
P'i-yu	See above	Diarrhea, dysentery hepatomegaly, splenomegaly	About 1.5 inch [to the side] from point below the 11th vertebra	See above
Shen-yu	See above	Backache, impotency preliminary ejaculation, incontinence	About 1.5 inch [to side] from point below the 14th [2nd lumbar] vertebra	See above
Chih-shih	See above	Acute back strain	3 inches [to side] from point below the level 14th [2nd lumbar] vertebra	Have patient in prone position. Locate point on same level as the "shen-yu."

Table 4-3-5. (Continued)

Acupuncture point	Meridian	Conditions treated	Location	Locating techniques
Yao-ch'i	Special point	Epilepsy	Two inches above the coccyx	Locate point with patient in prone position.
Ch'ang-ch'iang	The governing "tu-mo" meridian	Hemorrhoids, rectal bleeding, rectal prolapse, constipation, lumbago	Area just below tip of coccyx	Have patient in prone position. Locate point in fossa between the tip of coccyx and the anus.

Key:
1. Mai-pu (6701 2975)
2. Hsi-yen (5230 4190)
3. Tsu-san-li (6398 0005 6849)
4. Lan-wei-hsueh (7061 1442 4494)
5. Feng-lung (0023 7127)
6. Chieh-ch'i (6043 3305)
7. T'ai-ch'ung (1132 0394)
8. Pa-feng (0360 7364)
9. Ta-tun (1129 2415)
10. Yin-pai (7148 4101)
11. Wei-chung (1201 0022)
12. Ch'eng-shan (2110 1472)
13. Huan-t'iao (3883 6426)
14. Feng-shih (7364 1579)
15. Yang-ling-chu'an (7122 7117 3123)
16. Ling-hsia (7117 0007)
17. Lung-chung (5122 0022)
18. Hsuan-chung (2038 6945)
19. Kun-lun (2492 1510)
20. Ch'iu-hsu (8002 1072)
21. Tsu-lin-ch'i (6398 5259 3135)
22. Chih-yin (5267 7113)
23. Hsueh-hai (5877 3189)
24. Yin-ling-ch'uan (7113 7117 3123)
25. San-yin-chiao (0005 7113 0074)
26. T'ai-ch'i (1132 3305)
27. Yung-ch'uan (3196 3123)

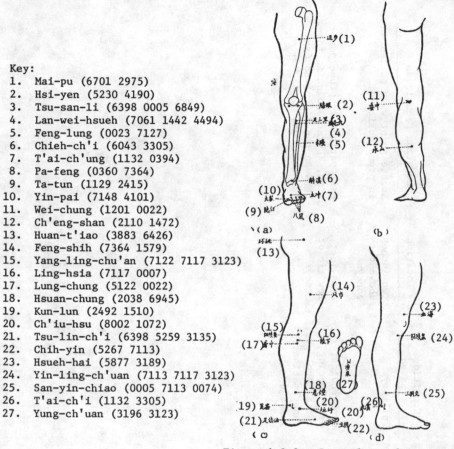

Figure 4-3-9. Commonly used acupuncture
points of the lower extremities.

(a) Anterior aspect
(b) Posterior aspect
(c) Lateral aspect
(d) Medial aspect.

Table 4-3-6. Acupuncture Points of the Lower Extremities

Acupuncture point	Meridian	Conditions treated	Location	Locating techniques
Mai-pu	New point	Post-infantile paralysis complications	Upper part of thigh, in front	Have patient in recumbent position, legs extended. Locate point 2.5 inch below the hip joint.
Hsi-yen	Special point	Stroke, beri-beri, arthralgia of knee	In depression along both sides of knee cap	Have patient bend knee (to right angle). Location point in depression outside the patella ligament below the patella
Tsu-san-li	Foot stomach meridian (tsu yang-ming wei ching)	Stomach ache, abdominal pain and distension, poor general health, indigestion	3 inches below the knee joint about a finger's width from outer edge of tibia	Ask patient to sit down with knee bent, and place his hand over his knee cap. The point is marked where the middle of finger stops.
Lan-wei-hsueh	Special point	Acute appendicitis	About 2 inches or so below the "tsu-san-li" point	Locate point along extension of imaginary line joining the "tsu-san-li" and "hsi-yen" points, about 2 inches down from "tsu-san-li" where pressure pain is felt.
Feng-lung	Foot stomach meridian (tsu yang-ming wei ching)	Constipation, cough with much mucus	On middle of anterior lateral aspect of leg, 8 inches above the external malleolus	Ask patient to sit with foot dangling. Locate midpoint of line between the "hsi-yen" and "chieh-hsi" points, cross over laterally a finger's width and locate the acupuncture point.

Table 4-3-6. (Continued)

Acupuncture point	Meridian	Conditions treated	Location	Locating techniques
Chieh-ch'i	Foot stomach meridian (tsu yang-ming wei ching)	Arthralgia of ankle, headache	Center of anterior aspect of ankle flexure, under edge of shoe lacings	Locate point at juncture between dorsal surface of foot and the leg in the transverse flexure in fossa between two sinews.
T'ai-ch'ung	Foot liver meridian (tsu chu'eh-yin kan ching)	Hernia, anuria, incontinence, gonorrhea, infantile convulsions	On dorsum of foot, in inter-metatarsal space between the big toe and second toe	Locate point in fossa between 1st and 2nd metatarsals.
Pa-feng	Special point	Beri-beri, swollen dorsum of foot	In all inter-digital spaces between toes, a total of 8 points	Locate points above the margin of interdigital "webs" between toes.
Ta-tun	Foot liver meridian (tsu chu'eh-yin kan ching)	Hernia, metrorrhagia, prolapse of uterus	Along lateral edge of big toe about 3 hairs away from base of nail	From base of big toenail at midpoint, extend posteriorly and laterally about 0.1 inch to locate point.
Yin-pai	Foot spleen meridian (tsu t'ai-yin p'i ching)	Epilepsy, menorrhagia, intestinal bleeding	Base of big toenail, inner side	Locate point about 0.1 inch from base of big toenail on side next to second toe.
Wei-chung	Foot bladder meridian (tsu t'ai-yang pang-kuang ching)	Lumbago, arthralgia of knee, acute fevers	In middle of popliteal space	Have patient in prone position. Locate point in fossa of popliteal artery.

Table 4-3-6. (Continued)

Acupuncture point	Meridian	Conditions treated	Location	Locating techniques
Ch'eng-shan	Foot bladder meridian (tsu t'ai-yang pang-kuang ching)	Vomiting and diarrhea, leg cramps, hemorrhoids	Behind leg at lower edge of gastrocnemius muscle where it meets soleus muscle	Have patient stand tiptoe with ankle elevated. Locate point in dimpled juncture of "L"-shape muscular formation [where gastrocnemius meets soleus to form tendon of Achilles].
Huan-t'iao	Foot gallbladder meridian (tsu shao-yang tan ching)	Arthralgia of back and knee, atrophy and paralysis of lower extremities	In hip joint area, in fossa behind joint	Have patient in lateral recumbent position, the leg on top bent and one below extended. Locate point at end of transverse flexure on lateral edge of hip joint.
Feng-shih	See above	Stroke-caused atrophy, arthralgia of thigh and knee	In middle of thigh, lateral aspect, 7 inches above knee	Have patient stand straight, both hands along sides and locate point at level indicated by tips of third finger.
Yang-ling	See above	Arthralgia of thigh and knee, hemiplegia, pain in chest and sides	Below knee, in front of head of fibula, opposite to the "yin-ling-ch'uan" on other side of leg	Have patient sit up, knees bent, feet dangling, and locate point in fossa over the anterior surface of the head of fibula.
Ling-hsia	New point	Deafness, cholecystitis, bile duct ascariasis	On lateral surface of leg	Locate point 2 inches below the "yang-ling-chu'an point.

Table 4-3-6. (Continued)

Acupuncture point	Meridian	Conditions treated	Location	Locating techniques
Lung-chung	New point	Deafness	On lateral surface of leg	Locate point 3 inches below head of fibula.
Hsien-chung	Foot gallbladder meridian (tsu shao-yang tan ching)	Pain in lower extremities -- leg, knee, foot	3 inches directly above the lateral malleolus	Locate point directly 3 inches above the lateral malleolus.
Kun-lun	Foot bladder meridian (tsu t'ai-yang pang-kuang ching)	Backache, epilepsy in children, swollen and painful ankle joints, heat stroke, paraplegia	In fossa just behind the lateral malleolus	Locate point between the lateral malleolus and the Achilles tendon. Point is opposite from the "t'ai-chi" point on medial aspect of leg.
Ch'iu-hsu	Foot gallbladder meridian (tsu shao-yang tan ching)	Fever, cough, dyspnea, pterygium, pain in chest and sides, swollen and painful heels, beriberi	In fossa below lateral malleolus	Locate point in fossa on outer edge of the toe extensor in lower edge of anterior part of the external malleolus.
Tsu-lin-ch'i	See above	Painful sides, breast abscess, temporal headaches	In depression between the 4th and 5th metatarsals	Locate depression in front of juncture between the 4th and 5th metatarsals.
Chih-yin	Foot bladder meridian (tsu t'ai-yang pang-kuang ching)	Pain in head and face. Sluggish labor (delivery). Abnormal fetal positions	On outside aspect of little toe, at base of nail.	Locate point 0.1 inch from corner of toenail base.

Table 4-3-6. (Continued)

Acupuncture point	Meridian	Conditions treated	Location	Locating techniques
Hsueh-hai	Foot spleen meridian (tsu t'ai-yin p'i ching)	Menstrual irregularities, pruritus	Locate 2 inches above inner border of patella	Same as location
Yin-ling	See above	Bloated abdomen, diarrhea, dysuria, arthralgia	On inner side of knee, in depression of foot and knee	Have patient bend knee. Locate point in fossa on inner side of tibia. Opposite to the "yang-ling ch'uan" point.
San-yin-chiao	See above	Dysmenorrhea, menorrhagia, leukorrhea in women, and premature ejaculation, gonorrhea and hernia in men	3 inches directly above the medial malleolus	Locate point 3 inches up from center of medial malleolus, on posterior margin of the tibia.
T'ai-ch'i	Foot spleen meridian (tsu shao-yin shen ching)	Malnutrition, cough, menstrual disorders	Behind the internal malleolus the ankle bone	Locate point in depression between the lateral-posterior aspect of medial malleolus, in position directly opposite that from the "kun-lun" point
Yung-ch'uan	See above	Aches and pains in head and neck, and foot. Also epilepsy	In depression anterior to sole of foot	Extend sole of foot posteriorly and locate point in middle of sole.

Moxibustion

Moxa cones or sticks prepared from dried and crushed moxa are often burned and smoked over acupuncture points of the body. This technique, called moxibustion, allows the heat generated to penetrate the skin and deeper muscle layers, and thereby attain the goal of disease prevention and treatment.

1. Moxibustion materials and their preparation.

   Materials: Powdered moxa (dried moxa leaves, crushed and sifted to remove impurities). Sometimes other substances are added (a mixture of crushed cinnamon, dried ginger, Carophyllus sp., Saussurea lappa, Angelica pubescens and anomala sp., Cynanchum atratum, realgar, myrrh, frankinsense, and piperitum, total weight 3 ch'ien, to be added to each stick).

   Preparation:
   a. Moxa cones: Place a small amount of powdered moxa on top of a smooth wooden board and use the thumb, index and middle fingers to mold the ingredients into a cone.

   b. Moxa sticks: Cut mulberry bark paper into rectangle (7 inches long by 6 inches wide). Place 20 grams of powdered moxa on each piece of paper. Smooth out, then rapidly roll up and seal.

2. Moxibustion technique.

   a. By moxa cones. Also called "mai-li-chiao," meaning granular (wheat) moxibustion. Here the cone is placed atop the acupuncture point and lighted. It is snuffed out when the patient feels the heat and some pain. Ginger or garlic slices, or salt, may be placed over site before lighting the moxa cone. This technique is called "ke-chiang-chiao," "ke-hsuan chiao," or "ke-yen-chiao," meaning moxibustion over (or separated by) ginger, garlic, or salt.

   b. By moxa sticks. Moxa sticks are lit here and placed over acupuncture point, as close to skin as possible, generally close enough for the patient to feel and tolerate the heat.

3. Illnesses suited for moxibustion treatment. Generally, suited for deficiency-type ailments, chill (cold dominating) ailments, and various types of chronic ailments.

4. Precautions.

   a. Make sure position taken by patient for treatment is an appropriate one. Just as different positions are assumed in acupuncture, depending on location of points, the same holds true for moxibustion therapy.

b. Prevent blister formation. If blisters are formed, use a fine "hao" needle to prick it open at base and let fluid drain out. Apply mercurechrome or gentian violet to prevent infection.

Ear Acupuncture Therapy

Ear acupuncture therapy is a method of treating disease by acupuncture (or massage, pressure, or application of other stimulation) performed on the pinna of the ear. This is one of the new acupuncture techniques; simple, easy to learn, quickly effective, and economical. It may be used as a form of acupuncture anesthesia, which makes it highly suitable for national defense (war preparedness) purposes.

1. Conditions suited for treatment. Not only does ear acupuncture treat various functional ailments, it can also treat many illnesses of an organic nature. According to reports, ear acupuncture can be the primary or supplementary means of treatment for at least 60 to 70 kinds of ailments. Widely used in clinical practice, it is most effective as an analgesic in treating various kinds of neuritis, traumatic soft tissue damage (pain), stomach spasms, intestinal cramps, dysmenorrhea, etc.

2. Delineation of regions of the ear (pinna). Practically all parts of the human body are represented by corresponding "representative zones" on the pinna of the ear. Distribution of these "representative zones" follows a definite pattern (Figure 4-3-10). When a certain part of the body undergoes pathologic change, pressure pain points (reaction points) often appear in corresponding zones on the pinna. A certain amount of stimulation applied to these pressure-pain points may, in turn, cure disease in the corresponding body part of organ. However, efficacy of treatment depends greatly on the precise accuracy with which the acupuncture site is pinpointed, since delineation of these representative zones is not absolute, and room must be allowed for individual differences. Sometimes, even in the same patient, the reacting zones shift a little for different ailments.

3. Technique.

a. How to locate reaction points on the pinna. The simplest method utilizes the blunt end of fine "hao" needles or the rounded edge of glass rod, or head of match, to carefully examine the pinna, using pressure. When a reaction point is pressed, the patient may cry out in pain, frown, or avoid contact. If many pressure pain points are found on the pinna at the same time, the most painful ones should be selected to be the important therapeutic acupuncture points.

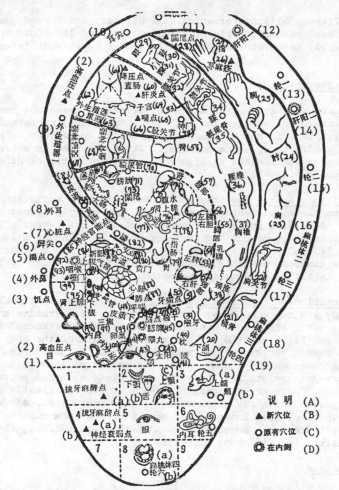

Figure 4-3-10. Mapped regions of the pinna

Legend: (A) Explanation   (C) Original acupuncture points
         (B) New acupuncture points   (D) Located on medial aspect

Zones in lobe

1. Tooth extraction anesthesia point   4. a. Tooth extraction anesthesia point
2. a. Mandible   b. Neurasthenia point
    b. Maxilla   5. Eyes
    c. Tongue   6. Inner ear wheel 5
3. a. Palate   7. --
    b. Cheek   8. a. Tonsils - 4   9. --
                                            b. Wheel 6

Key:

1. Eye
2. High blood pressure point
3. Hunger point
4. External nose
5. Thirst point
6. Screen (obstruction) point (p'ing-tien, 1456 7820)
7. Heart point
8. External ear
9. External genitals
10. Point of ear (ear lobe)
11. Tonsils
12. Yang-dominant liver one (kan-yang-I)
13. Wheel (cycle) 1
14. Yang dominant liver two (kan-yang-erh)
15. Wheel (cycle) 2
16. Tonsils, 2
17. Wheel (cycle) 3
18. Tonsils, 3
19. Wheel (cycle) 4
20. Jaw
21. Clavicle
22. Shoulder joint
23. Shoulder
24. Elbow
25. Wrist
26. Urticaria
27. Fingers
28. Appendix point (lan-wei tien)
29. Heel
30. Toes
31. Ankle
32. Knee joint
33. Wrist joint
34. Knee
35. Coccyx
36. Vertebrae, lumbar
37. Vertebrae, thoracic
38. Vertebrae, cervical
39. Larynx
40. Occiput
41. Apex (of head)

42. T'ai-yang
43. Forehead
44. Testicle
45. Parotid glands
46. Subcortex
47. Brain point
48. P'ing-ch'uan (1627 0820)
49. Brain stem
50. Toothache point
51. Neck
52. Right liver
53. Left spleen
54. Mammary gland
55. Chest
56. Left pancreas, right gallbladder
57. Abdomen
58. Buttocks
59. Shen-men (4377 7024)
60. Hepatitis point
61. Hypotensive (pressure lowering) point
62. External genitals 2
63. Urethra
64. Uterus
65. Wheezing
66. Hip joint
67. Sympathetic nerves
68. Sciatic nerve
69. Prostate gland
70. Ureters
71. Bladder
72. Large intestine
73. Appendix
74. Kidney
75. Ascites
76. Adrenal gland
77. Small intestine
78. Duodenum
79. Stomach
80. Cardiac orifice
81. Support (leverage) point (chih tien)
82. Diaphragm
83. Urethra
84. Rectum
85. Nerve organic function point
86. New eye

87. Esophagus
88. Heart and lungs
89. Pulmonary (lung) point
90. Bronchus
91. Trachea
92. Upper abdomen
93. Larynx
94. Ya-men (0800 7024)
95. Adrenal gland
96. Lower abdomen
97. Triple warmer (san-chiao)
98. Inner nose
99. Ovary
100. Endocrine glands

Key:
1. P'ing-chien (1456 1423)
2. External nose
3. Adrenal gland
4. Testicle
5. Pressure lowering groove
6. Abscess
7. Lower back
8. Middle back
9. Upper back

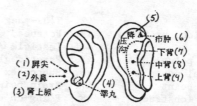

anterior view   posterior view

Figure 4-3-10. Mapped Regions of the Pinna (cont'd)

    b. Puncture technique. After acupuncture points on the pinna
have been selected, sterilize the area. Then take a slender
0.5-inch or 1-inch "hao" needle and insert vertically into
point, to a depth of .05 to 0.1 inch. Cartilage can also be
punctured. Judge the range and speed of needle twirling according to the patient's physique and condition, best to continue until a strong response is evoked. The needle may be
retained for 12-30 minutes. During this time, twirl the needle
every 5-10 minutes to intensify the stimulation. Or some moxa
may be burned next to the needle holder (needle warming or
"wen-chen") to provide heat stimulation. When necessary, the
needle may be retained for several hours. For certain chronic
and resistant disease, in order to maintain continuous stimulation, intradermal needles may be buried into ear acupuncture
points and left for about a week.

    4. Commonly seen illnesses treated by ear acupuncture therapy (Table
4-3-6)

Table 4-3-6. [sic] Ear Acupuncture Therapy Given to Commonly Seen Illnesses

Illness	Ear acupuncture points
Pains and aches over various parts of body (including sprains, bruises, inflammation of soft tissues)	Zones on the pinna map corresponding to painful parts, or other reaction points
Stomach ache	Zones for the stomach and subcortex
Neurasthenia (insomnia, forgetfulness)	Zones for the subcortex, forehead, inhibition, and forced concepts
Wryneck	Zones for the occiput and cervical vertebrae
Hiccups	Zone for diaphragm

Table 4-3-6 (Continued)

Illness	Ear acupuncture points
Pain in liver region	Zones for the liver, abdomen and stomach
Acute appendicitis	Zones for the large and small intestines
Constipation	Zones for the large intestine, and lower section of rectum
Asthma	Zones for the lung and adrenal glands, and the "p'ing-ch'uan" (wheeze relieving) point
Intestinal cramps	Zones for the large and small intestines
Sciatica	Zones for the buttocks, the coccyx, and the sciatic nerve
Tonsillitis	Zones of the larynx, mouth, and wheels 3, 4, 5, 6
Dysmenorrhea	Zones of the uterus and ovary
Hysteria	Zones of the subcortex, and inhibition
Toothache	Zones of the mouth, cheek and "p'ing-chien" (1456 1423) point

Fluid Puncture (Shui-chen)

Fluid puncture combines acupuncture with medicated fluids in a technique called acupuncture point injection therapy.

1. Classification of clinical methods.

   a. Small-dosage acupuncture point injection. Used for certain commonly seen or chronic illnesses, the amount of medication used for acupuncture point injection may be reduced to one-tenth to one-half that ordinarily used.

   b. Acupuncture point block. Used mostly for acute pain related to soft-tissue lesions. When the patient needs relief from pain, local anesthetic agents, tranquillizers or analgesics may be injected into the acupuncture point.

   2. Technique. In accordance with intramuscular injection requirements, sterilize skin over and around acupuncture point. Withdraw medicated solution into syringe, select a fine long needle and insert rapidly into point.

Table 4-3-7. Injection of Acupuncture Points in Commonly Seen Illnesses

Illness	Drug and dosage	Acupuncture point	Uses
Fever	Analgesin for injection 0.2-0.4 mm	"Ch'u-chih" and "ho-ku" points, singly	Emergency use to bring fever down
Headache	0.25-1% procaine solution	"t'ai-yang," "yin-t'ang", and "ho-ku" points	0.5-1 ml solution to each point, given daily for 5 days (one course of therapy)
Vomiting	5-10% dextrose parenteral solution	"Nei-kuan," "tsu-san-li" points	3-5 ml to each point, for emergency use, 1 to 2 times.
Asthma attack	0.1% adrenalin	"T'an-chung, "ch'uan-hsi" points	0.1-0.2% solution injected into each point, given during attack.
Pertussis	Streptomycin 25-50 mgm prepared in 0.5 ml solution	Ch'ih-tse	Given daily (5 days to a course), for two courses.
Bronchitis	1% procaine solution	T'ien-t'u	Daily injection 1 mgm for 5-7 days.
Trigeminal neuralgia	0.5-1% procaine solution	"Hsia-kuan," "ho-ku," "I-feng," "chia-che, "yang ling-chuan" points	Select two to three points each time for injection with 0.5-1 m of solution, every other day or daily. One course of 7 to 10 injections.
Facial paralysis	Vitamin B, 25 mgn	"Chia-che," "Ti-ts'ang," "yang-pai," "ying-hiang," and "ho-ku" points	Select 2 or 3 points each time, injecting 0.2-0.5 ml of vitamin into each point. Treatment given daily or every other day, a series of 10 treatments to a course of treatment.
Chronic rhintis	Vitamin B complex for injection	"Shang-hsing," "ying-hsiang," and "ho-ku" points	Select one acupuncture point each time for injection of 0.2-0.5 ml of vitamin. Treatment given on alternate days, a series of 15 treatments making up a course of therapy.

Table 4-3-7. (Continued)

Illness	Drug and dosage	Acupuncture point	Uses
Pulmonary tuberculosis	Streptomycin 0.1 gm	"Fei-yu" point	For patients treated with streptomycin, the daily dosage of 1 gm is reduced to 0.1 gm.
Stomach ache	0.5-1% procaine	"Chung-wan," "nei-kuan," "tsu-san li" points	(1) Inject 1-2 ml into each acupuncture point, once or twice in an emergency. (2) Inject 0.2-0.5 ml every other day, or twice a week. A series of 15 treatments is a course of treatment. (3) Inject 10-20 ml into each point every other day, for a total of 7 to 10 treatments which is one course of therapy.
Generally fragile health and poor appetite	Vitamin B complex injections	"Tsu-san-li"	See above
Acute back strain	Dextrose parenteral solution, 5-10%	Corresponding points on lumbar vertebrae that are painful on pressure and intervertebral spaces	See above
Sciatica	See above	"Huan-t'iao," "yin-men" points.	See above
Impotency	Vitamin B, 50-100 mgm, or testerone acetate 25 mgm	"San-yin-chiao," "shen-yu," "kuan-yuan"	Inject only one point every other day for a total of 15 times (a course of treatment).

Table 4-3-7. (Continued)

Illness	Drug and dosage	Acupuncture point	Uses
Incontinence	0.5-1% procaine solution	"Chung-chi," "san-yin-chiao."	Inject 0.2-0.5 ml into each point during each treatment given every other day. A total of 10 treatments make up a course of treatment
Neurasthenia	See above	"Nei-kuan," "san-yin-chiao" points	See above

Then slowly move needle [in place] up and down a few times until the patient experiences a full, numb or tingling sensation. Now slowly inject the medicated solution.

3. Injection of acupuncture point in commonly seen illnesses (Table 4-3-7)

4. Precautions

    a. Use fine long needle for injection. Do not twirl during insertion, though a small amount of needle movement (retraction) up and down is permissible.

    b. After needle is in place and the patient reacts to it, withdraw plunger of syringe slightly to see if needle hit blood vessel. If not, slowly inject the fluid in syringe.

    c. Before any procaine is used, check patient for sensitivity with a skin test. If negative, proceed with injection.

    d. Rotate acupuncture points selected for treatment. The same point should not be continuously used over a long period of time.

"Prick-open" Therapy (T'iao (2176) chih-liao fa)

1. Technique. Routinely sterilize the site or acupuncture point selected for "prick-open" treatment. First use a thicker needle to prick open the local surface skin tissue. Then prick the glistening white fibers of subcutaneous tissue, and break several scores of fibers with this "prick-open-and-rupture" technique. At this time the patient may feel some slight pain, but there is no bleeding. After the "prick-open" treatment, the local area is dabbed again with iodine and covered with adhesive dressing.

2. Conditions suited for treatment and selection of treatment points.

    a. For internal or external hemorrhoids, or mixed hemorrhoids: Select the proper "hemorrhoid" points on the patient's back (see "hemorrhoids"section) and continue with "prick-open" treatment.
Besides the "hemorrhoid" points, "prick-open" treatment can be used on certain acupuncture points, such as the upper, secondary, middle and lower "liao" (7539) points (located in the four openings in the sacrum alongside the 18th, 19th, 20th and 21st vertebrae). "Prick-open" only one acupuncture point at a time. The efficiency of pricking these acupuncture points is just as effective as pricking the "hemorrhoid" points.

    b. Granular (miliary) swellings. Locate small skin tubercles the size of grain, slightly raised above the skin. These little bumps are slightly red, and do not change "color" when pressed. Prick-open these swellings. Usually, pain at the affected "eye" dissipates a few hours after treatment.

c. Cervical lymph nodes. Locate the red and slightly elevated grain-size "tubercular points," whose coloring does not yield to pressure, on the lower corner of both shoulders and alongside both sides of spine. For disease affecting the left side, search for points on the right, and vice versa. If both sides are affected, locate points on both sides. After these "tubercular points" have been treated, the enlarged lymphatic nodes gradually dissipate after 30 to 40 days. If one course of treatment will not suffice, two or three more courses of treatment may be given.

Incision Therapy

1. Technique. After the area has been routinely sterilized, and anesthetized locally, use a surgical blade to make an 0.5-2 cm incision in the skin over acupuncture point. Extract the subcutaneous fatty tissue around the opening with a pair of hemostats, then move the blade handle around inside the base of incision to heighten stimulation and the patient experiences sensations of fullness, tingling, and numbness. Repeat 3 to 5 times. Then suture and dress cut. Remove stitches on third day.

2. Conditions suited for treatment and acupuncture point location.

a. Bronchial asthma. Use the "t'an-chung" points. If needed, repeat incision therapy, 7 days after the previous treatment at site 1 cm left or right of the "t'an-chung" point. Usually one to three incision treatments are necessary. The center of the surface over the first metacarpal below the index finger can also be a site for incision therapy.

b. Ascariasis in children. Use the "yu-fu" (7625 5215) point. This point is located on palm formed by intersection of line extended from interdigital space between the index and middle finger with the "ta-yu-chi" (1129 7625 7139) muscle near the center of the palm.

c. Chronic bronchitis. Use the "t'an-chung" and "fei-yu" points.

d. Chronic gastritis. Use the "shang-wan" and "chung-wan" points.

e. Peptic and duodenal ulcers. Give treatment at the "p'i-yu," "wei-yu," and "chung-wan" points. Any point that is effective for acupuncture therapy may be considered for incision therapy. However, care should be taken not to break any blood vessels.

3. <u>Precautions</u>

   a. Do not practice incision therapy in cases where the skin around the incision is infected or highly allergic, or in patients who are tired and hungry.

   b. Stop treatment if the patient feels dizzy and nauseated. Have patient lie down and observe any change in condition.

   c. To prevent infection, do not let the incision area get wet for at least a week following the procedure.

<u>Suture Implantation and Ligation at Acupuncture Point</u>

   Suture implantation at the acupuncture point site is a technique that anchors catgut in the acupuncture point and ligates it to maintain a continuous stimulation, and thereby attain the treatment goal.

   1. <u>Technique</u>.

   Place patient in a suitable position according to the acupuncture point selected. Routinely sterilize the area around site of procedure, drape with window sterile towels and anesthetize area with local 0.5-1% procaine infiltration before starting.

   a. <u>Suture implant method</u>. Insert catgut-threaded triangular round needle into skin about 1 cm from acupuncture points, through deeper soft tissues in an arced pattern, emerging 1 cm on the other side of point (the distance between insertion point and emerging point is about 2 cm). Gently stimulate skin around the point, allow enough catgut for loose ends and cut catgut. Allow skin to relax, and cover with sterile gauze.

   b. <u>Ligation method</u>. Make a small incision (about 0.5 cm [illegible] 1 cm) away from the acupuncture point, with a pointed surgical blade. Use mosquito forceps (inserted vertically) to separate the subcutaneous tissue and fascia layers until the patient experiences some tingling and full sensations. After this, bring a catgut-threaded round needle through the incision into subcutaneous tissue and out the other side of the point. Make one stitch and reinsert needle, going around the other side, for catgut to emerge at the incision opening. Tie two ends and cut loose ends. Plug knot into incision so it will not be exposed, and cover with gauze.

   2. <u>Conditions suited for treatment and location of acupuncture points</u>.

   Most commonly seen illnesses may be treated with this suture implantation technique. The principle of point selection is basically the same as that for acupuncture point selection, by tackling one to three points in one treatment. Besides the common points, sensitive and pressure pain points can also be selected. For example:

a. Post-infantile paralysis complications: the "huan-t'iao," "feng-shih," "tsu-san-li" and "hsien-chung" points.

b. Hypertension: "ch'u-chih," "ho-ku," "tsu-san-li," "san-yin-chiao," "t'an-chung" and other points.

c. Asthma: "ch'uan-hsi," "t'an-chung," "ju-chi," "chu-san-li" etc.

d. Epilepsy: "ta-ch'ui," "yao-ch'i" "feng-lung," "ho-ku," "shen-men" etc.

e. Peptic and duodenal ulcers: "chung-wan," "wei-yu," "tsu-san-li," or pressure pain points along both sides of the spine in back.

f. Enuresis: "ch'i-hai," "kuan-yuan," "chung-chi," "san-yin-chiao," "shen-yu" etc.

b. Backache, pain in thigh: "shen-yu," "chih-shih," "huan-t'iao," "yang-ling-chuan" etc.

3. Precautions:

a. Do not ligate shallow points on the skin along nerve and blood vessel passageways. Use only implantation over shallow skin surfaces. For points over the chest and back, be careful and avoid penetrating deeply and injuring blood vessels.

b. Though implantations may be repeated at the same point two to three times, allow at least 10 days between treatments.

c. Do not be alarmed after implantation and ligation if local reactions such as tingling, fullness, painful swelling, skin discoloration and limited motion in adjacent joints appear, if not accompanied by chills, fever and constitutional symptoms. Generally, the symptoms will subside after a few days.

d. Observe surgical asepsis for the operations. To prevent infection, do not leave the loose catgut ends exposed outside the skin surface.

e. This form of therapy is contraindicated for patients with active tuberculosis, serious heart disease, allergic skin reaction to procaine, and fever. Also excluded are females during pregnancy or menstrual periods.

Alkaline Therapy

Alkaline therapy is highly effective in treating Kashin Bek disease. It is definitely effective for treating endemic goiter, laryngitis, rheumatoid arthritis, and neurasthenia. The advantages of this treatment are an abundance of the medication used, low cost, simplicity of technique, and a great efficacy.

1. Drug preparation

   a. Powder: Place alkali chunks in porcelain enamel dish (do not let chunks come in contact with any metal utensils), and heat until melted. Filter the dissolved alkaline solution through four layers of gauze and bring to a boil again (do not stir). Continue boiling until all moisture has evaporated and the irrigating and volatile gas (hydrogen chloride) has dissipated. The alkaline fluid now changed from a dark brown fluid into a white crystal is the medicinal use alkali. Crushed into powder, the alkali is kept in a dry bottle to prevent deliquescence.

   b. Ointment

      (1) Filter the dissolved alkali chunks through four layers of gauze. Cool and stir in some raw straw ashes to form a soft ointment for use as poultice.

      (2) Add 2 gm of the powdered alkali to 10 gm of zinc oxide and mix well. This is 20% alkaline zinc oxide ointment which may be applied externally for skin diseases.

2. Dosage and use

   a. Powder preparation: For adults, 1 gm three times daily during the first 1-3 days. If there is no reaction, the dosage is increased to 2 gm three times daily. Depending on the patient's condition, the dosage sometimes may be increased to 3 gm three times daily. For children, the dosage is reduced accordingly. To take, place powder in bowl and add about 30-50 ml of warm boiled water to dissolve, and drink. Generally, it is best taken after meals, followed by a cup of warm water. Do not pour powder directly into mouth, as the mucous membranes of mouth may be burned.

   b. Ointment: Apply to affected parts, twice a day. Do not take internally.

3. Precautions:

   a. Watch for diarrhea (2 to 4 bowel movements a day or 6 to 8 in severe cases) and a burning sensation in the stomach. A few patients may experience nausea and vomiting. Mild reactions do not require any special treatment, but for severe reactions, reducing the dosage or stopping the drug will alleviate symptoms

b. During course of oral therapy, do not let patient eat or drink anything sour, hot, or sweet (brown sugar). Also contraindicated are soybean milk, cow's milk, etc.

c. Do not give powdered preparation to patients who have experienced hematemesis or rectal bleeding, to prevent massive hemorrhaging.

d. Conduct the extraction process (heating and boiling) outdoors, to prevent hydrogen chloride poisoning.

e. Keep powdered preparation in a dry place to prevent deliquescence which will lower drug activity.

Section 4. General Treatment Techniques

Checking Temperature, Pulse and Respirations (the "Three Checks")

There are certain physiologic limits to the temperature, pulse and respirations of a healthy individual which may undergo change during illness. Therefore, checking the reading of these vital signs is an important step in diagnosis.

1. Checking the temperature. The temperature of a normal person is usually between 36.5° to 37.5°C by mouth. The rectal temperature is generally 0.5 degree higher, while the axilla temperature is 0.5 degree lower. Thermometers are usually classed as oral (the tip is a long cylinder) or rectal (tip is a bulb). After use each time, the thermometer should be wiped clean, shaken down to register below 35°C, and soaked in a disinfectant solution.

a. To take oral temperature: Place thermometer under patient's tongue. Tell patient to keep mouth closed and breathe through nose. Keep in place for 3 minutes, then remove and read. For patients with mouth and nose ailments, and those who are unconscious or suffer from convulsions, do not take temperature by mouth. Wait 15 minutes before taking temperature of patients who have just exercised, or eaten or drunk hot or cold food or drink.

b. To take rectal temperature: Have patient lie on side with knees bent. Gently insert lubricated rectal thermometer into anus to a depth of about 1 1/2 inches. Hold the exposed end of thermometer to prevent dropping or breaking. Remove after 3 minutes and read the temperature. This method used more often in infants and in patients who are critically ill or comatosed.

- 140 -

c. To take axillary temperature: Have patient lie on back. Place
oral or rectal thermometer in armpit, and ask patient to cross
arm over chest and hug thermometer. After 5 minutes, remove
and read. As this method is not too accurate and it requires
a longer time to take, it is not used much ordinarily.

2. Pulse. The pulse rate of healthy individuals ranges between 60-80
times per minute, slower in older people and faster in children, and accele-
rated considerably after exercise. Take a patient's pulse after he has had
some rest. Put his forearm in a comfortable and steady position, and place
fingertips of the 2nd, 3rd, and 4th fingers over the radial artery. When the
pulse beat is felt, start counting for 30 seconds. Multiply this number by 2
to obtain the pulse rate per minute. If the radial pulse is not detectable,
try feeling for the pulse of the common carotid artery at the neck, or that
of the shallow temporal artery, or that of the dorsal artery of foot.

3. Respirations. Respirations of healthy individuals are counted at
rate of 16 to 18 times a minute. Check a patient's respirations when he is
sitting or lying down quietly, and observe his breathing by the rise and fall
of his chest or abdominal wall, equating one rise-and-fall movement as one
respiration. When the patient's breathing is shallow and undetectable, place
a small wisp of cotton next to his nose, and observe and count movements of
the cotton being blown on.

Checking Blood Pressure

The sphymomanometer commonly used for checking blood pressure employs
a mercury column for the readings. There is also another type that employs
a meter. When either style is used, make sure the instrument is in a level
and steady position.

1. Procedure

a. Allow patient to first rest for a few minutes (critical cases
the exception). Have him sit down or lie down, upper arm exposed, elbow extended, palm face up. Make sure the arm, the
heart and the "0" reading of the mercury column are all on the
same level.

b. Loosen the air valve at neck of rubber bulb, to expel all air
in the sphymomanometer. Smooth out the pressure cuff before
wrapping it around the upper arm about 3 inches above the
elbow. Connect cuff tubing to the instrument.

c. Locate the brachial pulse over the elbow and place stethoscope
over it. Put on [physician] the ear pieces.

d. Tighten the air valve. Squeeze the bulb until the pulse beat
is no longer heard (make the mercury column rise up over 160-
200mm). Then release the air valve gradually and let the

mercury column drop slowly. Watch the mercury column readings and changes in pulse beat sounds.

e. When the first pulse beat is heard as a distinct "tung," note reading on the mercury column in mm and register this as the systolic pressure. Follow drop in the mercury until the strong beat suddenly weakens and becomes lost, and note the reading then as the diastolic pressure.

f. Record the blood pressure reading in a fraction, the systolic pressure reading as the numerator and the diastolic pressure reading as the denominator. If the patient's systole is 120, and diastole is 80, it should be registered as 120/80 mm on the mercury column.

g. After the blood pressure has been checked, loosen the air valve and unwrap the cuff. Fold and put back in instrument box with rubber bulb and other attachments. Close box to keep the glass reading tube from being crushed.

2. Precautions

a. Before taking blood pressure reading, check sphymomanometer for damage and air leakage.

b. Expel all air in instrument and make sure the mercury is down to "0" before each blood pressure check.

c. Make sure readings for systole and diastole are heard clearly, otherwise, repeat the blood pressure check.

Cold Compresses

Cold compresses cause capillary constriction which in return reduces local congestion, and exert heat-dispelling, temperature-lowering, hemostatic and antiphlogistic action.

Generally, gauze (or towel) immersed in iced or cold water are wrung dry and applied externally over affected area. Ice bags can also be used. Change compresses every 5 minutes over a 30-minute period. Dry skin after each 30-minute treatment.

When cold compresses are used to lower the body temperature, place them on forehead, under the arms, or in the groin etc.

- 142 -

Hot Compresses

Hot compresses cause capillary dilation, relax local muscles, and exert an antiphlogistic and analgesic action. They may be applied by the following methods:

1. __Hot water bottle__. Fill with hot water and place over affected area. If a hot bottle is not available, use a camping canteen. Or stir-fry salt, rice, or polishings until hot and empty into cloth bags immediately for use as hot compresses.

2. __Wet hot compresses__. Immerse gauze or towel in hot water. Remove and wring out excess moisture before placing over affected part. Change every 5 minutes during a 30-minute treatment period.

When hot water bottle or moist hot compresses are used, protect skin against burns, especially in infants and unconscious or paralyzed patients.

3. __Hot water sitz bath__. Improves local blood circulation and reduces inflammation around the anus and the external genitals. Have patient sit in tub containing warm water or a warm 1:5000 potassium permanganate solution. Warm water should be added as necessary to maintain bath temperature. Each sitz-bath treatment should last for about 20 minutes. Avoid providing overly hot water which will scald the skin. Make sure the local areas are dried thoroughly after bath. If the patient has a dressing over wound, remove dressing before sitting patient in bath.

Allergy Tests

Injections of substances such as penicillin, procaine, tetanus antitoxin may cause allergic reactions such as urticaria, weak rapid pulse, nausea, irregular breathing and even shock. For this reason, allergy tests should be made first to prevent accidents. Give injections only if results are negative. If test results are positive, do not give injection, but desensitize patient first before giving the drug.

1. __Penicillin Sensitivity Test__.

The strength of penicillin used for skin test should contain 100 or 200 units of penicillin per cc.

__Preparation of penicillin in 100-unit (per cc) strength__. Inject 2 cc of injection-use water into bottle containing 200,000 units penicillin powder. After mixing thoroughly, take out 0.1 cc solution and place in another sterile bottle. Now inject 2 cc of injection-use water into this bottle, and withdraw 0.1 cc after mixing, for placement into still another bottle. Add injection-use water to make 5 cc. This will now meet the concentration requirements for each cc.

Procedure for intradermal sensitivity tests:

    a. Clean skin on medial aspect of forearm, 2 inches above the wrist, with 75% alcohol.

    b. Withdraw 1 cc (100 units) of the solution into a sterile syringe, expel air, inject 0.1 cc (10 units) intradermally, resulting in a local wheal.

    c. Use the same technique and inject 0.1 cc of normal saline intradermally on same part of opposite forearm for comparison purposes (this step used mostly on positive cases).

    d. Do not apply pressure after injection. Wait 20 minutes before observation of results.

    e. After drug injection, if the local part becomes red and hard and the wheal exceeds 1 cm in diameter, while the saline injection area shows no change, the reaction is said to be a positive one. If the wheal does not become red or larger after injection, the sensitivity test is negative.

2. Procaine sensitivity test

    a. Dilute the procaine solution to a 0.25% solution.

    b. Follow the same procedure used for the penicillin sensitivity test, including the same amounts injected, observation of results.

3. Tetanus antitoxin sensitivity test.

    a. Dilute 0.1 cc of tetanus antitoxin (1500 units to each cc) to make 1 cc.

    b. Follow the same procedure used for the pencillin sensitivity test, including the same amount injected, observation of results, etc.

4. Sensitivity test precautions.

    a. Do not repeat procaine skin tests, if it had been done once in the past.

    b. Repeat penicillin sensitivity test each time that it is prescribed, whether for oral use, eye drops, or external use.

c.   Be aware that in some patients who show a negative skin test, an allergic reaction can still take place after drug injection. For this reason, always observe patient for 15 minutes after injection before letting him go.

d.   If allergic shock occurs, immediately give patient a subcutaneous or intramuscular injection of 1:1000 adrenalin 1 cc, and adopt other emergency measures.

e.   For patients who need tetanus antitoxin, but are positive to the intradermal tetanus antitoxin test, use a desensitizing method for injections as follows:

(1)   Inject once every 20 minutes.

(2)   Give first injection, 0.05 cc of 1:20.

(3)   Give second injection, 0.05 cc of 1:10.

(4)   Give third injection, 0.1 cc of original antitoxin.

(5)   Give fourth injection, 0.5 cc of original antitoxin.

(6)   Give remaining amount in one injection.

(7)   If a reaction occurs after any sequence in the above series, wait 30 minutes before giving next injection. No change in dosage.

Injection Technique

1.   ## Drug Extraction Technique

For a drug contained in a glass ampoule, sterilize the exterior, and break it at neck. Holding a syringe in the right hand, and the broken-open ampoule in the left hand, draw drug solution into syringe held in right hand. For a drug solution contained in a rubber-stoppered bottle, first remove the metal cover over the stopper, then sterilize the stopper. Before plunging syringe in to withdraw solution, retract plunger slightly and let some air into syringe. Then insert needle and inject air into bottle, after which withdraw the wanted amount of drug solution.

If a drug is in powder form, it must first be dissolved with a suitable amount of water and drawn into syringe by technique just described.

2. Procedure and Precautions

    a. Select the proper syringe and pay attention to surgical asepsis
        procedure.

    b. Be aware of the indications and contraindications for injection.
        Doublecheck drug, dosage, patient, and procedure. If drug
        quality has changed or sediments are seen, do not use.

    c. After routine sterilization of injection site, and before in-
        troducing needle, be sure all air has been expelled from
        syringe.

    d. After needle is in place, and before drug is injected, retract
        plunger of syringe slightly to see if any blood is returned.
        If this is seen in a subcutaneous or intramuscular injection,
        do not inject drug, but withdraw needle and start again. If
        blood is returned in an intravenous injection, wait awhile to
        make sure needle has entered the vein before proceeding with
        injection.

    e. Make sure the needle is inserted and withdrawn quickly. If the
        patient feels pain during injection, or the drug being injected
        is irritating, inject slowly.

    f. After injection, wash and sterilize syringe and needle.

3. Injection Routes and Technique

    a. Intradermal injection: Commonly used for sensitization tests,
        preventive inoculations (Calmette's vaccination), and local
        anesthesia. The site for sensitization tests is generally on
        the inner aspect of the forearm about 2 inches above the wrist.

        Clean (sterilize) skin area with alcohol (not iodine). Use a
        sterile 1-ml syringe and a short needle. After drawing up the
        drug solution, expelling air, inject needle into skin (slant
        side of needle tip up) at a 15-20 degree angle, push plunger
        and inject the proper amount of solution until a skin "bump"
        is seen. Do not apply pressure after injection.

    b. Subcutaneous injection: Used mostly in first aid when medi-
        cation cannot be taken by mouth. The injection site is usually
        on the outer side of the upper arm where there is more flesh.

        After routine sterilization of injection site, introduce needle
        subcutaneously at a 30° angle (with the skin), and slowly in-
        ject drug solution. After injection, apply pressure with a
        dry cotton ball a while.

c. <u>Intramuscular injection</u>: Given to patient lying in the lateral recumbent or prone position with buttocks exposed. Select the upper outer quadrant of one side for the injection site (See Figure 4-4-1).

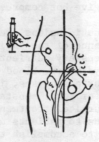

Figure 4-4-1. Intramuscular Injection.

After routine sterilization of the injection site, stabilize and stretch the skin over injection site with the left thumb and middle and index fingers. Holding syringe in right hand, the needle at right angle to the skin, quickly insert needle into muscle (do not insert for the whole length). Use the left thumb and index finger to stabilize head of needle and retract syringe slightly. If no blood is drawn, then inject slowly. After injection, quickly remove the needle, and massage part with an alcohol sponge and apply local pressure.

If the site selected for injection is hard or red and inflamed, change to the other side. If both sides are sore, select the deltoid muscle in the upper arm for the injection site. If pain or hardness appears after injection, apply hot compresses to the sore area.

d. <u>Intravenous injection</u>. The vein located in the elbow space is generally selected. In obese patients or small children with a good amount of subcutaneous fat, the vein might be difficult to locate in the elbow. If several attempts prove unsuccessful, select some other more easily detected shallow vein (such as the femoral vein) for injection.

Just before injection, the patient rolls up his sleeve, clenches his fist and extends his forearm for a tourniquet or manual pressure to be applied to the upper arm to facilitate prominent distension of the vein. Following routine cleansing of skin with an antiseptic, extraction of medication, and expulsion of air in syringe, place the left index finger and thumb over the elbow space, and feel for the vein and stabilize it, while the needle in the right hand is inserted, level side up, into the vein from atop or parallel to it. Once some blood escapes into the syringe, lift the needle slightly, move it forward a little more, then stabilize it. Loosen the tourniquet and inject medication. If a local hematoma or phlebitis appears after the injection, give hot compresses.

e. <u>Infusions</u>. Intravenous infusions are often given to maintain the acid-alkaline balance of the patient's body fluids, and to supplement it with necessary nutrients, fluids etc. They are suited for use in dehydration, blood loss, shock, and/or alkali intoxication due to various causes, in serious infections, in stimulating excretion of toxic substances, in various surgical procedures and post-surgical treatments, in supplying nutrients and certain medications to patients unable to eat (or eat adequately), in order to accomplish the purpose of treatment.

(1) <u>Puncture site</u>. Generally the elbow space is the site most commonly selected for venous puncture, though other sites over the wrist, the backs of the hand and foot where shallow veins are easily located and the saphenous vein in the ankle are acceptable. Among infants, the sagittal sinus is frequently used. If it is possible to estimate the number of times the patient will need repeated fluid replacements, arrange so the venous puncture will start at the most distal vein, and as the puncture site gradually works its way up, it will gradually increase the number of times this particular vein is used.

(2) <u>Procedural technique</u>. Use a sterilized fluid transfusion bottle, connected distally to the rubber tubing, Murphy's drip, and needle. Let small amount of injection fluid run through transfusion bottle and tubing and clamp. Empty rest of injection fluid into transfusion bottle and hang on I.V. stand. Take needle in right hand, open clamp and let injection fluid flow out to expel air. Clamp. Open the small tube in the drip so that the fluid surface in the drip and the drip will maintain a specific distance. Open and close the small side tube. The puncture technique is the same as that for venous puncture determining when needle has entered vein, and opening clamp upon evidence of blood escaping into tubing. If passage through the needle is unobstructed, fluid in the drip will continue dripping with regularity. At this time, place a piece of sterile gauze over the needle to protect it, and fix with adhesive tape or a splint. Also adjust clamp to regulate rate of drip. During the course of intravenous therapy, take note of the patient's reaction and make sure the infusion passageway is clear.

Another intravenous infusion technique uses the solution in its original bottle. In this setup, clean the bottle cap with antiseptic, then insert the infusion tubing, needle and clamp in place, and hang on I.V. stand. Proceed as described above.

(3) Precautions

(a) Note the rate of infusion flow is 60 drops/minute for adults, and 30-40 drops/minute for infants and small children. Increase or decrease when necessary, depending on the patient's condition. Old people and persons with heart ailments should have drip adjusted at slower rate.

(b) Best not to give intravenous fluids to patients with heart failure, pulmonary edema, serious pneumonia and high blood pressure. Avoid intravenous fluids, particularly those containing salts, for patients with seriously impaired renal function and ascites.

(c) Make sure intravenous fluids are given at room temperature, best not to be warmer than 34°C.

(d) Stop the intravenous when the patient experiences chills, palpation, continuous coughing and other unfavorable reactions. If necessary, give subcutaneous injection of 1:1000 adrenalin 1 ml.

Local Infiltration Anesthesia

When local anesthesia is given, the anesthetic agent is injected to tissues in a certain part (the operative area) of the patient's body to cause numbness in the nerve endings and temporary loss of pain sensation locally, so that an operative or exploratory procedure can be carried out smoothly.

1. Preoperative preparation

a. Relieve patient of worries before giving his anesthetic. Put him in a comfortable position for muscles to relax.

b. At about 45 minutes or 1 hour before anesthesia administration, give patient an intramuscular injection of phenobarbital 0.1 gm or Dolantin [Demerol] 50-100 mg, to increase patient's tolerance to the local anesthetic.

c. To prevent anaphylactic shock, perform a procaine sensitivity test on patient beforehand.

2. Anesthetic agents and amounts used

Generally procaine in strengths of 0.25%, 0.5%, or 1% is used. However, the amount of procaine used at one time should not exceed 1 gm.

On most occasions when this drug solution is used, 3-6 drops of adrenalin (1:1000) may be added to each 100 ml. However, the amount of adrenalin given during the whole operation should not exceed 1 ml. Do not use adrenalin if the patient has hypertension, hyperthyroidism, atherosclerosis, diminished cardiac function, skull and brain damage.

3. Procedure

First prepare the skin. After routine cleaning with an antiseptic, draw anesthetic solution into a syringe. Inject slowly, from surface to deeper layers, infiltrating the intra-derma, the subcutis, and muscle by layers. The extent and depth of infiltration depends on the requirements of the particular operation.

First inject intradermally, causing the local skin area to form a small wheal and the skin surface to look like a tangerine. Following this, continue injecting along margin of wheal in direction of incision to form a second, a third, and a series of wheals running the length of the anticipated incision.

After the superficial wheals have been raised, infiltrate the subcutaneous and deeper tissues layer by layer. When injecting the anesthetic solution, be sure to retract plunger of syringe slightly to check on the presence of blood and avoid injection of anesthetic into blood stream. Inject slowly, to avoid untoward accidents.

4. Precautions

a. Do not use infiltrate anesthesia for inflamed areas.

b. Stop injection immediately when a toxic reaction occurs.
   Note: Signs of a toxic reaction are nervous tension, talkativeness, dyspnea, palpitation, a rising blood pressure or dizziness, drowsiness, slow reflexes, slight drop in blood pressure, bradycardia, slow respirations etc.

Incisions

The purpose of making incisions is to expose tissues or promote drainage, etc.

Before making an incision scrub the skin clean (shave off hair, if any). Follow routine procedures for surgical asepsis and anesthetic use (general or local anesthesia, depending on the operation site).

Before the operation, be sure to have a good understanding of the local anatomy -- the sequence and thickness of tissue layers exposed in the operation site, blood vessel and nerve distribution, and location of important organs, to avoid unnecessary injury while the incision is being made.

Normal skin tissue shows a certain amount of tension, and the direction of tension receptivity corresponds to the lines on the skin. Consequently, wherever possible, make the incision to correspond to the direction of these lines, particularly on the face, neck and other exposed areas. For example, the lines on the forehead are horizontal lines, and incisions made here should be horizontal or transverse incisions.

When an incision is made, post-healing function of the area must be considered. It is best to avoid incisions made on load-bearing areas. Incisions made over joints must be planned so that post-healing scar contracture will not affect function of the part. Consequently, the incision made on a flexing surface must correspond to the transverse coordinate of the limb. The tissues must be opened layer by layer, best based on the direction of tissue fibers, to facilitate post-operative restoration of function.

The incision is made where it is easiest to expose the disease lesion, the length of incision determined by operation requirements. If the incision is too long, it causes unnecessary injury, too short, inadequate lesion exposure and inconvenience to the surgical procedure. Moreover, excessive stretching of skin on both sides of the incision causes trauma in a way that affects healing.

Make sure the incision made is clean cut and uniform in depth. The operator holds the blade in right hand, between thumb and rest of fingers or with the index finger placed over back of blade, and his left hand is used to stretch skin on the incision site. Or he may be assisted by other personnel. The incision at both ends should be as deep as that in the middle, and not like a funnel. The angles formed by blade and skin during the procedure are generally 90° at blade insertion, 45° while cutting, and 90° on blade extraction-removal. Usually, after the skin and subcutis have been incised, and sterile gauze is placed around the incision to separate and protect the skin, another blade is used to make incision of deeper tissues in proper sequence along fascia coverings. However, be sure to avoid injury to blood vessels and nerves. Muscle may be separated in direction of muscle fibers with blade holder, hemostat or the fingers, all the way to both ends of incision. If necessary, cut muscle fibers. When cutting open the peritoneum, watch out and not injure any of the organs in the peritoneal cavity. Most operating surgeons use toothed forceps to pick up the peritoneum, while his assistant also picks it up with curved hemostats about 1 cm away on the opposite side. Repeat again, and make a small incision and probe scissors into the peritoneum to ascertain the presence of organic adhesions. Extend the index and middle fingers into the deeper aspect of the peritoneum and cut to both ends of the incision.

Suturing

After tissues have been cut, they should be sutured to facilitate early healing of the incised wound.

1. Suture needles and sutures

    a. Suture needles. Needles ordinarily used are classified in two categories: triple-edged cutting needles and round needles. The cutting needles are grouped further as straight or curved needles that are suited for sewing together tough tissues such as skin. Round needles are usually curved, and are suited for suturing together soft tissues such as muscles, tendons, peritoneum etc.

    b. Sutures. Suture ordinarily used are classified into nonabsorbable sutures and absorbable sutures.

        Non-absorbable sutures include silk thread, alloy steel wire, nylon thread etc. Silk thread comes in various sizes, and it is strong, even and soft. It is easy to handle for ligating and tissue reaction to it is mild. However, it is not absorbable. When the ligated wound is infected, the suture knots are frequently the cause of non-closure.

        Alloy steel wire does not rust, and tissue reaction to it is slight. Available in different sizes, it is also soft, pliable and strong. Coarse wire is often used in tension-reducing sutures for fixing fractures; fine wire, for suturing muscles and tendons.

        Nylon thread is strong, sturdy and smooth, and tissue reaction to it is slight. Commonly used for sewing blood vessels together.

        Absorbable sutures consist of plain catgut and chromic catgut. Plain catgut is not chemically treated after manufacture, and it usually loses its tensile strength after 3 days inside tissues, and becomes soft and gradually absorbed after a week. Chromic catgut has been chemically treated with a chromic solution that increases its strength and delays its absorption by tissues for several weeks.

2. Suturing precautions

    a. Make sure that facing edges of tissue layers being sewn together approximate each other. Do not leave space in the wound, as they may result in hematomas or fluid collections or sources of infection.

b. Make sure the thickness of tissue layers approximate each other. The skin surface should not be pitted or twisted.

c. Do not pull sutures too tight or too loose when sewing. Too tight sutures may affect healing, and too loose sutures may delay ultimate wound closure.

3. Suturing technique

Commonly used are interrupted sutures and continuous sutures.

a. Interrupted sutures. Insert needle into skin at point about 3-8 mm from edge of wound and have it come out from opposite side at an approximate point. The needle and suture should take a course perpendicular to the skin surface or slightly deviated away from the edge of cut while passing through the various tissue layers to ensure that more of the underlying tissues are embraced by the suture, and post-suture drop of the wound closure will not occur. This technique is often used for suturing skin, subcutaneous tissues, muscles, tendon coverings etc.

b. Continuous suture. Commonly used for sewing up the peritoneum.

Stitches Removal

Stitches are usually removed 5-7 days after surgery. The timing cannot be determined mechanically, as readiness for stitches to be removed depends on many factors such as the nature of the incision, suture tension, type of sutures used, tissue capacity for wound closure etc. Generally speaking, sutures on the head and neck may be removed in an interrupted pattern 3 or 4 days after the operation, and the rest to be removed after another one or two days. Sutures on the trunk and the four extremities are usually removed during the 6th or 7th day after operation. Generally, wound healing is slower in patients suffering from malnutrition or delibilitating disease. For them, removal of stitches should be delayed.

Before the stitches are removed, clean the skin routinely with an antiseptic. Use forceps to pick the knot up to pull out part of suture buried in the skin. Cut with scissors at this spot, and gently pull the suture out. Clean with antiseptic again. Cover with sterile gauze and anchor with adhesive strips.

Wound Debridement

Wound debridement must be carried out before a wound becomes infected. Generally, this should be done no later than 12 hours after sustained injury. Its purpose is to remove dirt and excise dead tissue to facilitate early wound healing.

Before debridement is carried out, be sure to correct systemic conditions such as shock, hemorrhage and dehydration. To prevent against tetanus, give patient an intramuscular injection of tetanus antitoxin 1500 units (after a sensitivity test).

Select the form of anesthesia to be used according to the requirements and capabilities available at the time.

After the anesthetic has been given, pack the wound with sterile gauze and shave off all hair on skin surrounding the wound. Clean with ether or petroleum, then repeat with soapy water two or three times. Now, remove the gauze plug and wash wound lightly with soapy water and physiologic saline. Make sure that every necrotic corner and depression are cleaned. After this, paint area with iodine or alcohol (or tincture of merthiolate or mercurochrome, making sure they do not flow into the wound. Cover area with sterile towels. Now observe strict surgical aspesis and cut to remove dead tissue, leaving a fresh new "sterile" wound.

After preoperative preparations have been completed, change into a fresh sterile gown and gloves. Now wash the wound with warm saline, trim off necrotic tissue and about 2-3 mm along edges of the wound, making sure that hemostasis for the freshly cut edges is adequate (depending chiefly on pressure from saline packs or hemostats, and avoiding ligation of bleeding points and retention of foreign matter as much as possible. Then suture (See "Suturing Technique"). If tendon and nerve injuries and fractures are also present, reduce and fix fracture at the same time. After operation, give suitable amount of antibiotics to prevent infection.

Changing Dressings

The purpose for changing dressings is to keep the wound clean to facilitate healing.

1. Precautions

    a. Know the condition of the wound in order to select proper drugs and dressings for treatment.

    b. Before changing the dressing, the physician should wash his hands and put on a face mask. Surgical asepsis must be observed when the dressing is being changed.

    c. Sterilize all instruments used -- such as scissors, forceps, dressings, dishes, dressing solutions etc. Do not mix them up, but arrange them in usage sequence.

- 154 -

d. First change dressings on the clean wounds, then on infected wounds. Note size and depth of wound and the presence of granulation tissue. Remove all foreign matter, suture knots, sequestrum, shrapnel, necrotic tissue etc. that may be found in wound. Change the drainage strip if one is used.

e. Handle healthy granulation tissue gently (such tissue is usually red, and firm, with edema or bleeding).

f. Stress surgical asepsis even more when handling wounds infected by the tetanus bacillus, Bacillus welchii, and Pseudomonas aeruginosa. Burn the infected dressings.

2. Procedure

a. Take off the outside bandage and dressing by hand. Use forceps to handle dressing next to the wound and any drains used. Note the color, odor, and amount of secretion present, if any.

b. Use alcohol sponge to lightly wipe skin around the wound. Then use a sterile cotton ball soaked with sterile physiological saline to lightly wash the wound. Do not rub hard, nor use an already used cotton ball to go over the already washed wound area, as this may cause infection.

c. If the wound is deep and secretions are heavy, flush with physiologic saline. If there is much necrotic tissue, irrigate with cusol or other disinfectant solution. If there is not much secretion, use a wrung dry saline sponge to mop up the wound secretion. Remove fibrin, necrotic tissue, and pus.

d. Trim excessive or unhealthy granulation tissue. When the granulation tissue is edematous, use a wet hypertonic saline compress on it (change wet compress every 4-6 hours).

e. Use sterile vaseline gauze dressings to cover most wounds. Use a drain when necessary. Place additional gauze over initial coverings, and fasten with adhesive tape over bandage.

f. Clean all utensils and instruments used for this procedure. Do not throw utensils away, nor get them mixed up.

3. Selection of external-use drugs.

a. Vaseline gauze. Protects granulation tissue. Its removal is painless when dressings are changed. Generally suited for clean wounds.

b. Nitrofurazone (furacin), 1:5000.
    Exhibits broad range of antibacterial activity. Suited for
    use with infected wounds.

c. Eusol. That is a solution of bleaching powder and calcium
    borate. Antibacterial and well tolerated [by tissues]. Par-
    ticularly effective for treating gas gangrene. Often used on
    wounds with much pus secretion and necrotic tissue.

d. Physiologic saline, 0.9%. Protects tissues, but exhibits no
    antibacterial activity.

e. Isoniazid or streptomycin solution. May be used on tuberculous
    wounds.

f. Phenoxyethyl alcohol 2.2%. May be used on suppurative
    Pseudonomas aeruginosa contaminated wounds.

g. Certain Chinese medicinal herbs and preparations that exhibit
    antibacterial and tissue soothing properties. Consult Chapter
    7 on their external use.

Nasal Feeding

Nasal feeding is used when patients cannot take food or medications by
mouth, and it is necessary under certain conditions, for the medication to
pass through the gastrointestinal tract.

1. Procedure

    a. Have patient in sitting or recumbent position.

    b. Lubricate tip of nasogastric tube with some liquid paraffin,
        and clamp other end of tube. Insert tip of tube through one
        nostril into nasal passageway, and ease it slowly into the
        stomach (noted when 60-cm mark on tube reaches nostril).
        After tube is in place, place its external end in water and
        release clamp. If no bubbles are seen when patient is breath-
        ing, this proves nasogastric tube is in the esophagus or
        stomach. If the water keeps bubbling, this means the tube
        is placed into the respiratory tract by mistake, and should
        be removed immediately before starting all over again.

    c. After the nasogastric tube has entered the stomach, fasten
        it onto cheek with adhesive tape.

    d. Connect the exposed end of tube to a 50-cc syringe. Pour in
        a small amount of warm boiled water to check patency of tube.

If no obstruction is found, continue to pour in fluid nourishment. After the feeding, flood with some more boiled water to rinse out the tube and prevent obstruction. If the nasal tube is used only once that day, remove after feeding.

e. If more nasal feedings are to be given that day, do not remove tube, but cover the open end with some gauze, clamp tube, and fasten down the end of tube until use next time.

2. Precautions

a. Before giving patient any nasal feedings, be sure to check his nose, throat and oral cavity for obstructions. If patient has false teeth, they must be removed.

b. Do not use nasal feedings on patients with esophageal varices or esophageal obstructions.

c. Remove nasogastric tube immediately while it is being inserted, if patient coughs and shows breathing difficulty and cyanosis. This means tube has entered respiratory tract by mistake. Try inserting tube again.

d. If patient requires several nasal feedings daily, change nasogastric tube every 24 hours if possible. When necessary, tube may be left in place for 3-4 days. When the tube is changed, introduce via the other nostril.

e. Do not feed patient liquids that are too hot or too cold. Medications given via nasogastric tube must be dissolved.

Gastric Lavage

Gastric lavage is performed to wash out toxic and other harmful substances from the stomach.

1. Gastric lavage procedure

a. **Lavage by mouth**. Simple procedure, suitable for conscious patients.

Have patient drink about 5000 cc of the lavage solution. Then depress base of patient's tongue, and tickle his pharynx with a wisp of cotton or a feather, to make him vomit and bring up the lavage solution. Repeat several times, until all toxic substances in stomach have been removed.

b. <u>Lavage by gastric tube</u>. Before the stomach is washed out, put patient at ease to obtain his cooperation. Then continue as follows:

(1) Have patient in a lateral recumbent or sitting position, his head tilted forward. Drape a rubber or plastic sheeting in front of him. Have water bucket ready.

(2) Lubricate tip of gastric tube, then introduce into his mouth, and insert slowly while patient swallows (to the 50 cm mark on tube, which indicates tube has reached the stomach). Check proper placement of tube with same technique described for the nasogastric tube. If the tube is in the stomach, then raise the outside end of tube about 30 cm higher than patient's head and slowly pour in about 500 cc of the lavage solution (less for infants). Then lower tube to empty fluid in stomach out into bucket. If there is no fluid returned, squeeze the rubber bulb (at midsection of tube) a few times to force fluid in the stomach out. Repeat this procedure several times until the fluid returned from the stomach is almost like that introduced.

(3) Remove gastric tube after stomach has been washed out. Have patient rinse out his mouth and rest.

2. <u>Precautions</u>

a. Keep the stomach contents washed out the first time for necessary (in case of poisoning) inspection.

b. Stop lavage procedure if the patient experiences pain or if the contents show blood.

c. Do not perform stomach washouts on patients with acute strong-acid or strong-base gastrointestinal hemorrhage, or esophageal or cardiac stricture or obstruction, or aortic aneurysm etc.

d. Select the proper gastric lavage solution, one that is determined by the causative poisoning substance. See under appropriate chapter for details.

Enema

The most frequently used kinds of enema are the following:

1. <u>Evacuation Enema</u>.

It is used to help the patient with stool evacuation in constipation, or in preparation for certain examinations (such as sigmoidoscopy) or surgery.

First ask patient to void before giving him enema. Have him lie in a left lateral recumbent position, with left leg extended and right leg bent forward, and buttocks exposed. Lubricate rectal tube and expel air in it. Bring enema can to bedside, about 100 cm above bed and regulate temperature of enema solution. Separate patient's buttocks with left hand, to locate the anus and insert rectal tube into anus with right hand, to a depth of 10-12 cm. Keep catheter in place with left hand, to prevent it from sliding out. Adjust clamp on tubing to regulate flow of enema solution which should flow in slowly. If patient feels pain in abdomen, stop for a few seconds before continuing. The rate of flow and amount of enema solution used can both be reduced. After all the solution has been given, remove catheter and have patient lie quietly for 5-10 minutes before attempting bowl movement.

Solutions ordinarily used for an evacuation enema are warm water, physiologic saline 2%, soap suds, etc., given in amounts of 500-1000 cc each time.

2. Retention enema.

Used mostly for introduction of drugs to be absorbed by the large intestine for their therapeutic action to be effected.

An hour before a retention enema is given, perform a rectal washout to clean out the large intestine of all fecal matter so the drug can be better absorbed. Its procedure is similar to that for an evacuation enema, except the buttocks must be raised while the enema solution is going in and a catheter is used instead of a rectal tube. A small amount of drug solution may be introduced through a funnel and low pressure. Drug solutions in amounts of 200-1000 cc must be introduced slowly by rectal drip. After the drug solution has been injected, tell patient to hold it to facilitate drug absorption.

Catheterization

Catheterization is used to relieve the patient of bladder distention or to obtain a clean specimen of urine for examination.

Observe strict asepsis when catheterizing a patient. Have patient lie in the recumbent position with thighs separated. Place rubber sheeting and towel under buttocks. For male patient first wash the penis and foreskin with physiologic saline. Then wash area around meatus of urethra, in an outward expanding motion, twice -- first with soapy water and cotton sponge, followed with sterile saline and cotton sponge. Cover with sterile towels, exposing only the meatus. For female patients, cleanse the external genitals in an upward-downward and from-inside-toward-outside swabbing motion, working from the vestibule out toward the minor and major labia, and the surrounding skin. Cover with cutout-hole sterile towel.

The physician puts on sterile gloves or fingers. Standing on the right side of patient, he picks up the clamped sterile catheter (No 12 or 12) with his right hand, moistens the tip section (for 3-4 cm) with liquid paraffin. While holding the penis with his left hand (in female patient, he separates labia with thumb and index finger of left hand to expose the urethral orifice), he inserts the catheter gently through the meatus. After the catheter is in place, the clamp is slowly released to allow discharge of urine. Or some of it may be returned for examination.

For patients suffering from retention of urine, a new acupuncture technique may be performed first to promote diuresis (see section on "Retention of Urine").

Artificial Respiration

To save the patient from respiratory arrest, one must be "calm, quick, and methodical" in providing first aid. Furthermore, one must exhibit an "attitude that is not afraid of exhaustion and continuous struggle," to persevere until the patient's breathing is restored to normal. Commonly used artificial respiration techniques are described as follows:

1. <u>Mouth-to-mouth respiration (Figure 4-4-2)</u>.

Loosen the patient's collar and trousers belt, and remove all false teeth, dirt, blood, and foreign matter from mouth. Pull out base of tongue from back of throat to assure a clear breathing passageway. Have patient lie flat on back, head tilted backward, and chin pointing upward. Separate patient's lips and cover with handkerchief or gauze. Take a deep breath (the physician), and pinch patient's nose, and place mouth closely over patient's mouth and blow forcefully at the same time. When patient's chest expands, stop and let go pinch on nose, and let chest contract on its own. Listen for return of air, and blow again, mouth-to-mouth. If no air return is heard, examine position of patient's head and chin again. If there are still secretions in the mouth, remove. Continue with mouth-to-mouth air blowing at rate of 12 times a minute. For children, at rate of 20 times a minute.

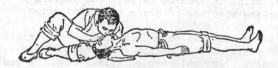

Figure 4-4-2. Mouth-to-mouth resuscitation technique.

This method is simple and effective, and does not affect any heart massage that may be performed simultaneously. Therefore, it is suitable for use with various types of respiratory arrest accompanied by fractured ribs or by cardiac arrest.

2. **Face-up chest-pressure method (Figure 4-4-3).**

Prepare patient for resuscitation as described in previous section, by cleaning mouth, pulling tongue up etc. Place patient on back, the back supported by some form of cushion so the shoulders and head would be lower, and turn patient's head to one side. Now facing the patient, straddle (the physician is the resuscitator here) him over thighs in a kneeling position. Bend both elbows and place both palms over patient's rib cage, fingers distributed naturally over ribs, the thumbs directed medially toward lower end of sternum and the four fingers spread out. Now channel weight of upper body (resuscitator's) into both palms causing your body to lean forward and increase pressure applied in patient's chest (do not use excessive pressure, to avoid damage to ribs or internal organs), forcing out air in the lungs. Pause for 2 seconds, ease up on pressure, relax both hands, and let body return to upright kneeling position, to allow natural expansion of patient's chest and entrance of air into lungs. After 2 seconds, repeat the procedure described, at the rate of 16-20 times per minute.

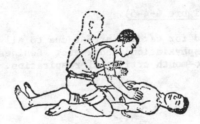

Figure 4-4-3. Face-up Chest-pressure Method.

This method is suitable only for asphyxiated patients. It cannot be used on patients with sustained chest injuries or those who need cardiac massage.

3. **Face-down back-pressure method (Figure 4-4-4).**

Prepare patient for artificial resuscitation as described in previous section. Place patient in prone position, one arm extended in front of head, the other bent and placed under head, the head turned to one side. Elevate abdomen with some sort of cushion. Now straddle (resuscitator) patient in kneeling position facing patient's head. Extending both arms, place palms on patient's back, thumbs next to the spine, fingers spread outwards over the ribs, the smallest finger pressing over the lowest rib. Tilt body slightly forward and direct pressure of body weight over patient's back, until both shoulders and palms are at right angles to each other. Maintain this posture for 2 seconds in order to push air out of patient's lungs. Then gradually return body (resuscitator's) to original upright position, to ease up pressure on patient's chest which expands naturally to allow air in. After 2 seconds, repeat above procedure, at rate of 16-20 times a minute.

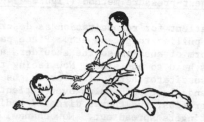

Figure 4-4-4.   Face-down Back-pressure Method.

This method is suited for cases of respiratory arrest caused by drowning or electrical shock, as it allows water to flow out. But this method
cannot be used simultaneously with heart massage.

External Cardiac Massage (Figure 4-4-5).

This method is suited for cardiac arrest due to all kinds of traumatic
injuries, electric shock, asphyxiation, shock etc. Besides immediate cardiac
massage, also start mouth-to-mouth artificial respiration.

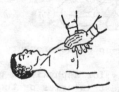

Figure 4-4-5.   External Cardiac Massage.

To carry out the massage, place patient flat on a hard board, lower his
head and point his chin upwards. Stand on one side of patient and place the
base of one (physician's) palm over the patient's sternum, the other hand over
it. Direct weight of your body toward both hands and apply pressure to the
sternum, causing it to be depressed 3-5 cm. Relax pressure immediately so
chest cage will expand. Continue and repeat procedure at rate of 60-70 times
per minute until the heart beat is restored.

Apply pressure evenly and forcefully, coordinating this technique with
mouth-to-mouth artificial respiration for effective resuscitation of patient.
The ratio of artificial respiration and heart massage should be coordinated
at a ratio of 1:4. If heart massage and resuscitation are effective, the
patient's coloring and lips will turn rosy red, the pupils will contract, and
the peripheral pulse can also be felt.

If the heartbeat is not restored after a period of heart massage, besides continuing with the technique, give an 0.5 cc intracardiac injection of 0.1% adrenalin or isopropylarterenol or other central nervous system stimulant. Continue until the heartbeat is restored, a distinct pulse is felt, and a blood pressure is maintained at 80-90 mm on the sphymo-manometer.

Note: Characteristics of true death

To save the lives of our comrades in time, do not easily let go the opportunity to provide resuscitation measures. For this reason, it is important to understand the characteristics of true death as described below:

1. Cat eyes. Use two fingers to pinch the patient's eyeball from both sides. If the patient is dead, the pupils are oval-shaped or cracked. Pupils of persons still alive do not change shape after being pinched.

2. A drop in body temperature to room temperature or that of the environment (cold corpse). Muscles after death harden and shrink, and joints become stiff (rigor mortis). Skin on dependent parts of the body show purplish red or purplish blue blotches (corpse lividity).

When any one of the two characteristics mentioned above is noted, it is an indication of true death.

Other features such as respiratory arrest or dilated pupils, loss of all reflexes etc., are not necessarily characteristics of true death. So in resuscitation work, do not give up easily and lose an opportunity to save a life.

Sterilization

Sterilization uses physical, chemical and pharmaceutical means to destroy bacteria on the body surface, in wounds, on instruments and utensils. Its purpose is to prevent the transmission of disease and infection, so that wounds can heal quickly and complications are reduced.

1. Common sterilization methods

   a. Boiling. Metal instruments, glassware, porcelain enamelware, rubber gloves, sutures, etc., may be wrapped with soap, rinsed in clear water before being wrapped in gauze and placed in sterilizer (with lid) and boiled. After water is boiling, the boiling should continue for another 10-15 minutes. Articles that have been in contact with tetanus and gas gangrene bacilli should be boiled for 4-5 minutes.

b. <u>Steaming</u>. This method uses the steam generated by boiling water to kill bacteria. Gauze, bandages, cotton, dressings, operating gowns, operating towels, etc., are sterilized by this method. These items are wrapped and placed on rack in a steam kettle which contains water and has a tight lid. After the water comes to a boil, lower the fire and continue steaming for about 2 hours. After this period, bank the fires, open lid for steam to dispel, and remove wrapped items for cooling and drying. Do not unwrap sterile articles before use to avoid their being rendered unsterile.

c. <u>Sunning (and airing)</u> Blankets and pillows used by the patient which are not boilable may be sunned and aired under strong sunshine. Turn frequently. Generally, this type of open-air treatment given for several hours will kill most surface bacteria.

d. <u>Burning</u>. Waste products that cannot be recycled, such as gauze, cotton, etc., used by patients with contagious disease should be burned. Face basin, dressing-use bowls and forceps, etc., may be flamed with 95% ethyl alcohol if they cannot be boiled in time. These items may be used after cooling.

e. <u>Drug and chemical treatment</u>. Certain instruments such as scalpels, scissors, plastic tubing or the patient's operative site which are not amenable to the aforementioned methods may be rendered bacteria-free by soaking in, or painting with chemicals. Drug solutions for soaking may be 75% alcohol or pure lysol solution, for 30 minutes. After these articles are taken out of chemical solutions, they should be rinsed in sterile boiled water or cold saline before use. Besides these, certain Chinese medicinal plants and their concoctions also have anti-bacterial properties. Some of these, such as <u>Ranunculus acris</u> <u>L</u>., <u>Berberis chengli</u> Chen, <u>Eucalytus nobusta Sm</u>, <u>Drosera Peltata</u> Sm. var <u>Lunata</u> Clarke, etc., may be used where appropriate.

2. <u>Disinfection of patient operative site</u>.

First shave off all hair over the operative site and the surrounding area. Paint skin over operative area with 2.5% iodine, in circular motion outward from the incision site. After iodine is dry, continue with 75% alcohol using same motion technique. Or paint twice with 1:1000 tincture of merthiolate in same manner. However, do not use iodine over mucous membrane areas and the scrotum, as these areas cannot tolerate its irritating properties.

3. <u>Simple operating room disinfection</u>

Though operating rooms found in the rural areas are simple and crude, it is still possible to perform successful operations in them. The disinfection tec nique first calls for a thorough dusting and cleaning of area, the walls and ceilings to be re-papered or given a coat of whitewash. To disinfect the air inside the operating rooms, some pure lactate may be steaming 2 hours before the operation. Dry moxa and some realgar can also be burned to fumigate the tightly sealed room. If there is a wood floor, scrub with 2% lysol. Close doors and windows to prevent bugs flying in. Operating room personal should best be fitted with special clothing and shoes, wear masks and hats, to prevent any contamination by loose ends of hair and saliva. The surgical team (surgeon and assistants) should wash hands, scrub with soapy water and soak in 75% alcohol (from fingers to elbow).

Preventive Inoculations

Preventive inoculations are also called "ta fang-l-chen," meaning injections received/given to prevent epidemic disease. The measure calls for inoculating certain vaccine onto the human body to produce immunity against certain diseases. It is an important technique used to promote the health goal of "prevention first."

Through a series of planned inoculations (See Table 4-4-1), the human body's immunity is strengthened to attain the goal of prevention and elimination of contagious and infectious diseases.

1. Types of preventive inoculation

    a. Active immunity. Causes the human body, after it has been inoculated with vaccine or toxoid, to produce by itself a somewhat longer lasting (for several years or longer) immunity to a certain disease.

    b. Passive immunity. Causes the human body, after it has been injected with an immune serum or antitoxin, to rapidly obtain a temporary (generally maintained for a month or less) immunity.

2. Precautions.

    a. Plan a vaccination program for the production team (brigade), based on the size of the team and prevailing epidemic conditions. When vaccinations are given, it is best to adopt a centralized mass approach, supplemented by individual vaccinations. Keep records.

    b. Before giving any vaccinations or inoculations, be sure to understand health conditions and know contraindications (see Table 4-4-1).

    c. Mobilize the masses, under the Party's leadership, and educate them on the importance of vaccination in disease prevention and in maintaining good health.

d. Practice strict asepsis and sterilization procedures. For smallpox vaccinations and Calmette's (BCG) vaccination, do not use iodine.

e. Place vaccine to be used in a cool dry place. Already opened bottles (ampoules) of live bacterial or live virus vaccine should be used up within a 2-hour period. Discard any vaccine that is not used up.

f. Be aware that after vaccination, individual reactions such as the following may appear.

   (1) Local reaction. A local red swelling may appear within 24 hours following vaccination. In severe cases, the local lymph nodes may become painful and swollen.

   (2) Systemic reaction. The important manifestation is a temperature rise, accompanied sometimes by headache, chills, nausea, vomiting, abdominal cramps and diarrhea.

Mild reactions generally do not need any treatment and the patient's condition returns to normal after a short while. Serious reactions, however, require close observation, and medical attention should be given when needed. In extreme individual cases, allergic reactions after vaccination may appear as anaphylactic shock. An injection of 1 cc of 1:1000 adrenalin for an adult may be given immediately in conjunction with other effective measures.

Table 4-4-1. Preventive Vaccines

Vaccine	Persons to be vaccinated	Method and frequency of vaccination	Dosage	Spacing interval	Booster and period of immunity	Contraindications
Calmette Guerin vaccine (BCG)	Newborn infants and children whose tuberculin tests are negative	(1) Oral method, 3 times; (2) Scratch method, once; (3) Intradermal injection, once.	Each time, 1 ml [orally]; one drop [scratch] or 0.1 ml [intradermal]	Every other day [by mouth, for 3 times]	Initially at 1 year, boosters at ages 4, 7, 10, 14 and 17 years; period of immunity between boosters 2 to 4 years.	Newborn, with following conditions, body temperature over 37°C (rectal), weight below 2.5 kg; persistent vomiting and pronounced indigestion; birth trauma; pyogenic dermatitis; systemic bullous eruptions; influenza etc. In children with following conditions: positive tuberculin test; x-ray finding of suspected tuberculosis; acute infection (including a convalescent period of 2 months)
Smallpox vaccine	Infants 2-6 months old, and others older who have not been vaccinated.	Lateral aspect of upper arm, 2 spots (2-3 cm apart) at initial vaccination, 1 spot in repeat vaccination. Scratch method, once, about 0.4 to 0.5 cm long.	Each vaccination 1 drop	Examination 1 week later. If reaction is negative for first vaccination, repeat.	Repeat vaccination every 6 years. Repeat during an epidemic. Repeat vaccination after contact with infections case. Duration of immunity: 3 to 4 years.	Contraindicated for patients with following conditions: acute infections, including convalescent period; systemic bullous eruptions and creeping dermatitis; heart or kidney disease, active tuberculosis; periodic fevers. After CGC vaccination, wait at least 1 month before giving smallpox vaccination. After smallpox vaccination, wait at least half a month before vaccination with other preparations.

Table 4-4-1. (Continued)

Vaccine	Persons to be vaccinated	Method and frequency of vaccination	Dosage	Spacing interval	Booster and period of immunity	Contraindications
Pertussis vaccine	Babies at least 3 months old	Lateral aspect of upper arm, given in series of 3 injections.	First injection, 0.5 ml; 2nd injection, 0.1 ml; and 3rd injection, 1.5 ml.	From 1-10 days	Booster given 1-3 years Immunity lasts for 1 to 3 years.	Contraindicated for acute infections and convalescent period, heart disease, active tuberculosis, serious malnutrition, serious indigestion.
Attenuated poliomyelitis vaccine	Two months old to 7 years	By mouth, 3 times	Sugar-coated pill, one pill each time. Type I (red), Type II (yellow) and Type III (green) liquid form, each time 0.1 ml.	Take Type I first, followed by Types II and III, in 1-month intervals.		Same contraindications that apply to pertussis vaccine.
Diphtheria toxoid	From age 8 months on	Lateral aspect of upper arm, hypodermic injection 3 times	First injection, 0.5 ml; 2nd injection, 1.0 ml; and 3rd injection, 1.0 ml.	In 1-month intervals	At ages of 3 to 4 years, and 7 to 8 years. Immunity lasts about 3 years.	Contraindications: (1) same as those for pertussis vaccine; (2) Patients who have Japanese encephalitis

Table 4-4-1. (Continued)

Vaccine	Persons to be vaccinated	Method and frequency of vaccination	Dosage	Spacing interval	Booster and period of immunity	Contraindications
Combination vaccine of pertussis vaccine, diphtheria toxoid	3 months to 6 years	Method same as that for previous entry, 3 times	First injection, 0.5 ml; 2nd injection, 1.0 ml; and 3rd injection, 1.0 ml	Interval of 4-6 weeks	Booster in 1-2 years. Immunity tests 2-3 years.	Same as that for diphtheria toxoid
Triple vaccine of pertussis vaccine, diphtheria toxoid and tetanus toxoid	Same as above	Method same as above	Injection of 0.5 ml each time	Same as above	Booster given every 1-2 years. Immunity lasts 2-3 years	Same as above.
Attenuated measles vaccine	Susceptible infants over 8 months old who have never had measles	Method same as above, and given once.	Injection of 0.2 ml each time.			Same as those for pertussis vaccine.

Table 4-4-1. (Continued)

Vaccine	Persons to be vaccinated	Method and frequency of vaccination	Dosage	Spacing Interval of immunity	Booster and period of immunity	Contraindications
Japanese encephalitis B vaccine	Between ages of 6 months to 12 years	Method same as that for previous entry, given twice.	Injection for those between 6-12 months of age, 0.25 ml each time; between 1-6 years old, 0.5 ml each time; and between 7 to 12 years old, 1.0 ml each time.	7 to 10 days	After complete series, booster given once the second year. Immunity lasts 1 year.	Same as those for typhoid, paratyphoid A & B combined vaccine
Triple bacterial vaccine of typhoid, paratyphoid A and B	Ages between 2 and 59 years old	Method same as that used in previous entries, given 3 times	Injection dosage for those between 2 and 6 years of age: first injection 0.2 ml; 2nd 0.4 ml, and 3rd, 0.3 ml. For those between 7 and 14 years old first injection, 0.3 ml; 2nd, 0.6 ml; and 3rd, 0.6 ml. For those over 15 years old; first injection, 0.5 ml; 2nd, 0.5 ml; and 3rd, 1.0 ml.	7 to 10 days	After completion of whole series, booster given annually. Immunity lasts 1 to 3 years.	Contraindicated in presence of acute infectious diseases and their convalescent periods, heart disease, liver and kidney disease, active tuberculosis, active rheumatism, severe hypertension, hyperthyroidism asthma, active gastric or duodenal ulcers, menstrual period (temporarily postponed), pregnancy, and women who were nursing mothers 6 months ago.

Vasectomy

As a male sterilization technique, the procedure is simple and does not affect health and the individual's sexual life. The procedure is described as follows:

1. Have patient lie in recumbent position. Shave off pubic hair. Wash scrotum, penis, and perineal area with soapy water and rinse with warm water.

2. Paint area with antiseptic solution of 1:1000 tincture merthiolate. Drape with sterile towels.

3. Feel for the vas deferens along anterior wall of scrotum. Pull it toward the lower wall of scrotum. Perform an infiltration block using 1-2 ml of 1% procaine, at the spot.

4. Make 1-cm incision (about) on scrotal wall. Dissect and expose the vas deferns.

5. Separate a 2-cm section of the vas deferns and lift out with hemostat. Pull two silk threads through space under the vas, about 1.5 cm apart. Tie each silk thread separately around the duct.

6. Cut section of vas deferens between the two silk ligations.

7. After bleeding has been controlled, suture incision.

8. Repeat procedure on vas deferens on other side. When done, cover both incisions with sterile gauze.

Precautions

1. Make sure bleeding is controlled, particularly that from artery adjacent to the vas deferens which may cause a postoperative hemotoma if hemostasis is not effective.

2. Avoid strenuous physical activity for the first two days after operation, to avoid any secondary hemorrhage.

3. Make patient aware that sexual intercourse the first few times after operation still require birth control measures.

4. Be sure that the ligated and resected vas deferens is correctly identified to avoid ligating other body parts by mistake.

Rectal Digital Examination

This technique that is used for examination during labor or for examination of the rectum, prostate or seminal vesicles may also be used as a diagnostic aid in acute abdomen cases and certain obstetrical and gynecological conditions.

Place patient in a left recumbent position, left leg extended and right leg bent (suitable for aged and weak patients). Or place patient in knee-chest position (suitable for examination of the prostate and seminal vesicle). Or have patient on back in recumbent position, both knees flexed (suitable for examination during labor). To examine the patient, put (the physician) finger glove on index finger, lubricate with liquid paraffin or glycerine, and press anus gently causing patient to bear down. Then insert finger into anus gently, using rotation motion. Note tension of the anus, smoothness of the rectum, presence of masses, stenosis, etc. Sometimes the method is combined with the rectoabdominal bimanual examination technique to better locate pain pressure points in appendicitis or gynecological conditions. When the finger is withdrawn, notice any mucous or blood on the glove.

CHAPTER V.   BIRTH CONTROL PLANNING

Section 1.   Significance of Birth Control Planning

Birth control planning is a momentous measure of national import and interest. It uses the scientific method to suitably determine the timing and frequency of human reproduction.

Section 2.   Promoting Late Marriage

If the young people talk about love, marriage and having children at too early an age, their energies will be dissipated, affecting their work and their study. Furthermore, from the standpoint of physical development, most young people do not attain all-round maturity until after 25 years of age. Premature marriage and procreation are not beneficial for the young and succeeding generation.

Section 3.   Contraception

Contraception is a technique employing scientific methods to prevent union of the spermatazoa and the ovum, so that conception is not possible within a certain time span. Several simple yet safe methods of contraception are as follows:

Chinese Herbs (effective to a certain extent)

1. Decoction prepared from tender sprouts of Pinus massoniana, 9 stalks (each about 5 inches (ts'un) long), and roots of white stipa, 1 liang, to be taken once after conclusion of menstrual period, for 5 months in succession. Effective as contraceptive for 3 years.

2. Preparation from roots of the following, 1 liang of each:

> Coniogramme japonica
> Dysosma auranticocaulis
> Paris polyphylla

Crush for juice, and take orally with cold boiled water during menstrual period, 3 times daily. The number of days the drug is taken depends on the length of the menstrual period. Effective as contraceptive for 8 months.

3. Preparation from flowers and roots (about 1-2 ch'ien) of Paris polyphylla. Crush and take in one dose with wine at end of menstrual period. Effective as a contraceptive for a year.

4. Decoction prepared from the following:

> Dates (from palm Trachycarpus excelsa), 5 liang
> Roots of bamboo Phyllostachys nigra, 2 liang
> White wine, 1 liang
> Brown sugar, 1 liang

Take at end of menstrual period, once a day for 3 days in a row. Decoction effective as a contraceptive for 1 year (if taken by women already 2-3 months pregnant, abortion may result).

Use of Condoms

A contraceptive device used by the male, it is simple to use, with good results. Its selection depends on the size of the erect penis. Before intercourse, the condom should be blown up to test for leaks. Then air at the tip should be expelled before fitting it on the penis. After ejaculation, and before the penis becomes completely soft, the condom should be removed by pulling at the opening, to prevent its retention in the vagina. Wash and clean after use. Dry, and check for breaks. Dust with talc, wrap and put away for later use.

Other devices, such as the diaphragm and the loop, are also effective. However they must be fitted for appropriate use.

Oral Contraceptives

At present, western contraceptive medicines are based primarily on hormones used to control ovulation. Their use follows a regimen described as follows:

1. Progesterone, 1 tablet taken nightly beginning on 5th day of menstrual period, for a total of 22 days, as one cycle.

2. Duosterone, used in the same manner as progesterone.

Note: Precautions while on oral contraceptives.

> (1) Be sure to follow regimen prescribed for the cycle by taking a pill daily, for this approach to be effective.

> (2) Be aware that uncomfortable symptoms such as nausea, dizziness, weakness and distended breasts may be experienced upon first taking the drug, but will subside later on.

3. If a small amount of vaginal bleeding occurs after taking the drug, take another 1-2 tablets of ethinyl estradiol each evening. If bleeding is heavy, discontinue the pill, but use another method of contraception.

4. If menstruation does not occur after 22 days on the pill, begin the next cycle of pill-taking 7 days later.

5. Do not use such medications in the presence of liver disease or nephritis.

Section 4. Sterilization

Oral contraception or some other measure may be used by those who have had too many children too closely, or by those whose health does not recommend having more children, to terminate their reproductive capacity. This is called sterilization, that is, no more children born for the rest of their lives. Some of the more common sterilization measures are described below:

Chinese Herbs: of certain value

1. Fresh roots from the date palm, 3-5 liang, and hog large intestines, half chin.

First cook the date palm roots in water. Bring to boil. After 20 minutes add the hog large intestines. Continue cooking until the ingredients are tender, then remove roots and season with a small amount of sugar or salt. Eat the hog intestines and take the herb juices in one sitting after a menstrual period.

2. Preparations from the following, 2 liang each:
Upland sorghum (kaoliang)
Hydrocotyle rotundifolia
Ophtopogon Japonicus

Taken within two weeks post-partum. On the first day, crush Hydrocotyle rotundifolia for juice, mix with sweet wine and take orally. On the second day, prepare d coction from sorghum and water, and take with equal parts of wine. On the 3rd day, prepare decoction of Ophtopogon sp. and water, and take in 3 separate doses.

3. Preparation of the following:
Cuscuta japonica, 1 liang
Carpesium divaricatum, 1 liang
Anemone vitifolia, 5 ch'ien
Dysosma auranticocaulis, 5 ch'ien (may be increased to 1 liang for healthy individual)

Take first three ingredients and prepare decoction with water. Mix with Dysosma sp. crushed in 2 liang of water. Take once or twice after menstrual period.

4. Preparation of the following:
   <u>Alangium chinense</u>, 2 liang (3 liang if roots are thick)
   <u>Rhododendron molle</u>, 1 ch'ien (roots removed)
   Undiluted sweet wine 1/2 chin

Wash the two herbs clean and place in dish of sweet wine. Cover tightly and cook in steamer for 4 hours. Strain. Drink juice.

Start regimen around 45 days post-partum or one day before end of menstrual period. Can also be taken at other times. Take 1-2 tablespoons daily at bedtime for 7 days. (This prescription is also good for treating backache and pains in the thighs in gynecologic practice.)

General side effects of these herb medications are dizziness, and spots before eyes. Nausea and vomiting accompany overdosage. It is also seen in those whose health is deficient [anemic]. However, these symptoms will subside on their own after 2 or 3 days.

Surgery

Sterilization accomplished through surgical technique hardly affects the health and working capability in those who undertake the operation. It is equally satisfactory for males and females. In particular, vasectomy, performed on men, is a simple technique that should be given greater promotion.

1. <u>Vasectomy</u>. This surgical technique is simple and quick to perform. There is very little bleeding, and does not affect the individual working ability. Its practice should be widened. However, for a 3-month period following surgery, other contraceptive measures should still be taken during sexual intercourse, as some sperm are still retained in the seminal vesicle. (Consult section on "Therapeutics" for surgical procedure).

2. <u>Tube Ligation</u> (ligation of fallopian tubes). This technique can be done anytime after 24 hours post-partum, after artificial abortion, or after end of menstrual period.

Section 5. New Methods for Delivery of the Newborn

Because this concerns the health of two generations, we must perform this task with great seriousness. Some general facts on this new method of newborn delivery will be described.

Sensation When Childbirth is Imminent

For several days before labor (childbirth) is imminent, the pregnant woman often experiences irregular and intermittent uterine contractions (short duration contractions accompanied by longer intervals) accompanied by a feeling of heaviness in the abdomen. On the day before, or several hours before labor set in, a blood-stained mucous secretion is noted in the vagina. The interval of uterine contractions becomes increasingly shorter with a longer duration of contraction. This sensation is not as marked among multipara, women who have given birth several times, as it is among the primipara, those experiencing childbirth for the first time.

The Course of Childbirth

Because of the intensity of uterine contractions that push the amniotic fluid and the fetus toward the cervix of the uterus, the external os gradually becomes dilated. When the cervix is completely dilated, the amniotic fluid will rush out when the "water has broken." After the external os is completely open, the baby will pass through it on its way to the vagina, and for delivery outside the body. A few minutes after the baby has been delivered, because of the continuous uterine contractions, the placenta will be separated from the uterine wall and be expelled. After the placenta is expelled, bleeding follows. However, because of the intensity of the uterine contractions, the bleeding is generally not excessive.

Preparations for Labor and Delivery

Health workers should be diligent in their visits and pay attention to the following points:

1. Make sure all instruments, equipment and clothing needed for delivery are ready.

2. Teach the pregnant woman to fold, use, and sterilize perineal pads (steamed for 30 minutes in a steamer-pot).

3. Make sure the bed is firm and level, air and light in the room adequate.

4. Explain to the pregnant woman some of the sensations indicating birth is imminent.

5. Make sure that instruments and equipment such as scissors, forceps, gloves, kidney basins, etc., to be used by the midwife (or attending physician) have been boiled and sterilized. If there is enough time, give patient an enema, after which wash and clean the external genitals. If time is more pressing, wash the genitals immediately and pay strict attention to the course of labor and delivery procedure. If necessary, ask family members taught on previous visits, to come in as assistants.

Table 5-6-1. Stages of Labor

Stage	Course	Maximum normal duration
First stage (dilating stage)	Regular and periodic uterine contractions (labor pains)	24 hours
Second stage (placenta expulsion stage)	From expulsion of baby to expulsion of placenta	30 minutes

Procedures During First Stage

1. Prepare patient mentally for birth event, by dispelling anxieties and instilling confidence that delivery will be a normal one.

2. Doublecheck preparations made for labor and delivery.

3. See that pregnant patient eats and drinks properly, moves bowels and passes urine regularly.

4. Check fetal heartbeat and blood pressure at the appropriate time.

5. Examine patient by rectum (using finger) to check for the location of baby's head and the size of the cervical opening, to better grasp the progression of labor.

6. If the amniotic membrane has ruptured, or the cervix of the primipara is completely dilated, or the cervix of the multipara has dilated to about 3 cm [in diameter], wash the external genitals immediately with soap and water, followed by an antiseptic (using a 1% lysol solution to cleanse), the area to include the vulva, the labia minora and majora, the perineum and the inner aspect of the upper thigh, the pelvis and the perianal region. The midwife or physician attending the delivery observes the following procedure: scrub hands with soap and water, following with a 5-minute soak in 75% alcohol or an alcohol wipe, after which gloves are put on. Open the sterile obstetrical package, drape patient with sterile towels and be ready for delivery of baby.

Procedures During Second Stage

1. If the cervix is completely dilated, but the waters have not "broken," use forceps to carefully rupture the amniotic sac. OUCH!

2. Teach the pregnant patient how to carry out her breathing exercises to assist in the delivery.

- 178 -

* NOTE: FORCEP'S USED TO RUPTURE THE MEMBRANES IS A DRASTIC APPROACH. THEY WILL USUALLY BURST within the next few contractions

3. When the head of the baby is exposed, use [the midwife or physician]
the right palm, by separating the thumb and the four fingers, to support and
protect the perineum. Use four fingers of left hand to support the head, for
it to extend itself after bending forward, to prevent tearing of the perineum
(see Figure 5-6-1). When the head comes out, turn it to one side, that is
pulling the head of fetus downward and allow the fore-shoulder to appear
(Figure 5-6-2). Now pick up the head of fetus again and help in delivery of
the posterior shoulder (Figure 5-6-3). At this time, the perineum must still
be protected, until the whole baby is delivered.

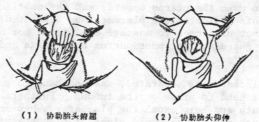

(1) 协助胎头俯屈   (2) 协助胎头仰伸

Figure 5-6-1. Assisting Delivery of Head of Fetus

Key: (1) Assisting head of fetus to bend forward
      (2) Assisting head of fetus to extend

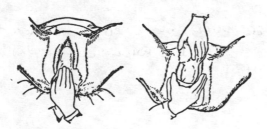

Figure 5-6-2. Assisting Delivery   Figure 5-6-3. Assisting Delivery of
of Fore-shoulder   the Posterior Shoulder

After the baby has been delivered, pick it up by both feet to allow
mucus in its throat to flow out. Or use a piece of gauze to wipe out mucus
in its mouth. If the baby has begun to cry, the umbilical cord may be severed
by first clamping the cord with two hemastats after which the cord is cut between the two clamps. Now tie cord once close to the "button." Make another
tie about 4 cm away. Then cut cord about 4 cm on distal side. If the tie is
tight and no bleeding is seen, apply iodine to the cut end. Wrap stub with
gauze, and use an umbilical bandage to keep it in place. After dressing
and wrapping baby, drop eyes with 1% silver nitrate, and flush with normal
saline.

*cord should be cut only after it has
stopped pulsing. (unless emergency such as
tight around babes neck)

- 179 -

** Pure Lemon Juice has been successfully used
in place of silver Nitrate.

Procedures During Third Stage

Generally, the placenta separates 10-15 minutes after the baby has been delivered. At this time, the uterus may become firm and hard, show lengthening out and rising upward, or the umbilical cord may show signs of descending. If the side of hand placed on the abdominal wall above the upper edge of the pubis symphysis can push the uterus upward, and the umbilical cord does not move up with it, this indicates the placenta has separated. Before the placenta has separated, do not use force to massage the uterus nor use force to pull the umbilical cord, to guard against post-partum hemorrhage and inversion of the uterus.

After the placenta has separated, use one hand to pull on the umbilical cord, and the other hand to press on the fundus. Furthermore, ask the patient to take a deep breath and help expel the placenta. When most of the placenta has come down through the vagina, hold sides of placenta with both hands, gently rotate and pull, to prevent any tearing and retention of placental membrane inside. After the placenta has been expelled, inspect carefully to see that the placenta and membrane are intact. Besides this, check the birth-passageway for tears and observe the mother and newborn infant closely for changes.

* NEVER "PULL" ON CORD OR PLACENTA !!
IT WILL COME OUT BY ITSELF.

CHAPTER VI. DIAGNOSIS AND TREATMENT OF COMMON DISEASES

Section 1   First Aid

The general principles of first aid as listed below must first be mastered:

1. <u>Save the dying and Aid the Injured</u>.

2. <u>Observe first aid in the following sequence</u>:
    a. First make sure that the breathing passageway of the wounded is clear and open, that hemorrhage and shock are arrested.
    b. Second, treat internal organ injuries.
    c. Third, treat fractures.
    d. Fourth, treat other wounds in general.

When providing first aid to wounds, note the following:

    a. Do not apply iodine on an open wound.
    b. Do not wash a wound with water (chemical and phosphorus burns being exceptions).
    c. Do not remove any foreign body from a wound.
    d. Do not try to return into place any protruding internal organ.

3. <u>Use every opportunity to speedily give first aid to, and transport the injured</u>.

4. <u>Work speedily as follows if a wounded person is discovered during the night</u>: Time is of the essence.

    a. If possible, ask the wounded patient how he feels.
    b. Examine the patient's body reflexes.
    c. Look for open wounds and the presence of sticky substances smelling like blood.

5. **Expose wounds as follows:**

   a. If the clothes can be removed, first remove clothing from the healthy extremities, then from the injured parts last. To dress the patient again, follow this same procedure in reverse.
   b. When the forearm or the leg is injured, roll up the sleeves or trouser leg.
   c. Under emergency conditions, cut clothing over the injured part for each of quick treatment, but do not expose too large an area.

The Four Basic Techniques

Hemorrhage Control

Loss of great amounts of blood within a short time will endanger the life of the injured, so every minute counts in rendering emergency treatment. Whenever bleeding from organs and tissues occurs within the body, that is internal bleeding. Whenever bleeding occurs on organs and extremities seen outside the body, that is external bleeding. External bleeding can further be classified as capillary, venous, or arterial. Capillary bleeding is seen as a small amount of blood oozing out. In venous bleeding, the outflow is a dull dark red. In arterial bleeding, the spurts are a bright fresh red, spilling in greater amounts. Certain types of internal bleeding require surgery to stop the hemorrhage. In the sections that follow, some of the more common techniques used to arrest external bleeding will be discussed.

1. **Using Chinese herbal drugs:**

   a. A pulverized mixture prepared as a pressure compress over bleeding point, consisting of equal parts of the following, roasted until yellowish-black: t'ien-pien chu (Aster trinervius), wu-pao hsieh (leaves of blackberry Rubus tephordes), tung-kao, huo-pa-kuo (pyracantha berries), and p'u-huang (Typha latifolia).

   b. Pulverized mixture of the following, for use as pressure compress over wound:

Tzu-chu ts'ao (Callicarpa pedunculata)	4 parts
Kang-nien (Rhodomyrtus tomentosa)	3 parts
San-ya (Evodia lepta)	3 parts

   c. Pulverized mixture of the following:

Chiang t'an (Ashes of ginger)	1 liang
Wu-ming-I (magnesium)	1 liang
Pai-chi (Bletilla striata)	1 liang
Chi-nei-chin	5 ch'ien
Rock sugar	1 ch'ien

Stored in airtight bottle, to be available for sprinkling over wounds before bandaging.

d. Pulverized ashes from coals of dried palm (minus coarse bark) stored for use when needed. For sprinkling over wounds (in treatment of open fractures with bleeding, to stimulate wound healing).

e. Burnt coals [ashes] of p'u-huang (Typhya latifolia) kept in bottle for use when needed.

2. <u>General method of bleeding control</u>: Bleeding from capillaries and small veins coagulate more readily [than arterial bleeding]. Place sterile gauze over wound and bandage.

3. <u>Digital pressure method</u>: Used generally for arterial bleeding. Apply digital pressure on the proximal side of the blood vessel, firmly against bone to temporarily arrest the blood flow. Usually the arterial pulse is felt over the pressure point.

Table 6-1-1. Pressure Technique Over Different Bleeding Points

Artery subjected to pressure	Pressure point	Scope of bleeding control
Facial artery	In fossa one-half inch in front of the mandibular angle, sometimes requiring pressure on both sides before bleeding is controlled.	Bleeding in face below the eyes and bleeding in the lateral oral cavity.
Temporal artery	One finger's breadth in front of the ear, right up against the temporomandibular joint.	Bleeding from the temple area and the scalp.
Common carotid artery	On posterior cervical spine alongside trachea where the common carotid artery branches into the external and internal carotid, but keep pressure off the trachea. Avoid applying pressure to both common carotid arteries at the same time. Do not keep pressure on for too long, to avoid brain damage.	Bleeding from the oral cavity, laryngo-pharynx, neck, and head.
Subclavian artery	Pressure at point one-third the way into the supraclavicular fossa, applied toward the first rib.	Bleeding from shoulder, axilla, and upper extremity.
Brachial artery	Pressure at point on mid-humerus within the inner marginal groove of the brachial triceps, applied toward the humerus.	Bleeding from the arm and forearm.
Axillary artery	Extension of injured arm toward back, keeping it as straight as possible and pulling it toward the intact arm with opposite hand placed over the wrist.	Bleeding from upper extremity.
Femoral artery	Pressure over pulsating point in groin, against the flat pubic bone.	Bleeding from lower extremity.

4. <u>Pressure bandaging</u>. Two kinds.

  a. Direct pressure to stop bleeding over wound.
  b. Indirect pressure at an extremity joint space such as the
     elbow space or the popliteal fossa. (Figure 6-1-1).

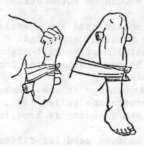

Figure 6-1-1. Indirect pressure bandaging to arrest hemorrhage.

  5. <u>Tourniquet use</u>. For massive bleeding in the four extremities,
place a rubber tourniquet on the upper (proximal) side of bleeding site,
and tie to top bleeding (Figure 6-1-2). Points to note in use of tourniquet.

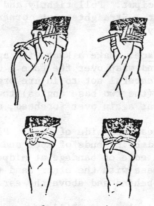

Figure 6-1-2. How to apply a tourniquet.

  a. Place a cloth pad between skin and tourniquet. Do not
     tie tourniquet directly on skin.
  b. Use proper amount of tension. Too tight a tourniquet will
     cause nerve damage. Too loose a tourniquet will not stop
     bleeding.
  c. Relax tourniquet slowly, once every hour, after it has been
     tied, to prevent gangrene of the extremity.
  d. Indicate very noticeably on tag to accompany patient during
     transport, <u>the time</u> tourniquet was applied.

- 185 -

Bandaging

Bandaging protects the wound, reduces infection, applies pressure to arrest bleeding, fixes fractures, and reduces pain.

The following points should be noted during bandaging.

1. Bandaging materials used are sterile.
2. Movements are familiar and quick.
3. Bandaging tension must be just right: too tight a bandage will affect the circulation, too loose a one will not keep dressing in place.
4. If a triangular bandage is used, make sure the edges are fixed, the corners are pulled taut, the center has enough of give, and the dressing is kept in place.

General bandaging techniques used for different parts of the human body are described below.

1. Bandaging of the head: Fold base of the triangular bandage (Figure 6-1-3) slightly, and place over forehead above the eyebrow, making sure the two base angles are just above both ears, crisscrossing over the apex of bandage at the occiput. Pull tightly and bring ends around to forehead in front and tie knot. Straighten out corner of bandage at back of head and tuck under neatly.

2. Bandaging of face. Make a knot with apex of triangular bandage and place over forehead and wrap over the face. Cut holes in bandage for eyes, nose and mouth (be careful not to injure organs of the senses). Then pull two ends of bandage (the two base angles) toward back, crisscrossing at occiput. Bring to front again over forehead, and tie knot.

3. Bandaging of head and side of face: Place one side of triangular bandage over forehead, and bring ends of apex and one base angle below and tie knot. Then pull base edge of bandage at midpoint upward with one hand while pulling remaining base with the other hand to wrap up forehead, tying the two together in knot behind and above the ear.

4. Bandaging of single eye: Fold triangular bandage into long strip about 4 fingers wide. Drape 2/3 of it over injured eye, bringing it around below ear and occiput over to area above opposite ear. Wind once around head over forehead and occiput. Tie knot over intact eye.

Key: (1) Base angle
     (2) Side
     (3) Apex angle
     (4) Base

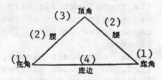

Figure 6-1-3. The triangular bandage.

5. <u>Bandaging of both eyes</u>: Fold triangular bandage into long strip about 6 fingers wide. Cover both eyes from front and crisscross ends in back over occiput. Bring ends around to forehead and tie knot.

6. <u>Bandaging of jaw</u>: Fold triangular bandage into long strip 4 fingers wide. Divide into thirds. Wrap bandage around jaw, bringing two ends up to top of head in front of both ears. Tie knot on top of head toward the front.

For bandage techniques mentioned above, handkerchiefs or a cloth cap may be used if no triangular bandage is available.

7. <u>Bandaging crown of head, lower jaw and both shoulders</u>. Because of the extent of the injury, a shirt may be used for bandaging. Place collar of shirt over forehead above eyebrows. Pull body of shirt toward back covering the ears, and button behind head at 2nd buttonhole. Now pull both sleeves down toward jaw, wrap around it and bring around to back of neck, and tie knot. Now tie a narrow bandage to corners of shirt and cover shoulders with shirt body in back, crisscrossing shirt-tails in front, and bring bandage ends under axillae to back over bottom edge of shirt and tie knot (Figure 6-1-4).

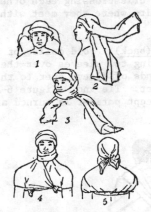

Figure 6-1-4. Using shirt to bandage crown of head,
jaw, and both shoulders.

8. <u>Bandaging of single shoulder</u>: Pull up shirt shoulders, turn collar under. Place shirt over injured shoulder, and pull sleeves over to other side of body from back and front. Tie knot. Then place elbow of injured shoulder before chest and wrap forearm with body of shirt, by pulling shirt tails toward opposite side of body from front and back. Tie knot. (Figure 6-1-5).

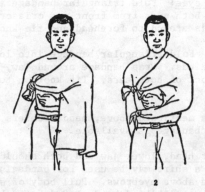

Figure 6-1-5. Bandaging single shoulder with shirt.

9. <u>Bandaging of both shoulders</u>: Fold collar over at level of shirt shoulders. Drape folded-over shirt over both shoulders from back. Bring both sleeves to front of chest crisscrossing each other. Bring ends of sleeve around to opposite armpits where they meet with shirt corners from the front. Tie knots.

10. <u>Bandaging of chest (back)</u>: Fold collar of shirt under, drape shirt in front of chest, bringing two sleeves over the shoulder and criss-crossing them behind. Bring ends of sleeve over to the axillae where they meet the bottom corners of shirt. Tie knot (Figure 6-1-6). The back is bandaged in similar manner, except patient is turned around.

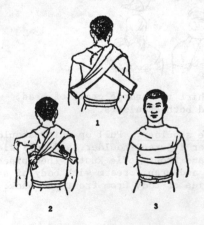

Figure 6-1-6. Bandaging chest with shirt.

11. <u>Bandaging of side of chest:</u> Turn shirt upside down and place collar over waist on injured side of chest. Bring two sleeves around to other side of body. Tie a knot. Grasp bottom of shirt by two corners, bring up along both sides of healthy shoulder. Tie knot over shoulder.

12. <u>Bandaging of chest and back:</u> Unbutton patient's shirt, over-lapping the front panels, pull shirt tighter. Insert belt strips into the 2nd and 4th buttonhole, pull and encircle back and chest. Tie knot. Then fold bottom of shirt upward. Attach tie to both front garment corners. Bring up over shoulders to middle of back where they tie a knot with the bottom of shirt. (Figure 6-1-7).

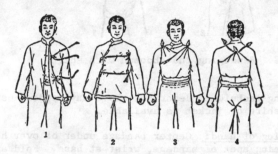

Figure 6-1-7. Bandaging chest and back using the injured's shirt.

13. <u>Bandaging the abdomen:</u> Take jacket and place collar against waist on one side, and bring sleeves over to other side of waist from front and back. Tie knot. Fold bottom of jacket (or shirt) up and wrap around thigh on covered side (Figure 6-1-8). A multi-strip bandage can also be used here.

<u>Note</u>: If abdominal organs are protruding, do <u>not</u> try to reinsert. Use sterile gauze to protect the extrusion, or cover the part with a clean small bowl before bandaging. Take care that the protrud-ing organ does not incure additional damage. Depending on the patient's condition, provide immediate emergency care or transport.

14. <u>Bandaging one buttock:</u> Take shirt (or jacket) and place bottom edge over waist of injured buttock. Pull corners over to other side and tie knot, with the inner side of shirt covering the injured buttock. Wrap the two sleeves around thigh on injured side, and tie knot.

15. <u>Bandaging of both buttocks;</u> Take jacket and cover buttocks with inner side facing injured part. Bring bottom edge of shirt around to front and tie knot. String bandage through sleeves individually for wrap-ing around thighs separately. Tie knots.

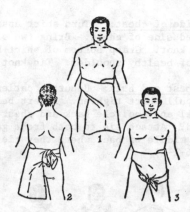

Figure 6-1-8. Bandaging the abdomen with shirt.

The bandaging techniques described above may be done using a triangular bandage if no shirt or jacket is available.

16. **Bandaging of hand:** Center bandage under or over hand, with patient's fingers facing apex of bandage, wrist at base. Fold apex over covering hand, crisscross the two base angles over or under the hand, circling around the wrist, and tie knot. A handkerchief or roller bandage can also be used instead.

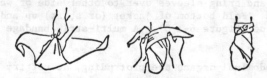

Figure 6-1-9. Wrapping hand using triangular bandage.

17. **Bandaging the foot:** Incline foot along one edge of triangular bandage. Wrap one side around ankle and tie knot. Wrap other base angle around foot and bring up to ankle. Tie knot. Bandage is shaped like a shoe.

18. **Arm sling:** Place triangular bandage flat against chest, apex facing elbow of injured arm. Band arm 90° placing forearm over bandage. Then bring up lower tip of bandage to cradle the arm. Extend both ends of bandage over shoulder behind neck and tie knot. Fold remaining apex angle over elbow and secure with safety pin or tie down with tape (Figure 6-1-10).

Or triangular bandage can be folded over to make wide bandage for cradling forearm. Bring ends up behind neck and tie knot (Figure 6-1-11).

Figure 6-1-10. Large arm sling.   Figure 6-1-11. Small arm sling.

Note: Bandaging methods most commonly used

1. Circular bandage: For stabilizing the roller bandage so it will not slip off easily, make the first winding on a slant downward, then go over with 2nd and 3rd windings. Then with each turn, make a fold a reverse spiral to return bandage to a working circular motion as the windings go one on top of the other. After winding has been completed, secure with safety pin or adhesive tape. Or, split the end of bandage and [twist split sections to keep from splitting further] and tie to fasten.

2. Spiral bandage: First make 2-3 windings with a roller bandage, after which, continue to unroll the bandage while making the upward windings, each one to cover one-third to two-thirds of the previous winding.

3. Spica (fan-shape) bandage: Used mostly for bandaging joints, employing centrifugal technique. That is, unroll the bandage in figure of "8" motion, first around part below the joint, then coming down to part below the joint, then going back up again, etc.

4. Four-tailed (headed) bandage: Cut two ends of the bandage, thereby making it a four-tailed bandage. Use mostly to bandage up injuries sustained on the jaw, nose, forehead, and occiput.

Immobilization

Immobilization of fractures with splints or other hard objects will keep the fracture from further displacement and subsequently, additional damage to muscle tissue, nerves, blood vessels. Splinting also reduces patient suffering and complications while facilitating transport of the injured.

1. General Principles

a. Select splint of proper width suited to the fractured part. Its length must also be appropriately longer than the broken bone. In absence of splints, use bamboo poles, wooden poles, boards, doors, etc., as substitutes.

b. Immobilize and fix the fracture immediately, but do not use too much pressure as to injure skin and muscles. The ties or bandages must not be too tight or too loose, fixed below and above the fracture site.

c. For compound fractures, check the wound and stop bleeding first. Cover with sterile gauze before immobilizing fracture.

2. Immobilization of different fractures

a. Fracture of clavicle: For fracture of one side (clavicle) only, using a large sling will be sufficient. For fracture of both clavicles, place a T-shaped splint behind the injured's back, then bandage both shoulders and waist to the splint.

b. Fracture of humerus or forearm: Place a splint of suitable length and width laterally alongside the fracture, and secure with bandage above and below the fracture. Then flex arm 90° and support with small sling.

c. Fracture of femur or leg: Take two splints and place them medially and laterally to the injured limb. Secure in several places. Make sure that the length of splint is longer than the broken bone (must extend beyond two joints at least, for the lateral splint).

If no splint or other substitutes are available, tie the intact limb and the fractured limb together. Plug the space in between limbs with cotton or other soft material. Secure the fixation with several bandages from the ankle up to the thigh. This method is suitable for fractures of the thigh bone or bones of the leg.

d. Fracture of the spine: Such an injury is more serious. Place the injured (lying down) on a stretch or door right away, inserting a small cushion in small of back between the thorax and lumbar spine. Keep the injured immobilized to prevent further damage.

Transport

The purpose of transport is to move the injured to a safety zone -- to a hospital or first aid station, for further treatment. For this reason, the logistics of transport emphasize proper and quick movements involving quick assistance, quick transport, using the proper methods and tools with great agility. During transport, particularly under battle conditions, the revolutionary spirit of "saving the dying and aiding the injured in carrying out the humanism of revolution" must be exuded.

Several frequently used methods of handholding and stretcher transport will now be described.

1. Supporting method
2. Carry-support method
3. Back-carry method
4. Chair method (Figure 6-1-12)
5. Pull-cart method (Figure 6-1-13)
6. Figure of "8" strap transport method
7. Circular strap transport method (Figure 6-1-14)
8. Wooden pole transport method
9. Crawling-on-side method of transport (Figure 6-1-15)
10. Carrying pole method of transport
11. Samples of stretcher substitutes (Figure 6-1-16)

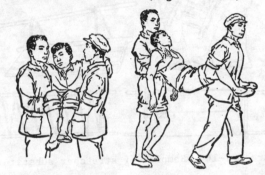

Figure 6-1-12. Chair method of transport   Figure 6-1-13. Pull-cart method
of transport

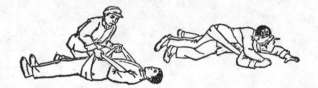

Figure 6-1-14. Circular strap method of transport.

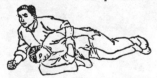

Figure 6-1-15. Crawling-on-side method of transport

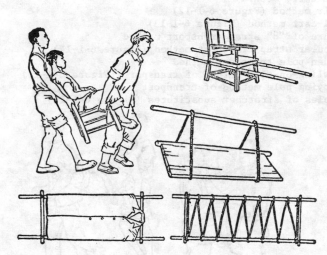

Figure 6-1-16. Samples of stretcher substitutes

Treatment of Burns

Burns may be caused by high-temperature solids, boiling water, steam, boiling oil, flames, or chemicals, which inflict damage on the human body.

In light burn cases, symptoms may only be local redness, blistering, and pain. In severe cases, particularly extensive burns, shock may occur.

In the treatment of burns, many innovations have originated in China. Many serious cases with burns covering over 90 percent of the body surface have recovered.

Estimate of Burn Surface

1. **Palmar method:** The surface covered by the palm of patient, with fingers held close together, comprises 1 percent of his total body surface (Figure 6-1-17)

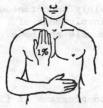

Figure 6-1-17. The palmar method.

2. **New Nine-Division Method:** Suited for adults (Figure 6-1-18).

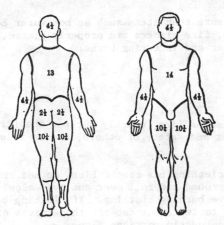

Figure 6-1-18. New Nine-Division Method

Estimate of Burn Depth (Table 6-1-2)

Table 6-2-2. Classification of burn depth

Depth of classification	Extent of damage	Clinical symptoms
First degree (erythema)	to the cuticle	Erythema, pain, supersensitivity
Second degree (blistering)	to the corium	Blistering, damage area wet and moist, red at base (shallow second-degree), pale and white, showing small bleeding points (deep second-degree), and pain.
Third degree (eschar)	Includes the whole skin layer and possibly subcutaneous involvement of muscle and bone.	No blistering, dryness. Area white or charred, exposing subcutaneous venous thrombosis, some pain, though sensation frequently lost.

Prevention

1. Strengthen education programs in fire prevention and occupational safety.

2. Make sure that places storing strong acids and alkalis and flammable materials are supplied with safety equipment (such as water tanks, sandbags, fire extinguishers).

3. Make sure that items such as hot water bottles, rich cooker, boiling water kettle, fire cinders are properly placed, to prevent small children knocking them over and incurring burns.

First Aid

1. In case of fire, quickly put out the fire at its source, to protect the lives and safety of others, and to reduce material loss to the nation.

2. When clothing has caught fire, do not run aimlessly, but throw yourself on the ground and roll over and over slowly to put the flames out. Or, quickly remove burning clothing. If clothing becomes stuck to the skin do not use force to tear, but cut off those parts of clothing not stuck. Leave the adhered-to-skin portions alone.

3. For acid and alkali burns, besides removing the clothing, flush burn area with water, or soak affected part in a clear water bath. Alkali burns may be neutralized with a weak acid solution such as a 1-2 percent acetic acid solution or a 5 percent ammonia chloride solution. For phosphorus burns, apply a wet cloth or a wet sodium bicarbonate compress over the affected area.

4. To prevent further infection and to protect the injured surface, use first aid wraps, triangular bandages, handkerchiefs, available clothing that is still fairly clean, or sheets to rapidly bandage the damaged surface, avoiding wherever possible any blisters that have formed.

5. To prevent shock in patients with a large burn surface, give them a special drink prescribed for burn cases (solution of 0.3 gm salt, 15 gm sodium bicarbonate, 0.005 gm phenobarbital in 100 ml water).

6. Be on the alert for asphyxia occurring in cases with burns of the respiratory tract. In an emergency situation, a thick pin may be inserted directly into the trachea to maintain an open airway.

Treatment

1. Using Chinese herbs

    a. Solution: (for burn cleaning and wet compresses) prepared from the following:

Mao-kuo suan-p'an-tzu	5 ch'ien
Kung-pan kuei	5 ch'ien
Chin-yen-hua (honeysuckle)	1.5 ch'ien
Nan-t'ien-chu (or Huo-hsieh shih-ta-kung-lao)	1.5 ch'ien
Water	1500 ml

    Cook and simmer above ingredients in water until concoction is reduced to 1000 ml.

    Dusting agent from same herbs prepared in the following pro- portions:

Mao-kuo suan-p'an-tzu	35%
Kung-pan kuei	35%
Chin-yen-hua (honeysuckle)	15%
Nan-t'ien-chu	15%

    Mix and pulverize above ingredients. Steam-sterilize and use the dried powder for sprinkling over injured burn area.

b. Mixture of

Tung oil tree blossoms	4 liang
Tung oil	1 chin

Pick blossoms from tung-oil tree and soak in tung oil, (Make
sure blossoms are fresh and clean, and not wet nor dry.)
the longer, the better. Store in cool place above ground.
When burns are treated with this tung-oil mixture, apply on
burn surface using a duck feather that has been immersed in
boiling water. Apply frequently [about 10-20 times daily]
to keep the burn surface from drying out.

c. Hu-chang ken in one of following forms:

(1) Juice of fresh root crushed, for application over burn
(2) Powder, obtained from root with bark peeled, roasted and
    pulverized, for sprinkling over burn
(3) Concoction for taking by mouth

2. General and symptomatic treatment

a. For 1st and 2nd degree burns over a small area. Apply a paste
   prepared from aged calcium oxide and 95 percent alcohol several
   times a day. Or equal parts of huang-lien (Coptis chinensis)
   and ti yu pulverized, for sprinkling over burned surfaces.

b. For burns with large blisters. After using a sterile needle
   to break them, cover with vaseline gauze and bandage. Change
   dressings after 4 days. To dry the raw areas and aid in eschar
   formation, gentian violet 2-4 percent may be used. For the
   head and face and the perineal area, use exposure therapy.

c. Observe aseptic procedures whenever contact is made with the
   patient, whether changing dressings or giving treatment.

d. Alleviate pain. All Chinese herbs used are generally analgesic.
   If pain is severe, I. M. dolantin [demerol] 50 mg may be given.
   If necessary, use morphine (exception being burns of the head
   or respiratory tract).

e. Replace fluid loss. Generally, give saline by mouth. For
   serious cases, give I.V. drip of 5-10 percent dextrose in
   normal saline.

f. Prevent infection. For burns incurred under contamination
   conditions, give one dose of tetanus antitoxic serum 1500 I.U.
   If necessary, prescribe penicillin, tetracyline, or chloromycetin etc.

g. **Maintain nutrition**. Whenever possible, give nourishment by mouth. If necessary, use nasal feeding.

3. **For cases of extensive and deep burns**, including those patients with shock symptoms. Note the following points if hospitalization is necessary.

   a. Give preliminary shock treatment and transfer patient to hospital after his condition has stabilized. Avoid jarring movements to patient during transport.

   b. Watch patient's blood pressure, pulse, and respiration closely. Be sure to keep the airway patent.

Section 2   Other Medical Emergencies

In medical emergencies, the onset is sudden and acute. If not treated right, damage and deformity or death may take place within a very short period of time. For this reason, barefoot doctors must have a strong sense of political responsibility, adhere to Chairman Mao's admonition to "save the dying and aid the injured in our practice of revolutionary humanism," and do all they can in giving first aid, quite aware that every minute counts.

Various emergencies will be discussed here. Also consult under respective sections for treatment of fever, hemorrhage, acute abdomen, infantile convulsions etc.

Drowning

Drowning is due to the great amount of water introduced into the body system via the mouth and nose and flooding of the respiratory passages and lungs that prevent oxygen absorption. Though the water introduced this way may not be very much, spasms in the trachea frequently cause asphyxia, anoxia and coma. If first aid is not provided in time, death will rapidly ensue. In drowning of a short duration, the lips may be cyanosed, the eyes watery and lids swollen. In drowning of a longer duration, the face of the victim is cyanosed, extremities are cold, and unconsciousness, or even respiratory and cardiac arrest, may be present.

Prevention

1. Encourage collective swimming, strengthen group leadership, and enforce safety measures. Persons just learning how to swim should not go into deep water.

2. Teach water safety. Check swimming area regularly, and see that children not venture off by themselves to play in water along edges of ponds, rivers and lakes.

3. Make sure that all boats are equipped with lifesaving equipment.

First Aid

1. <u>Drain water</u>. Remove bits of grass and dirt in the victim's mouth and nostrils. Loosen up collar and shirt, and place patient in prone position. Using both hands, lift patient at waist, and let his head face down for water in stomach and lungs to be drained, to restore patency of airway (Figure 6-2-1).

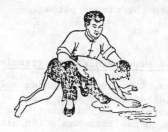

Figure 6-2-1. First aid to the drowning victim.

2. <u>Give artificial respiration, if breathing has stopped</u>. Pull the victim's tongue out to prevent it from obstructing the airway. Then give artificial respiration, using the back pressure arm lift method to be maintained continuously in conjunction with mouth-to-mouth resuscitation, until the victim can breathe by himself. If the patient's heart beat is also weak or arrested, coordinate resuscitation with external cardiac massage.

3. <u>Keep patient warm</u>. Give oxygen if needed.

4. <u>Give acupuncture treatment</u>, in accordance with <u>New Methods of Acupuncture Therapy</u>.

Use strong stimulation on joints jen-chung, yung-ch'uan, nei-kuan, kuan-yuan, retaining needle 5-10 minutes. After patient has awakened, give him some strong tea or sweetened ginger brew.

5. <u>Other</u>

a. For victims with shallow respirations, give an injection of nikethamide if needed; and for those with a weak heart beat, give an injection of caffeine sodium benzoate or epinephrine if needed. Treat victims with cerebral edema, the result of anoxia experienced over a longer period of time, with isotonic glucose or mannitol.

b. Give injection of penicillin to forestall pneumonia.

Electrical Shock

Electric shock may be caused by contact with electricity [via wires] or by lightning strike. The consequence of electric shock is frequently immediate loss of consciousness or even death in severe cases. After contact with live electricity, the victim may show muscular spasm, pallor, cyanosed lips, drop in blood pressure, weakened or loss of heart beat, respiratory arrest, and different degrees of burn injury on the electricity contact site.

Prevention

1. Educate the masses on electrical safety. Do not use wet hands or wet cloth to contact the electrical device. Light switches should be installed in higher locations, and wherever possible, they should be pulling switches.

2. Inspect electrical equipment routinely. Repair damages in time. When making repairs, first cut off power supply and take safety precautions. It is best to wear rubber shoes or use insulating devices while working.

First Aid

1. Quickly cut off electrical source, such as turning off a switch. Or take insulators such as any dry or flat wood pole, bamboo pole, rope etc., to push victim away from the electric source. Under most conditions, the first aider must not use hands to directly push the victim.

2. If breathing in the shock victim is arrested, first loosen his collar, pull out his tongue and start artificial respiration which may stretch over a long period of time, sometimes over 10 hours non-stop. Do not give up easily. If his heart has stopped beating, or the heart sounds are almost inaudible, and pulse is weak and irregular, immediately conduct external heart compression. Remember to keep patient warm.

3. Practice new acupuncture technique, by strong stimulation of the "jen-chung," "nei-kuan," "yang-ling-ch'uan" points, continuing the stimulation all the while the needles are retained.

4. Use other methods, such as intramuscular injections of alkali of shan-keng-ts'ai, caffeine sodium benzoate, nikethamide etc. Do not use injections of epinephrine. For local burns, concentrate on prevention of infection, and treatment of symptoms.

Heat Stroke

Heat stroke is commonly referred to as "fa sha" by the local populace. It is induced by long exposure to sun, or by working under high temperatures.

In the early stage, its manifestations are headache, dizziness, "spots" before eyes, fatigue, nausea, vomiting, and hidrosis. Later developments may include high fever, increased pulse, and respirations, flushed face, perspiration mechanism break-down or even excessive perspiration, facial pallor, muscular spasms (throughout the four extremities), and pain.

Prevention

1. Proper scheduling of working hours in hot weather. Be sure to have a shady and cool place for lunch and rest breaks. Wear light-colored or white clothing when working outdoors. Wear straw hat.

2. Drink slightly salted water instead of tea. Or substitute tea with one of the following brewed concoctions.

a.	Mei-hsieh tung-ch'ing	1 liang
b.	Chin-yen hua	1 liang
	Hsiang-no	1 liang
	Chung lo-po-tou	1 liang
c.	Huang-ching leaves	

3. Take preventive of ch'ing-liang yu (or oil) [clear-cooling oil] with 10 drops of water.

4. If sudden dizziness, sudden cessation of perspiration, or increased bradycardia are noted when working under high temperature, take off immediately to a cool shady spot, and rest.

First Aid

1. Move victim immediately to cool shady spot, loosen clothing and trousers waist. Place cold compress on forehead, fan and massage the four extremities. Give cool tea or slightly salted water to drink.

2. Kua-sha (skin-scrape) massage:

   a. Kua-sha technique (See "Folk Treatments")

   b. Forcefully grasp-massage the "ho-ku," "nei-kuan" and "jen-chung" points. After the victim has come to, separately massage the "wei-chung," "tsu-san-li," "feng-ch'ih," "chien-ching" points 15 to 20 times.

3. Apply new acupuncture technique: For those who have fainted, prick the "shih-hsuan" until it bleeds. Then apply medium or strong stimulation to "ne-chung," "yung-ch'uan," "ch'u-ch'ih."

4. Give Chinese herbs:

   a. For early symptoms, give jen-tan and "Lu-I" powder with 10 drops of water.

b. For emergency use (suitable for heat stroke fainting), blow
a small amount of the following pulverized mixture into nose:

Ya-tsao	2 ch'ien
Hsi-hsin	2 ch'ien
Chang-nao (caomphor)	5 fen

c. (For nausea and fainting in heat stroke), give victim a mixture
of rice crushed with tse-lan leaves and combined with rice
rinse water.

d. A 3-ch'ien dose of the following pulverized mixture, taken with
boiled water (for abdominal cramps in heat stroke):

Roots of ma-tou-ling	1 liang
Wa-erh t'eng	1 liang

e. (For heat stroke fainting), give victim a suitable amount of
juice crushed from mu-ching leaves, mixed with red alum
(hung-fan) water.

f. For internally shut-off heat stroke in which the body is hot,
perspiration is absent, and the victim has fainted, gave tzu-
hsueh tan or tzu-chin-ting. If it is an externally releasing
syndrome with continuous perspiration, pallor, clammy hands
and feet, immediately give hei-hsi tan (ready-to-take drug)
or a ginseng-aconitum concoction (tang-shen 5 ch'ien, processed
fu-tzu 3 ch'ien).

5. If necessary, provide symptomatic relief with analgine, chlorpromazine, caffeine, coramine etc. Serious cases, after initial treatment, should
be hospitalized for further follow-up.

Fainting

Fainting is a sudden and temporary loss of consciousness due to an
inadequate blood supply to the brain. Simple fainting occurs in presence
of intensely emotional states, fright, acute pain, poor health, sudden activity after long period of bed rest, standing in erect position overly long,
sudden rise from squatting position, fatigue, heat, stress or pregnancy. In
certain patients with a history of heart disease, hypertension, toxemia of
pregnancy, acute hemorrhage, or central nervous system illnesses, black spots
before eyes and sudden keeling over may occur. However, this symptom must be
distinguished from coma, shock, and low blood sugar.

First Aid

1. Put victim flat on back, head slightly lower. Loosen up his
clothing. Keep warm.

- 203 -

2. Use new acupuncture technique: apply strong stimulation to the "jen-chung" point, but prick "shao-shang" point sufficiently until it begins to breath." Or, use fingers to pinch the "jen-chung," "ho-ku," and "kun-lun" points.

3. Blow a little t'ung-kuan san [a powder] into nose to cause sneezing.

Shock

Shock is a constitutional reaction of the body to irritation by certain etiological factors which frequently provoke acute peripheral circulatory failure and oxygen hunger in the tissues. The chief manifestations are dizziness, spots before eyes, apprehension, clammy sweating, pallor, cold hands and feet, rapid and weak pulse, blood pressure drop, listless or restless expression, and even coma. Etiological factors that frequently cause shock are traumatic hemorrhage, hemoptysis, hematemesis, postpartum bleeding, spleen rupture, rupture in ectopic gestation, toxic pneumonia, toxic bacterial dysentery, septicemia, epidemic meningitis, biliary tract infections, acute gastroenteritis intestinal obstruction, large-surface burns, extensive soft tissue avulsion, compound fractures, external brain injuries, allergic reactions to penicillin, streptomycin or procaine, insecticide and food poisoning, heatstroke, myocardial infarction etc.

Prevention

Carefully examine and check for all diseases and etiological factors that can easily cause shock. For example, if the patient is found to be restless and apprehensive, perspiring clammily, with pulse increased and blood pressure dropping consider the likelihood of these symptoms as pre-shock manifestations, and take emergency measures immediately, to prevent onset of shock and subsequent complications.

First Aid

1. At the same time that anti-shock measures are being taken, attempt to find the cause and treat in time. If it is a massive hemorrhage, stop bleeding immediately. If it is the result of infection, strengthen antibacterial and toxin elimination measures.

2. General treatment

    a. Place patient in recumbent position, his head lower than his feet (brain injuries the exception). Keep warm, and try not to move patient whenever possible.

    b. Observe changes in condition closely, with particular attention to the blood pressure, respiration, pulse, facial coloring, amount of urine passed, and mental state.

3. With new acupuncture therapy technique apply moderate acupuncture stimulation to points "jen-chung," "nei-kuan," and retain needle. Activate needle every 4 or 5 minutes. Use needling technique with moxibustion over "ch'i-hai" and "pai-hui" points.

4. With Chinese herbs

    a. Concoction of
       Ch'ai-hu   3 ch'ien
       Pai-shao   3 ch'ien
       Chi-shih [acorns]   2 ch'ien
       Licorice   1 ch'ien
       (This prescription is good for any yang-deficient ailment by fever headache, thirst, and a sinking and slippery pulse.)

    b. Concoction of
       Unprocessed fu-tzu [aconitum]   3 ch'ien
       Dry ginger   2 ch'ien
       Licorice   1 ch'ien
       (This prescription is suitable for yin-deficient ailments characterized by cold hands and feet, aversion to cold, a weak and sinking pulse).

    c. Concoction prepared from 1-3 ch'ien of ginseng; or ginseng 2 ch'ien to processed fu-tzu [aconitum] 3 ch'ien. (This prescription is suited for seriously ill patients with pallor, dizziness, dyspnea, listlessness, cold extremities, protracted hidrosis, and a weak pulse. The ginseng in prescription may be substituted with tang-shen 5 ch'ien).

5. Other

    a. Intravenous drip of 5 percent dextrose in saline. Or use norepinephrine to raise blood pressure.

    b. For patients suffering from toxic shock or unstable blood pressures even with use of hypertensors, consider using hydro-cortisone 100-200 mg daily, 8-10 mg per kg in small children, given by intravenous drip.

    c. Correction of acidosis, with intravenous drip of 5 percent destrose 500 ml, to which 100 cc of 11.2 percent sodium lactate solution is added.

       Fluid supplements and blood transfusions should not be given too rapidly or in excessive amounts, to prevent complications.

    d. Prevention of infection with penicillin and other antibiotics.

Poisonous Snakebites

Injury from poisonous snakebites is an emergency frequently encountered in rural areas of southern China in the summer and fall. The upper jaw of the poisonous snake contains a venom gland which secretes the venom. After a snake bite has occurred, the venom is injected into the human body via the snake's fangs, resulting in a series of intoxicating symptoms, the worse of which are life-threatening.

In the beginning, the site of the snakebite swells rapidly and becomes numb. Or acute pain is felt locally, followed by erythema, purplish gangrene in extreme situations with an oozing of thin serum due to the bite. The edema develops rapidly proximally, with adenopathy in nearby lymph nodes. The victim may experience dizziness, nausea, vomiting, abdominal cramps, diarrhea, epistaxis, urinary incontinence, weakness and numbness of limbs, etc. In serious cases, petechial appear on skin, together with other critical symptoms such as diplopia, drowsiness, blood pressure drop, pupil dilatation, clenched jaw, respiratory and swallowing difficulties, spasms convulsions of all four limbs, swelling in the corneal arch, tongue fur purplish black etc.

Based on variations in the manifestations described, most snake bites may be classified into three types: <u>neurotoxic</u> (manifested by central nervous system symptoms appearing after bites by chin-huan [golden ring] and yen-huan [silver ring] snakes), <u>hemotoxic</u> (characterized by blood poisoning symptoms following bites by chu-hsieh ch'ing [bamboo-leaf green] and wu-pu [five-step] snakes), and <u>mixed</u> (characterized by a combination of neurotoxic and hemotoxic symptoms appearing after bites by snakes of the Elapidae such as cobra and coral snakes). Several frequently seen poisonous snakes are shown in Figure 6-2-2.

Prevention

1. Educate the masses on the prevention and care of poisonous snake-bites and promote a poisonous snake eradication program.

2. Observe environmental health practices for areas surrounding dwellings. Sprinkle powdered lime or plants or crushed parts of cucumber or shan-tou-ken (<u>Ardisia crenata</u>) indoors.

3. Wear boots, stockings and long trousers when moving through snake-infested areas. When walking around at night, use a staff to prod along in front to scare snakes off path.

4. Chinese herbs, taken to develop immunity to snake venom.

Pai-wei   1.5 liang
Pai-t'ou weng   1.5 liang
Hsu-chang-hsing 1.5 liang
Tu-hsing   1 liang
Pa-chiao-lien   1 liang

(handwritten annotations: Bai Wei — Pai-wei Cynanchum stratum; Bai Tou Weng — Pai-t'ou weng Pulsatilla; Hsu-chang-hsing Pycnostelma miliuva; Pa-chiao-lien 8 corned lotus / Berberis)

94 Lieh-hsieh ch'u-hai-t'ang
    [split-leaf begonia]   1 liang
Ch'ien-chin teng Stephania   5 ch'ien
I-tien hsueh Stephania   1 liang

Dry and pulverize the above ingredients. Prepare and take 3 times during year (best during late spring or early winter) 7-10 days apart, at bedtime (Mix 4 ch'ien of pulverized mixture with a small amount of wine to which ashes from a small piece of cloth and 3 drops of cockscomb blood have been added). For children and women reduce dosage accordingly. Boiled water can also be used instead of wine to wash the powder down. Not recommended for children under 12 years of age, pregnant women, and women during their menstrual periods. If this regimen is followed, protection lasting one year against poisonous snake-bites is acquired. This regimen followed 3 years in a row (a combination of 9 doses) will confer lifelong protection against poisonous snakes and snake venom.

First Aid

1. Allay victim's fears and restlessness in order to keep venom spread to minimum.

2. If the snakebite is located on any limb, immediately tie a tourniquet on the proximal side of bite (Figure 6-2-3), to prevent the venom from entering into the body's general circulation. (However the rope or tourniquet must be relaxed every 30 minutes for several seconds, and the injured limb is lowered, to prevent gangrenes). After this, use a clean small knife to open up the bite (bite impressions for various snakes shown in Figure 6-2-4), and lift out the fangs. Apply pressure along sides of bite to force out venom. At the same time, wash bite with rice water and use cupping technique over bite to draw out the poisoned blood. A match lit over the bite can also be used to dissipate the toxic effect of the venom. In extreme emergency, sucking bite by mouth can also be used. (Make sure no breaks or sores are in the nucous membrane of mouth, and the contents are spit out as sucking progresses and not swallowed. Rinse mouth repeatedly with clear water after sucking).

3. Use new acupuncture therapy technique: At the "pa-hsieh" and "pa-feng" points of the injured limb place triple-edged needle parallel to skin and insert in upward direction into skin to a depth of 1 cm. Quickly extract needle and return injured limb to a dependent position. Then massage gently in an up-to-down direction to force out blood containing the venom. If the swelling does not subside, continue treatment 2 to 3 times a day.

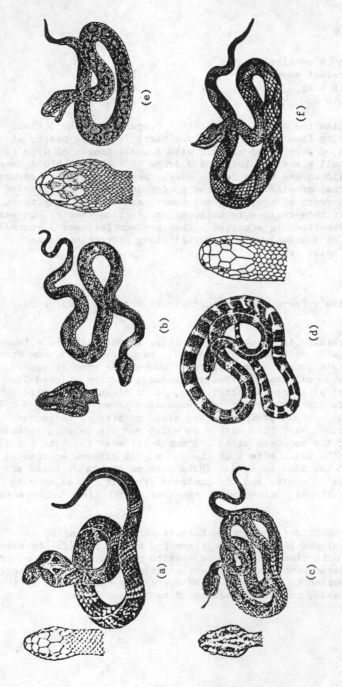

Figure 6-2-2. Some poisonous snakes found in South China

Key: (a) Yen-ching she (Cobra)
     (b) Lao-t'ieh she
     (c) Chu-hsieh ch'ing she [bamboo-leaf green snake]
     (d) Yen-huan she [silver-ring snake]
     (e) Fu she (viper)
     (f) Wu-pu she [Five-step snake]

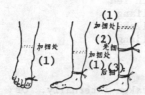 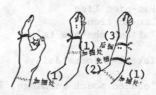

Figure 6-2-3 a. Location in bites on   Figure 6-2-3 b. Location in bites
    the lower extremity   on the upper extremity

Key: (1) Additional tourniquet (3rd)   (1) Additional tourniquet (3rd)
      (2) First tourniquet   (2) First tourniquet
      (3) Second tourniquet   (3) Second tourniquet

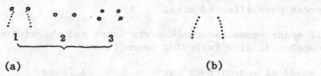

         (a)   (b)

Figure 6-2-4. Snakebite impressions

Key: (a) For poisonous snakes
      (b) For nonpoisonous snakes

    4. Use Chinese herbs.

        a. Cucumbers in suitable quantity prepared as follows: Soak fresh
           cucumbers in fresh human urine for 7 days and night. Remove
           and place on rooftops for 7 days and night to dry. Then wrap
           in cloth and store for later use, or carry around on body for
           emergency use. When needed, crush by chewing, and apply around
           affected part.

        b. Extract for painting over bite, prepared as follows: Mix
           honeysuckle leaves, she-mei (Indian strawberry Duchesnea
           indica), chin-wa-erh (Carpesium divaricatum) in suitable
           amounts with cold water. To use, paint from proximal side
           of bite toward bite, 5 times daily. If swelling and pain do
           not subside or constitutional symptoms appear, take about
           half a bowl of this juice extract by mouth, simultaneously
           with external treatment.

c. Concoction from the following:

Ch'ih-hsieh I-chih-hua	3 ch'ien
Pan-pien lien	1 liang
Lan-ho lien	1 liang
Pai-hua she-she ts'ao	1 liang

Take 1-2 doses daily.

d. Tobacco pouch washings, 2-3 bowlfuls taken internally. Or apply a tobacco grease compress over affected part.

e. Concoction of pan-pien lien 4-8 liang (half this amount for the dried herb) to be taken in 3 doses. Concoction can also be used for painting area around bite.

f. Ch'iang-wei mei and lu-pien ching, 4 liang of each, crushed and soaked in rice rinse-water, juice of which is taken internally. Juice also used for rubbing affected limb, in up-to-down direction. Medication is also used as paint or compress over affected area.

g. If snake venom has reached the heart and the victim becomes comatosed, give following concoction:

Leaves of wan-nien-ch'ing	2 liang
Leaves of chrysanthemum	2 liang

Stir mix with water while adding an appropriate amount of lacquer-wax (hsi-la, urushial?).

Or, a small amount of hsiung-huang (realgar) powder mixed with several crushed garlic sections in appropriate amount of water may be given victim instead. If snake venom has paralyzed the throat and eating is impossible, give juice crushed from shih-hu-t'o   2 liang.

h. If bite becomes infected, treat with poultice crushed from the following fresh herbs:

Wu-chiu	1 liang
Leaves of nan wu-wei-tzu	1 liang
Kang-mei	1 liang
Leaves of chin ying-tzu	1 liang

Crush herbs and use as poultice over bite.

i. Chi te-sheng [brand] snake pills to be taken internally or used externally for dressing. Dosage: Take 5 tablets by mouth, immediately. Also melt tablet with warm boiled water or saliva to render into thin liquid for dressing over wound and surrounding area.

5. Besides these measures, procaine block may be used, according to patient's condition, with fluid supplements for flushing out poisonous toxins, or with antibodies to prevent and control infections.

Gas Intoxication

Incomplete combustion of coal or charcoal may produce carbon monoxide. In the wintertime when a stove is lit for warmth and ventilation is poor, gas intoxication (carbon monoxide poisoning) can easily occur.

In the early stages of intoxication, the victim generally experiences discomfort, dizziness, weakness, nausea and vomiting, tinnitus, facial flushing then pallor. If intoxication worsens, respiratory difficulty, muscular cramps, coma, and even death may set in.

Prevention

1. Put coal stove outdoors at bedtime to avoid large amounts of gas produced during inadequate combustion being retained indoors.

2. Check chimney for obstruction during the winter and open windows to allow good air ventilation.

First Aid

1. Open windows immediately and move victim to a well-ventilated area. Unbutton clothing, but keep victim warm. If breathing becomes shallow or arrested, give artificial respiration immediately.

2. Use new acupuncture technique, applying strong stimulation to the "ho-ku," "nei-kuan," and "jen-chung" points, and retaining needle 20 to 30 minutes.

3. Crush raw radishes for juice and make victim take in quantities.

4. Give symptomatic treatment through selective use of dextrose, nikethamide, caffeine or 1 = 1000 epinephrine, according to different conditions.

Organic Phosphate Insecticide Poisoning

Organic phosphate insecticides frequently used are 1605 [parathion] 1059 [Systok] ti-pai-ch'ung [Propanil], le-kuo [rogor] DPUP etc. These highly effective insecticides are very toxic with respect to humans and animals. Because of lax management and improper use, acute intoxication may result through absorption via the respiratory and gastrointestinal tracts and the skin. Generally, a few hours after contact with such insecticides, central nervous system and gastrointestinal symptoms will suddenly appear. Toxic symptoms may be classified as light, medium and severe.

Light intoxication symptoms: Dizziness, headache, no appetite, nausea, vomiting, hidrosis, weakness.

Medium intoxication symptoms: Besides the above symptoms, excessive salivation, abdominal pain, diarrhea, tetany, excessive hidrosis, dysphasia, slight pupillary contraction, mental cloudiness.

Serious intoxication symptoms: Additional coma, incontinence of urine and feces, tachycardia, increased blood pressure, marked pupillary contraction, respiratory and circulatory failure in extremely serious cases, culminating finally in death.

Prevention   (See section "Agricultural Production Hygiene")

First Aid

1. Remove the intoxicated victims from the immediate area quickly. Take off contaminated clothing and wash with soap and water (do not use hot water and alcohol). If insecticide has been taken internally by mistake, poke throat with fingers to stimulate vomiting (or give 2-4 percent soda solution as emetic to stimulate gastric lavage). If the toxic substance has entered the eyes, irrigate with clear water immediately.

2. **Use of Chinese herbs**

   a. Kuan-tsung 1 liang, crushed and flushed by cool boiled water through a gauze sieve. Give victim the foamy strained solution to induce vomiting and diarrhea.

   b. Pulverized yeh pao-ho leaves, 1-2 ch'ien each time given with cold boiled water, will neutralize phosphorus toxicity and treat food poisoning at the same time.

   c. She-mei and raw mung beans, 2 liang of each, crushed and steeped in cold boiled water. Extract later for juice, and give internally.

   d. Juice extracted from crushed herbs listed as follow:

Ta-hsueh t'eng (bold vine)	5 ch'ien
Nan-wu-wei tzu	5 ch'ien
Kuang mu-hsiang	5 ch'ien
Rock sugar	1 ch'ien
Wu chiu, crushed	8 liang

   Pulverize first four ingredients, then mix with juice of crushed "wu-chiu," divide into three doses and give to patient accordingly. This prescription will also neutralize various types of insecticide intoxication.

3. New Acupuncture therapy

    Use needle technique on "tsu-san-li," "ho-ku," and "nei-kuan"
points, and apply strong stimulation. For serious cases, needle every half
hour.

4. Other treatment

    Depending on the severity of the intoxication, give atropine by
mouth, by subcutaneous injection, or massive (2-3 mg each time), repeated
(every half hour) intravenous injection, until consciousness is restored.
In serious cases, this may be used in conjunction with phosphate detoxifi-
cation therapy.

    For victims with respiratory difficulty, initiate artificial respira-
tion and give oxygen.

    In the presence of respiratory and circulatory failure, give intra-
muscular injection of lobeline or coramine.

    For cramps, give intramuscular injection of phenobarbital 0.1 gm.

Pesticide Intoxication

    Besides the organic phosphorus insecticides described in the previous
section, DDT, hexachlorophene (666), cresol etc. are other insecticides frequently used. If they are used improperly or taken by accident, intoxication
may result.

Table 6-2-1. Symptoms of intoxication for several pesticides

Pesticide	Symptoms
DDT	Congestion and light erosion in mucous membrane of throat, nausea and vomiting, abdominal cramps and diarrhea, muscular tremor, coma, respiratory arrest leading to death
666 (Lindane, benzene hexachloride)	Tetany, coma, liver and nervous system damage
Phenol-based intoxi-cation	Odor of phenol in breath, burning sensation in throat and stomach, nausea, vomiting, abdominal pain, hematuria, albuminuria, ischuria, blood pressure drop, coma.

    The important manifestations of intoxication are central nervous sys-
tem and gastrointestinal symptoms. Because of local irritation, DDT and 666
can further provoke conjunctivitis and dermatitis.

<u>Prevention</u>   (See "Agricultural Production Hygiene")

<u>First Aid</u>

1. Using Chinese herbs

   a. Raw eggs 10-20 mixed with powdered alum, taken to induce vomiting and emptying of stomach.

   b. Concoction of following herbs taken as purgative.

Tang-kuei	1 liang
Ta-huang (rhubarb)	1 liang
White alum	1 liang
Fresh licorice	5 ch'ien

   c. For neutralizing 666 intoxication

      (1) Roots of wu-chiu crushed and mixed with second rice rinsing. Give to victim by mouth.

      (2) Concoction of

Ta-huang (rhubarb)	1 liang
Fang-feng	1 liang
Licorice	1 liang

2. For dermatitis, washing with warm soapy water. Then apply zinc oxide ointment locally. For other local symptomatic treatment, consult relevant chapters and sections.

Lei-kung T'eng Poisoning

Lei-kung t'eng (<u>Tripterygium wilfordii</u>), also called "huang-t'eng ken," "shui-mang ts'ao," "san-ling hua," "ts'ao ho-hua," "huang-l'a hua," "nan-she ken," "lan-ch'iang ts'ao," "tuan-ch'iang ts'ao," etc., contains a strong neurotoxin. Intoxication symptoms such as burning pain in mouth and throat, excessive salivation, nausea and vomiting, abdominal pain, etc., usually appear within half an hour of taking this herb. Following this, dilated pupils or even blindness, drooping eyelids, dizziness, dysphasia, cold clammy hands and feet, muscular weakness or cramps, swallowing difficulties and finally coma, may be manifest. Finally, bradycardia followed by tachycardia, and irregular respirations, if not treated immediately, may culminate in respiratory failure and death.

<u>Prevention</u>

Lei-kung t'eng is used for external purposes to eliminate and eradicate pests. Do not take by mistake. A specific person should assume responsibility for its storage and use.

- 214 -

First Aid

1. Immediately give victim solution of salt mixed with boiled water. Then perform gastric lavage using strong tea. Tickle throat to induce vomiting.

2. Use Chinese herbs

   a. Concoct feng-wei ts'ao 1 chin and give to victim by mouth.

   b. Crush wu-chiu one-half chin stirred in rice rinse-water. Give extracted juice to victim frequently and continuously.

   c. Concoct the following:

Yen-hua (honeysuckle)	1 liang
Lien-ch'iao (forsythia)	5 ch'ien
Fang-feng	1 liang
Licorice	3 ch'ien
Mung beans	1 liang

   Cook until beans are done. Give by mouth, immediately.

   d. Crush roots of mi-hou t'ao (Actinidia Chinensis) 1 liang.

   Give juice to victim. Or, crush 10 or more chin of yung ts'ai and give juice continuously and frequently.

3. Other:

   For abdominal pain, give atropine. In presence of respiratory arrest, give artificial respiration. For respiratory and circulatory failure, alternate intramuscular injections of sodium benzoate caffeine with those of coramine every one-half to two hours.

Food Poisoning

The causes of food poisoning may be bacterial, vegetative or animal. Poisoning resulting from the consumption of rotten or spoilt food is an example of bacterial poisoning; that resulting from consumption of poisonous mushrooms, ginkgo nuts, sprouting potatoes, almonds etc., of vegetative poisoning; and that resulting from consumption of globefish and certain crabs, of animal poisoning.

Food poisoning frequently occurs simultaneously in people who have eaten food originating from the same source. The chief manifestations are vomiting, diarrhea, dehydration and other symptoms of acute gastroenteritis. Central nervous system symptoms may also be present leading to respiratory paralysis and death in serious cases.

Prevention

Measures are generally identical to those used for acute gastroenteriti
Additionally, note following points:

1. Make sure food is cooked well. If contents of canned food are spoilt or show change in quality, do not eat.

2. Do not eat gingko nuts, poisonous mushrooms, globefish, etc.

3. Have veterinarian check out sick animals before slaughtering them for food.

First Aid

1. Consult relevant chapters and sections on how to induce vomiting, and how to perform stomach and rectal washouts. General treatment here is like that for acute gastroenteritis. Bed rest and attention to keeping warm are important. Give serious cases parenteral fluids.

2. Use new acupuncture technique (same as that for treating acute gastroenteritis).

3. Use Chinese herbs

    a. Concoction of
Mung beans	1 liang
Licorice	3 ch'ien

       Crush and cork for 10 minutes or more. Give liquid and sediments to patient.

    b. Pulverize yeh pai-ho 5 ch'ien and add alum 5 fen. Mix with boiled water and have patient take by mouth.

    c. Crush 4 liang of wu-chiu and blend well with one bowl of rice rinse-water. Strain and give patient juice. Or, to portulaca one-half chin or honeysuckle leaves 1 chin add a handful of dirt. Place in jar, and crush. Take juice extract, let settle then give to patient.

4. Other

    a. For abdominal pain and serious vomiting, give 0.5 mg atropine subcutaneously. In cases of mushroom poisoning, atropine is furthermore a poison neutralizer.

    b. For cramps, give intramuscular injection of phenobarbital 0.1 g

    c. For collapse, give intramuscular injection of epinephrine
1:1000, 0.5-1 ml.

    d. For respiratory difficulty and cyanosis, give subcutaneous
injection of nikethamide 1 ml. Repeat when necessary.

Bones Stuck in Throat

Fish bones (or small prickly bones) are the chief culprits that get
stuck in the tonsils, sides of the throat, or base of the tongue. Frequently,
a prickly pain and sensation of a foreign body presence after eating are felt.

First Aid

1. Illuminate throat with flashlight. Push tongue down with tongue
depressor or chopstick to expose prickly bone. Remove with long forceps.
If the foreign body is deeply imbedded, use some other method to remove bone.

2. Using Chinese herbs

    a. Pulverize whole herb of yeh pai-ho (hua ts'ao). Mix with
boiled water and give to patient to sip.

    b. Concoct:

Wei-ling-hsien	5 ch'ien
Rock sugar	5 ch'ien

Mix with a little huang-chiu [yellow wine]. Give to patient
and have him gargle before swallowing. Take two doses.

The two methods described are also suitable when other foreign materials such as bamboo toothpicks, metals etc., are caught in the throat.

Section 3   Common Symptoms

High Fever

The causes of fever are numerous and those that should be clinically
differentiated are certain infectious diseases, parasitical infestations,
internal medical ailments, or malignancies etc. (See Table 6-3-1).

Types

In the practice of traditional Chinese medicine, the symptomatic treatment of high fever is based on its manifestation as wind-chill(feng-han),
fever (wen-ping), feverish intoxication (jeh-tu), or internal fever (li-jeh).
This condition is generally manifested as chills or fever, in varying degrees,
described as follows:

Table 6-3-1   Differential Diagnosis of High Fever

Disease (Illness)	Onset of illness	Symptoms	Physical findings
Upper respiratory tract infection	Sudden onset. History of chills.	Stuffy nose, coryza, general malaise, cough	Congested throat. Nasal secretions present.
Lobar pneumonia	Onset acute	Coughing, chest pain, rust-colored sputum	Moist rales may be heard; sound of breathing diminishes, speech accelerated.
Lung abscess and bronchiectasis	History of respiratory tract infections	Chest pain, coughing, purulent sputum, which shows 3-layer separation inside container.	Moist rales possibly heard; fingers clubby if disease of long duration.
Tuberculosis	Onset insidious, though sudden in small children	Coughing, recurrent afternoon fever which drops to below 37°C in the morning, hidrosis, weight loss, poor appetite, insomnia.	Fine rales possibly heard in tuberculosis cases; percussion pain over kidney region in renal tuberculosis
Rheumatism	History of tonsillitis and skin infections	Large joints red, swollen, hot and painful (of migrating nature); sweating, palpation, circular red patches, small subcutaneous nodes.	Increased heart rate, lowered heart sounds or murmurs heard in region of heart valves.
Urinary tract infections		Urinary frequency, dysuria, chills	Percussion pain over kidney region, pressure pain over suprapubic region.
Measles	History of measles epidemics usually occurring during winter-spring	Coughing, running nose and tearing	Red buccal membrane showing spots, exanthem first appearing as maculo-papular rash, starting from neck, then spreading to face, body, and extremities.

Table 6-3-1 (Continued)

Disease (Illness)	Onset of illness	Symptoms	Physical findings
Measles	History of measles epidemics usually occurring during winter-spring	Coughing, running nose and tearing	Red buccal membrane showing spots, exanthem first appearing as maculo-papular rash, starting from neck, then speading to face, body, and extremities. After fever has subsided, skin desquamation takes place.
Scarlet fever	Onset acute and history of contact; occurring mostly during winter-spring.	Sore throat	Congested throat exanthem scarlet red, small maculo-papular rash that blanch upon pressure. Pale lips, strawberry tongue, skin peeling in large patches.
Epidemic meningitis	Likely to occur during winter-spring	Headache, projectile vomiting, coma	Dull red petichiae, neck rigidity, Kernig's sign positive, sole scratch test positive.
Epidemic Japanese B encephalitis	Likely to occur during summer-fall	Headache, vomiting sleepiness, delirium	Neck resistance present; possibly positive Kernig's sign and sole [foot] scratch test.
Typhoid	Onset slow, history of contact	Gradual temperature rise, continuous high fever 1 week later; nausea and vomiting possibly present; expression dull and listless.	Hepatosplenomegaly, roseola, relatively slow pulse.
Infectious hepatitis	History of contact	Poor appetite, nausea and vomiting, weakness, upper abdominal discomfort, appearance of jaundice upon temperature drop in some cases.	Hepatomegaly, pressure pain felt over liver region, urine dark tea-colored and foamy, the foam also dark.

Table 6-3-1 (Continued)

Disease (Illness)	Onset of illness	Symptoms	Physical findings
Leptospirosis	Likely to occur in summer-fall, history of contact with infected water.	Chills and muscular aches throughout body, particularly pronounced in the gastrocnemius muscle of the leg; sometimes bleeding and jaundice.	Pressure pain obvious over the gastrocnemius; possibly hepatosplenomegaly.
Acute schistosomiasis	History of contact with infected	Fever over long duration, coughing, diarrhea.	Hepatomegaly, pressure pain, spleen possibly palpable.
Malaria	History of mosquito bites	Course of rigors, fever, sweating and temperature drop in tertian or quartan pattern	Possibly splenomegaly and anemia
Septicemia	History of infection	Headache, chills, frequently accompanied by nausea, vomiting and diarrhea.	Subcutaneous bleeding points, hepatosplenomegaly, pressure pain, slight jaundice
Various malignant tumors		Fever over a long period of time, ineffective antibiotic therapy, rapid loss of weight	Lymphadenopathy and hepatosplenomegaly possible, anemia.
Acute mastitis	Mostly in primiparas	Painful breasts, chills	Cracked nipples, local redness, swelling, burning and pain.
Puerpural fever	3-5 days post-partum	Chills, unpleasant odor to lochia	Pressure pain over and alongside uterus

Wind-chill: High fever, chills, coryza, flat taste in mouth, tongue normal and thin-coated, pulse usually floating.

   Fever: Generally expressed as high fever, non-aversion to chills, dryness in mouth, tongue red and thinly coated yellow, pulse rapid.

   Feverish intoxication: High fever, sore throat, mouth dryness or skin rash, tongue red and coating thin.

   Internal fever: High fever, hidrosis, excessive thirstiness, tongue red and coating yellow, constipation, even delirium.

Treatment

   1. Bed rest and fluids. If necessary when the patient cannot take fluids by mouth, give intravenous fluids. Place patient on nourishing and easily digestible diet. Keep his bowels open.

   2. New needle puncture treatment. Apply strong stimulation to "ta-chiu," "ch'u-ch'ih," "ho-ku," and "shao-shang" points, once a day. Use a triple-edged needle on the "shao-shang" and puncture until it bleeds.

   3. Skin-scrape "kua-sha" technique. Scrape both sides of spinal column using a soup spoon and soapy water (or vegetable oil), starting from the ta-chu down to the coccyx, until skin becomes purplish. It has a definite effect on lowering fever.

   4. Chinese herbs.

        a. For wind-chill. Dissipate wind (flatus) and dispel chill with
           the following concoction:
           Ma-huang (ephedra)   1 ch'ien
           Kuei-chih (cinnamon sticks)   1 ch'ien
           Hsing-jen (almonds)   3 ch'ien
           Licorice   1 ch'ien

        (Suitable for external signs of exposure in wind-chill ailments).

        b. For fever. Relieve fever with an acrid-cool concoction con-
           sisting of following ingredients:
           Honeysuckle   5 ch'ien
           Lien-ch'iao (Forsythia suspensa)   4 ch'ien
           Nui-pang tzu   3 ch'ien
           Cicada molting   1 ch'ien
           Po-ho (mint)   1 ch'ien
           Ching-chieh   1.5 ch'ien
           Chieh-keng   1.5 ch'ien
           Licorice   1 ch'ien

        (Usually taken in early stage of fever)

- 221 -

c. For _feverish intoxication_. Clear fever and neutralize toxicity with one of following concoctions:

(1) Feng wei ts'ao   1-2 liang
    Jen-tung t'eng (Lonicera
                  vine)   1-2 liang

(2) Pan-lan ken   1 liang
    Ta-ch'ing hsieh   1 liang
    Yen-hua (honeysuckle
            flowers)   1 liang
    Lien-ch'iao
      (Forsythia suspensa) 5 ch'ien

d. For _internal fever_. Clear (purify) the internal organs and purge fever with the following concoction:

Gypsum   2 liang
Chih-mu   3 ch'ien
Kan-ts'ao (licorice)   2 ch'ien
Unglutinous rice   1 ladle
Ta-huang (rhubarb)   3 ch'ien
  (if constipation present)
Yuan-ming powder   2 ch'ien
Niu-huang
  "heart-clearing" pill 1 pill
  (if delirium present)

5. Other

a. Analgine 0.5 gm by mouth or intramuscular injection.

b. Aspirin compound 1 tablet by mouth.

c. Phenothiazine 25 mg by mouth or intramuscular injection (used on restless patients running high temperature).

d. Treating cause of fever. Cold compresses may be used for symptomatic treatment.

Headache

Headache is a frequently noted symptom, and illnesses causing headache are quite numerous. Besides those listed in Table 6-3-2, other causes of headache are farsightedness, astigmatism, papillitis, laryngitis, malaria, schistosomiasis, hypertension, althero sclerosis, hysteria, neurasthenia, epilepsy, etc.

Table 6-3-2. Differential Diagnosis of Headache

Disease (Illness)	Symptoms	Physical Findings
Post-concussion complication(s)	Loss of consciousness for few minutes after injury, followed by dizziness, headache, etc. after patient has regained consciousness which may persist for several months or years.	Noticeable signs frequently absent
Epidemic Japanese B encephalitis	Occurring frequently during summer and autumn seasons, accompanied by fever, headache, projectile vomiting, and with development of disease other symptoms such as restlessness, coma and convulsions.	Neck rigid, Kernig's test positive, sole [foot] scratch test positive.
Epidemic encephalomyelitis	Occurring frequently during winter-spring seasons, onset acute, with high fever, excrutiating headache, projectile vomiting, and rapid progression into coma.	Neck rigid, Kernig's sign positive, foot [sole] scratch test positive, scattered petechial over chest and abdomen area, with purpuric blotches all over body in serious cases.
Purulent meningitis	May occur any time during year. Fever, headache, vomiting. Frequently has history of lobar pneumonia or otitis media.	Neck rigidity present. Kernig's sign, and sole (foot) scratch test both positive.
Tuberculous meningitis	May occur any time during year. Fever, headache, vomiting. Frequently has history of tuberculosis. Course of illness long, coma appearing in late stage.	Neck rigid. Kernig's sign and sole (foot) scratch test both positive.
Subarachnoid hemorrhage	May occur anytime during year. History of high blood pressure. Headache, vomiting, generally afebrile, coma not often seen.	Physical findings same as above
Glaucoma	Eye pain and headache, reduced vision, rainbow-hued halo around lights noted. Nausea and vomit-possibly present. Onset insidious in chronic cases, with no clinical manifestations	Corneal edema, pupils enlarged, in elliptical shape

Table 6-3-2 (Continued)

Disease (Illness)	Symptoms	Physical Findings
Iridocyclitis	Pain in eyes, photophobia, lacrimation, reduced vision	Congestion increasingly severe closer to the cornea, purplish red, pupils contracted, light reflex lost.
Acute otitis media	Severe pain, excrutiating in serious cases [of infection], with throbbing sensation and possibly fever. Intermittent pus drainage in chronic cases over long period.	Pus drainage in external auditory meatus. Otoscopi examination shows congestion or rupture.
Chronic rhinitis	Nasal obstruction and coryza, both nostrils simultaneously or alternately stopped up, usually intermittent, frequently more severe in the dormant positions. Sense of smell possibly impaired, parched and painful throat.	Congestion in nasal mucous membrane.
Chronic paranasal sinusitis	Nasal discharge excessive, sense of small impaired, dizziness, feeling of distension in head, and dull headache	Purulent nasal discharge. Post-nasal discharge sometimes caught in posterior wall of throat
Tonsillitis	Pain in throat accompanied by fever, chills, and arthralgia.	Tonsils enlarged, congested, with white secretions.
Temporal headache	Severe headache felt on one side; when severe, accompanied by vomiting which relieves headache. In absence of attack, patient normal. Its incidence quite possibly arrested after middle age.	No positive physical findings.

Types

According to the location of the headache and accompanying symptoms, exposure headaches, liver yang-dominant headaches, kidney deficient headaches are some of the more common types seen.

Exposure headache. Headache and fever are present. With chill (han) dominance, other symptoms are an absence of perspiration, flat taste in mouth and a tight pulse. With heat (jeh) dominance, other symptoms are hidrosis, dry mouth, sore throat or enlarged tonsils, and rapid pulse.

Liver yang-dominant headache. Generally the type that occurs during exhaustion or after fits of anger, accompanied by insomnia, restlessness, thin tongue fur, and a full pulse.

Kidney-deficient headache. Symptoms are dizziness, tinnitus, blurred vision, backache, thin-coated tongue fur, a fine thready pulse.

Treatment

1. New acupuncture therapy, for

   a. Frontal headache. At "yin-t'ang," "shang-hsing," and "ho-ku" points.

   b. Temporal headache. At "t'ai-yang," "wai-kuan," and "tsu-lin-ch'i" points.

   c. Occipital headache. At "feng-ch'ih," "hou-ch'i" points.

   d. Apical [top of head] headaches. At "pai-hui," "t'ai-ch'ung" points.

2. Massage therapy

   a. First press the "yin-t'ang," "ts'an-ch'u," and "t'ai-yang" points with enough pressure to loosen up these points. Then follow with the wiping massage technique, going from the "yin-t'ang" to the "shang-hsing," and from the "yin-t'ang" to the "t'ai-yang," a total of 20-30 times for each wipe.

   b. Wipe-massage from the "t'ai-yang" to "feng-ch'ih" points, 30 to 50 times on each side, after which grasp-massage the "feng-ch'ih" and "chien-ching" points (applying strong stimulation) 20 to 30 times. Finally repeat the wiping-massage regimen, going from the "yin-t'ang" to the "ts'an-ch'u" to the "t'ai-yang" points for a total of 10 times.

   Treat daily in this manner once or twice.

3. Chinese herbs

   For exposure headache (See under section for epidemic influenza).

   For liver yang-dominant headache. Treatment should quiet the liver and quell the wind with remedies such as one of the following:

a. Concoction of
   Lung-tan ts'ao (gentiana   3 ch'ien
   Chrysanthemum flowers   3 ch'ien
   K'ou-t'eng (Uncaria sinensis)   4 ch'ien
   Tu-li (oyster shell), precooked   1 liang
   Magnetite, precooked   1 liang
   Ch'uan-kung (Conioselinum
                 unuitlatum)   1.5 ch'ien
   Hsia-ku ts'ao (Brunella uulgaris) 4 ch'ien

b. Ta-ch'ing ken (roots)   1 liang
   Eggs   3

   Cook together. Eat as food.

For kidney deficient headaches. Treatment should nourish the yin and
supplement the kidneys, with remedies such as one of the following:

a. Chi-chu ti-huang (Rehmannia glutinosa) pill (patent medicine),
   3 ch'ien each time, taken with salted boiled water, 2-3 times
   daily.

b. Concoction of
   Tang-shen (Campanumaea pilosa)   3 ch'ien
   Shu-ti (processed ti-huang   3 ch'ien
   Shan-yao (yam)   3 ch'ien
   Shan chu-yu (Cornus officinalis)   2 ch'ien
   Tu-chung (Eucommia ulmoides)   3 ch'ien
   Tang-kuei (Angelica sinensis)   3 ch'ien
   Kou-chi (Lycium chinense)   3 ch'ien

4. Other

a. Aspirin compound, 1 tablet, 3 times daily. Used generally
   for most headaches.

b. Phenergan, 25 mg each time, 3 times daily.

c. Treating cause of headache.

Dizziness

Dizziness is frequently manifested in a visual blurring of images and
a sense of disbalance, with oneself and external objects going around in circles. In mild cases, one only feels unsteady on one's feet, without the feeling of going around in circles. This is called "t'ou-yun" in contrast to the
more severe "hsuan-yun" (dizziness).

In certain diseases of the chest, ear, cardiovascular or central nervous systems, dizziness does occur. (See Table 6-3-3).

Types of Dizziness

According to the different nature of the dizziness experienced, the clinical types most often seen are usually associated with a stagnation in sputum and moisture, an abnormal rise in liver yang-dominance, and energy and blood deficiencies. Types of dizziness are classified as follows:

Due to sputum and moisture stagnation. Symptoms are a dizzy heavy-headedness, uneasy feeling in the chest, nausea, vomiting and spitting (of saliva), white and greasy tongue coating, a slippery pulse.

Due to abnormal rise in liver yang-dominance. Symptoms and restless-ness, ill temper, insomnia, a dry and bitter taste in mouth, white or slightly yellow tongue fur, full pulse.

Due to energy and blood deficiencies. Symptoms are facial pallor, absence of mental sparkle, palpitation, tinnitus, spots before eyes, a flat taste in mouth, thin tongue coating, weak pulse.

Treatment

1. New acupuncture therapy. Apply medium stimulation to "nei-kuan," "fend-ch'ih," "pai-hui," "t'ai-ch'ung," and "san-yin-chiao" points.

2. Massage therapy. Follow technique described under "Headache."

3. Chinese herbs.

For dizziness due to sputum and moisture stagnation. Dissipate the sputum and resolve the moisture, with remedies such as the follow-ing:

a. Concoction of
Processed pan-hsia   3 ch'ien
Toasted pai-shu   3 ch'ien
T'ien-ma   3 ch'ien
Fu-ling   3 ch'ien
Ch'en-p'i (orange peel, dried)   2 ch'ien

b. Concoction of
Processed pan-hsia   3 ch'ien
Dried orange peel   1.5 ch'ien
Fu-ling   3 ch'ien
Tender bamboo shoots   3 ch'ien
Chih-shih (acorns)   1.5 ch'ien
Huang-lien (Coptis chinensis)   1 ch'ien

For dizziness due to abnormal rise in liver yang-dominance.
Balance the liver and quell the yang, with remedy such as the
following concoction:

T'ien-ma	3 ch'ien
K'ou-t'eng (Uncaria sinensis)	4 ch'ien
Mother-of-pearl (precooked)	1 liang
Magnetite (precooked)	1 liang
Hsia-ku ts'ao	4 ch'ien
Lung-tan ts'ao (gentiana)	3 ch'ien
Yeh chiao t'eng	5 ch'ien

For dizziness due to simultaneous energy and blood deficiencies
[anemia]. Aid the wind and supplement the blood with remedies such
as the following:

a. Concoction of

Ta-hsueh t'eng (Sargentodoxa cuneata)	1 liang
Kang-nien kuo	1 liang
Li-chih, edible fruit dried (litsi nephelium)	5 ch'ien
Lung-yen, edible fruit dried (litsi longana)	5 ch'ien
Tang-shen	5 ch'ien
Dates (meat)	3 ch'ien

b. Extract of shan chi-hsueh t'eng prepared as follows: Cut up
3 chin of shan chi-hsueh t'eng, add water, and cook slowly
until well done. Strain, and cook liquid some more until liquid
is reduced to 500 ml. Take with a small amount of rice wine,
3 times a day, 15-20 ml each time. The chief benefit of this
prescription is its blood-building properties.

c. Shih-ch'uan ta-pu yuan [Most complete building (blood) pill]
(patent medicine). Take 3 times daily, 3 ch'ien each time.

4. Other

Tranquillizers may be given. If vomiting continues, phenothiazine
12.5 mg may be given intramuscularly. Also hypertonic dextrose
solution given intravenously.

Treat cause of dizziness.

Appendix: Seasickness (Carsickness)

For some individuals, riding in an automobile or travelling by boat is
enough to bring on symptoms such as nausea and vomiting, gastric discomfort,
listlessness, increased or slowered pulse rate, blurred vision, clammy sweating, and even fainting. This phenomenon is referred to as carsickness or
seasickness.

Table 6-3-3. Differential Diagnosis of Dizziness

Disease (illness)	Symptoms	Physical findings
Hypertension	Dizziness, headache, feeling of fullness in head, palpitation, increased severity of headache after excitement, increased blood pressure.	Blood pressure reading over 140/90 mm, enlarged heart possibly displaced to left, murmurs heard over apex during systole
Neurasthenia	Dizziness, headache, tinnitus, spots before eyes, poor memory, inability to concentrate, insomnia, and other ill-defined symptoms.	No obvious physical findings
Hysteria	History of repeated recurrences, manifested by irregular convulsions, dizziness, and ability to remember what happened after attack. No incontinence of urine or feces	No noticeable positive positive physical findings.
Epilepsy	Loud cry heard at onset of attack, with loss of consciousness. Whole body goes into convulsive spasms, foaming at mouth, loss of bowel and urinary control. Post-attack dizziness and headache, nervous exhaustion	Pupils dilated during attack
Anemia	Facial pallor, dizziness and spots before eyes, tinnitus, palpitation	Conjunctiva under eyelids and tips of fingers pale
Otogenic vertigo (Meniere's disease)	Sudden dizziness occurring with a feeling that external objects and the victim are going around in circles, nausea and vomiting, sweating, and mental confusion in serious cases	Nystagmus
Brain tumor	Headache and dizziness becoming progressively severe, often accompanied by stubborn vomiting; in certain cases patient can lie only on one side and appear unsteady on his feet	Nystagmus
Carsickness, seasickness	Occurring when riding in automobile or sailing on ship, accompanied by nausea and vomiting, dizziness.	

Seasickness (or carsickness) is due primarily to a disturbance in the function of the vestibular nerve which serves to maintain the body's equilibrium.

Because of differences in the physical makeup of different individuals, the speed and severity of the reactions produced will vary among them. To prevent such symptoms from occurring, when travelling by car or boat, keep eyes on some distant non-moving object. Do not close eyes, or follow movement of moving vehicle. Maintain air ventilation in the car or boat, and not let air become hot and humid. If seasickness or carsickness does occur, use needle-puncture, or pinch-pull with fingers the skin over the "nei-kuan" point. (Many individuals prone to carsickness will use needle puncture at the "nei kuan" upon boarding vehicle, as a preventive measure.) Or, use ch'ing-liang yu [a "cooling" camphorated oil somewhat like Vicks or Mentholatum?], ch'ing-liang yuan, or chlorpromazine, or tincture of belladonna as preventive measures.

Coughing

Coughing is a symptom frequently associated with diseases of the respiratory system. Besides respiratory tract ailments that cause coughing, others are associated with cardiac failure and acute infectious diseases under certain conditions. (Table 6-3-4).

Types of Coughing

According to different manifestations of the coughing (etiology, complications, physical makeup of patient, and season), coughing is clinically considered mostly as wind-chill, wind-heat, dry-heat, sputum-moisture, and deficiency types.

Wind-chill (feng-han) cough. The sputum is loose. Other symptoms are a stuffy nose, running nose, chills and fever, thin and white fur on tongue.

Wind-heat (feng-jeh) cough. Sputum is more difficult to bring up during coughing spell. Fever, a parched mouth, sore throat, thin and yellow fur on tongue, slippery pulse may be other symptoms.

Dry-heat (tsao-huo) cough. Cough dry and unproductive. Mouth, lips and throat all dry, tip of tongue red.

Sputum-moist (t'an-shih) cough. Sputum mostly thick and tenacious, rasping heard in throat, chest tight, and breathing rapid.

Deficiency (hsu) cough. Coughing intermittent. Facial pallor present, as are a flushed face, shortness of breath, weakness, sometimes hemoptysis or blood-streaked sputum, or feverish hands, feet and heart. Pulse deficient, tongue red and uncoated.

Table 6-3-4 Differential Diagnosis of Cough

Disease	Symptoms	Physical findings
Upper respiratory tract infections	Sudden onset accompanied by coughing, stuffy nose, running nose, chills, fever (some patients do not have fever symptoms)	Nasal secretions present, throat congested
Bronchitis	In acute cases, coughing present with some sputum brought up, and often accompanied by fever; in chronic cases, condition more serious in cold weather, and lets up in warm weather	Dry and moist rales heard
Bronchial asthma	Severe coughing, generally worse at night, accompanied by respiratory difficulty, inability to lie flat, and coughing up a white foamy sputum when attack about to subside.	Whistling sounds heard over lungs
Bronchiectasis	Purulent sputum may be brought up over long period of chronic coughing, particularly profuse during change of position; sputum frequently blood-streaked or hemoptysis may be present	A few dry or moist rales heard over lungs
Bronchial carcinoma, lung cancer	Occurring in individuals over middle age, characterized by non-expectorant cough, blood-streaked sputum, pain in chest, rapid loss of weight	Malignancy symptoms appearing during late stage
Lobar pneumonia	Onset sudden, accompanied by chills, high fever, continuous coughing, and following development of disease, the appearance of rust-stained sputum and more noticeable pain in chest	Bronchial breathing sounds and moist rales heard over affected lung, marked increase in leukocyte, neutrophil, and granulocyte count

Table 6-3-4 (Continued)

Disease	Symptoms	Physical findings
Lung abscess	High fever, large quantities of yellow or green purulent sputum which separates into three layers upon settling; lobar pneumonia when not treated in time may develop into a complicating lung abscess	Moist rales heard over lungs
Pulmonary tuberculosis	Characterized by flushed face, recurring fever, poor appetite, hidrosis, dull pain in chest, sputum regularly blood-streaked or bloody	
Pertussis (whooping cough)	Seen mostly in children, characterized by spells of continuous coughing that ends with a characteristic whoop, much like the last sound of a cock's crow	Dry rales sometimes heard over lungs
Cardiac failure	Characterized by history of heart disease, coughing, dyspnea, inability to lie down flat, sputum pinkish	Lips purplish and cyanotic, moist rales heard over both lungs, tachycardia, murmurs sometimes heard
Diphtheria	Fever, coughing coarse and croupy, similar to dog's bark. In serious cases, laryngeal obstruction may occur, accompanied by respiratory difficulty, stridor, cyanosis, and extreme restlessness	Milky white or greyish white pseudomembrane over the pharynx, trachea, or tonsils -- not easily removed. Will bleed superficially if force is used to detach this covering

Treatment

1. New acupuncture therapy. Apply medium stimulation to needle puncture performed over the "ch'ih-tse," "feng-lung," "fei-yu" points, once a day. Cupping by "pa-huo-kuan" may be done over the "fei-yu" point.

2. Chinese herbs

   a. Wind-chill cough. Treatment emphasizes deflating the wind to dispel the chill with one of following preparation:

      (1) Concoction of
          Tzu-su   3 liang
          Ch'ien-hu   3 liang
          Ching-chieh   2 ch'ien
          Pan-hsia (processed)   3 ch'ien
          Chieh-keng   3 ch'ien
          Orange peel, dried   2 ch'ien
          Licorice   1 ch'ien

      (2) Preparation of
          Shu-ch'u ts'ao (whole plant 5-8 ch'ien, steeped in boiled water for one hour. Take warm.

      (3) T'ung-hsuan li-fei yuan (patent medicine). Take one or two pills each time, once or twice daily. Take with boiled water.

   b. Wind-heat cough. Treatment directed to clearing fever and resolving the sputum, with concoctions such as the following:

      (1) Concoction of
          Ma-huang (ephedra)   1.5 ch'ien
          Hsing-jen (almonds)   3 ch'ien
          Gypsum   1 liang
          Licorice   1 ch'ien

      (2) Concoction of
          Mulberry leaves   3 ch'ien
          Chrysanthemum flowers   3 ch'ien
          Hsing-jen (almonds)   3 ch'ien
          Licorice   1 ch'ien
          Chieh-keng   2 ch'ien
          Lien-ch'iao (Forsythia suspensa) 3 ch'ien
          Mint   1 ch'ien
          Lu ken (roots of bulrush) 1 liang

      (3) Concoction of
          Leaves of p'i-p'a (loquats), fuzz removed   1 liang
          Mulberry leaves   1 liang
          Ch'e-ch'ien ts'ao (Plantago)   1 liang

   c. Dry-heat cough. Treatment directed toward clearing the dryness, and moisturizing the lungs, with preparations such as the following:

- 233 -

(1) Concoction of
   Sha-shen   4 ch'ien
   Kuan-yin tso-lien   2 ch'ien
   P'i-p'a (loquat) leaves   5 ch'ien

(2) Concoction of
   Mulberry leaves
   Hsing-jen (almonds)   3 ch'ien
   Leaves of p'i-p'a (loquat), hairs removed 3 ch'ien
   Mai-tung   3 ch'ien
   Sha-shen   3 ch'ien

(3) Preparation of ch'uan-pei (Fritillaria roylei) and p'i-
   p'a in a patented medicine, 2 spoonsful each time, two or
   three times a day.

d. <u>Sputum-moist cough</u>. Treatment should warm-dry the moisture
   and resolve the sputum, with preparations such as the following:

(1) Concoction of
   Ma-huang (ephedra)   1.5 ch'ien
   Hsing-jen (almonds)   3 ch'ien
   Processed pan-hsia   3 ch'ien
   Orange peel, dried   2 ch'ien
   Fu-ling   3 ch'ien
   Pai-shu   3 ch'ien
   Hou-pu   2 ch'ien
   Licorice   1 ch'ien

(2) Preparation of
   Tsao-chia (shelled, toasted and
                    pulverized)   5 fen
   Ta-ts'ao (dates)   3

(3) Chi-hung yuan (patent medicine). Two pills to be taken
   each time, once in the morning, and once at night, with
   boiled water.

e. <u>Deficiency cough</u>. Treatment concentrates on supplementing
   and benefitting the pulmonary energy.

(1) Concoction of pai-ho (lily) 1 liang cooked with ta-ts'ao
   (date) 1 liang, and eaten.

(2) Concoction of 3 ch'ien each of
   Tang-shen
   Pai-ho
   Huan-tung hua

- 234 -

(3) Mixture of
   Unglutinous rice (cooked into thin gruel)   2 liang
   Extract of crude ti-huang (<u>Rehmannia glutinosa</u>),
     soaked in boiled water, crushed, and
     extracted for juice   1 small cup

   Mix well, and take warm. (This prescription is used for
   hemoptysis, and feverish hands and feet and heart.)

3. <u>Other treatments</u>

   a. Licorice compound, 10 ml each dose, 3 times daily. If sputum
      is tenacious and not easily coughed up, add ammonium chloride.

   b. Anti-tussive (Ti-ke), 10 ml each time, 3 times daily.

<u>Note</u>: Since coughing performs an expectorating function to bring up
sputum, do not use cough sedatives carelessly. The emphasis is on treating
cause of illness.

                          Dyspnea

    When a patient experiences dyspnea, he is not getting enough air and
shows various signs of laboring to relieve this air hunger. For example, the
nasal nares are pinched in the effort, the mouth is open and gasping, and
there are changes in the number, depth, and regularity of the respirations.
In severe cases, the patient is frequently forced to assume a sitting or semi-
recumbent position to make breathing easier. When anoxia is severe, cyanosis
may set in. Besides respiratory tract illnesses that provoke dyspnea, others
are certain heart failure conditions or intoxicating illnesses (Table 6-3-5).

<u>Treatment</u>

    1. <u>Maintaining patency of respiratory tract</u>. Suction sputum out with
rubber tubing attached to 50-ml syringe. In case of emergency, start mouth-
to-mouth sputum suction, and administer oxygen when needed.

    2. <u>New acupuncture therapy</u>. Apply needle puncture of medium stimu-
lation intensity over the "t'ien-tu," "t'an-chung," "nei-kuan" points, (for
healthy individuals, strong stimulation may be used) once daily.

Table 6-3-5. Differential Diagnosis of Dyspnea

Disease (illness)	History of illness	Symptoms	Physical findings
Bronchial asthma	History of recurring attacks	Respiratory difficulty the primary symptom at onset, accompanied by coughing and coughed-up foamy sputum	Whistling sounds heard over both lungs
Asthmatic bronchitis	History of bronchitis	Coughing, yellow sputum, accompanied by fever, chills	Scattered wheezes heard over both lungs; also fine moist rales heard sometimes
Emphysema	History of chronic cough and bronchial asthma	Coughing and shortness of breath over a long period	High pitch clear sounds heard on percussion of lungs, breathing sounds low, heart sounds light; sometimes accompanied by a barrel chest
Lobar pneumonia	Onset acute. No history of dyspnea	Coughing, pain in chest, high fever, rust-colored sputum coughed up	Dull sounds emitting during percussion of affected side, with moist rales heard sometimes, and increased quiver in speech
Pleural effusion	History of tuberculosis frequently found	Coughing, pain in chest, and fever	Lowered breathing sounds heard over affected side, solid sounds heard on percussion, and lowered quiver in speech

Table 6-3-5 (Continued)

Disease (illness)	History of illness	Symptoms	Physical findings
Cardiac failure	History of heart disease	Cyanosis, palpitation, edema, restlessness	Moist rales may be heard over both lungs, rapid heart beat, liver enlarged, lower limbs edematous
Hysteria	Related to nervous factors	Shortness of breath, numbness or convulsions of hands and feet	No positive physical findings

3. **Chinese herbs**

   a. Generally consult section on "Asthma" to provide symptomatic treatment.

   b. Use the following homemade preparation consisting of 3 ch'ien of ya-tsao [legume of Gleditschia japonica?] shelled, crushed and concocted into extract for local treatment of air passageway. Draw extract into pipette and drop 20 drops onto patient's throat. Observe to see how patient coughs and bring up sputum. If not satisfactory, drop some more medication until the plug of mucus is brought up and breathing is easy again. (This prescription is suitable for loosening up tenacious mucus and tight breathing in patients with laryngeal obstruction.)

4. **Other**

   a. Tranquillizer: Phenergan 12.5-25 mg, given by mouth or intramuscular injection, three times daily.

   b. Aminophylline 0.1 gm, three times daily, by mouth. In emergency give aminophylline 0.25 gm added to 20 ml of 50 percent dextrose intravenously. Or add same amount (0.25 gm) to 500 ml of 50 percent dextrose and give by intravenous drip.

   c. Coramine 0.375 gm given intramuscularly or intravenously. Repeat when necessary.

   d. Treatment of cause. If cardiac failure is the cause, give a digitalis preparation; if a lung infection, a suitable antibiotic etc.

   e. If breathing stops, start artificial respiration immediately.

Chest Pain

Chest pain is a common symptom associated with chest diseases, such as those affecting organs contained in the chest cavity -- the heart, lungs, pleura, esophagus, and the vascular and neural pathways (Table 6-3-6).

Types

According to different manifestations, chest pain is usually classified into lung-heated (fei-jeh), energy stagnation (ch'i chi), blood-clotting (hsueh yen), moist-hot (shih-jeh) etc., types.

Table 6-3-6 Differential Diagnosis of Chest Pain

Disease	Symptoms	Physical findings
Intercostal neuritis	Stabbing pain felt along the inter-costal network of nerves over the chest, frequently heightened during coughing and deep breathing	No obvious positive physical finding
Fractured rib(s)	History of trauma, pressure pain over fracture site, hematoma	Noticeable crepitus heard
Herpes zoster	Location of herpes following dis-tribution of intercostal nerves, spreading from back to front, pain extremely severe	Herpes forming belt pattern
Pneumothorax	Onset of chest pain sudden, accom-panied by dyspnea, air hunger, cyanosis	Breathing sounds over affected side lower-pitched, percussion evoking a high clear sound, bronchus dis-placed toward healthy side
Pleurisy	Onset insidious, chest pain in-creased on coughing and during breathing; fever, coughing, and dyspnea present sometimes	Sounds on affected side dull on percussion, breathing sounds low-ered, and speech vi-bration weakened
Lobar pneumonia, lung abscess, pulmonary tuber-culosis, bronchial carcinoma and lung cancer	See Table 6-3-4 on differential diagnosis of cough	
Angina	History of heart disease. Seen mostly among the middle-aged and the aged. Feeling of pressure in area of heart during attack. Pain radiating to left-shoulder and arm, sometimes accompanied by cold sweat	

Table 6-3-6 (Continued)

Disease	Symptoms	Physical findings
Myocardial infarction	Excruciating pain felt suddenly over region in front of heart, usually in evening, accompanied by a drop in blood pressure, facial pallor, cold sweat, cold and clammy extremities and other symptoms of shock	
Pericarditis	Pain in pre-cardial region, accompanied by fever, cold sweat, and exhaustion. Dyspnea and coughing sometimes present	Tachycardia, and sound of pericardium rubbing heard

Lung-heated type. Mostly a burning pain in the chest, accompanied by coughing, spitting of yellow sputum, fever, chills, a thin white coating on tongue, and rapid pulse.

Energy-stagnation type. Pain that is felt on expansion of chest and sides, coming at regular intervals, characterized by belching, fur on tongue thin-white or absent, slow pulse.

Blood-clotting type. Stabbing pain generally felt in chest and sides, with petechial spots on tongue, irregular pulse.

Moist-hot type. Pain in chest and sides, characterized by a reddish-brown urine, red and furry white-yellowish tongue, slippery and rapid pulse.

Treatment

1. New acupuncture therapy. Use strong stimulation with the needle technique from the "nei-kuan" point penetrating the "wai-kuan" and "yang-ling" points. Puncture in this manner once a day.

2. Massage therapy. Knead-massage over the "t'an-chung" point. Combine knead-massage with the press-rotate technique over the "kao-meng-yu" for 1-2 minutes.

3. Chinese herbs

   a. For lung-heated chest pain. Treatment is directed toward clearing the pulmonary heat [or fever], with a remedy such as the following concoction:
      Honeysuckle blossoms   5 ch'ien
      Forsythia suspensa   5 ch'ien
      Kua-wei   4 ch'ien
      Pei-mu (Frittillaria roylei)   3 ch'ien

- 240 -

Fresh roots from reeds (with knots   2 liang
    removed)
Tung-kua-tzu   2 liang
Seeds of I-tz'u   5 ch'ien
Fresh yu-hsing ts'ao   1 liang
Chieh-keng   2 ch'ien
T'ing-li tzu   3 ch'ien

b. For <u>energy-stagnation chest pain</u>. Treatment should concentrate
   on correcting the energy, with concoctions such as the following:
   (1) Concoction of
        Wu-pu-ch'a   5 ch'ien
        Orange peel, old   2 ch'ien
        Kua-wei   3 ch'ien
        Pan-hsia, processed   2 ch'ien
        Hsiang-fu   3 ch'ien
        Yu-chin   2 ch'ien
        Hsuan-fu hua   3 ch'ien
        Chih-ho (acorn shells)   2 ch'ien

   (2) Concoction of
        Chin-ling-tzu   3 ch'ien
        Yen-hu-so   4 ch'ien
        Kuang-mu-hsiang   1.5 ch'ien
        Hsiang-fu, processed   3 ch'ien
        Yu-chin   3 ch'ien
        Chih-ho   1.5 ch'ien

c. For <u>blood-clotting chest pain</u>. Treatment should stimulate
   blood circulation and resolve the clots, with concoction such
   as the following:
   Tan-shen   5 ch'ien
   Tang-kuei   5 ch'ien
   Ling-chih (bat droppings)   3 ch'ien
   P'u-huang   3 ch'ien
   Ch'ih-yao   3 ch'ien
   T'ao-jen (kernel of peach)   2 ch'ien
   Toasted licorice   1 ch'ien

d. For <u>moist-hot chest pain</u>. Treatment should clear fever and demoisturize with remedies such as the following:
   (1) Concoction of
        Crude ti-huang   5 ch'ien
        Tang-kuei   3 ch'ien
        Tan ts'ao   3 ch'ien
        Shan-chih   3 ch'ien
        Huang ching   3 ch'ien
        Tapioca   4 ch'ien
        Tse-hsieh   4 ch'ien
        Che-ch'ien-tzu   4 ch'ien

(2) Local application of shang-shih chih-t'ung (analgesic moisture-counteracting plaster) to local region.

4. Other

a. Selective use of pain relievers such as analgine, "yu-sa-t'ung.

b. Local 10 percent procaine block to treat localized pain, quite effective for intercostal neuritis.

c. Immediate hospitalization and emergency care of chest pain is suspected to be caused by angina, myocardial infarction or pneumothorax. Time is of the essence. Even more important is treating the cause of chest pain.

Vomiting

The symptoms of vomiting, besides those traceable to diseases and ailments of the digestive system may also be due to certain diseases of the central nervous system (Table 6-3-7).

Table 6-3-7. Differential Diagnosis of Vomiting

Disease	Symptoms	Physical findings
Cancer of the esophagus	Progressive worsening of condition from possible intake of soft food to inability to tolerate liquid food, until water cannot even be swallowed in the final stages. Seen usually in older individuals. Emaciation present. A nauseous and painful sensation experienced (by patient) behind the sternum	
Chronic gastritis	Upper abdominal pain, a burning and full sensation felt after eating, poor appetite, halitosis, belching	Pressure pain sometimes felt over epigastrium
Gastric ulcers	Pyloric obstruction caused by ulcers characterized by obvious vomiting with chronic, regular, periodic epigastric pain	Pressure pain over epigastrium, swishing sound heard with pyloric obstruction
Gastric perforation	Sudden and acute epigastric pain frequently occurring after a full meal. History of ulcers	Abdominal muscles tensed up like board, boundary of hepatic murmur dissipated

- 242 -

Table 6-3-7 (Continued)

Disease	Symptoms	Physical findings
Cancer of the stomach	Occurring in older individuals, with progressive emaciation, noticeable vomiting during pyloric obstruction phase	Mass felt in epigastrium upon palpation, clavicular lymphadenopathy present, occult blood in stool over long period
Acute infectious hepatitis	Fever, nausea, vomiting, aversion to greasy foods, jaundice sometimes appearing with drop in body temperature, urine reddish tea brown	Some hepatomegaly and pressure pain present. Conjunctiva yellow
Intestinal obstruction	Abdominal pain, intermittent, constipation, vomitus containing bile or fecal-like matter	Tenderness over abdomen, peristaltic waves visible
Epidemic encephalomyelitis	Sudden high fever, headache, projectile vomiting, petechial spots, coma, convulsions, incidence in winter-spring	Neck rigid, Kernig's sign and Babinski's sign (sole-of-foot scratch test) positive
Epidemic Japanese B encephalitis	High fever, headache, vomiting, restlessness, coma, incidence of disease occurring in summer/fall.	Neck sometimes rigid, and Kernig's sign and Babinski's sign sometimes positive
Vomiting of pregnancy	Nausea and vomiting in normally menstruating women 2 months after sudden cessation of menstruation	

Types

On the basis of different conditions surrounding the vomiting, the types frequently seen are cold vomiting (han-ou), heat vomiting (jeh-ou), deficiency vomiting (hsu-ou), and salivary vomiting (yin-ou).

Cold vomiting: Caused mostly by exposure to cold, the vomitus usually contains undigested food, or clear fluid. Mouth is not dry, and patient shows a liking for warmth and an aversion to cold. Or the abdomen may experience mild cramps, and the patient likes heat and some pressure over the area. Pulse mostly sunken and delayed.

Heat vomiting. Mostly due to summer heat, the vomiting occurs as soon as the food is ingested, becoming increasingly worse. Patient prefers cold to heat, mouth is dry, urine brown and scanty, pulse rapid, and fur on tongue yellow.

Deficiency vomiting. Due mostly to overeating, this type of vomiting occurs with regularity. The onset is insidious and course of disease lengthy. However, chest is not painful or distended, and patient prefers warmth to coolness. Tongue fur is thin and white, pulse sunken and thready, or sunken and weak.

Salivary vomiting. Because of mucus saliva in the body system, vomiting occurs frequently. The vomitus is frequently saliva. Mouth is dry. No desire is felt for drinking water, as drinking water provokes the vomiting reflex. Nausea and dizziness are present, tongue fur greasy and white, pulse slippery and rapid.

Treatment

1. New acupuncture therapy. Apply moderate stimulation to needle puncture of the "nei-kuan" point in upward direction, twirling for 2 minutes. For abdominal pain, apply needle technique to the "tsu-san-li" also.

2. Chinese herbs.

    a. For cold vomiting. Dispel cold to stop vomiting is suggested, using the following remedies:

        (1) Mixture of

Juice of fresh ginger	1 cup
Juice of tzu-su leaves	1 cup

Take with warm boiled water.

        (2) Concoction of

Processed pan-hsia	3 ch'ien
Dried orange peel	1 ch'ien
Juice of fresh ginger	1/2 spoonful

    b. For heat vomiting. Clear fever (heat) to stop vomiting with the following:

        (1) Concoction of

Roots of fresh bulrushes	1 liang
Fresh bamboo shoots	1 liang

        (2) Concoction of

Szechuan lotus	1.5 ch'ien

Divide into two doses, and take with one-half spoonful of fresh ginger juice.

c. **For deficiency vomiting.** Warm and supplement the stomach with the following:

    (1) Concoction of
Tang-shen	3 ch'ien
Processed pan-hsia	3 ch'ien

    (2) Concoction of
Toasted ginger	1 ch'ien
Pai-shu	3 ch'ien
Tai-che-shih	4 ch'ien

       [substitute hematite?]

    (3) Hsiang-sha Lu-chun yuan
       (patent medicine),   2 ch'ien
    each time taken by mouth, twice daily.

d. **For salivary vomiting.** Dispel the saliva to stop vomiting with the following:

    (1) Concoction of
Processed pan-hsia	3 ch'ien
Fu-ling	3 ch'ien
Fresh ginger	2 ch'ien

    Take twice a day.

    (2) Concoction of roots of I-tz'u   2 liang, boiled down to concentrate. Take continuously until vomiting is stopped.

    (3) Hsiang-sha yang-wei yuan (patent medicine). Take 3 ch'ien each time, three times daily.

3. **Other**

a. Belladonna compound tablets, three times daily, 1-2 tablets each time.

b. Tranquillizer phenothiazine 12.5 - 25 mg each time, three times daily.

c. For severe vomiting accompanied by dehydration, give intravenous drip, 1000-2000 ml of 5 percent dextrose or saline to which is added 1000 mg of vitamin C.

Diarrhea

As a symptom, diarrhea is characterized by loose frequent stools.
Besides digestive tract ailments that may cause diarrhea, certain infectious
diseases, parasitical infestations, tumors or intoxications can also cause
diarrhea (Table 6-3-8).

Table 6-3-8. Differential Diagnosis of Diarrhea

Disease	Symptoms	Physical findings
Bacterial dysentery	Aversion to cold, presence of fever, abdominal pain, diarrhea, tenesmus, mucopurulent and bloody stools	Pressure pain over lower left abdomen
Amebic dysentery	Low grade or no fever at all, diarrhea, no obvious sign of urgency to stool, and no tenesmus. Bean-sauce like stool, frequently emitting characteristic odor	Pressure pain over lower right abdomen
Acute gastroenteritis	History of unsanitary eating habits or of frequent exposures (to chill), vomitus gassy and sour-smelling, watery stools, sense of relief often felt after defecation	Pressure pain over epigastrium or area surrounding umbilicus
Food poisoning (due to Salmonella, Staphylococcal organisms)	Frequently a history of eating in-adequately cooked crabs, spoilt fish and meat and other unsanitary eating habits. Others eating the same food showing the same symptoms, seen as vomiting, diarrhea, watery stools, sometimes accompanied by fever and colic around the umbilical region	
Indigestion	Caused usually by improper feeding in infants, and chronic disease of the gastrointestinal tract in adults undigested food particles seen in stools	Emaciation, anemia, malnutrition
Schistosomiasis	History of contract with contaminated waters, diarrhea generally mild, stools sometimes purulent and bloody, hepato-splenomegaly present, fever and urticaria in acute cases	

Table 6-3-8 (Continued)

Disease	Symptoms	Physical findings
Intestinal tuberculosis	Frequently a history of tuberculosis, abdominal distension, diarrhea and constipation alternating, right lower abdominal pain usually occurring after meals, relieved after defecation.	Pressure pain over right lower abdomen
Cancer of the colon, cancer of the rectum	Occurring usually among the middle-aged and above, accompanied by anemia, weight loss, bloody stools, sometimes small stools in cancer of the rectum	Tumor mass palpable in cancer of the colon. In cancer of the rectum, a hard and irregular mass possibly felt on digital examination.
Chronic colitis	Duration long, symptoms light, white mucus in stools, abdominal pain increased before bowel movement and relieved after defecation.	No obvious physical findings

Types

Based on the causes of diarrhea and its clinical manifestations, diarrhea is generally classified into cold (han) diarrhea, heat (jeh) diarrhea, wet (shih) diarrhea and deficiency (hsu) diarrhea.

Cold diarrhea. Stools resemble duck droppings, not too smelly, possibly containing undigested particles. Other symptoms are an aversion to cold, spitting of clear saliva, clear urine and length urinary stream, mouth unparched. Fur of tongue white, pulse weak and slow.

Heat diarrhea. Stools resemble thin porridge, odor offensive, accompanied by burning sensation in the anus on defecation. Other symptoms are an aversion to heat, dryness and bitter taste in mouth, an inclination for cold drinks, and yellow urine passed. Fur of tongue yellow, pulse rapid.

Wet-(watery) diarrhea. Diarrhea that results from working in damp places or in the rain over a long period of time, characterized by watery stools, abdominal distension, "gassy" rumblings in abdomen, scanty urine, sallow complexion, nausea, no appetite, and feeling of weightiness. Fur of tongue white and greasy, pulse slippery.

Deficiency diarrhea. Duration of diarrhea somewhat longer, physical condition weakened. Stools resemble rice rinse water, or watery and containing undigested food, or characterized by urge to move bowels at daybreak, or by unconscious movement of bowels in severe cases. Complexion sallow, extremities weak, and spirits poor. Pulse usually sunken and fine.

Treatment

1. New acupuncture therapy. Medium stimulation to needles placed into "t'ien-shu," "ch'i-hai, " and "tsu-san-li," points, once a day. Or use moxibustion around umbilical region for 10 minutes.

2. Chinese herbs.

 a. For cold diarrhea. Warm the central organs and stop diarrhea with the following remedies:

  (1) Concoction of
Pai-shu (atractylis ovata)	3 ch'ien
Dry ginger	1 ch'ien

  (2) Concoction of
Dry moxa leaves	1 bunch
Rice (stir-fried toasted brown)	3 ch'ien

  Mix with 3 ch'ien of brown sugar before taking by mouth

  (3) Fu-tzu [Aconitum fischere] li-chung yuan (patent medicine). Take 1 ch'ien each time, 3 times daily.

 b. For heat diarrhea. Clear the fever to stop the diarrhea, with the following remedies

  (1) Concoction of
Roots of ko-ken	3 ch'ien
Huang-lien (Coptis chinensis)	2 ch'ien
Huang-ch'ing	2 ch'ien
Licorice	1 ch'ien

  (2) Concoction of
Lu-tou (mung bean)	2 liang
Che-ch'ien-tsao	1 liang

  (3) Fresh pepperweed (la-liao ts'ao) 1 bunch, in concoction

 c. For wet diarrhea. Resolve the moisture to stop the diarrhea with the following:

(1) Pulverize
     Tsang-shu   1 liang
     Che-ch'ien tsao   1 liang

     Take 2 ch'ien of the mixture each time, stirred in
     some boiled water

(2) Concentrated concoction of
     Alum   1.2 ch'ien
     Black or green tea   1.2 ch'ien

     Take for three successive days, 3 times a day.

(3) Lu-I san (patent medicine). Take 3 ch'ien each time,
     two times a day.

  d. For deficiency diarrhea. Warm and supplement the stomach-
spleen with the following remedies.

(1) Stir-fry brown and pulverize
     Wu-wei tzu   2 liang
     Wu chu-yu   5 ch'ien

     Mix with crushed date meats to form pills. Take 2-3
     ch'ien each time. Or mix with dry tangerine or orange
     peel and concoct. Take twice daily.

(2) Concoction of
     Pai-shu   3 ch'ien
     Shan-yao   3 ch'ien

     Add 4 ch'ien of rock sugar to concoction. Take in one
     dose.

(3) Ssu-shen (the four gods) yuan (patent medicine). Take
     3 ch'ien each time, twice daily.

  3. Diet (food and drink). Give rice congee rice soup, noodles and
other easily digested pasta. Encourage patient to drink more boiled salt
water. If dehydration is evidenced, encourage fluid supplement.

Constipation

When the conducting function of the large intestine is disturbed, and
fecal matter retained in the intestines over a longer period becomes so dry
and hard that a bowel movement is not possible within a 48-hour period. The
condition is called constipation.

Diseases causing constipation are numerous. For example, chronic emphysema bronchial asthma, obesity, ascites, abdominal tumor, hemorrhoids, malnutrition among the aged, consumptive or chronically febrile illnesses etc. Sedentary activity or pregnancy are also likely causes of constipation.

Types

Because the causes of constipation and their clinical manifestations vary, the commonly seen types are classified as hot constipation (jeh-pi), cold constipation (han-pi), gassy constipation (ch'i-pi), and bloody constipation (hsueh-pi).

Hot constipation. The stools are hardened, and the bowels will not move. Mouth is dry, lips are black, breath is unpleasant, or mouth tastes bitter, face is flushed, and body feels hot. Abdomen is distended and painful, urine scanty and brown, fur on tongue yellow or yellow and dry, and pulse slippery and solid.

Cold constipation. No bowel movement lips pale, mouth not dry, no appetite, intermittent abdominal pain, cold hands and feet, urine clear and voluminous. Fur on tongue white, and pulse sunken and slow.

Gassy constipation. No bowel movement, abdominal distension painful. Belching and abdominal flatus present, discomfort relieved upon release of gas. Pulse tight, tongue fur white.

Bloody constipation. No bowel movement, stools tarry, abdomen distended and painful, restlessness present, no desire for water though mouth dry. Tongue purplish red, pulse jumpy.

Treatment

1. New acupuncture therapy. Apply medium-intensity stimulation to needle puncture performed over "ch'ang-ch'iang," "yang-ling ch'uan" points. Treat daily.

2. Chinese herbs.

a. For hot constipation. Clear fever and open bowels with following remedies:

   (1) Give concoction of
       Ta-huang   4 ch'ien
       Salt peter (Glaubers' salt)   2 ch'ien

   (2) Give ch'ing-ning yuan (patent medicine) 2-3 ch'ien at a time, twice daily.

   (3) Give sesame oil one-half cup to be mixed with rice rinse water.

(4) Apply poultice over the "ch'i-hai" point, prepared from three large snails, crushed, to which 3 fen of salt are added.

b. <u>For cold constipation</u>. Warm up the passageway and open up the bowels.

(1) Prepare extract obtained from steeping

Su-tzu	1 liang
Sesame seeds	5 ch'ien

Crush ingredients and extract juice. Cook with rice to make gruel.

(2) Give pan-liu yuan (patent medicine) [contains some sulfur?] 5 fen, once a day.

c. <u>Gassy constipation</u>. Correct "energy" dissipation and open up bowels.

(1) Toast 1 liang of ts'ao-ch'ueh-ming and give with honey.

(2) Give concoction of

Almonds	3 ch'ien
Kuo-wei skins	4 ch'ien
Pan-ta-hai	3 ch'ien

d. <u>For bloody constipation</u>. Nourish the blood and lubricate the intestines.

(1) Give concoction of

Tang-kuei	3 ch'ien
Huo-ma-jen	3 ch'ien

mixed with 5 ch'ien of honey, in one dose.

(2) Give concoction of

Black sesame seeds	1 liang
T'ao-jen [peach kernel]	5 ch'ien
Chi-shih [acorns]	1.5 ch'ien

3. Other

a. Give I-ch'ing-sung [laxative] or phenolphthalein, 1-2 tablets, at bedtime.

b. Give 50 percent magnesium sulfate by mouth, 10-40 ml.

c. Give 15-30 ml liquid paraffin at bedtime.

d. Besides eliminating cause of constipation, give enema when
    needed. Or insert a small soap suppository into anus to
    promote evacuation of bowels.

Abdominal Pain

A characteristic of acute abdominal pain in what is called an "acute
abdomen," is its sudden onset and rapid development, sometimes requiring immediate surgical treatment. Besides diseases of the digestive system that
may cause abdominal pain, other conditions such as pneumonia, kidney colic,
drug intoxication, or certain pelvic ailments in women can also cause abdominal pain (Table 6-3-9).

Characteristics of abdominal pain vary according to the etiology, and
the site, nature and symptoms of the pain. In differential diagnosis, one
must clearly recognize the actual nature of illness through the phenomenon
of abdominal pain. "All conclusions are the end results of investigation
and not its forerunner." Only by careful examination combined with possible
and necessary laboratory tests in an analytical study in depth, can we obtain
an early accurate diagnosis.

Treatment

1. Before diagnosis is clarified.

    a. Observe patient's general condition closely, checking his
        temperature, pulse, blood pressure etc., and changes in nature
        of local symptoms such as abdominal pain, pressure pain, the
        severity and extent of muscular tension, etc.

    b. Depending on the patient's condition, take proper measures to
        restrict diet, administer parenteral fluids, propping patient
        in semi-recumbent position, prevent infection, counteract
        shock and so forth.

    c. For pain, use needle puncture on "tsu-san-li," "yang-ling-
        ch'uan," "t'ai-ch'ung," "ho-ku" and other points. If "acute
        abdomen" symptoms are absent, tincture of belladonna or atropine
        can also be used to prevent pain. If the diagnosis is unclear,
        do not use morphine type drugs.

If, after a period of close observation, and the patient's condition
does not show any improvement, or if it becomes worse, have the patient taken
to hospital for further examination.

2. After the diagnosis is clarified, provide proper treatment, based
on different etiological factors. (See related sections).

Table 6-3-9. Differential Diagnosis of Abdominal Pain

Disease	Disease onset and history	Site of abdominal pain	Nature of abdominal pain	Abdominal symptoms	Other symptoms
Acute appendicitis	Gradual onset	Beginning in upper abdomen or around umbilicus, shifting gradually to lower right quadrant	Continuous pain accompanied by slight increase in paroxysmal pain	Localization of tenderness and pain in right lower quadrant, muscular tension present	Slight rise in body temperature, accompanied by nausea and vomiting
Acute cholecystitis and cholelithiasis	Onset frequently sudden, usually on evenings after a diet of greasy foods	Middle or right epigastrium	Continual or periodic colicky pain radiating toward the right shoulder	Tactile tenderness over right epigastrium, muscles tense, percussion pain frequently present over liver, gallbladder sometimes palpable.	High fever accompanied by chills, nausea, and vomiting, and possibly jaundice
Bile duct ascariasis	Onset sudden. Has history of taking an anthelmentic recently	Right lower part of the xiphoid of the sternum	Recurring acute colicky pain, a "drilled-through-the-top" feeling	Slight degree of tenderness and rebound tenderness felt under the Xiphoid on the lower right	No fever in early stage. Chills, high fever, nausea and vomiting (sometimes vomiting up ascaris) accompanying infections of the bile ducts.

Table 6-3-9 (Continued)

Disease	Disease onset and history	Site of abdominal pain	Nature of abdominal pain	Abdominal symptoms	Other symptoms
Acute perforation of peptic and duodenal ulcer	Sudden onset, frequently after a full meal. History of ulcers often accompanied by women	Upper and mid-abdomen rapidly involving the the whole abdomen	Continual stabbing pain	Considerable tactile tenderness abdominal muscles tense, liver hard and murmurs over boundary of liver dissipated	Body temperature drops during state of shock, showing obvious rise 6-12 hours later, accompanied by nausea and vomiting.
Acute intestinal obstruction	Onset sudden, history and surgery of extra-peritoneal hernia possible	Arising usually from mid-abdomen	Intermittent colicky pain	Tenderness and distension present, sometimes intestinal type, peristaltic rushes strong, bubbly and metallic sound present	No fever in early stage, though bile and fecal fluid may be vomited. No bowel movements, no flatus expelled via anus.
Acute pancreatitis	Sudden, usually following gluttonous consumption of food and drink, sometimes accompanied by shock	Upper abdomen	Continuous acute pain, usually radiating toward back	Horizontal tenderness, slight muscular rigidity, abdominal distension in severe cases	Fever occurring 2-3 days later, with nausea and vomiting

Table 6-3-9 (Continued)

Disease	Disease onset and history	Site of abdominal pain	Nature of abdominal pain	Abdominal symptoms	Other symptoms
Renal colic	Sudden. Past history of hematuria	Upper abdomen or sides [at waistline]	Intermittent acute colicky pain, usually radiating toward external genitals along medical aspect of thigh, accompanied by painful micturition	Slight tenderness, though percussion pain over kidneys definite	Chills and fever, nausea and vomiting accompanying infection
Intestinal parasites	Gradual. History of ascaris expulsion positive in many cases	Peri-umbilical area	Intermittent colicky pain	Tenderness not felt over definite area, no noticeable abdominal distension, sometimes knotted belt-like mass caused by ascaris felt.	Nausea and vomiting possible
Acute gastroenteritis	Sudden onset, usually with history of ingesting food less than clean	Whole abdomen	Intermittent colicky pain	Tenderness not localized, rigidity usually lacking	Chills and fever usually seen, vomiting occurring before onset of abdominal pain, the severity of abdominal pain lessened after stools have been passed.

Table 6-3-9 (Continued)

Disease	Disease onset and history	Site of abdominal pain	Nature of abdominal pain	Abdominal symptoms	Other symptoms
Lobar pneumonia	Sudden, accompanied by symptoms of respiratory in-fection	Upper abdomen	Continual pain, ac-companied possibly by chest and shoulder pain that is heightened by deep breathing	Tenderness over epigas-trium	Chills, high fever
Acute salpingitis	Onset gradual, ac-companied often by increased leukorrhea. Usually occur-ring during or after menstrual periods.	Lower abdomen	Continual pain, frequently accom-panied by low back pain.	Site of ten-derness some-what lower, but frequent-ly symmetrical	Chill and fever
Rupture of ectopic gestation	Onset sudden, frequently ac-companied by shock. History of menstrual period overdue. Also history of sterility for many years.	First on one side of lower abdomen, developing to generalized abdomen pain later on	Continuous pain, frequently radia-ting toward shoulder	Marked tender-ness over one side of lower abdomen, but muscular rigidity slight. Shifting dullness some-times present	

Jaundice

Jaundice is present when the patient's sclera (the whites of his eyes) and skin becomes yellow. Commonly seen diseases that cause jaundice, besides certain liver and gallbladder diseases, are certain intoxicating or biliary obstruction conditions (Table 6-3-10).

Types

According to differences in the manifestation of jaundice, the most common types are moist-heat or fever (han-jih), cold-damp (han-shih), or sluggish blood/energy (hsueh-yen ch'i-chi) jaundice.

Moist-heat jaundice. The jaundice coloring is bright and fresh, fever is present, and the urine is concentrated, like tea. Tongue fur yellow and oily-looking, pulse rapid and tense.

Cold-damp jaundice. Jaundice coloring is dull, appetite is poor, stomach nauseous or abdomen bloated, stools thin. Tongue fur white and oily, pulse slow and tense.

Sluggish blood/energy-related jaundice. Jaundice remains with patient over long period, acute pain felt in upper right abdominal region. Tongue fur is thin and spotted with petechiae.

Treatment

1. New acupuncture therapy. Strong stimulation to "tan-yu," "t'ai-ch'ung," "chih-yang," points during acute phase, moderate stimulation during chronic phase, once daily. After jaundice has subsided, give needle therapy every other day.

2. Chinese herbs

   a. For moist-heat jaundice. Clear fever and resolve moisture with one of the following:

   (1) Concoction of
Yen-ch'en (artemesia)	1-2 liang
Hei-shan-chih (gardenia)	3 ch'ien
Crude ta-huang (added later)	5 fen - 1.5 ch'ien
Huang-pai (phellodendron)	3 ch'ien

   Adjustable method: In presence of nausea and a white-coated oily tongue, add the following herbs to concoction

Tse-hsieh, replacing huang-pai	3 ch'ien
Chu-ling	5 ch'ien
Hou-pu	1 ch'ien
Hai-chin-sha (in cloth bag)	1 liang

- 257 -

Table 6-3-10 Differential Diagnosis of Jaundice

Disease/ailment	Symptoms	Physical findings
Infectious hepatitis	Seen mostly in children and young adults, history of contact with hepatitis, fever, nausea, vomiting, poor appetite, aversion to greasiness frequently present, pain in upper right abdomen, weakness.	Slight hepatomegaly, liver soft and tender.
Toxic hepatitis	History of drug intoxication, for example, to phosphorus, zinc etc.; poor appetite, nausea and vomiting generally seen, and gradual subsiding of jaundice upon drug discontinuance.	Tenderness over liver.
Liver cirrhosis	History of hepatitis or schistosomiasis, weakness, weight loss, poor appetite	Hepatomegaly, liver hard, vascular "spider" markings, possible ascites
Cholecystitis, cholelithiasis	Fever or chills, regular periodic or sudden colicky pain radiating toward the right shoulder and back, repeated appearance of jaundice.	Marked tenderness over right upper abdomen, gallbladder palpable.
Favism	History of horsebean consumption in large quantities, headache, nausea, aching pains in extremities, fever, anemia. Occurring usually during season when horsebeans mature.	Hepatosplenomegaly, tenderness.
Rice fever (leptospirosis)	Occurring from May through August during season of rice harvest; history of working in paddy fields; symptoms being fever, rheumatic ache pain in legs, congestion or petechial noted in skin and mucous membranes throughout body.	Liver and spleen possibly enlarged, tenderness marked over gastrochemius muscle.

Table 6-3-10 (Continued)

Disease/ailment	Symptoms	Physical findings
Liver abscess	History of amebic dysentery or septicemia, fever, tenderness over liver region, jaundice, etc.	Hepatomegaly, marked tenderness, ultrasonic examination an aid to diagnosis
Carcinoma of liver	Increasing jaundice, progressive weight loss, seen usually in older persons	Progressive hepatomegaly, liver felt to be hard and tubercular on surface, ascites possibly present.

----

      (2) Concoction of 1 liang each of yen-ch'en kao (artemesia) and dandelions.

      (3) Concoction of wu-chiu (allium species), 2 liang of the whole plant.

  b. For cold-damp jaundice. Warm the "cold" and resolve the moisture with one of the following remedies:

      (1) Concoction of

Yen-ch'en	1-2 liang
Roasted pai-shu	3 ch'ien
"Toned-down" slices of fu-tzu (cooked first)	1-3 ch'ien
Dry ginger	1 ch'ien
Licorice	1.5 ch'ien

      (2) Chin-ch'ien tsao 2 liang, in concoction. Very effective against obstructive jaundice (that not caused by cancer).

  c. For sluggish blood/energy related jaundice. Correct energy flow and dissipate clots (stagnation) in circulation with one of following:

      (1) Concoction of

Ch'uan-shan-chia (cooked first)	5 ch'ien
Ma-pien ts'ao (verbena)	1 liang
T'u-fu-ling	5 ch'ien
Pan-pien-lien	1 liang
Shih-chien-ch'uan	1 liang
Ch'ai-hu (browned with vinegar)	3 ch'ien
Processed hsiang-fu (fu tzu)	3 ch'ien

        (2) Concoction of
            Roots of stipa (mao)   1 liang
            Tan shen   5 ch'ien
            Yen-ch'en (artemesia sp.)   3 ch'ien

     3. Other methods. Besides treating illness at its cause, give vita-
mins and glucose as general supportive measures. If necessary, give parenteral fluids. Frequently used liver-building and liver-protective drugs include the following.

        a. Furfuramide. Take 2-5 gm each time, 3-4 times daily to ward
           off diabetic coma.

        b. "Kan-t'ai-le." Take 1 gm 3 times daily in cases of hepatitis,
           liver cirrhosis, intoxication hepatitis etc.

        c. Glucose powder. Take 2-4 spoonfuls 4 times a day.

                              Ascites

     When the fluid content in the abdominal cavity exceeds normal levels,
the condition is called ascites or "water tympanum" by the common people.
Some cases are manifested as abdominal distension only; others are seen as
abdominal distension combined with a generalized edema of the whole body.
Besides certain liver, heart, and kidney diseases which cause ascites, other
conditions which may cause ascites are certain parasitical infestations, peritonitis, malnutrition or right heart failure etc. (Table 6-3-11). Ascites in
female patients should be differentiated from a large ovarian tumor. Do so by
percussion of the abdomen with the patient lying down flat. If the distension
is caused by an ovarian tumor, percussion of the frontal abdomen shows a dullness of the lateral sides, a tympanic sound. If distension is caused by ascites
the frontal abdomen presents a tympanic sound, and the lateral sides, murmurs.

Types

     On the basis of ascites manifestations and the physical makeup of dif-
ferent patients, ascites may be classified as abnormal-solid (hsieh-shih) and
normal-deficient (cheng-hsu) for symptomatic treatment.

     Abnormal-solid ascites. Characterized by a mostly healthy physique,
urine dark and red and urination [pattern] short, and constipated bowels.
Fur of tongue yellow, pulse sunken and rapid.

     Normal-deficient ascites. Characterized by a mostly thin physical
build, watery bowel movements, and weakness of extremities. Fur of tongue
thin, pulse thready.

                              - 260 -

Table 6-3-11 Differential Diagnosis of Ascites

Disease/ailment	Symptoms	Physical findings
Liver cirrhosis, carcinoma of liver	See "Differential Diagnosis for Jaundice."	Late stage schistosomiasis.
Late stage schistosomiasis	See "Differential Diagnosis of Hepatosplenomegaly."	
Filariasis	Recurrent fever, with lymphoadenitis and lymphangitis, chyluria and possibly ascites.	Elephantiasis, hydrocele, ascites fluid milky white
Acute and chronic nephritis, malnutrition	See "Differential Diagnosis of Edema"	
Tuberculous peritonitis	Seen mostly in children and young adults, fever, hidrosis, emaciation, history of pulmonary tuberculosis frequently positive.	Abdomen soft and plastic, pressure pain present; ascites fluid frequently cloudy yellow or light pink
Right heart failure	Frequently a history of heart disease, dyspnea, cyanosis, fullness or dull pain in upper abdomen region.	Protruding jugular vein, pulsation marked, hepatomegaly, pressure pain and lower-extremity edema.

Treatment

    1. New acupuncture therapy. Apply medium amount of stimulation to puncture of points "p'i-yu," "shen-yu," "tsu-san-li," "yang-ling-ch'uan," and "san-yin-chiao," once daily.

    2. Chinese herbs.

        a. For abnormal-solid ascites. Purge to channel fluid removal with the following remedies.

        (1) Crush the root bark of "kan-sui" (Euphorbia sieboldiana) into fine powder. Take 1 ch'ien each time at early morning on an empty stomach, with some boiled water (See "Late-Stage Schistosomiasis")

(2) Concoction of ma-pien ts'ao (common verbena), taken once a day. Depending on the severity of clinical symptoms, add suitable amounts of pan-pien-lien, (Lobelia radicans) pan-chih lien (Scutellaria barbata) t'ien-chi-huang or pai-hua she-she ts'ao (white-flowered snake tongue grass) etc. (This remedy is effective for ascites caused by liver cirrhosis.

(3) Concoction of

Fu-shui ts'ao	
Whites of leeks	2 liang
Fresh ginger peel	3 ch'ien
	1 ch'ien

Avoid salt intake (Used for ascites caused by various etiological factors).

(4) Mix and crush to fine powder

Kan-sui	3 ch'ien
Sha-jen	3 ch'ien

Add crushed leeks. Add water to form paste and apply to umbilicus as poultice. Dress and apply bandage.

b. For normal-deficient ascites. Regulate nourishment and promote diuresis with following concoction:

Tang-shen	5 ch'ien
Toasted pai-shu	4 ch'ien
Fu-ling	3 ch'ien
Dried gourd scrape	2 liang
Barley	8 ch'ien

For anemic patients with facial pallor, add tang-kuei and tan-sheng 3 ch'ien each.

c. For yang-deficient types with cold extremities, add sliced fu-tzu, toasted, 3 ch'ien and dried ginger one.

c. Other

Use dihydrothiazide [a diuretic] or hypertonic dextrose selectively. Pay attention to treatment of cause. Take care with paracentesis procedures. Do not perform too often nor let fluid flow out too rapidly.

Edema

Edema is caused by excessive fluid accumulation in body tissues.

Edema is further classified as generalized or localized. Generalized edema is usually caused by diseases of the heart, liver, kidneys and endocrine glands or by malnutrition. Localized edema is usually due to venous or lymphatic obstruction, infection or allergic conditions (Table 6-3-13).

Types

According to the manifestations of edema, edema may further be classified as wind-watery (feng-shui), watery-damp (shui-shih), moist-hot (shih-jeh), and yang-deficient (yang-hsu) types.

Wind-water edema. Characterized by swollen eyelids and face which later spreads to whole body, and accompanied by chills, fever, arthralgia, coughing and some wheezing, diminished micturition. Tongue coating thin, pulse floating.

Watery-damp edema. Characterized by "pitting" [when pressed] diminished urinary output, nausea, headache, aversion to wind, and fatigue of extremities. Tongue coating white and oily, pulse slow.

Moist-hot edema. Characterized by localized edema, local parts generally erythematous and hot. Tongue fur thin, pulse rapid.

Yang-deficient edema. Characterized by generalized edema, accompanied by facial pallor, poor appetite, cold extremities, aversion to cold, or anhidrosis with some wheezing. Tongue tasting flat, pulse sunken and slow.

Treatment

1. New acupuncture therapy. Apply medium stimulation to needles placed in "tsu-san-li," "yin-ling ch'uan," and "san-yin-chiao" points, once daily. For edema of head and face, add "jen-chung" to points needled, for upper-extremity edema, add "ch'u-ch'ih" point; for swollen ankle, add "tsu-lin-li." For deficiency conditions, use acupuncture on "p'i-yu" and "shen-yu" and "ch'i-hai" points.

2. Chinese herbs.

    a. For wind-watery edema. Dissipate the wind and stimulate fluid circulation with the following concoction:

Toasted ephedra	3 ch'ien
Unprocessed gypsum	1 liang
(crush and cook first)	
Fresh ginger	3 slices
Licorice	1.5 ch'ien
Burnt pai-shu	3 ch'ien

Table 6-3-13 Differential Diagnosis of Edema

Disease	Symptoms	Physical findings
Acute nephritis	Onset sudden, involving eyelids and spreading to whole body; rise in blood pressure, proteinuria and hematuria with large amounts secreted; history of boils and other inflammatory/infective conditions	Generalized edema
Chronic nephritis	Onset gradual, recurring repeatedly, history of acute nephritis in some cases; fatigue, backache, poor appetite.	"Pitting" edema, possibly rise in blood pressure, possible manifestations of edema.
Heart failure	History of heart disease, dyspnea, fullness or dull pain over upper abdomen, dependent edema most marked at evening, gradual decrease of edema if disease improves.	Protrusion of jugular veins, pulsation marked, possible hepatomegaly and tenderness, heart enlarged, murmurs and arrhythmia, tachycardia, "pitting" edema (when part is pressed).
Liver cirrhosis	Onset gradual, ascites and dependent edema in lower extremities more noticeable, fatigue, weight loss, poor appetite, history of hepatitis and schis likely.	Hepatosplenomegaly, liver hard, vascular "spiders" seen, liver polmate, veins alongside abdominal wall protruding, shrinkage in liver size during late stages.
Malnutrition	History of ankylostomiasis and iron-deficiency anemia; dizziness, fatigue, tinnitus, sallow complexion; gradual generalized edema possibly present.	Coloring under eyelids and nailbeds pale. Other signs of anemia possibly present.
Edema of pregnancy	Hypertension appearing in final stage of pregnancy accompanied by edema and albuminuria.	

Table 6-3-13 (Continued)

Disease	Symptoms	Physical findings
Angioneurotic edema	Sudden appearance of edema following ingestion of certain foods or drugs, seen most often on eyelids and face, fever possibly present.	Patches of hives possibly seen
Poisonous snakebite	History of poisonous snakebite, local swelling appearing after bite, and extending rapidly in direction of the heart; fever, diplopia, drooping eyelids possibly present; coma in serious cases	Snakebite markings over wound, or retention of fangs in tissues.
Cellulitis	Redness, swelling, heat, and pain appearing in localized skin area; usually occurring on extremities or neck; fever possibly present.	Lymphadenitis in nearby lymph glands, tenderness, and numerous pus-filled boils.
Filariasis	See "Differential Diagnosis of Ascites"	

b. For watery damp edema. Reach the "yang" and promote diuresis with the following concoction:

Cinnamon sticks	3 ch'ien
Pai-shu	3 ch'ien
Fu-ling	5 ch'ien
Chu-ling	5 ch'ien
Tsu-hsieh	5 ch'ien
Bark of white mulberry	1 liang
Bark of ta-fu	1 liang

c. For moist-hot edema. Clear fever and promote diuresis with the following:

    (1) Concoction of

Hai-chin sha	1 liang
Corn silks	4 ch'ien
T'ien-pien chu	1 liang
T'ien hu-lu	1 liang

(2) Concoction prepared from one or two of the following
     1-1.5 liang each.
     Roots of mao-ken
     (Imperata arundinaceae)
     Skin of tung-kua
     (Winter melon)
     Corn silk
     Hai-chin-sha
     Che-ch'ien ts'ao
     Pan pien lien
     Hsieh-hsia chu

d. For yang-deficient edema. Warm the yang and promote diuresis
    with concoction, prepared from the following:

Fu-tzu (cook first)	3 ch'ien
Dried ginger	2 ch'ien
Burnt pai-shu	3 ch'ien
Fu-ling	3 ch'ien
Chu-ling	5 ch'ien
Tse-hsieh	5 ch'ien

If energy is also deficient, add the following:

Tang-shen	3 ch'ien
Huang-ch'i	3 ch'ien

If backache and scantiness of urine exist, add to the basic
concoction:

Hu-lu pa	3 ch'ien
Pa-chi-t'ien	3 ch'ien

3. Other treatment combining traditional Chinese and western medicine
directed toward etiological factors.

Use of diuretics is chiefly suited for generalized edema.
Dihydrothiazode [?] or hypertonic glucose may be used.

Besides this, for patients with more obvious edema, prescribe
salt-free or low-sodium diet.

Hepatosplenomegaly

In healthy individuals, the liver and spleen are generally located below the rib margin and cannot be palpated.

However, in certain disease conditions, the liver and spleen are both enlarged simultaneously. In some diseases, only the liver or the spleen is enlarged. Diseases presenting with hepatomegaly primarily are hepatitis, liver abscess, liver carcinoma etc. Those presenting primarily with splenomegaly are malaria, schistosomiasis, typhoid, etc. (Table 6-3-12).

In children under three years of age and certain individuals of long lean build without any complaints, a soft liver may be palpable, but this does not necessarily indicate disease.

Types

On the basis of its manifestations, hepatosplenomegaly is mostly seen in two types -- energy-stagnant (ch'i-chi) hepatosplenomegaly, and blood-clotting (hsueh-yen) hepatosplenomegaly.

Energy-stagnant type. Liver and spleen are both enlarged, generally as soft masses, characterized by pain over both sides. Fur of tongue is thin, pulse tense.

Blood-clotting type. Liver and spleen are both enlarged. Much tenderness felt upon pressure. Patients generally present a dark complexion showing obvious vascular "spiders" and capillary congestion. Tongue is purplish, coating thin.

Treatment

1. New acupuncture therapy. Apply medium stimulation to needle puncture at "nei-kuan," "tsu-san-li," "yin-ling-ch'uan," "san-yin-chiao," "t'ai-ch'ung" points. Puncture from the "nei-kuan" to the "wai-kuan," from the "yang-ling-ch'uan" to the "yin-ling-ch'uan," once daily.

2. Chinese herbs

   a. For energy-stagnating hepatosplenomegaly. Treatment should stimulate energy circulation and clear the "lo" passages with the following remedies:

   (1) Concoction of
       Tan-shen (salvia multiorrhiza)   1 liang
       Ch'uan-chien (melia sp.)   3 ch'ien

Table 6-3-12 Differential Diagnosis of Hepatosplenomegaly Commonly Seen in
Hunan Province

Disease	Symptoms	Physical Findings
Hepatitis, liver cirrhosis, liver abscess, carcinoma of liver	See "Differential Diagnosis of Jaundice"	
Liver congestion	History of heart disease and cardiac failure, dyspnea, cyanosis, distension or dull pain over epigastrium	Distended jugular veins with marked pulsation, heart enlarged with possibly murmurs heard, hepatomegaly with tenderness felt upon pressure
Late-stage schistosomiasis	History of residing in endemic lakeshore areas, contact with infected waters	Liver and spleen both enlarged, liver hard, granular nodes felt on liver surface, vascular "spiders" possibly present, varicose veins along abdominal wall, abdomen distended, with obvious ascites present.
Malaria	Chills and fever, latter subsiding after perspiring. Pattern present. Bouts occurring every other day (tertian, malaria), or every two days (quartan malaria); Pattern not evident in malignant malaria.	Extent of splenomegaly determined by length and severity of illness, finding of malarial parasites in the blood, and jaundice appearing sometimes.
Typhoid, para-typhoid	Usually seen in summer-spring, characterized by continuous fever, poor appetite, lethargy, relatively slow pulse, rose-colored rash	Slight hepatosplenomegaly, soft, tender.
Leukemia	Long period of fever, anemia, weakness, tendency toward bleeding	Hepatosplenomegaly, abnormal cells found in blood, slight enlargement of lymph nodes throughout body.

Table 6-3-12 (Continued)

Disease	Symptoms	Physical Findings
Thrombocytopenic purpura	Subcutaneous petechial or purplish patches in greater distribution on extremities than on trunk.	Splenomegaly, thrombopenia, tourniquet test positive
Lymphoma	Recurrent fever, chills, weakness, hidrosis, weight loss.	Generalized lymphadenopathy, splenomegaly

(2) Concoction of

Fresh and dried orange peel	3 ch'ien
Processed hsiang-fu (cyperes rotandus)	3 ch'ien
Huo-hsiang (Agastache sp.)	3 ch'ien
Chieh-keng (Platycondon sp.)	2 ch'ien
Tan-shen (Salvia sp.)	4 ch'ien

b. For blood-clotting hepatosplenomegaly. Treatment should stimulate blood circulation to break up clots with following remedies:

(1) Concoction of split-leaf begonia (lieh-hsieh ch'iu-hai-t'ang) prepared fresh from the whole plant 1-2 liang.

(2) Concoction of

T'ao-jen (peach kernel)	3 ch'ien
Ti-pi ch'ung	5 ch'ien
Hung-hua	1.5 ch'ien
Hsuan-fu-hua	2 ch'ien
Wu-ling-chih	3 ch'ien
Ch'uan-kung (conioselinum unvittaltum)	1.5 ch'ien
Pai-shao (Paenia sp)	3 ch'ien
Yen-hu-so (Corydalis sp.)	3 ch'ien
Ch'uan-chien (Melia sp.)	3 ch'ien

To correct energy deficiency, add 3 ch'ien each of tang-shen, tang-kuei, and pai-shu to the concoction.

3. Treatment of etiological factors (See related sections.)

Backache

Backache is a commonly seen symptom. It is usually caused by twisting, strain or sprain in the back muscles, by diseases of the urinary tract, or by inflammatory conditions within the pelvis. The patient generally feels the backache himself, particularly severe when the local part over-exerts and the pain easing up somewhat with rest. Very often the pain becomes more severe in face of cold weather or weather changes.

Types

Clinically, the types of backache most frequently seen are cold-damp (han-shih) backaches and kidney-deficient (shen-hsu) backaches.

Cold-damp backache. Usually the back feels cold and aching at the same time, accompanied by a heavy feeling. The pain is such that it is difficult even to turn over. The tongue is coated white and oily, pulse is sunken.

Kidney-deficient backache. The backache is characterized by a weak wobbly feeling in the back and lower extremities, usually worse after strenuous activity, and ameliorated by rest. Tongue color is pale, and pulse is sunken and thready.

Treatment

1. New acupuncture therapy. Apply medium stimulation to needles inserted into "shen yu," "wei-chung" "k'un-lun," "A-shih" points, once a day. Burning moxa or cupping may be used after needling.

2. Ear puncture. Insert needle into tender points on pinna of the ear at its lumba-sacral and kidney designations, and retain needle for 15 minutes. Repeat every day. Or the buried-needle technique can be used.

3. Chinese herbs.

   a. For moist-damp backache. Treatment should dissipate the cold (han), and promote diuresis, to warm the meridians and clear the "lo" passageways, using the following remedies.

      (1) Concoction of O-pu-shih ts'ao 1 liang taken with a little white wine. Mix dregs from concoction with some wine and use as rub over back.

      (2) Powder of yao-chu hsiao (pulverized) 1-3 ch'ien each time, mixed with white wine, twice daily.

      (3) Rice gruel prepared from cocoction of tzu-ssu tou, minus dregs, cooked with glutinous rice.

      (4) Wu-chi san-yuan (patent medicine), 3 ch'ien each time, three times a day.

(5) Hot compress of crushed cotton boll seeds dry roasted

b. For <u>kidney-deficient backache</u>.
Treatment should warm and supplement the kidney's yang energy with the following remedies.

(1) Concoction of kou-ku   1-2 liang
(<u>Ilex cornuta</u>)

(2) Concoction of
Tu-chung   4 ch'ien
Ch'ing mu-hsiang   2 ch'ien
Pu-ku-chih   4 ch'ien

(3) Concoction of
Processed ti-huang (shu-ti)   4 ch'ien
Tang-kuei   4 ch'ien
Shan-yu jo   4 ch'ien
Wu-chia-p'i   4 ch'ien
Niu-hsi (<u>Achyranthes</u> sp.)   3 ch'ien
Tu-chung   3 ch'ien
Fu-ling   3 ch'ien
Hsu-tuan (<u>Dipsacus</u> sp.)   3 ch'ien
Pai-shao (<u>Pacnia</u> sp.)   3 ch'ien

4. Treatment of etiological factors

Hemoptysis

Hemoptysis is hemorrhaging from the trachea, bronchi, and lung tissues. The blood is coughed up, frequently accompanied by an itching in throat and the smell of fresh blood. The blood is generally bright red or frothy, or mixed with sputum. Differential diagnosis of diseases commonly associated with hemoptysis is listed in accompanying table (Table 6-3-14)

Types

According to manifestations of hemoptysis, the most frequently seen types are energy counteracting (ch'i-ni), yin-deficient (yin-hsu), feverishly intoxicating (jeh-tu), and blood-clotting (hsueh-yen) hemoptysis.

<u>Energy-counteracting hemoptysis</u>. Symptoms are coughing, dyspnea, repeated hemoptysis bringing up fresh red blood or bloody sputum. Fur on tongue is white and thin, pulse is tense and slippery.

<u>Yin-deficient hemoptysis</u>. Symptoms are mostly weight loss, recurring afternoon fevers, "deficient" sweating in the evening, fresh red blood or blood-streaked sputum coughed up, mouth parched. Tongue looks pinkish, pulse is deficient [weak?] and rapid.

Table 6-3-14 Differential Diagnosis of Hemoptysis

Disease	History	Hemoptysis and coughing up sputum	Signs
Pulmonary tuberculosis	Possibly weakness, underweight, recurring afternoon low-grade fever, hidrosis etc., or unclear symptoms	Blood bright red, or as blood-streaked sputum; usually dry cough; after cavity formation, sputum amount increased, becoming purulent	Sometimes fine moist rales heard, or respiratory sounds lowered in pitch
Bronchiectasis	History of coughing over long period with sputum expectorated, and repeatedly recurring lung infections, or a history of repeatedly recurring hemoptysis	Mouthfuls of fresh blood or blood found in sputum, or accompanied by profuse amounts of sputum that looks purulent and smells unpleasant.	Scattered moist rales usually heard in lower chest and back.
Lung abscess	History of foreign body suction, coma, vomiting, post-oral surgery infective material suction; high fever, weakness, loss of appetite, or chest pain and dyspnea	Sputum bloody or containing large quantities of fresh blood, sputum frothy in beginning, becoming purulent later on, unpleasant odor more intense	Possibly unclear or breathing sounds over site of lesion becoming low-pitched, with moist rales heard, after cavity formation, hollow sounds heard.
Heart failure	History of heart disease; dyspnea, palpitation, cyanosis, inability to lie down flat possibly noticed.	Large amounts of pink frothy sputum	Signs of cardiac failure seen. Moist rales heard extensively over base of lungs or over the whole lung field.

Feverishly intoxicating hemoptysis. Symptoms are hemoptysis, accompanied frequently by fever, an unpleasantly smelling sputum coughed up, parched mouth and constipation. Fur on tongue is yellow, pulse rapid.

Blood-clotting hemoptysis. Coughing, dyspnea, clots of blood coughed up and cyanosed lips. Pulse is sunken and rapid.

Treatment

1. New acupuncture therapy. Use moderate amount of stimulation on needles inserted in "ju-chi," "ch'ih-tse" "tsu-san-li," and "lieh-ch'ueh" points.

2. Chinese herbs.

General treatment: Give concoction of mao-ken (Imperata cylindrica) 2 liang, with 1 ch'ien of powdered pai-chi.

a. For energy-stagnating hemoptysis. Treatment should lower the energy level and prevent bleeding with a concoction prepared from

Fresh crude ti-huang	5 ch'ien
(sheng-ti or Rehmannia glutinosa)	
Su-tzu	3 ch'ien
Tan-p'i	3 ch'ien
Roots of hsi ts'ao (Rubia cordifolia)	5 ch'ien
Bwint (Thuja orientalis) tse-pai	4 ch'ien

b. For yin-deficient hemoptysis. Treatment should nourish the yin to stop bleeding with the following remedy:

Mao ken (roots)	3 ch'ien
Hsi ts'ao (roots)	3 ch'ien
Ta-huang (rhubarb)	2 ch'ien
Leaves of tse-pai (Thuja sp.)	2 ch'ien

Burn to ashes. Mix and pulverize. Give 5 ch'ien each time, downed with fresh juice of crushed nelumbo or turnip-radish.

c. For feverish intoxicating hemoptysis. Treatment should neutralize toxin and promote pus drainage, using the following concoction:

Ju-hsing ts'ao	1 liang
Chieh-keng	5 ch'ien

d. For blood-clotting hemoptysis. Treatment should stimulate blood circulation and resolve clots using concoction prepared from the following:

```
Tan-shen                          5 ch'ien
T'ao-jen (peach kernelt)          3 ch'ien
Hung-hua (carthamus)              2 ch'ien
Su-tzu                            3 ch'ien
Burnt knots of nelumbo root       5 ch'ien
Mai-tung                          3 ch'ien
```

3. Other

   a. If the patient is tense, prescribe phenobarbital. For cough-
      ing, give a licorice compound; for heart failure, provide a
      cardiac stimulant.

   b. First aid in asphyxiation. If asphyxiation results from exces-
      sive hemoptysis (which provokes respiratory tract obstruction
      and tracheal or bronchal spasm, place patient immediately in
      a head-low feet high position. Slap his back gently so blood
      obstructing the passageway can be coughed up, and clear clots
      inside his mouth. If an emergency, use mouth-to-mouth resusci-
      tation, if necessary to suck out blood clots and sputum.

   c. If shock appears as result of large scale hemorrhage, take
      proper measures to arrest bleeding and counteract shock.

Epistaxis

Nosebleeds are also called "epistaxis." Diseases causing nosebleeds
are chiefly trauma, influenza and colds, diseases of the blood, hypertension,
liver cirrhosis, uremia, atrophic rhinitis, deviated septum, tumors or foreign
bodies in nose, vicarious menstruation in females.

Types

According to the manifestations of epistaxis, the most common types are
classified as lung-heated (fei-jeh), stomach-heated (wei-jeh), and liver-fire
(kan-huo) epistaxis.

Lung-heated epistaxis. Characterized by a dry mucous membrane, a dry
cough with little sputum coughed up. Tongue is red, pulse slippery and rapid.

Stomach-heated epistaxis. Characterized often by halitosis, thirst,
drinking water in quantity, constipation. Fur on tongue is yellow and oily,
pulse rapid and solid.

Liver-fire epistaxis. Characterized frequently by headache, dizziness,
restlessness, pain over both sides [lumbar region] and in vicarious menstruation, some abdominal pain. Fur on tongue is thin, pulse tight and rapid.

Treatment

1. **New acupuncture therapy.** Needle-puncture the "ta-chui," and "shang-hsing" points until they bleed a little.

2. **Local treatment**

   a. Take ashes from hair burnt or burnt shan chih (gardenia) pulverized and blown into nares.

   b. Apply cold compresses to forehead, using two washcloths immersed in cold water alternately and wrung dry, for 2-3 minutes each time.

   c. If bleeding from anterior septum of nose, use pressure alongside both nares to stop bleeding.

   d. Soak cotton balls in 1-2 percent solution of epinephrine or 1 = 1000 adrenalin solution and plug into bleeding anterior nare to promote vascular constriction and arrest of bleeding. If no drugs are available, a simple pledget of cotton or cloth can be used as plug.

3. **Chinese herbs**

   a. **For lung-heated epistaxis.** Treatment should clear heat build up in lungs, with concoction prepared from the following:

Bark of sang-pai (white mulberry)	4 ch'ien
Ti-ku p'i	3 ch'ien
Crude ti-huang (sheng-ti)	1 liang
Mao-ken (Imperata cylindrica)	1 liang
Mai-tung (Liriope sp.)	3 ch'ien
Huang-chin (Scutellaria baicalensis)	2 ch'ien

   b. **For stomach-heated epistaxis.** Treatment should clear heat buildup in stomach with concoction prepared from the following:

Crude ti-huang (sheng ti)	1 liang
Unprocessed gypsum	4 ch'ien
Chih-mu (Anamarrhena sp.)	3 ch'ien
Mai-tung	3 ch'ien
Niu-hsi (Achyranthes sp.)	3 ch'ien
Shan chih (gardenia)	3 ch'ien
Tan-chu hsieh (leaves)	3 ch'ien

   c. **For liver-fire epistaxis.** Treatment should purify the liver and purge the fire with concoction prepared from the following:

Lung-tan ts'ao (gentian)	3 ch'ien
Crude ti-huang (Sheng-ti)	5 ch'ien
Huang-ch'ing (Scutellaria sp.)	2 ch'ien
Shan-chih (Gardenia sp.)	3 ch'ien
Hsien-he ts'ao	1 liang

For vicarious menstruation: add 3 ch'ien each of tang-kuei, ch'ih shao, and niu-hsi to the above ingredients.

4. Other

In presence of excessive bleeding, take measures to prevent shock by administering 50 percent dextrose solution intravenously. Or depending on the patients' condition, use a hemostatic agent such as hsien-he ts'ao. Additionally, pay attention to treatment of etiological factors.

Hemetemesis and Tarry Stools

Frequently, hemetemesis and tarry stools are due to bleeding in the upper digestive tract (esophagus, stomach and duodenum). Before an attack of hemetemesis, there usually is some discomfort felt in the epigastric region, accompanied by nausea or dizziness. The vomitus is bright red or purplish brown, in bloody fluid or clot form. The stools, on the other hand, are black, like tar. For diseases that are commonly associated with hemetemesis and tarry stools, consult table 6-3-15.

Types

According to manifestations of hemetemsis, the frequently seen types are stomach-heated (wei-jeh), and liver-fired (kan-jeh).

Stomach-heated hemetemesis. Characterized by burning sensation in stomach, precordial pain, vomitus a dull red or containing food residues, generally associated with an earlier history of gastric disorders. Tongue is red, the fur yellow and oily, the pulse slippery and rapid.

Liver-fire hemetemesis. Generally characterized by a bitter taste in mouth, distension and pain in both sides, tension and impatience, restlessness, bad temper, fitful sleep, dreams and nightmares. Condition of tongue is red, pulse tight and rapid.

Treatment

1. General

   a. Absolute bed rest if bleeding is in large amounts. Try to move patient as little as possible.

Table 6-3-15 Differential Diagnosis of Hemetemesis and Tarry Stools

Disease	Bleeding condition	History and symptoms	Physical findings
Ulcers	Hemetemesis or tarry stools, tarry stools more commonly seen, with varied amount of bleeding.	History of pattern of regular pain in epigastrium, repeated attacks, or history of belching and acid eructations.	Possible tenderness over epigastrium
Liver cirrhosis (varicosities of fundus of stomach and esophagus)	Chiefly noted as hemetemesis, blood bright red, in excessive amounts.	History of hepatitis, schistosomiasis or alcoholic dissipation, discomfort over epigastrium, poor appetite, pain in region of liver, abdominal distension, weakness, etc.	Vascular "spiders" noted on skin surface, modular liver, hepatosplenomegaly positive, varicosities on abdominal wall, ascites present
Cancer of the stomach	Tarry stools seen continuously	Poor appetite, upper abdominal distress, pain following ingestion of food, nausea and vomiting, occurring mostly among those over 40 years of age.	Rapid weight loss, emaciation, tumor mass felt over epigastrium, lymphadenopathy over the clavicle, ascites condition poor.
Cancer of the esophagus	Mostly hemetemesis, in small amounts	Progressive dysphagia, pain behind sternum, xyphoid specifically, age of patient frequently above 50 years.	Weight loss, poor condition.

c. Withold food and drink from patient with severe hemetemesis, but allow fluids for patient who only shows tarry stools. Under certain conditions, fluid supplements should be given.

d. Give concoction prepared from hsien-he ts'ao (agrimonia pilosa) 2 liang, or tzu-chu hsieh 1 liang. If hemetemesis is excessive and patient shows pallor, cold clammy extremities, clammy sweating, thready pulse, give concoction prepared from Korean ginseng as emergency measure (Substitute with tang shen 1 liang if Korean ginseng is not available).

2. Chinese herbs

   a. For heated stomach. Treatment should clear fever to arrest bleeding with one of following remedies:

      (1) Powder crushed from equal parts of
          Leaves of tse-pai (Thuja orientalis)
          Pai-chi (Bletilla striata)
          Take 2 ch'ien each time, twice daily, mixed with boiled water.

      (2) Concoction from
          T'su-hsin t'u (stove ashes)   2 liang
             (concocted brew)
          Crude ti-huang (sheng-ti)   5 ch'ien
          Fresh ti-yu   4 ch'ien
          Huang-ch'ing charred   4 ch'ien
             (Scutellaria baicalensis)
          Pai-chi (Bletilla sp.)   3 ch'ien
          Pai-shu, roasted   2 ch'ien

   b. For liver fire. Treatment should calm (quiet) the liver and stop bleeding, using

      (1) Powder, pulverized from
          Hua-hui shih   3 ch'ieh
          Pai-chi (Bletilla sp.)   3 ch'ieh
          Divide in two doses and take with boy's urine.

      (2) Concoction of
          Chih-tzu (gardenia sp.) charred   3 ch'ien
          Lung-tan ts'ao (gentian)   3 ch'ien
          Hsien-he ts'ao   5 ch'ien
          P'u-huang (Typha latifolia)   2 ch'ien

3. Others

    a. Tranquillizer such as phenobarbital to tense and nervous patients, to prevent shock.

    b. Agrimonine used judiciously to arrest bleeding. Thromboplastin can also be used.

If all treatments described above remain ineffective after trial, the patient should be hospitalized and considered for surgery.

Rectal Bleeding

Rectal bleeding, as a term, refers to the presence of blood in the stools. Coloration of the bleeding may be a bright or dark red, a characteristic symptom indicative of bleeding in the lower digestive tract. Diseases commonly considered as causes of rectal bleeding and the differential diagnosis of rectal bleeding are described in Table 6-3-16.

Types

According to differences in the nature of the rectal bleeding and in the manifestation of body symptoms, most commonly seen are the moist-heat (shih-jo) and cold-deficient (hsu-han) types of rectal bleeding.

Moist-heat rectal bleeding. Characterized by the bleeding usually appearing before the bowel movement, blood a bright red, and accompanied by difficult defecation, scanty urination (yellow), mouth dry with no inclination toward drinking water, nausea. Tongue fur is yellow and oily, pulse slippery and rapid.

Cold-deficient rectal bleeding. Characterized usually by bleeding following bowel movement, blood dull red, and accompanied by facial pallor, cold hands and feet, poor appetite and nervous exhaustion. Tongue is pink, pulse slow and weak.

Treatment

1. New acupuncture therapy

    a. For rectal and anal bleeding, strong stimulation to needles placed at "ch'ang-ch'iang," "ch'eng-shan" points, once or twice daily.

    b. For rectal bleeding due to systemic disease. Medium stimulation to needles placed in "ta-chui," "tsu-san-li," "ch'u-ch'ih," "san-yin-chiao" points, once daily. For tenesmus, include "ti'ien-shu," "ch'ang-ch'iang" points; for fever, add "feng-ch'ih" point.

Table 6-3-16 Differential Diagnosis of Rectal Bleeding

Disease	Symptoms	Physical findings (signs)
Anal disorders (hemorrhoids, anal fissure, anal fistula, anal prolapse)	Blood bright red, coating the stools or appearing after stools as drops of blood, pain following bleeding in anal fissure.	Diagnosis confirmed by rectal examination.
Bacterial dysentery, amebic dysentery, schistosomiasis, tuberculosis of intestines, cancer of colon, cancer of rectum	See "Differential Diagnosis of Diarrhea"	
Intestinal intussusception	Seen mostly in infants under 2 years of age, characterized by spasmodic abdominal pain and vomiting, small amount of rectal bleeding resembling brown bean sauce.	Mass in abdomen palpable.
Typhoid complicated by bleeding	Continual high fever accompanied by nausea and vomiting, poor appetite, lethargy, rash, slow pulse, rectal bleeding appearing 2-3 weeks after onset of illness, facial pallor	Hepatosplenomegaly, soft to feel, possible tenderness, blood pressure drop following bleeding.
Upper digestive tract bleeding (rupture of esophageal varix, bleeding peptic or duodenal ulcer)	See "Differential Diagnosis of Hemetemesis and Tarry Stools"	Tenderness over upper abdomen in ulcer cases, hepatosplenomegaly in rupture of esophageal varices, vascular "spiders," nodular liver, distended veins over walls of abdomen.
Leukemia	Fever of long duration, anemia, weakness, a tendency to bleeding, (such as epistaxis, bleeding gums, rectal bleeding)	Hepatosplenomegaly, generalized superficial lymphoadenopathy.

Table 6-3-16 (Continued)

Disease	Symptoms	Physical findings (signs)
Thrombocytopenic purpura	Subcutaneous petechiae, or cyanotic blotches, distributed inequally, more on extremities than on trunk, anemia.	Splenomegaly, tourniquet test positive
Aplastic anemia	Anemia, facial pallor, subcutaneous bleeding, rectal bleeding, hematuria, weakness, fever following repeated infection.	

---

2. Chinese herbs

   a. For moist-heat rectal bleeding. Treatment should clear fever
      and cool the blood with one of following:

      (1) Concoction of root bark from hsiang-ch'un shu (Cedrela
          sinensis)

      (2) Concoction of
          Crude ti-huang (sheng-ti)   5 ch'ien
          Ti-yu, charred   3 ch'ien
          Huai-hua (blossoms from   3 ch'ien
            Sophora japonica) burnt
          Leaves of tse-pai (Thuja   5 ch'ien
            orientalis)

   b. For cold-deficient rectal bleeding. Treatment should warm and
      supplement, to arrest bleeding with one of following:

      (1) Concoction of:
          Pai-shu, roasted   3 ch'ien
          Ti-yu, charred   3 ch'ien
          Ginger, toasted   1 ch'ien
          Licorice, toasted   1 ch'ien

      (2) Concoction of:
          Tang-shen (Campanumaea sp.)   3 ch'ien
          Huang-ch'i (Astragalus sp.)   3 ch'ien
          Pai-shu, roasted   3 ch'ien
          Seeds of dates   4 ch'ien
          Dry ginger (toasted brown and   1 ch'ien
            black)
          Yuan-chih, burnt   2 ch'ien

- 281 -

(3) Kuei-p'i yuan (patent medicine), 3 ch'ien each time, twice daily with some boiled water.

3. Combination traditional Chinese and western medicine to treat cause. Symptomatic treatment can be carried out with judicious use of agrimonine and thrombloplastin etc.

Hematuria

Normal urine does not contain blood. If red cells are found in the urine, the condition is called hematuria. If the amount of blood in the urine is minute and cannot be detected by the naked eye, a microscope is needed to see it. Diseases that cause hematuria and differential diagnosis of hematuria are described in Table 6-3-17.

Types

According to differences in the manifestation of hematuria, most commonly seen are the solid-form (shih-cheng) and deficient-form (hsu-cheng) types.

Solid-form hematuria. Characterized by hematuria, possibly mixed with small blood clots, urine frequently yellow, burning sensation in urethra, mouth dry and bitter, moodiness, distended abdomen and sides, coating of tongue is yellow, pulse tight and rapid.

Deficient-form hematuria. Characterized by hematuria, though the urinary stream is clear and uninterrupted and the urinary tract does not experience any burning sensation. Noted also are dizziness and "spots before eyes," backache and pain in knees, weakness of extremities, or poor appetite. Tongue is pink, pulse deficient and rapid.

Treatment

1. New acupuncture therapy. Apply medium stimulation to needles inserted into the "shen-chi" (alongside bone on both sides of the "ming-men" point), "kuan-yuan," "san-yin-chiao."

2. Chinese herbs

   a. For solid-form hematuria. Treatment should clear fever and arrest bleeding, using one of following remedies:

   (1) Concoction of:
Crude ti-huang	5 ch'ien
Hsiao chi (cirsium)	5 ch'ien
Bamboo leaves	5 ch'ien
Shan-chih (gardenia sp.) toasted	3 ch'ien
Mu-t'ung	2 ch'ien
Licorice sticks	2 ch'ien

Table 6-3-17 Differential Diagnosis of Hematuria

Disease	Symptoms	Physical Findings (signs)
Tuberculosis in the urinary system (kidney, T.B. bladder)	History of tuberculosis. In T.B. kidney, only symptom may be hematuria. In T.B. bladder, other symptoms, in addition to hematuria are dysuria, frequency of urination, urinary urgency.	
Stones in the urinary system (renal calculi, ureteral calculi, vesical calculi)	Hematuria following renal colic which radiates to genitals and inner aspect of thigh; sudden urinary mid-stream cut off seen more often in vesical calculi.	Gravel-like stones of various sizes possibly eliminated with urine, percussion tenderness over kidney region.
Tumors of urinary system	Non-painful hematuria in beginning; pain arising later with tumor growth or uteral obstruction by blood clot	
Trauma to urinary system	History of trauma, bloody urine frequently seen	
Acute and chronic nephritis	Hematuria frequently accompanying acute nephritis, characterized by acute onset, edema spreading from eyelids to rest of body, blood pressure rise; hematuria seen less often in chronic nephritis which is characterized by repeated edema flareups.	
Acute and chronic pyelonephritis	Acute sumptoms such as fever, chills, pain over sides, urinary urgency and frequency seen in acute pyelonephritis; may also occur in chronic pyelonephritis.	Percussion tenderness possibly noted over kidney region
Systemic diseases (leukemia, aplastic anemia, purpura etc.)	See "Differential Diagnosis of Rectal Bleeding"	

(2) Concoction of
     Shui-yang-mei (roots)   3 liang
     Hai-chin-sha (roots)   3 liang
     Man-t'ien hsing   1 liang
     Mao-ken (Imperata cylindrica)   2 liang

(3) Concoction of
     Chin-ch'ien ts'ao (fresh)   3 liang
     Hai-chin-sha (fresh)   1 liang
     Chi-nei-chin   3 ch'ien

     (This concoction is suited for cases with colicky pain
     or those patients who passed stones in their urine.)

b. For deficient-form hematuria. Treatment should nourish body
    to extract the blood (eliminate bleeding), using one of fol-
    lowing remedies:

(1) Concoction of
     Crude ti-huang (shu ti)   4 ch'ien
     Shih-hu (Dendrobium nobile)   4 ch'ien
     Niu-hsi   3 ch'ien
     Huang-pai (Phellodendron sp.)   3 ch'ien
     Chih-mu   3 ch'ien

     (This prescription suited for patients with rheumatoid
     arthralgia in back and knees.)

(2) Concoction of
     Chih-ts'ai, 8 ounces   2 liang
      (Shepherd's purse)
     Chi-shih-t'eng   1.5 liang

     (This prescription is suited for cases of kidney tubercu-
     losis)

(3) Concoction of
     Huang-ch'i (burnt)   5 ch'ien
     Tang-shen   3 ch'ien
     Burnt pai-shu   3 ch'ien
     Orange peel, dried   1.5 ch'ien
     Ch'ai-hu   1.5 ch'ien
     Sheng-ma   2 ch'ien
     Burnt licorice   1 ch'ien
     Hsiao chi   5 ch'ien

     (This prescription suited for patients with weak stomachs
     and poor appetite.)

3. Other

Hemostatics such as agrimomine, vitamin K etc., may be used.

If the hemorrhage continues even after treatment, take patient to hospital for emergency treatment. At the same time, pay attention to treatment of the cause.

Pruritus

Pruritus or itching is commonly seen in skin diseases. It is also a symptom of certain systemic diseases such as allergies or jaundice. In some cases, the itching is intolerable, in that it recurs and is particularly severe at night. In the beginning, the pruritus is the only symptoms and there is very little skin damage. However, pigmented scabs could be produced by the incessant scratching.

Types

On the basis of conditions surrounding the itching, the commonly seen types of pruritus may be categorized as wind-heat (feng-jo), moisture-heat (shih-jo), and anemic (hsueh-hsu) types.

Wind-heat pruritus. The site of itching is not definite, and bleeding follows scratching. It is usually dry, accompanied by localized redness, restlessness and thirstiness.

Moisture-heat pruritus. Sites of itching are specific and localized weeping, pain, and dryness of mouth are noted.

Anemic Pruritus. Generally of a longer duration, it is characterized by a dry flaky skin, and a dry stool.

Prevention

Avoidance of alcoholic beverages and highly seasoned foods. Refrain from scratching, washing with soapy water or application of ointments. If the pruritus is caused by other disease, the important contradictions must be grasped. Take active measures to control systemic illness.

Treatment

1. New acupuncture therapy. Apply strong stimulation to "ch'u-ch'ih," "hsueh-hai," "san-yin-chiao" points, once a day. For itching all over the body, apply needle puncture to point on view behind the ear until it bleeds.

2. Chinese herbs

    a. For wind-heat (fever). Treatment should control the wind to
    clear the fever, using one of the following remedies:

        (1) Concoction of
             Ta-ch'ing hsieh (leaves)   5 ch'ien
             K'ou-teng   3 ch'ien
             Mint   1.5 ch'ien
             Licorice   1 ch'ien

        (2) Ching-chieh   3 ch'ien
             Fang-feng   3 ch'ien
             Mulberry leaves   3 ch'ien
             Prickly chi-li (Tribulus terrestris) 3 ch'ien
             Sheng-tu (crude ti-huang)   4 ch'ien
             Huang-ch'ing   2 ch'ien
             Wild daisies   5 ch'ien

        (3) Concoction for bathing itching areas, consisting of
             Lu-lu-t'ung   ⎫ in suitable
             Ts'an-sha (silkworm droppings) ⎬ amounts
             Leaves of mugwort   ⎭

             (This prescription is also suited for moist-heat and
             anemic types of pruritus.)

    b. Moist heat. Treatment should clear fever and promote diuresis,
    using one of following remedies.

        (1) Concoction of
             Lu-I san (patent medicine)   1 p'kt
             Che-ch'ien ts'ao (plantago sp.)   5 ch'ien

        (2) Concoction of
             K'u shen   3 ch'ien
             Huang-pai (phellodendron sp.)   3 ch'ien
             I-mi (barley)   3 ch'ien
             Fu-ling   3 ch'ien
             Ts'ang-shu   2 ch'ien
             Che-ch'ien-tzu (plantago)   5 ch'ien
             Pai hsien-p'i   4 ch'ien

    c. For anemia. Nourish the blood and break up wind (flatus),
    using the following remedies:

        (1) Concoction of
             Ho-shou-wu   5 ch'ien
             Ch'ing-chu (Piperbetle)   5 ch'ien
             Ma-ch'ih-hsien (portulaca)   5 ch'ien
             Prickly chi-li   3 ch'ien
             Ching-chieh (Nepeta japonica)   3 ch'ien

- 286 -

(2) Concoction of

Shu-ti (processed ti-huang)	3 ch'ien
Tang-kuei	5 ch'ien
Chi-hsueh t'eng	5 ch'ien
Pai-shao (Palnia sp.)	3 ch'ien
Mummied silkworms	3 ch'ien
Cicada moltings	1.5 ch'ien

(3) Cured lard (shu-chu yu) for external application

Section 4   Common Infectious Diseases

Epidemic Influenza

Epidemic influenza is an acute respiratory tract infection caused by the influenza virus, and characterized by its potent epidemic nature and rapid transmission. Symptoms generally are headache, stopped-up nose, caryza, sneezing, aversion to wind and cold, fever, sore throat, congestion, aches over body, weakness etc. In some cases, abdominal pain, diarrhea, and pneumonia symptoms are also noted. However due to the climate and differences in the human physique, influenza is generally of the wind-chill (feng-han) and wind-heat (feng-jo) types.

Wind-chill influenza. Patient does not prespire and mouth is not dry. Pulse is floating and forceful, fur on tongue thin and white.

Wind-heat influenza. Patient perspires. Mouth is dry. Pulse is floating and rapid, fur on tongue thin and white or thin and yellow and dry.

Prevention

1. Public health education programs. Cultivate good health practices by not spitting anywhere and wiping nose on anything. Moreover, do not cough or sneeze in the face of another individual.

2. When an epidemic prevails, gargle with salt water daily.

3. Take Chinese herb concoction prepared from following:

Leaves of huo-hsiang	1 liang
Leaves ot tzu-su	1 liang
Leaves of huang-ching	1 liang
Mint	5 ch'ien
Water	4 chin

Boil until fluid is reduced to 2 chin, enough for 10 persons, 2 doses per person. To be taken once in the morning and once in afternoon.

Treatment

1. <u>New acupuncture therapy</u>. Apply medium stimulation to needles inserted in "ho-ku," "feng-ch'ih," "ch'u-ch'ih," points, once daily. Cupping
technique can also be used over "ta-chui," "fei-yu" and "wai-kuan" points.

2. <u>T'ui-na massage</u>.

For headache, massage the "t'ai-yang," push-massage the "yin-t'ang,"
spot-massage the "ho-ku," and grasp-massage the "feng-ch'ih." For stopped-
up noses, use both index fingers to pinch the "ying-ch'un," twice a day.

3. <u>Chinese herbs</u>

a. For <u>wind-chill influenza</u>. Treatment should stimulate warmth
to promote perspiration, and air and dispel wind-chill influenza, using the
following remedies:

(1) Concoction of:
Ts'ung-pai (white onions), fresh   5 cloves
Mild salted black beans   3 ch'ien
Fresh ginger   3 slices

(2) Concoction of
Tzu-ssu   5 ch'ien
Fresh ginger   5 slices

(3) Powdered roots of chieh-ts'ao, 1-3 ch'ien each time, taken
with some boiled water, twice a day.

b. For <u>wind-heat influenza</u>. Treatment should stimulate coolness
to promote perspiration, dispel flatus and clear fever.

(1) Yen-ch'iao chieh-tu yuan (patent medicine), a detoxifying
pill, to be taken twice daily, 1-2 pills each time.

(2) Concoction prepared from
Leaves of huang-ching   1 liang
T'ien-pien chu   1 liang
Lu-pien ching (<u>Serissa foetida</u>)   1 liang

(3) Crushed fresh shih-hu-t'o (coriander) in a small amount
used to pack one nostril.

Measles

Measles is called "ch'u-ma-tz" [meaning rash coming out] or "sha-tzu"
by the local populace. It is a highly infectious disease caused by the
measles virus, and usually occurs in the winter and spring. Small children

between the ages of 6 months and 5 years are most susceptible. When the measles first appear, it should be differentiated from hives. The measles rash usually appears after 3 or 4 days of fever, coughing, and coryza, the papules about size of a mustard seed, perceptible to touch. Moreover, pinhead size white spots are seen on the buccal membrane opposite to the first molar. In German measles, the fever only lasts a day, after which the rash appears and the fever subsides in severity. Size of the rash varies, and disappears after 1 or 2 days. The buccal membrane also does not display the spots noted in measles.

Course of Infection

The course undertaken by a bout of measles may be divides into three stages, the incubation period, the rash-appearance stage, and the convalescent stage.

Incubation period. At the onset, the patient experiences chills and runs a fever, accompanied by coughing, sneezing, yawning, stopped-up nose, coryza, red eyes, restlessness, and a cold ear auricle striped red on the dorsal surface. Two or three days after onset, pinhead-sized white spots (called Kopkik's spots formerly) are detected on buccal membrane, a sign that is characteristic of measles.

Rash appearance stage. The measles rash usually appears first behind the ears and around the neck, spreading gradually to the face, chest, back, hands and feet, until it covers the whole body. At this time, the fever is quite high. In the beginning the rash is a purplish red, and well-defined like mustard seeds, but with more of the rash appearing, these eruptions merge into patches which change slowly to a dull blackish coloring. After about 2 or 3 days, the rash has appeared completely. The hacking cough now sounds hoarse, the throat becomes sore, and the patient does not want to eat. Fur on the tongue is yellowish white, the pulse full and rapid.

Convalescent stage. The rash recedes gradually, the earlier patches fading before the later ones. Desquamation, much like bran, sets in. Rash-faded areas frequently leave a pinkish tinge. The fever falls by lysis.

Prevention

1. Early discovery and isolation of patient. Since the sputum, nasal discharge and lacrimations of the sick child all contain measles viruses, towels, clothing, and linens used by the patient should be washed and aired out in sunshine. Boil and disinfect fomites and other utensils.

2. Chinese herbs

   a. Pulverized tzu ts'ao (Lithospermum erythrorhizon) 1 ch'ien each time, to be taken every 7 days for a total of 3 times.

b. Chopped nan-kua (pumpkin) vine (about 3 ts'un long) concocted into strong brew, to be taken in two doses, once
in morning, and once in afternoon, for 3 days in a row.
Discontinue for 5 days, then repeat regimen for a total of
3 cycles (this formula suited for use in summer and fall).

c. Kuan-ts'ung (Cyrtomium fortunei) 4 ch'ien in concoction.
Take one dose (4-ch'ien concoction) daily for 3-5 days in
succession.

Treatment

1. Rest and quiet. Keep room warm (but not hot) and well-ventilated.
Force fluids and give patient easily digestible food. Pay attention to
cleanliness of mouth, nose and eyes. Best to wash affected parts with a weak
saline solution.

2. New acupuncture therapy

For headache and high fever during the incubation period, needle-
puncture the "lieh-ch'ueh" and "ch'u-ch'ih" points; for high fever during the
rash appearance stage, needle-puncture the "ho-ku" and "ch'u-ch'ih" points;
and during the convalescent stage, needle-puncture the "tsu-san-li" and "nei-
kuan" points. For tonsillitis complications, needle the "t'ien-tu," and
"shao-shang" points until they bleed a little; for pneumonia complications,
use cupping technique over the "fei-yu" point.

3. Chinese herbs

a. For measles during the incubation period and the early stage
of rash appearance, stimulate cooling to "erupt" [to bring
out] the rash with one of the following remedies:

(1) Concoction of
Yuan-t'o ts'ai (coriander)   2 liang
Tzu-p'ing   2 liang

Bathe skin with concoction. Stimulates rash eruption.

(2) Concoction of
Sheng liu (Tamarix sp.)   5 ch'ien
Liu-hsieh pai-ch'ien   5 ch'ien

(3) Concoction of
Ching-ch'ieh   1.5 ch'ien
Mint   1 ch'ien
Honeysuckle blossoms   1.5 ch'ien
Forsythia suspensa   2 ch'ien
Niu-pang-tzu   1.5 ch'ien
(not to be used with vomiting
and diarrhea)
Cicada molting   1 ch'ien

Modifications of prescriptions. In winter, omit honeysuckle and forsythia, but add su hsieh (leaves) 1 ch'ien and fang-feng, 1.5 ch'ien. In summer, omit ching-ch'ieh, but add tan ch'u-hsieh, 1.5 ch'ien. For severe diarrhea and "non-eruption" of rash on face, add k'o-ken (Pueraria japonica) 1.5 ch'ien. For severe vomiting and "non-eruption" of rash over lower extremities, add ch'ien-hu 1.5 ch'ien.

b. During the rash appearance stage, clear and lower fever and resolve toxins with one of following remedies:

(1) Concoction of
Honeysuckle blossoms   2 ch'ien
Forsythia suspensa   2 ch'ien
Sheng-ti (crude ti-huang)   3 ch'ien
Ch'ih-shao (water chestnut)   2 ch'ien
Mulberry bark (root)   3 ch'ien
Ti-ku-p'i (Lycium chinense)   2 ch'ien
Mint   5 fen
Cicada molting   8 fen

(2) Yen-ch'iao chieh-tu yuan (patent medicine), a detoxifying pill -- 1 or 1/2 tablet, taken with boiled water, 3 times a day.

c. During convalescent stage, clear fever to promote salivation, with one of the following:

(1) Concoction prepared using fresh roots of rushes, 1 liang, and a little rock sugar, to be used as tea.

(2) Concoction of
Ti-ku-p'i   3 ch'ien
Sha-shen   3 ch'ien
Mulberry root bark   3 ch'ien
Chih-mu (Anemarrhena sp.)   1.5 ch'ien

For treatment of various complications, see related sections on their treatment.

Chickenpox

Chickenpox is caused by the chickenpox virus, and it is spread by contact. It generally occurs in the winter and spring, mostly among small children between the ages of two and six. Symptoms noted at onset are fever, cough, coryza, headache, and the appearance of reddish lesions which turns into bean-shaped vesicles inside a day or two. The priorities in appearance of the rash vary, for discrete lesions, vesicles, and crust formations can all be seen simultaneously. After scabs over the lesions have been shed, no marks are left. Fur of tongue of patient is white and thin, and pulse is floating, slippery, and rapid.

Prevention. Quarantine the sick child until all scabs have fallen off.

Treatment

1. Chinese herbs. Clear fever, moisturize, and detoxify system with remedies such as the following:

a. Concoction of

Hai-chin-sha (root)	1 liang
Yeh chu-hua (wild daisy)	3 ch'ien
Fu-ling (Smilax) bark	3 ch'ien
I-jen (Job's tears)	3 ch'ien

b. Concoction of

Chin-yen (honeysuckle blossoms) hua	3-5 ch'ien
P'u-kung ying (dandelion)	3-5 ch'ien
T'u-fu-ling (Smilax sp.)	3-5 ch'ien
Licorice	1 ch'ien

c. Concoction of

Chin-yen hua (honeysuckle)	3 ch'ien
Forsythia	3 ch'ien
Talc	3 ch'ien
Phellodendron	3 ch'ien

2. No scratching, to prevent vesicles from breaking and incurring secondary infection. If vesicles are broken, paint with 1 percent gentian violet.

Pertussis

Whooping cough is called "t'ien hsiao-lun," "tun-ke," "lu-su ke" all describing some aspect of the whooping cough. It is caused by the Hemophilus pertussis, and is transmitted by air and dust. As a common contagious disease seen among children, pertussis can occur at any time during the year, though more frequently in late winter and spring. At onset it resembles the grippe or influenza, with slight coughing, low-grade or no fever, coryza and sneezing as predominant symptoms. After about a week, the coughing appears in paroxysms accompanied by cyanotic lips. The sick child coughs until he cannot catch his breath and vomits milk, food or a large amount of mucus before it stops. Sometimes he even coughs up fresh blood. However, this type of coughing presents a characteristic whoop that climaxes a coughing spell when the patient tries to catch his breath and emits this sound that resembles the end of a cock's crow. Facial edema and ulcers at the base of the tongue are often present. Generally, after 5 to 6 weeks, or even as long as 2 to 3 months in some cases, the patient's condition will improve.

Types

Clinically, pertussis is described as lung-cold (fei-han), lung-hot (fei-jo) or lung-deficient (fei-hsu).

Lung-cold pertussis. Characterized by low-grade fever, white sputum, and poor appetite. Pulse is floating and slow, fur of tongue white, and fingertips pale.

Lung-hot pertussis. Characterized sometimes by epistaxis, blood-streaked sputum or fresh blood coughed up, and a parched mouth. Pulse is slippery and rapid, fur of tongue yellow and dry, and fingertips cyanotic.

Lung-deficient pertussis. Characterized by a shorter frequency and duration of the coughing spasms. The coughing lacks vigor, sputum is scanty, and patient's lips are pale. Tongue is pink, the pulse is deficient, and fingertips appear bloodless.

Prevention

1. Quarantine of patient until all symptoms have disappeared.

2. Injections of pertusis vaccine to all infants over 3 months of age, a total of three injections. Give 0.5 ml in the first injection, and 1 ml each in the remaining two, at 7-10 day intervals. After this, give a booster of 1 ml each every year or every two years. All vaccines are given subcutaneously.

Treatment

1. New acupuncture therapy. Apply medium stimulation to needles placed in "t'ien-tu," "feng-lung," "t'ai-yuang," once a day. Use cupping technique over the "fei-yu" point.

2. Massage therapy

Massage. Over the "feng-ch'ih" and "chien-ching" points massage with a grasping motion, over the "fei-yu" with a pressing motion, in light, quick and gentle movements. Then use both hands to massage the "t'an-chung" point in an effort to ease the pulmonary energy [breathing]. If the child has been ill for a long time and the spleen is deficient, have the child lie down flat on his back and massage the "chung-wan."

3. Chinese herbs.

    a. For lung-cold pertussis. Treatment should loosen up and dispell wind-chill (feng-han), using one of following remedies:

(1) Concoction of pai-pu (Stemona sp.) 3 ch'ien, to be taken 5-8 days successively.

(2) Concoction of
Ma-huang (ephedra)   8 fen
Almonds   3 ch'ien
Licorice   1 ch'ien

(3) Infusion of ta-suan (garlic) 3 ch'ien, allowed to steep in cold boiled water for 10 hours. Strain and sweeten with sugar (garlic with purplish-tinged bubblets best).

b. For lung-hot pertussis. Treatment should clear fever, resolve mucus, and stop coughing with remedies such as the following:

(1) One chicken gallbladder (gallbladder from other domestic fowl or animal also suitable) to be taken with some sugar. For a one-year child, give one-fourth of a gallbladder each time, a 2-year-old, half a gallbladder; and a 5-year-old, a whole gallbladder. Follow this regimen once a day for 4-5 days.

(2) Cooked mixture of
Ju-hsing ts'ao (Houttuynia cordata) fresh 2 liang
Mung beans   4 ch'ien
Rock sugar   1 liang

To be eaten, once a day, for 4 days.

(3) Concoction of
Fresh leaves of tse-pai (Thuja orientalis) 4 ch'ien
Shih-hu-t'o, fresh   4 ch'ien

Add a little brown sugar before consumption.

(4) Concoction of
O'-pu-shih ts'ao   5 ch'ien
Pai niu-hsi   5 ch'ien
T'ien-pien chu (Aster trinervius) 5 ch'ien
Sweet wine

c. For lung-deficient pertussis. Treatment should nourish the lungs to stop coughing, using remedies such as the following:

(1) Concoction of
Tang-shen (Campanumaea pilosula) 3 ch'ien
Szech'uan pei-mu (Fritillaria roylu) 1.5 ch'ien
Pai-pu (Stemona sp.)   1.5 ch'ien

If the sick child feels parched and wants to drink water, and his pulse is thready and fingertips are pink, then replace tang-shen in the concoction with sha-shen 3 ch'ien.

(2) Fritillaria roylei treated eggs.
How to prepare: Crush 1 ch'ien of Szechu'an pei-mu into powder. Then very gently break a hole in shell of uncooked egg, and insufflate the powdered pei-mu into egg. Seal hole with wet paper and steam-cook egg on top of rice. Feed treated eggs to patient twice a day, one egg in the morning, and one in the evening.

4. Western medicines

Tetracyline, terramycin, or chloramphenicol prescribed within two weeks of onset, in which case the medication would be quite effective. Prescribed after two weeks may be less effective.

Diphtheria

Diphtheria, also called "pai hou-lung" (white throat), "li-hou feng" is an acutely infectious disease caused by the diphtheria bacilli, transmitted chiefly by air droplets. Its incidence is greatest in late fall and early winter, particularly among infants. At onset, the only symptoms are a low-grade fever, headache, and cough which may easily be mistaken for signs of a cold. However, a redness in the throat appears very rapidly, the throat is covered by a thin greyish-white membrane which spreads rapidly, and is easily seen alongside and behind the throat. The white membrane is not easily removable. If force is used, bleeding results. At this time, the patient experiences chills, runs a fever, feels great pain when he tries to swallow breathes with difficulty, and the nares of the nose heaves like bellows, the voice is hoarse, and the cough is a coarse croup. When he breathes, a buzzing rasp is heard. The tongue is generally red, the pulse is thready, and in infants, the fingertips are cyanosed and do not react to pressure. Serious cases may present with tachycardia pulse irregularity, facial pallor, cold extremities, cyanotic fingertips and lips, smoke-grey nostrils, and other signs of toxic myocarditis.

In making a diagnosis, diphtheria should be differentiated from the following diseases:

Tonsillitis. Characterized by fever and sore throat. The exudate does not extend beyond the tonsils, and any whitish membrane-like substance is easy to wipe off without any bleeding.

Thrush. Seen usually in weak nursing infants. The "ulcer" is frequently on the inner buccal surfaces and on the tongue surface. In serious cases it is seen over the trachea as a shallow white membrane that looks like curdled milk.

Ulcerative angina. Characterized by an unusual halitosis, and distribution of numerous painful ulcers on the gums, buccal and tracheal membranes that make blowing air and speech movements difficult, because of the pain. The ulcerated surfaces are covered by a greyish-yellow exudate that bleeds easily when wiped.

Prevention

Isolation of patient for immediate treatment. Also report case.

2. **Chinese herbs**

    a. Concoction of t'u niu-hsi (root)   1 liang

    b. Banana (root)   1 liang

    c. Concoction of
       Ch'ing-kuo (olive)   1 liang
       Pai ko-pai [radish]   1 liang

    Drink as would tea. Or just eat 4 liang of fresh radishes daily.

    d. Concoction prepared from
       T'u niu-hsi   1 chin
       Pan-lan (root)   8 liang
       Leaves of maize   4 liang
       water   30 chin

    Simmer until 25 chin remains. Give 3 liang each time, three times daily for 3 days in a row.

Treatment

1. **New acupuncture therapy**. Apply strong stimulation to needles placed in "lieh-ch'ueh," "t'ien-tu," "ho-ku," "jen-chung" points. Or use triple-edged needles on "shao-shang" and "chung-ch'ung" points until they bleed a little. Needle treatments are to be given once daily.

2. **Chinese herbs**. Treatment should clear fever, detoxify and nourish the yin, with remedies such as the following:

    a. Concoction of t'u nui-hsi <u>Achyranthes bidentata</u> (root). For a 5-year-old, 1 liang; 10-year-old 1.5 liang; 14-year-old, 2 liang; and adults, 3 liang.

    b. Concoction of chu-sha ken 1 liang. For infants, give a proportionately reduced dose, and continue medication until cured.

c. Concoction of

Sheng-ti (crude ti-huang)	5 ch'ien
Hsuan-shen (Scrophularia sp.)	5 ch'ien
Tan-p'i	2 ch'ien
Ch'ih-shao (water chestnut)	2 ch'ien
Honeysuckle blossoms	3 ch'ien
Forsythia suspensa	3 ch'ien
Szech'uan pei-mu (Fritillaria sp.)	1.5 ch'ien
Cicador molting	1 ch'ien
Licorice	1 ch'ien
Peppermint	5 fen

d. Emetic consisting of hog bile 75 percent and garlic 25 percent. Then mix two mackerel (ch'ing ju) gallbladders with 1 ch'ien of gypsum, and crush into fine powder. Use to insufflate throat.

e. Insufflating powder, consisting of the following, crushed fine:

Wang-kua [cucumber]	1 ch'ien
Chin-kuo lan [golden dates]	1 ch'ien
Ch'ih-hsieh I-chi hua	1 ch'ien
Mint	5 fen
Rock sugar	2 fen

f. Plaster prepared from

Pa-tou (Phaseolus sp.)	5 fen
Chu-sha (cinnabar)	5 fen

Mix and sprinkle on plaster backing. Apply plaster to mid-brow [between eyebrows] area. Leave for 8 hours, then remove. Caution: Be sure plaster does not get into eyes.

3. Western medicines

a. Diphtheria antitoxins. For mild cases, give 10,000-20,000 units; moderately serious cases, 20,000-60,000 units; and for serious cases, 60,000-100,000 units. In the early stage, the antitoxin is given all at once in an intramuscular injection, after prior skin test. In serious cases, half of the antitoxin may be given intramuscularly, and the other half intravenously.

b. Chloramphenicol in large doses. Also provide supportive therapy with hypertonic glucose, vitamin B, and parenteral fluids, when necessary.

Infantile Paralysis

Infantile paralysis, also called "poliomyelitis" is an acutely infectious disease affecting the central nervous system. It is caused by the poliomyelitis virus introduced into body via the digestive tract. It usually occurs in the summer and fall. At onset, the symptoms are fever, coughing, diarrhea, headache, hidrosis, general discomfort and no appetite. After about a week, the symptoms subside, and another set of symptoms appear, with fever, headache, drowsiness, vomiting, and stiffness of neck. Another characteristic symptoms also appears -- muscular pain. Infants do not wish to be held, and cry when touched. At this time, the temperature begins to drop, and muscular paralysis sets in. The patient cannot walk or he feels very weak. The paralysis may be seen on one or both sides, usually affecting the lower extremities. Left untreated, the extremities will undergo atrophy and change, and pose further complications.

Prevention

1. Isolation of patient, and disinfection of his fomites and excreta, using bleaching powder.

2. Preventive vaccine of live attenuated viruses for children of suitable age, to increase their resistance.

Treatment

1. New acupuncture therapy. For paralysis of upper extremities, needle "ch'u-ch'ih" penetrating the "shao-hai," "ssu-tou" penetrating the "tien chung," "wai-kuan" penetrating the "nei-kuan," and the "ho-ku" penetrating the "lao-kung."

For paralysis of the lower extremeties, needle the following points, using strong stimulation: the "huan-t'iao," "feng-shih," "tsu-san-li," "chueh-ku," "wan-pu," and the "yang-ling-ch'uan" penetrating the "yin-ling-ch'uan." Needle puncture once daily, combined with moxibustion.

2. Massage therapy

    a. For upper-extremity paralysis, with the patient in sitting position:

    Rolling technique: practiced in the following sequence from the "ta-chui"→"chien-ching"→"chien-yu"→"ch'u-ch'ih"→"ho-ku" back and forth, for 5 minutes; on the spinal column (from the cervical vertebrae to the 5th thoracic vertebrae) for 5-10 minutes, using light gentle movements.

    Grasping technique (na-fa): Performed on the medial and lateral surfaces of the upper extremities.

b. For lower-extremity paralysis: patient in recumbent position, flat on his back.

   Rolling technique: Practiced on the waist down to the anterior and posterior surfaces of the affected limb, paying attention to correction of joint deformity.

   Rubbing technique: Practiced on waist and affected lower limb, until warm.

   Grasping technique: Practiced on the medial and lateral surfaces of affected limb down to ankle.

3. Chinese herbs

   a. For early stage preceding paralysis. Treatment should dissipate gas (wind) and resolve moisture, with one of following remedies:

      (1) Concoction of
          K'o-ken (Pueraria sp.)   3 ch'ien
          Tsang-shu (Atractylis ovata)   2 ch'ien
          Huang-pai (Phellodendron sp.)   2 ch'ien
          Niu-hsi   2 ch'ien
          Ch'in-chiu (Justicia sp.)   2 ch'ien

      (2) Concoction of
          Fang-chi (Sinomenium acutum)   3 ch'ien
          Pai-shu (Atractylis ovata)   1.5 ch'ien
          Huang-ch'i (Astragalus sp.)   1.5 ch'ien
          Ch'in-chiu (Justicia gendarussa)   2 ch'ien
          Wei-ling-hsien (clematis)   1 ch'ien
          Licorice   5 fen
          Large dates   3
          Fresh ginger   2 slices

   b. For paralytic stage: Should supplement energy, stimulate blood circulation, and strengthen bones and sinews, with following remedies.

      (1) Hu-t'i yuan (patent medicine), 2 ch'ien each time, three times a day.

      (2) Concoction of
          Cinnamon sticks   1 ch'ien
          Pai shao (Paenia albiflora)   2 ch'ien
          Tzu-wan (Aster tataricus)   2 ch'ien
          So-yang   2 ch'ien
          Licorice   1 ch'ien
          Fresh ginger   3 slices
          Large dates   5

4. Western medicines

If the paralysis occurred within a year's time, consider using hydrobromic "chia-lan-t'a-min."

Pulmonary Tuberculosis

Pulmonary tuberculosis is called "fei-lao" by the common people. It is a chronic infectious disease caused by the tuberculosis bacilli, transmitted via the respiratory tract. Persons with delicate health are most susceptible to the disease. Its clinical manifestations are cough, hemoptysis, feverish hands and feet, recurring afternoon fever, pain in chest and on back, night sweats, weakness of extremities, mental exhaustion, etc.

Types

Tuberculosis is generally seen with a pulmonary yin-deficiency (fei yin-hsu) or with a pulmonary energy-deficiency (fei ch'i-hsu).

Pulmonary yin-deficient tuberculosis. Characterized mostly by cough, dry parched throat, thick yellow sputum, blood-streaked sputum, or fresh bloody sputum, rosy cheeks every afternoon with feverish hands and feet, night sweats, restlessness, dark yellow urine, bitter taste in mouth, thirst, dry stools, emaciation, weakness, reddish tongue, and a fine rapid or deficient rapid pulse.

Pulmonary energy-deficient tuberculosis. Characterized by facial pallor, weakness of four extremities, mental exhaustion, dizziness and backache, pain in chest and back, poor appetite (feeling distended whenever a little more than usual is eaten), peristaltic noises, loose stools, clear and voluminous urine passed at great frequency, cold hands and feet, clammy perspiration at the slightest exertion, aversion to wind, and thin and white sputum. Fur on tongue is thin, white and moist, the tongue itself tender and pink, pulse deficient and weak, or sunken-fine and slow.

Prevention

1. Instruct people not spit anywhere on ground or floor. When coughing or sneezing, cover mouth and nose. Burn the patient's sputum. It is best to keep eating facilities for the patient separate, and boil chopsticks and dishes after use. Utensils that cannot be boiled should be aired in sunshine frequently.

2. Vaccinate newborn infants with BCG (Bacillus Calmette-Guerin).

Treatment

1. New acupuncture therapy. Use moderate stimulation on "ta-chui," "fei-yu," "kao-meng," "ch'ih-tse," "t'ai-yuang," and "tsu-san-li" points,

in once-a-day treatments. It is sufficient to select 2 to 3 points each time for needling.

2. <u>Injection of acupuncture points</u>.

For patients who need to be given streptomycin injections, inject the streptomycin into the "fei-yu" point. This way, the dosage can be reduced to 0.1-0.2 gm daily.

3. <u>Chinese herbs</u>

a. For <u>pulmonary yin-deficient tuberculosis</u>. Treatment should nourish the yin and moisturize the lungs with remedies such as the following:

(1) Concoction of fresh ai-ti ch'a (<u>Ardisia japonica</u>) 1 liang.

(2) Extract, prepared by concocting
Processed ti-huang   4 liang
Crude ti-huang   4 liang

With half wine and half water to which honey is finally added. Given twice a day, 1 liang each time.

(3) Concoction of
Pai-ho (lily)   5 ch'ien
Crude ti-huang   3 ch'ien
Hsuan-shen (<u>Scrophularia</u> sp.)   3 ch'ien
Chekiang pei-mu (<u>Fritillaria</u>
                    <u>verticillata</u>)   3 ch'ien

(4) Powder prepared by burning following into coals:
Mao ken (cogongrass, roots)   3 ch'ien
Hsi ts'ao (roots of <u>Rubia cordifolia</u>) 3 ch'ien
Ta-huang (rhubarb)   2 ch'ien
Tse-pai leaves (<u>Thuja orientalis</u>)2 ch'ien

Fine powder is then wrapped in paper and allowed to stay on ground overnight for huo-tu (toxic effects remaining from the burning process) to be dissipated. When given for cough, 5 ch'ien should be mixed with crushed juice of nelumbo root or radish. (Suited for patients with hemoptysis).

(5) Powder prepared from dried slices of
Huai-shan yao   4 liang
Pai-chi (<u>Bletilla</u> sp.)   2 liang

To be taken 3 times a day, 3 ch'ien each dose, sweetened with sugar, and downed with rice gruel or boiled water.

b. For <u>pulmonary energy-deficient tuberculosis</u>. Treatment should supplement and restore pulmonary energy with remedies such as the following:

(1) Kuei-p'i yuan (patent medicine), 3 ch'ien each dose, three times a day.

(2) Lu chun-tzu yuan (patent medicine), 3 ch'ien each dose, three times a day.

(3) Pai-pai kao

<u>To prepare:</u> Cook together

Pai-pu	30 chin
Szechu'an pei-mu	3 chin
(Fritillaria roylei)	
Wheat sprouts	3 chin

Then filter concentrate and add powder prepared from 5 chin of pai-chi, then honey to form extract consistency. Remove from fire, cool, fill jars and seal for later use. For adults, dosage is 15 ml each time, by mouth, three times a day.

4. <u>Western medicines</u>

On the basis of different conditions, prescribe isoniazid, streptomycin, p-amino-salicylate singly or in combination. Keep in mind the possibility of drug tolerance when certain drugs are used over a long period of time.

Epidemic Parotitis

Epidemic parotitis, called "mumps" or "hsia-mo wen" or "ts'ou-erh feng" by the native populace, is caused by an epidemic mumps virus. It is an acute infectious disease frequently seen in small children, transmitted chiefly through droplet infection in the air. Its incidence is greatest among children between ages of 5 and 9 years, during the winter and spring seasons. At onset, pain is felt frequently on one side of jaw in front of ear, accompanied by fever. After one or two days, the other side will become involved. The swelling over the angle of jaw grows larger very rapidly, becomes hard, and the pain and fever become more severe. The patient feels general malaise and has no appetite. Moreover, the pain is heightened if he tries to open his mouth to eat. In severe cases, there is retching, drowsiness etc. Others may be complicated by meningitis or orchitis. This disease is generally classified as a heat-toxic type, with mild or severe symptoms.

Mild parotitis. Characterized by a swollen jaw, no change in coloring, dizziness, chills, coryza. Pulse is floating and rapid, fur on tongue unchanged.

Severe parotitis. Characterized usually by swelling and pain over parotid gland area, erythematous skin, fever, and thirst. Pulse is bounding and rapid, and fur on tongue is yellow.

Prevention

Avoid contact with sick child.

Treatment

1. Pay attention to oral hygiene. Force fluids.

2. New acupuncture therapy. Use medium stimulation on needles inserted in the "I-feng," "chia-che," "ch'u-ch'ih," and "ho-ku" points. Treat with needle puncture once a day.

3. Moxibustion. Thoroughly soak a piece of wick in vegetable oil (tea oil, vegetable oil, or tung oil is satisfactory). After lighting it, quickly flame it over the "chiao-sun" point, once each on left and right sides, until a "ch'a" sound is heard.

4. Chinese herbs

    a. For light cases. Treatment should evoke coolness and neutral-
        ize the toxin, using the following remedies:

        (1) Concoction of
            Honeysuckle blossoms   5 ch'ien
            Forsythia suspensa   3 ch'ien
            Hsia-ku ts'ao (Brunella vulgaris) 5 ch'ien
            Chiang ts'an   3 ch'ien
              (mummied silkworms)
            Snake molting   5 fen
              (toasted and crushed fine)

        (2) Poultice for local application, prepared from
            Ma-ch'ih-hsien (portulaca), fresh 2 liang
            Flour   suitable amount
            Crush and mix to proper consistency for local application.

        (3) Poultice prepared from 2 liang each of ju-hsing ts'ao
            (Houttuynia cordata) and dandelions, crushed. Apply
            locally to face.

    b. For severe cases. Treatment should clear fever and neutralize
        toxins, with remedies such as the following:

        (1) Concoction of roots from pan-lan-ken (Strobilanthes sp.)
            2 liang in a little water.

        (2) Concoction of
            Leaves of ta-ch'ing   1 liang
            Forsythia suspensa   5 ch'ien
            Ch'ih-hsieh I-ch'ih hua   2 ch'ien
             (Paris polyphylla)

        (3) Paste for local application, prepared from sifted quick
            lime mixed with tung oil. Apply twice daily.

        (4) Root of ch'ih-hsieh-I-chih-hua crushed and mixed with
            vinegar for local compress.

        (5) For complications of orchitis, concoction of
            Ts'a-chiang ts'ao (sorrel)   1 liang
            Chu-hsieh ch'ai-hu   5 ch'ien
             (Thoroughwax sp.)
            This concoction can also be used to bathe the scrotum.

Epidemic Encephalomyelitis

Epidemic encephalomyelitis called "liu-nao" is an acute infectious disease caused by the meningitis diplococcus which is transmitted via the respiratory tract. It is seen mostly among small children and adolescents, during the winter and spring seasons. Onset of illness is preceded one or two days by sneezing, coryza, cough, and headache much like that in one coming down with a cold. This is followed by sudden fever and chills, excruciating headache, neck rigidity (bulging of fontanels in infants), vomiting, restlessness, drowsiness, or general malaise, appearance of possible petechial and cerebral irritation in what is called the "ordinary type." If high fever presents at onset accompanied by delirium, quickened respirations, neck rigidity, projectile vomiting, convulsions, dilated pupils, and even septicemia or shock, this is the "fulminating type." This disease is much like the "spring fever"(ch'un-wen) or "winter fever" (tung-wen) described by traditional Chinese medicine practitioners. According to course of illness, there are three stages:

Chills phase. Characterized by chills and fever, headache, gradual neck rigidity, red throat, vomiting, aches in four extremities, a white and thin or oily fur on tongue, and a floating and rapid pulse.

Feverish stage. Characterized by high fever, excruciating headache, sore throat, hidrosis or anhidrosis, thirst, drowsiness, restlessness, delirium, a more rigid stiffening of neck, a fur on tongue changing from white to yellow, pulse full and rapid.

High fever stage. Characterized by high fever, coma, delirium, stiff rigidity of neck and four extremities, a distended gerontotoxon, upward rolling of eyes, tight gritting of teeth, purpural spots or petechial all over body. Tongue is red, pulse full and rapid, or sunken and rapid.

Prevention

1. Isolate and treat patients accordingly. The wards should be well-ventilated. During the epidemic season, infants and small children should avoid public places.

2. Mobilize the masses in a broad cleanliness and hygiene program to wash and air frequently their mosquito nettings, pillows, blankets, clothing etc.

3. Chinese herbs

    a. Concoction of a proper amount of chi-ts'ai (Shepherd's purse)

    b. Concoction of 5 ch'ien of kuan-ts'ung (Crytomium fortunei)

4. Preventive doses of sulfathiazole 4 gm daily for adults, 100 mg/kg/day for infants, for a total of 3 days.

Treatment

1. <u>New acupuncture therapy</u>. Apply strong stimulation to needles inserted in "jen-chung," "pai-hui," "shih-suan" points (prickly-puncture latter
until it bleeds), in once-a-day treatments. If the neck is stiff, include
the "ta-chui" point; if patient is restless, add the "yung-ch'uan; if vomiting present, add the "nei-kuan" point, and for much sputum, add the "fung-lung"
point.

2. <u>Chinese herbs</u>

    a. For the <u>chills phase</u>. Treatment should promote coolness to
       surface with the following concoctions:

        (1) Concoction of

Mulberry leaves	3 ch'ien
Chrysanthemums	2 ch'ien
<u>Forsythia suspensa</u>	3 ch'ien
Mint	1.5 ch'ien
Chieh-keng (<u>Platycodon</u> sp.)	3 ch'ien
Licorice	1 ch'ien
Almonds	3 ch'ien
Lu-ken	4 ch'ien

        (2) Concoction of

Honeysuckle flowers	5 ch'ien
<u>Forsythia suspensa</u>	3 ch'ien
Nui-pang-tze	3 ch'ien
Chieh keng	3 ch'ien
Mint	1.5 ch'ien
Licorice	1 ch'ien
Bamboo shoots	3 ch'ien

    b. For the <u>feverish stage</u>. Treatment should clear the fever and
       resolve the toxins, with remedies such as the following:

        (1) Concoction of

Quick lime	1 liang
(precooked for 20 minutes)	
Licorice	1.5 ch'ien
Chih-mu	3 ch'ien
Rice	1 ladle
Honeysuckle flowers	3 ch'ien
Forsythia	2 ch'ien

        (2) Extract from concoction of

T'ien-ch'ing ti-pai	1 chin
Lu-pien ching (<u>Serissa foetida</u>)	1 chin
Quick lime	0.5 chin
Water	3 chin

Cook for 4 hours. Remove sediments and strain. Cook
again, reducing fluid to 480 ml. Adult dosage 30-40 ml,
four times a day.

c. For <u>high-fever stage</u>. Treatment should clear fever and cool
the blood with remedies such as the following:

(1) Concoction of
Rhinoceros horns   2 ch'ien
  (Buffalo horns may be substitute)
Crude ti-huang   5 ch'ien
Hsuan-shen (<u>Scrophularia</u> sp.)   3 ch'ien
Chu-hsieh ch'uan-hsin   2 ch'ien
Mai-tung (<u>Liriope graminifolia</u>)   3 ch'ien
Tan-shen (<u>Salvia multiorrhiza</u>)   2 ch'ien
Huang-lien (<u>Coptis chinensis</u>)   1 ch'ien
Honeysuckle blossoms   2 ch'ien
Forsythia   2 ch'ien

(2) Concoction of
Rhinoceros horns   2 ch'ien
  (May be replaced by buffalo horns)
Crude ti-huang   5 ch'ien
Pai-shao (<u>Paenia albiflora</u>)   3 ch'ien
Tan-p'i   2 ch'ien

3. <u>Western medicines</u>. According to patient's condition, prescribe
sulfadiazine, chloramphenicol, or penicillin judiciously.

In the presence of shock, for adults administer 500 to 1,000 ml of
5 percent dextrose in normal saline by intravenous drip. For infants, administer 5 percent dextrose with saline at rate of 10-20 ml/kg/each time, by
intravenous injection.

In presence of acidosis, administer 5 percent soda bicarbonate solution
in suitable amount by intravenous injection or fast intravenous drip.

Bacterial Dysentery

Bacterial dysentery is an infectious disease of the gastrointestinal
tract caused by the dysentery bacilli. Its incidence is greatest during the
summer months and early fall because of inadequate attention to food and
drink sanitation, by eating cold fruits and vegetables without adequate washing, or eating food contaminated by flies. It is characterized by passage of
red and white stools (purulent-bloody stools), at a frequency of 10 to 20
times during the day, accompanied by great tenesmus at the same time. Abdominal cramping generally located in the lower left abdomen and tenesmus are
its important characteristics.

Types

According to differences in the manifestation of dysentery, it is generally seen as feverish dysentery (jo-li), epidemic dysentery (I-li), and deficiency dysentery (hsu-li).

Feverish dysentery. Characterized by red and white globs in the stool, defecation is uncomfortable, accompanied by abdominal cramps and tenesmus. Urine is scanty and brown, taste in mouth is bitter, and chills and fever are sometimes present. Pulse is rapid, fur on tongue yellow.

Epidemic dysentery. Characterized by acute onset, high fever, chills, vomiting, halitosis, inability to eat, severe abdominal cramps, frequent (over 20 times a day) bowel movements that contain blood and mucus or just bloody liquid. In severe cases, drowsiness, coma, convulsions, confusion are also evident. Pulse is rapid and solid, fur on tongue yellow and oily.

Deficiency dysentery. Characterized by the chronic nature of the ailment, of such long duration that the patient's body has weakened. The appetite is poor, and bowel movements contain globs of mucus, resembling fish brain in some instances. Or the fecal matter may contain undigested food particles that were passed involuntarily. Abdomen experiences cramps. Chills are also felt. Pulse is rapid and deficient, tongue is without fur.

Prevention

1. Actively promote the Patriotic Health Movement for the masses to grasp the proper techniques for environmental health and excreta management.

2. Intensify health education propaganda, and present the four "must's" and the three "do not's". The four "must's" are: 1) Must thoroughly eliminate flies; 2) Must wash hands before meals and after defecation or urination; 3) Must wash and scald vegetables and fruits if they are to be eaten raw; 4) Must report the onset of dysentery, for early treatment and timely disinfection of excreta. The three do not's are: 1) Do not defecate anywhere; 2) Do not eat spoilt or unclean food; and 3) Do not drink water that has not been treated.

3. Thoroughly treat the germ carriers and patients with chronic dysentery. Locate these patients early, and isolate them for proper treatment.

Treatment

1. New acupuncture therapy. Use medium stimulation on needles inserted into the "t'ien-shu," "tsu-san-li," and "ho-ku" points in once-a-day treatments. In presence of fever, add the "ch'u-ch'ih" and "ta-chui" to the puncture points. For tenesmus, include the "yin-ling-ch'uan." For vomiting, add the "nei-kuan."

2. <u>Chinese herbs</u>.

    a. For <u>feverish dysentery</u>. Treatment should clear fever and
       channel out the stagnant, using the following remedies:

       (1) Concoction of

Ching-chieh	3 ch'ien
Fang-feng (<u>Siler divoricatum</u>)	3 ch'ien
K'o-ken (<u>Pueraria</u> sp.)	3 ch'ien
Huo-hsiang (<u>Agastache rugosa</u>)	2 ch'ien
Lu-pien ching (<u>Serissia foetida</u>)	5 ch'ien
I-chih-huang-kua	5 ch'ien
Chieh-keng (<u>Platycodon</u> sp.)	2 ch'ien
Licorice	1 ch'ien

          (This prescription is effective in the early stage of
          dysentery when fever, chills, headache, and general aches
          are present)

       (2) Concoction of jen-hsien, 1 liang. Take with 4 liang of
          crushed portulaca

       (3) Concoction of shui yang-mei (<u>Adina rubella</u>) 1 liang.

       (4) Anti-dysentery powder, prepared by pulverizing

Huang-ching-tzu	2 liang
(dry-roasted till brown)	
Chiu-ch'u (browned)	2 ch'ien

          Add granulated sugar 1 liang. Mix and ready for use.
          Dosage is 2-3 ch'ien, three times a day.

    b. For <u>epidemic dysentery</u>. Treatment should clear fever and de-
       toxify patient's system, with remedies such as the following:

       (1) Concoction of shui-yang-mei (<u>Adina rubella</u>)

       (2) Concoction of

Pai-t'ou-weng (anemone) roots	3-5 ch'ien
Chin-wa-erh roots	3-5 ch'ien
La-liao-ts'ao (pepperweed)	3-5 ch'ien
Shui-ssu, roots	3-5 ch'ien
Pai niu-tan (whole plant)	3-5 ch'ien

       (3) Concoction of

Dried pan-li-ch'iu (chestnut)	1-2 liang

(4) Tzu-chin-ting (patent medicine), 2-5 fen each dose crushed and dissolved with boiled water, for patients who are drowsy, comatosed, or confused.

c. For deficiency dysentery. Treatment should warm and nourish the body and antidiarrheals should be used to arrest the dysentery, using the following:

(1) Anti-dysentery powder [pill], described under b(4).

(2) Concoction of
La-liao ts'ao (pepperweed)	5 ch'ien -1 liang
Ma-pien ts'ao (verbena sp)	5 ch'ien-1 liang
She-mei (Indian strawberry)	5 ch'ien

(3) Concoction of
Burnt huang-ch'i (Astragalus henryi)	4 ch'ien
Wu-mei (black prune)	2 ch'ien
Dried ginger	1.5 ch'ien

3. Western medicines

Depending on the patient's condition, consider prescribing li-teh-ling (furazolidone) sulfaguanidine, and for seriously ill patients, chloramphenicol, syntomycin, tetracyline, etc.

These drugs are mostly used singly by themselves, but depending on the circumstances, they can also be used in combination.

Amebic Dysentery

Amebic dysentery is caused by the parasitical presence of the Endamoeba histolytica in the large intestine of the human body. In their life cycle, amebas present themselves at different times as trophozoites and as cysts. After the trophozoites become encysted, these cysts are expelled from the body via the stools to contaminate food. When people ingest cyst-contaminated food, the cysts change into trophozoites in the lumen of the human intestines, and cause amebic dysentery. Its incidence is usually sporadic, onset slow with low fever or no fever, accompanied by pain in the right lower abdomen. Frequency of defecation is usually less than 10 times, but the volume is large, with blood and mucus (like bean sauce) mixed in. The stools also have a very unpleasant odor. This disease should be differentiated from bacterial dysentery and other colitis conditions, on the basis of history, symptoms, site of abdominal pain, consistency of stool, and microscopic examination.

Prevention

Identical to that for "Bacterial Dysentery."

Treatment

1. **New acupuncture therapy**. Use moderate stimulation on needles placed once a day at the points: "t'ien-shu," "kuan-yuan," and "tsu-san-li." For patients with fever at onset, include the "ch'u-ch'ih" and "ho-ku"; for chronic cases, use moxibustion also over the "kuan-yuan," "chi-chung" (with intervening layer of salt between moxibustion and point).

2. **Chinese herbs**. Treatment should clear fever, detoxify poisons, and resolve stagnation, with remedies such as follows:

   a. Concoction of ya-tan-tzu (Brucea javanica) with shell removed, 15 placed inside rubber pouch or wrapping of meats of longana fruit cooked with roots of pai-t'ou-weng (anemone) and water, to be taken 3 times daily.

   b. Snake molting (burnt to ashes), 1 ch'ien each dose, to be taken with light brown sugar syrup, three times a day.

   c. Concentrated concoction of feng-wei ts'ao, 3 liang, to be taken with a little granulated sugar.

   d. Concoction of
Bark of peach tree	3 ch'ien
Pai-t'ou weng (anemone)	5 ch'ien
Root bark of ch'un (Cedrela sinensis)	5 ch'ien

3. **Western medicines**.

   a. To **kill the trophozoites**. Depending on the patient's condition, consider selective use of chloroquine, emetine, etc. Chloroquine can also be used for amebic abscess when accompanied by high fever and hepatosplenomegaly with obvious tenderness.

   b. To kill the amebic cysts. Carbosone is effective for chronic cases and amebic cysts but less effective toward the trophozoites. Generally, treatment for amebic dysentery calls for a drug that kills the trophozoites, followed by one specific for cysts.

Typhoid

Typhoid is also called "intestinal fever." An acute infectious disease of the intestinal tract caused by the typhoid bacilli, it occurs mostly in the summer and fall. The onset is insidious, much like a cold or influenza in the beginning, with poor appetite, nausea, and abdominal distension. It is also characterized by low-grade fever which rises gradually, recurring every afternoon though it drops a little in the morning, but never back to normal. About a week after disease onset a light purplish rash called "rose spots" appears on the chest and abdomen. When pressed, the color fades. The patient is rather listless, the pulse may be slow (pulse not rapid in presence of high fever), and the liver and spleen slightly enlarged. In serious cases, the patient may be delirious or stuporous. Intestinal bleeding is one of the common complications. If the hemorrhage is massive, other symptoms such as facial pallor, dizziness or even fainting, sudden temperature drop, rapid pulse, and tarry stools may appear. If the patient further feels severe pain in the lower right abdominal region and shows signs of nausea, vomiting, and a rapid thready pulse, then an intestinal perforation should be suspected. This disease should be differentiated from malaria, pulmonary tuberculosis, and acute schistosomiasis. Traditional Chinese medicine differentiates typhoid into moisture-heat retaining (shih-wen nei-liu) and fever ills condensing (jo-hsieh nei-chieh) types as the most common.

Moisture-heat-retaining typhoid. Characterized by continuous fever, general malaise, hidrosis, dry mouth, no inclination to drink more water, scanty urine, constipation, achy and heavy-feeling extremities. Fur on tongue white and oily or yellow and oily, pulse floating and slow.

Fever-ills condensing typhoid. Characterized by continuous high fever, great thirst and desire for water, parched lips, absence of saliva. Fur on tongue yellow and caked, sides of tongue prickly red, pulse rapid, and patient condition is serious.

Prevention

1. Attention to food and water sanitation. Do not drink untreated water. Eliminate flies.

2. Initiate a broad program of typhoid and paratyphoid inoculations, early discovery of patients, and early isolation and treatment.

3. Disinfect patient excreta. Cover urine and stools with lime. Eating utensils should be sterlized by boiling.

Treatment

1. New acupuncture therapy. Apply medium stimulation to needles placed in "ta-chui," "ch'u-ch'ih," "ho-ku," "yin-ling-ch'uan" points, once every day.

2. Chinese herbs.

    a. For moisture-heat retaining typhoid. Treatment should resolve
    moisture and clear fever, using remedies such as the follow-
    ing

        (1) Concoction of
            Yin-ch'en (artemesia)   5 ch'ien
            Talc   5 ch'ien
            Fu-ling   4 ch'ien
            Lien-ch'rao (Forsythia sp.)   3 ch'ien
            Pei-mu (Fritillaria sp.)   3 ch'ien
            She-kan   3 ch'ien
            Mu-t'ung   3 ch'ien
            Pai tou-k'ou (Amomum costatum)   5 fen
            Ch'ang-p'u (Acorus sp.)   8 fen
            Leaves of huo-hsiang   2 ch'ien

        (2) Concoction of
            K'ou-jen (seeds of Amomum costatum) 2 ch'ien
            Bamboo leaves   3 ch'ien
            T'ung ts'ao (Tetrapanax papyrifera) 3 ch'ien
            Hou-pu (Magnolia officinalis)   3 ch'ien
            Talc   5 ch'ien
            Almonds   3 ch'ien
            I-jen (Seeds of Job's tears)   6 ch'ien
            Processed pan-hsia   3 ch'ien

    b. For fever-ills condensing typhoid. Treatment should moderate
    the chill and clear fever, using remedies such as the follow-
    ing:

        (1) Concoction of
            Ts'ang-shu (Atractylis ovata)   3 ch'ien
            Gypsum   1 liang
            Chih-mu   5 ch'ien
            Licorice   2 ch'ien
            Glutinous rice   1 scoopful

        (2) Shen-hsi tan (patent medicine). For adults, one pill
            each time; for children, a suitably reduced dose.

        (3) Concoction of
            Crude ti-huang   8 ch'ien
            Mai-tung   5 ch'ien
            Yu-ch'u (Polygonatum officinalis) 5 ch'ien
            Sha-shen   3 ch'ien
            Pai-shao (Paeñia albiflora)   4 ch'ien
            Licorice   1.5 ch'ien

- 313 -

Tortoise shell	6 ch'ien
Turtle plate	6 ch'ien
Tu-li (oyster)	5 ch'ien

(This prescription is suited for cases in which the fever remains high, the yin is deficient and dehydration is great, and the patient is delirious at night.)

c. For <u>intestinal bleeding</u>. Treatment should nourish the yin, clear fever, and stop the bleeding, with the following remedy:

(1) Rhinoceros antlers, 2 ch'ien and take with some water. (Buffalo horns may be used as substitute)

(2) Concoction of

Crude ti-huang	5 ch'ien
Pai-shao	3 ch'ien
Tan-p'i	3 ch'ien

3. <u>Western medicines</u>

a. <u>Syntomycin</u> or <u>chloramphenicol</u> taken 4 times a day, dosage reduced 48 hours after temperature has been stabilizing and discontinued 3 days after temperature has come down [to normal]. The whole course of treatment generally takes about 14 days.

b. <u>Fluid supplements</u>. For serious cases, intravenous drip of dextrose with saline and addition of Vitamin C, depending on condition.

If complications of intestinal bleeding or intestinal perforation set in and emergency measures prove ineffective, take the patient to hospital immediately for further treatment.

<u>Note</u>: Clinical manifestations of paratyphoid are similar to those for typhoid, except they are less severe, and duration of illness is shorter. But treatment remains the same.

Infectious Hepatitis

Infectious hepatitis is an acute infectious disease caused by the hepatitis virus, usually transmitted via the digestive tract. At onset, the patient's appetite is poor and he shows symptoms such as an aversion to greasy foods, nausea, vomiting, abdominal distension, or slight epigastric pains, general weakness. Or, chills, fever, headache, stopped-up nose may accompany the onset of illness. Auscultation of the abdomen reveals hepatomegaly and tenderness.

Those cases in which jaundice occurs are referred to as "jaundiced infectious hepatitis." Where symptoms are fever, a bitter taste in mouth, thirst, a noticeably bright jaundice of sclera and the whole body (orange-colored), apprehension and restlessness, dark scanty urine, thick coat of yellow fur on tongue, and a rapid and forceful pulse, it is called yang jaundice (yang huang-cheng). Where the symptoms are a dully yellow skin and yellowed whites of the eyes without fever and parchness, a distended abdomen, loose stools, a thick oily coating of fur on tongue, a pink tongue, and a slow pulse, the hepatitis is called yin jaundice (yin huang-cheng). However, many patients do not show any jaundice at all and these cases are called "non-jaundiced infectious hepatitis."

Prevention

1. Initiating a broad program of health education. Pay attention to food and drink sanitation and the purification (disinfection) of drinking water. The goal should be a general observance of clean lines and hygiene, and the washing of hands before meals to be practiced by all.

2. Proper treatment and disposal of the hepatitis patient's excreta, by sprinkling a layer of lime over the waste matter and covering tightly with lid. As for fomites such as dishes, chopsticks etc., used by the patient, boil in clear water for 20-30 minutes.

3. Chinese herbs in concoction, prepared from the following:

Soybeans or mung beans	1 liang
Leaves of ta-ch'ing (Clerodendron sp.)	5 ch'ien
Licorice	1 ch'ien

Treatment

1. New acupuncture therapy. Moderate stimulation to "tan-yu," "tsu-san-li," "t'ai-ch'ung," points, once daily. When fever is present, also needle "ho-ku" and "ch'u-ch'ih" points.

2. Chinese herbs

    a. For yang jaundice cases. Treatment should "embitter" the cold (han) and clear fever, using the following remedies:

        (1) Concoction of

Yin-ch'en (artemesia capillaris)	1 liang
Dandelions	1 liang

        (2) Concoction of

Ti-erh ts'ao	2 liang
Yin-ch'en (Artemesia sp.)	1 liang
Hsia-ku ts'ao (Brunella vulgaris) or ma-pien ts'ao (verbena)	5 ch'ien

(3) Concoction of
    Yin-ch'en (<u>Artemesia</u> sp.)   1 liang
    Yu-chin   2 ch'ien
    Ch'ih hsiao-tou   5 ch'ien
       (<u>Phaseolus angularis</u>)

(4) Concoction of mei-hsieh tung-ch'ing (roots and leaves)
    2 liang in water.

b. For <u>yin-jaundice cases</u>. Treatment should strengthen the spleen and resolve moisture, using the following remedies:

(1) Concoction of
    Tsang-shu (<u>Atractylis ovata</u>)   4 ch'ien
    Dried orange peel   2 ch'ien
    Processed pan-hsia   1.5 ch'ien
       (<u>Pinella ternata</u>)
    Yin-ch'en (<u>artemesia</u>)   5 ch'ien

(2) Concoction of
    Hou-pu (<u>Magnolia</u> sp.)   4 ch'ien
    Tang-shen (<u>Campanumal pilosula</u>) 3 ch'ien
    Pai-shu (<u>Atraetylis ovata</u>)   1.5 ch'ien
    Ch'ai-hu (thoroughwax)   2 ch'ien
    Hsuan-hu-so (<u>Corydalis ternata</u>) 1.5 ch'ien
    Chi-nei-chin   2 ch'ien

c. For <u>non-jaundice cases</u>. Treatment should loosen up the liver and rectify energy flow, using the following remedies

(1) Concoction of
    Tan-shen (<u>Salvia multiorrhiza</u>) 4 ch'ien
    Hsia-ku ts'ao (<u>Brunella vulgaris</u>)3 ch'ien
    Ti-erh ts'ao (<u>Hypericum japonicum</u>) 5 ch'ien
    Chin-ch'ien ts'ao   5 ch'ien
    Shih-ta-kung-lao   3-5 ch'ien

(This prescription is suited for chronic hepatitis)

(2) Concoction of

    Ch'ai-hu (thoroughwax)   3 ch'ien
    Huang-ch'ing   3 ch'ien
    Hsiang-fu (<u>Cyperes rotandus</u>) 3 ch'ien
    Processed pan-hsia   3 ch'ien
    Tan-shen   5 ch'ien
    Fresh licorice   1 ch'ien

3. Western medicines

Liver-conserving drugs such as vitamin B complex, vitamin C or glucose etc., may be given accordingly.

Epidemic Encephalitis B

Epidemic encephalitis B is called "yueh-nao" for short. It is an acute infectious disease caused by the encephalitis B virus that is transmitted by mosquitoes. It is frequently epidemic in the summer and fall, occurring in the old and young, males and females. The onset is acute, characterized by a sudden very high rise in temperature accompanied by headache, vomiting, convulsions, and in most cases, signs of cerebral irritation such as neck rigidity and positive reactions to Brudzinski's and Kernig's signs, and the plantar reflex. In severe cases, the patient rapidly becomes confused, lethargic or stuporous, his breathing slowed or irregular, and his lips cyanosed. Or his breathing may stop suddenly and the patient dies. In some cases, aphasia or paralysis may remain as complications following recovery. This disease must be differentiated from heat stroke, falciparum malaria, epidemic meningitis, purulent or tuberculous meningitis.

In traditional Chinese medicine theory, this disease falls within the scope of "summer moisture" (shu-shih). Generally speaking, it can be divided into the following four stages.

Exposure summer moisture (wai-kan shu-shih), which is characterized by high fever, headache, restlessness, and neck rigidity. The fur on tongue is thin and red, the pulse is slippery and rapid.

Fever penetration into heart (jo jih hsin-pao), characterized by high fever, cramps, coma, and cyanosed lips. The pulse is full and rapid, the fur on tongue yellow, or brownish and dry. The tongue itself is red.

Summer moisture retained internally (shu-shih nei-liu), characterized by a continuous low-grade fever, nausea, no appetite, and parchness with no desire to drink water. Fur on tongue is white and oily, the pulse is slippery and slightly fast.

Prevention

1. Promoting the Patriotic Health Movement, with particular attention to eradication of and protection against mosquitoes indoors and outdoors (See "Pest Eradication to Eliminate Disease") and timely isolation and treatment of affected patients.

2. Chinese herbs, using concoction of
   Leaves of huo-hsiang (Agastache rugosa)   5 ch'ien
   Leaves of shih ch'ang-k'u (Acorus sp.)   3 ch'ien
   Wild chrysanthemums   1 liang
   Pan-lan-ken (Strobilanthes sp.), whole plant 1 liang

Treatment

1. __New acupuncture technique__. Needle puncture to "ta-chiu," "ch'u-ch'ih," "ho-ku" and "t'ai-ch'ung" points until some bleeding is seen. Add "shih-hsuan" to points needle-punctured, when high fever and convulsions are also present. When coma is present, add "jen-chung," "yun-ch'uan," "nei-kuan" points. Where there is much mucus and sputum, add the "ch'ih-tse" and "feng-lung"; and when there is headache, add the "t'ai-yang" point. Use strong stimulation to these points, once daily.

2. __Umbilical compress__ prepared from an eviscerated toad preserved in 1 ch'ien of powdered realgar and a little alcohol (or urine). Use two or three toad compresses in succession. (also applicable for other high fevers).

3. __Mud pack treatment__. Break up clods of dirt into fine pieces. Spread on ground and build up to 5 ts'un. Place bamboo mat over dirt and place sick child on the mat. Leave him there until his body temperature drops to about 38°C. Or use clean yellow dirt mixed with well water to make a mud pack. Place pack on chest of the sick child.

4. __Chinese herbs__

    a. For exposure summer-moisture type (of epidemic encephalitis B). Treatment should clear summer heat and resolve moisture, with remedies such as the following:

        (1) Concoction of

Huo-hsiang (<u>Agastache rugosa</u>)	3 ch'ien
P'ei-lan	3 ch'ien
Mild salted soybeans (tou-shih)	3 ch'ien
Shan-chih (<u>Gardenia florida</u>)	1.5 ch'ien
Lu-I powder	6 ch'ien
Leaves of ta-ch'ing (<u>Clerodendron cyrtophyllum</u>)	5 ch'ien

        (2) Huo-hsiang cheng-ch'i yuan (patent medicine). Take 3 ch'ien each time, three times a day.

    b. For __summer moisture fever type__. Treatment should clear fever and promote moisturization, with remedies such as the following:

        (1) Concoction of

Lu-pien ching (<u>Serissa foetida</u>)	5 ch'ien
T'ien-pien chu (<u>Aster trinervius</u>)	5 ch'ien
Ya-chih ts'ao	3 liang
Ch'i-hsieh I-chih hua (<u>Paris polyphylla</u>)	3 ch'ien

(2) Concoction of
    Hai-chin-sha   3 ch'ien
    Violets   5 ch'ien
    K'ou t'eng (Uncaria Rhynchophylla) 3 ch'ien
    Honeysuckle flowers   3 ch'ien
    Chrysanthemums   2 ch'ien
    Gypsum   1 liang
    (crushed and precooked 20 minutes before use)

(3) Concoction of
    Honeysuckle flowers   3 ch'ien
    Forsythia   3 ch'ien
    Chrysanthemums   3 ch'ien
    Mountain gardenia   3 ch'ien
    Salted soybeans   2 ch'ien
    Fresh roots of rushes   1 liang
    Leaves of ta ch'ing (Clerodendron sp.)   5 ch'ien

c. For fever-penetration-into-heart type. Treatment should be
    tranquillizing, using remedies such as the following:

    (1) Special concoction of pan-lan-ken (Strobilanthes flaccidi-
        folius) prepared as follows: To 1 chin of pan-lan-ken
        add 2000 ml water and concoct until fluid measures only
        1000 ml. Add 1500 ml water to a second batch [of pan-lan-
        ken] and concoct until only 600 ml remains. Mix both
        concoctions and keep in thermos bottle. Give adult patient
        20-25 ml of concoctiong every two hours, day and night.
        For children, reduce dosage accordingly.

    (2) Concoction of leaves of ta-ch'ing, 1 liang, given every
        3 hours until fever subsides.

    (3) Niu-huang ch'ing-hsin yuan (patent medicine), 1 tablet
        twice a day.

    (4) Concoction of
        Hearts of lotus flowers   1 ch'ien
        Bamboo leaves (tender inside leaves) 2 ch'ien
        Hearts of forsythia   2 ch'ien
        Hsuan-shen (Scrophularia sp.)   3 ch'ien
        Hearts of mai-tung (Liriope sp.) 3 ch'ien
        Tips of rhinoceros horns   2 ch'ien
        (if none available, buffalo horns may be used)

        If patient has much mucus, add 5 teaspoonfuls of chu-li
        (bamboo drippings) to each dose.

d. For summer-moisture-retained-internally type. Treatment should clear fever and resolve moisture, with remedies such as the following:

(1) Concoction of
    Crude ti-huang   5 ch'ien
    Mai-tung (Liriope sp.)   3 ch'ien
    Forsythia   3 ch'ien
    Ch'ing kao (artemesia sp.)   3 ch'ien
    Huang-lien (Coptis chinensis)   8 fen
    Pi-yu san   6 ch'ien

    After the moisture has been eliminated, concentrate on reducing the fever and nourishing the yin, using concoction of
    Hsuan-shen (Scrophularia sp.)   5 ch'ien
    Mai-tung (Liriope sp.)   3 ch'ien
      (including hearts)
    Crude ti-huang   4 ch'ien

5. Western medicines

a. To lower temperature: Give intramuscular injections of analgene 0.5 gm.

b. To stop convulsions: Give 5-ml intravenous injection of 10 percent sodium amytal slowly; in small children, reduce dosage accordingly.

c. For respiratory difficulties: Give 0.25-0.375 gm of nikethemide by intramuscular or intravenous injection.

d. For patients comatosed over a long period of time, provide intravenous fluid supplements of 10 percent dextrose, vitamins C or B.

Besides these measures, large amounts of penicillin can be given intravenously, based on the patient's condition.

Malaria

Malaria, called "ta-pai-tzu" by the local populace is an infectious disease caused by the malarial parasite. The gametocytes, malarial parasites in the blood of the malaria patient, are transmitted into the body of [anopheles] mosquitoes when these mosquitoes feed on infected patients. In the mosquito, these gametocytes develop into numerous sporozoites. Then when these mosquitoe bite other people, these sporozoites are transferred into the blood stream of new patients and transported to the liver where they develop and invade the red cells, thereby causing the clinical signs of chills and fever in varying recurring patterns.

This disease is characterized by chills, high fever, sweating, and a definitely timed onset. The attacks may occur daily, or every other day (tertian malaria), or every three days (quartan malaria). Sometimes the attacks are characterized by severe chills and moderate fever, or by mild chills and high fever. Untreated over a period of time, the patient's face becomes sallow and yellowish, and a hard mass is felt under the left rib margin (splenomegaly). According to the patient's condition and the severity of the attack, malaria may be classified as a solid-type disease (shih-cheng) or a deficiency-type disease (hsu-cheng).

Solid-type malaria is characterized by a feeling of chest discomfort, parchness of mouth (which may also be absent), general uneasiness, retching or vomiting and spitting of mucus, presence of perspiration. Pulse is usually full, and fur on tongue is a thin yellow coating. Untreated over a period of time, abdominal distension and splenomegaly will be discernible.

Deficiency-type malaria is characterized by a facial sallowness or pallor, listlessness and lethargy, dyspnea, anorexia and weakness, lack of energy, and susceptibility to malaria after working hard, with chills and fever difficult to delineate. Pulse is generally deficient, tongue pink and uncoated.

Prevention

1. Protection against and eradication of mosquitoes (see "Pest Eradication to Eliminate Disease").

2. Initialling active measures to treat the sick. During epidemic seasons, provide prophylactic medication.

Treatment

1. New acupuncture technique. Apply needles 1-2 hours before attack to the "ta-chui," "nei-kuan," and "chih-yang" points. Using strong stimulation.
GV 14   PC 6   GV 7 thoi
2. Chinese herbs

    a. For solid type malaria. Treatment in beginning emphasizes neutralizing action, and forestalling attacks in later stages, with remedies such as the following:

        (1) Concoction of

Ch'ai-hu (thoroughwax)	3 ch'ien	Bupleurum
Pan-hsia (Pinellia ternata)	3 ch'ien	Pinellia
Tang-shen (Campanumaea sp.)	3 ch'ien	Codonopsis
Huang-ch'ing (Scutellaria baicalensis)	2 ch'ien	Scutellaria
Gypsum (add if fever high)	1 liang	Gypsum

- 321 -

(2) Concoction of

Leaves of huang-ch'ing (<u>Scutellaria</u> sp.)	5 ch'ien
Ch'ing-kao (artemesia)	2 ch'ien

The two prescriptions just given exert a neutralizing and moderating effect.

(3) Concoction of

Ch'ang-shan (<u>Dichroa febrifuga</u>)	3 ch'ien
Betelnut	3 ch'ien
Hou-pu (<u>Magnolia officinalis</u>)	3 ch'ien
Ts'ao-kuo (<u>Amomum medium</u>)	1.5 ch'ien
Tangerine peel	1.5 ch'ien
Dried orange peel	1.5 ch'ien
Licorice	1 ch'ien

For patients who are weakened by repeated attacks and prolonged illness, add

Ho-shou-wu (<u>Polygonum multiflorum</u>)	3 ch'ien
Tang-shen (<u>Campanumaea</u> sp.)	3 ch'ien

This prescription forestalls malaria attacks.

(4) Concoction of

Tortoise shell (toasted)	4 ch'ien
Peach kernel	4 ch'ien
Ch'ai-hu (thoroughwax)	2 ch'ien

(This prescription is suitable for chronic cases where splenomegaly is present.)

b. For <u>deficiency-type malaria</u>. Treatment should supplement the deficiency and eliminate malaria, using remedies such as the following:

(1) Concoction of

Processed ho-shou-wu (<u>Polygonum multiflorum</u>)	1 liang
Fresh ginger	3 ch'ien
Large dates	10

(2) Concoction of

Tang-shen	5 ch'ien
Tortoise shells	5 ch'ien
Black prunes	2 ch'ien

c. <u>External treatment</u>. Suitable for both solid-type and deficiency-type malaria.

    (1) Crush 1 liang of leeks, add dash of salt, and mix well. Use as compress over "nei-kuan" point 3 hours before onset of malarial attack.

    (2) Crush into powder 3 fen of pepper and 1 ch'ien of cicada molting. Mix with some rice to form a ball. Apply over "hsin-ch'u" point.

    (3) Pulverize equal parts of ts'ang-shu (<u>Atractylis ovata</u>), pai-ch'ih (<u>Angelica anomala</u>), ch'uan-kung (<u>Conieselinum unvittatum</u>), and cinnamon sticks. For each application, wrap 1 gm of powdered mixture inside piece of thin silk or cloth and tie securely, size of packet small enough to be plugged comfortably into nostril. Keep plugs inside nostrils for at least 4 hours, until sweating sets in following a bout of malarial chill and fever. Do not remove during attack. Repeat treatment daily or every other day until 3 days have lapsed after final attack. Store this medication in airtight jar as it loses its action rapidly.

3. <u>Western medicines</u>

    a. <u>Treatment during malaria active phase</u>. Combination therapy may be used in the radical treatment of new cases or those undergoin relapses. (See Table 6-4-1).

    b. Treatment during arrested stage. To completely root out the source of infection, it is best to give another course of drug therapy for patients without signs of disease for the past two years, at some time between October and February of the following year. (See Table 6-4-2).

Table 6-4-1.　Treatment During Malaria Active Phase

Unit = tablet

药物 (1)	氯化喹啉、伯氨喹啉混合疗法 (2)									奎宁、伯氨喹啉混合法 (3)			
	氯化喹啉 0.25克/片 (4)				伯氨喹啉13.2毫克/片 (5)					奎宁 (6) 0.3克/片		伯氨喹啉 (7) 13.2毫克/片	
年龄及剂量 (8)	第一日	第二日	第三日	总量	第一日	第二日	第三日	第四日	总量	每日	总量	每日	总量
2 岁以下 (15)	1/2	1/4	1/4	1	1/2	1/2	1/2	1/2	2	1	4	1/2	2
3～5岁 (16)	1	1/2	1/2	2	1	1	1	1	4	2	8	1	4
6～10岁 (17)	2	1	1	4	2	2	2	2	8	4	16	2	8
11～15岁 (18)	3	1½	1½	6	3	3	3	3	12	6	24	3	12
16 岁 (19)	4	2	2	8	4	4	4	4	16	9	36	4	16
疗程 (20)	连服 3 天 (21)				连服 4 天 (22)					连服 4 天 (22)			
服法 (23)	第1～3天二药同服，第4天单服 伯氨喹啉，每天一次顿服 (24)									二药同时服，奎宁每日二至三次分服，伯氨喹啉每天一次顿服 (25)			

Key:　(1)　Drug
　　　(2)　Combination therapy using chloroquine and primaquine
　　　(3)　Combination therapy using quinine and primaquine
　　　(4)　Chloroquine 0.25 gm/tablet
　　　(5)　Primaquine 13.2 mg/tablet
　　　(6)　Quinine 0.3 gm/tablet
　　　(7)　Primaquine 13.2 mg/tablet
　　　(8)　Age and dosage
　　　(9)　First day
　　　(10)　Second day
　　　(11)　Third day
　　　(12)　Total [dose]
　　　(13)　Fourth day
　　　(14)　Daily
　　　(15)　Two years and below
　　　(16)　3-5 years
　　　(17)　6-10 years
　　　(18)　11-15 years
　　　(19)　16 years
　　　(20)　Course of therapy
　　　(21)　Taken 3 days in a row
　　　(22)　Taken 4 days in a row
　　　(23)　Mode of medication
　　　(24)　Both drugs are taken simultaneously the first three days, primaquine only is taken on the 4th day; all in single daily doses.
　　　(25)　Both drugs are taken simultaneously; the quinine taken in daily divided (2 or 3 times) doses, the primaquinine, in single daily doses.

Table 6-4-2. Arrested Stage Treatment of Malaria

Unit = tablet

药物及 年 剂量 (1) (10)	第 一 天 (2)		第 二 天 (3)		第 三 天 (4) 伯氨喹啉	第 四 天 (5) 伯氨喹啉
	乙胺嘧啶 (6)	伯氨喹啉 (7)	乙胺嘧啶 (8)	伯氨喹啉 (9)		
(11) 2 岁以下	1	1/2	1	1/2	1/2	1/2
(12) 3~5 岁	2	1	2	1	1	1
(13) 6~10 岁	4	2	4	2	2	2
(14) 11~15 岁	6	3	6	3	3	3
(15) 16 岁以上	8	4	8	4	4	4

(16) 注: 乙胺嘧啶每片6.25毫克，伯氨喹啉每片13.2毫克。

Key: (1) Drug and dosage   (11) Two years and under
      (2) 1st day   (12) 3-5 years
      (3) Second day   (13) 6-10 years
      (4) 3rd day - primaquine (14) 11-15 years
      (5) 4th day - primaquine (15) 16 years and over
      (6) Pyrimethamine   (16) Note: Each tablet of pyrimethamine
      (7) Primaquine   is 6.25 mg; each tablet of prima-
      (8) Pyrimethamine   quine is 13.2 mg.
      (9) Primaquine
     (10) Age

Leptospirosis

Leptospirosis, also called "rice fever," is caused by the leptospira.
The source of infection is frequently water collected in rice fields that is
contaminated by excreta from diseased field mice, and the leptospires enter
the human body by skin penetration. Because this disease occurs during the
busy planting and harvesting seasons, accompanied frequently by hepatosplenomegaly, it must be differentiated from typhoid, malaria, and infectious hepatitis.

The onset of leptospirosis is acute, with sudden chills and fever that
frequently remains high, nausea, vomiting, headache, general myalgia, pre-
tibial pain and tenderness, hemorrhage in skin and mucous membranes together
with bleeding points of varying sizes, and possibly hemoptysis, epistaxis.
In serious cases, the patient may be delirious and jaundiced.

This disease falls within the scope of fevers and epidemic intoxications, in traditional Chinese medicine, and is seen clinically as fever-
dominant or moisture-dominant types.

The fever-dominant type of leptospirosis is characterized by headache, body aches, fever, chills, or fever without chills, thirst (frequently), desire for water, restlessness, dark yellow urine, hidrosis, red tongue, and a thin white fur coating on a dry tongue. Pulse is bounding and rapid or tense and rapid.

The moisture-dominant type of leptospirosis is characterized by a heaviness and giddiness of the head, chills and fever, or chills more severe than fever, mouth parched but not desiring water, chest discomfort, and anhidrosis. The fur on tongue is thick, white and oily. Pulse is slow.

Prevention

1. Eradication of field mice. Add lime or straw ashes to disinfect patient's urine.

2. Chinese herbs, using

   a. Concoction of ku-shan-lung (vine), 5 ch'ien, to be taken once a day for three days.

   b. Treatment of rice paddies with scattering of hsiang-tse-lan (Eupatorium adoratum), chopped, or sprinkling of lime.

3. Prophylactic vaccine. Initial inoculation of leptospirosis vaccine 1 ml given subcutaneously, followed a week later by a 2-ml injection.

Treatment

1. Bed rest, forced fluids, and parenteral fluids, if necessary. In severe cases, give intravenous drip of 10 percent dextrose or 4 percent glucose with saline, 2000-3000 ml daily, as a measure to protect the liver and kidneys.

2. Chinese herbs

   a. For fever-dominant leptospirosis. Treatment should clear fever and detoxify poisons with the following concoction:

Honeysuckle blossoms	5 ch'ien
Forsythia	4 ch'ien
Niu-pang-tzu	3 ch'ien
Mint	1 ch'ien
Kuan-tsung (Cyrtomium fortunei)	5 ch'ien
Artemesia	1 liang
Mung beans	1 liang
Licorice	1.5 ch'ien

If epistaxis is present, also add the following to concoction

Crude ti-huang	5 ch'ien
Ch'ih shao (red waterchestnut)	
Fresh p'u-huang (_Acorus_ sp.)	3 ch'ien

b. For <u>moisture-dominant leptospirosis</u>. Treatment should clear fever and promote moisture elimination, using concoction such as the following:

Artemesia	1 liang
Talc	5 ch'ien
Fu-ling	4 ch'ien
Forsythia	4 ch'ien
Pei-mu (_Fritillaria_ sp.)	2 ch'ien
She-kan	3 ch'ien
Che-ch'ien-tzu	3 ch'ien
Pai tou-k'ou (_Amomum_ sp.)	8 fen
Huo-hsiang	2 ch'ien
Ch'ang-p'u (Acorus sp.)	1 ch'ien

3. <u>Western medicines</u>. Penicillin 600,000 units is generally given intramuscularly, four times a day. When necessary, the initial dose may be doubled. If the patient is sensitive to penicillin, aureomycin may be used, 3-4 gm daily. Given here is the adult dose. For children, reduce dosage accordingly.

Tetanus

Tetanus is an acute infectious disease caused by the tetanus bacillus which is frequently found in manure. Any wound contaminated by dirt or rust is an opening for tetanus bacilli invasion into the human body to cause disease. Generally, the disease does not manifest itself until a few days after the initial injury (such as happens with battle wounds and stab wounds). The chief symptom is the periodic and rigid spasmodic contraction of the muscles. Symptoms at onset are chills, headache, facial myalgia, loss of mastication "power" etc. Spasms begin with the muscles of mastication which result in the patient presenting a sardonic grin, teeth gritted together tightly [lock-jaw] and it is impossible to eat. Because of spasms in the cervical muscles, neck rigidity, opisthotonos, and swallowing difficulties appear. Each spasm lasts from several seconds to several minutes, easily provoked by slight stimulation such as noise, light or moving the patient. Untreated, the patient becomes weakened, and spasms of the respiratory muscles will cause asphyxia and death. The patient's mind remains clear until death.

<u>Prevention</u>

1. Attention to occupational and production safety to cut down on the chances for puncture wounds and cuts to occur.

2. Wherever possible, practice of a tetanus toxoid inoculation program.

Treatment

1. Care of wound: When suspected signs of tetanus appear, clean out the wound if it has not been properly done.

2. Put patient in a quiet bedroom and wipe off and clean his mouth and upper respiratory tract of secretions. Burn all soiled dressings.

3. New acupuncture technique. Needle the "chia-che" penetrating the "ti-tsang," and also the "ho-ku" and "t'ai-ch'ung" points using strong stimulation, twice a day.

4. Chinese herbs. Treatment should be directed toward eliminating wind to ease the spasms, and clearing fever to detoxify, using remedies such as the following:

a. Concoction of
Cicada moltings   5 ch'ien - 1 liang
Scorpion   3-5 ch'ien
Centipede   3-5 ch'ien
Fresh aconite   1.5 ch'ien
Liang-mien-chen   5 ch'ien - 1 liang
Ko-ken (Pueraria matsumura)   5 ch'ien - 1 liang

Prescription modification:
For high fever, add
 Forsythia suspensa   5 ch'ien
 Coptis chinensis   3 ch'ien

If cough is productive, with much sputum, add
 Pei-mu   5 ch'ien
 Chieh-keng   4 ch'ien
 Peel of kuo-wei   5 ch'ien

When urine is dark yellow and there is dysuria, add
 Pai mao-ken   1 liang
  (white congongrass)

For constipation, cook
 Ta-huang (rhubarb)   1 liang
 Yuan-ming-fen (Glauber's salt)   1 liang
in 800 ml water and use for enema.

b. Concoction of

Cicada moltings	1 liang
T'ien-nan-hsing	2 ch'ien
T'ien-ma	2 ch'ien
Scorpion	1.5 ch'ien
Roasted chiang-ts'an (silkworms)	3 ch'ien

Before drinking concoction, give patient 5 fen of chu-sha (vermillion) taken with some yellow wine. If jaw is locked, consider using nasal feeding. If patient starts perspiring in hands and feet, this is a good sign. Otherwise, the prognosis is poor.

c. Concoction of

Mulberry twigs	5 ch'ien - 1 liang
Ti-lung	3 ch'ien
Mu-kua [papaya]	5 ch'ien
Pei-mu (Fritillaria sp.)	5 ch'ien
Pai-shao (Paenia albiflora)	5 ch'ien
Tang-shen	8 ch'ien
Huang-ch'i (Astragalus sp.)	1 liang
Ho-shou-wu	1 liang
Mai-tung (Liriope graminifolia)	5 ch'ien
Fu-ling	5 ch'ien

(This prescription is suitable for use during resolution and recovery phases).

5. Western medicine

a. When suspected signs of tetanus appear, immediately give patient tetanus antitoxin 30,000 to 60,000 units added to 5 percent dextrose solution by slow intravenous drip. If symptoms cannot be controlled, consider sending patient to better-equipped hospital for treatment.

b. Use 10 percent formaldehyde, sodium amytal, or dolantin to keep patient quiet.

Rabies

Rabies, also called "hydrophobia" is an acute infectious disease caused by the rabies virus. This disease can be transmitted by a rabid dog bite or open-wound contact with saliva of a rabid dog. At onset, signs are a mental apathy, headache, slight fever, restlessness, apprehension, disturbed slumber, dryness in mouth, nausea, painful urination, and a painful numbness over wound if it has already healed. One or two days later, mania, sensitivity to wind, sound and light are noted. Very slight stimulation is enough to cause convulsions and wild movements. In the beginning, there is an aversion to drinking water, but later on, any mention or sight of water is enough to cause laryngeal spasms. In the final stage, the patient quiets down, paralysis appears, the respirations become weak, and death ensues.

Prevention

1. Impoundment and destruction of rabid and wild dogs. Strengthen management of domestic dogs. Most rabid dogs show neck stiffness, the head, ears and tail all droop, and they can only run forward in one direction, unable to turn back to see what is happening behind. Rabid dogs caught and destroyed should be burned.

2. When a victim is bitten by a dog, but not sure if it is rabid, the first step is proper treatment of the wound and injection of rabies vaccine.

Treatment

1. Cleaning wound. Examine wound carefully to determine scope and depth of bite. Wash with generous amounts of soapy and clear water. Deep wounds may be cauterized by a carbolic acid concentrate. If necessary, the wound may be opened up some more.

2. Rabies vaccine. Administer series of vaccine injections in time. The dosage is 2 ml of vaccine given subcutaneously in the abdomen or other site, daily for 14 to 21 days. If the bite is on the head, face, or neck, or if the victim is a child, the haste is even more urgent. In these instances, the injections are given twice daily for the series to be completed within 5 to 7 days.

3. <u>Chinese herbs</u>

    a. Juice of fresh wan-nien-ch'ing (<u>Rohdea japonica</u>) 5 ch'ien obtained from crushing the whole plant (including roots). Wrap crushed plant in gauze and extract juice by wringing the gauze.

    b. Concoctions of the following, twice a day:

Fresh ti-yu	1 liang
Fresh roots of bamboo tzu-chu (<u>Phyllostachys nigra</u>), fresh	2 liang
Tang-shen	3 ch'ien
Chiang-huo	3 ch'ien
Tu-huo	3 ch'ien
Ch'ai-hu (Thoroughwax)	3 ch'ien
Ch'ien-hu	3 ch'ien
Chi-he (acorn shells)	2 ch'ien
Chieh-keng (<u>Platycodon</u> sp.)	2 ch'ien
Szechwan unvittatum	1.5 ch'ien

- 330 -

```
Mint                                          1 ch'ien
Licorice                                      3 ch'ien
Fresh ginger                                  3 slices
```

Or, roots of tzu-chu may be boiled in water, and the concocted juice used to steam eggs for eating.

Both of these prescriptions are suitable for use in the early stage of the illness.

c. Pulverized mixture of
```
    Centipede                                 1 ch'ien
    Scorpion                                  1 ch'ien
```

Take with warm boiled water.

d. Fleshy root covering of yuan-hua (Daphne genkwa), with surface corium and woody pith removed, roasted and pulverized. Take 1 ch'ien each time with boiled water. Stools passed following this medication are watery and contain black masses of occult blood. Repeat medication every other day until stools passed are a normal yellow-brown.

The two prescriptions given above are suitable for use during the mania and spasmodic stage.

Section 5   Parasites

Schistosomiasis

Schistosomiasis is a disease caused by parasitism of the schistosoma [Schistosoma japonicum] in the portal venous system of the human body. The ova are expelled with passage of feces and they hatch into larvae outside the human body. The larvae then penetrate into bodies of oncomelania snails in which they develop into cercariae. Upon separation from the snail, the cercariae swim freely in water. On encounter with man or animal, the cercariae penetrate their skin and travel to the liver via the blood circulation. Development in the liver is rapid, and the almost mature schistosomes are shifted over to the mesenteric veins where they complete their development, establish a foot-hold and produce ova. Examination of stools from infected persons will show the ova.

Prevention

1. Oncomelania snail eradication. Measures include burying, manure-composting, reclamation planting, burning, and chemical eradication (See section "Snail Elimination" in Chapter 2).

2. <u>Excreta management</u>. If managed properly, ova will be destroyed (see Section "Excreta Management, Chapter 2).

3. <u>Protection</u> and proper management of <u>water supply source</u> (see "Drinking Water Sanitation, Chapter 2).

4. <u>Chinese herbs</u>

    a. Before going into the water, apply tea oil or rub smartweed all over extremities. After coming out of the water, rub limbs with tieh-ma-pien ts'ao (verbena sp.)

    b. After working in infected waters, take concoction prepared from huang-mieh [brown bamboo strip?] sweetened with brown sugar.

5. Active program of therapy for patients.

A. Acute Schistosomiasis

Acute schistosomiasis usually occurs in patients infected for the first time. Victims who have come in contact with infected waters usually come down with the disease in about a month. The season of greatest incidence runs from May through September. The onset of illness is acute, accompanied by fever, chills, hidrosis, cough, muscular and joint pains, hepatomegaly, etc. After onset of illness, culture of stool from infected patient for schistosoma larva is usually positive. This disease must be differentiated from malaria, typhoid, dysentery, septicemia, tuberculosis, etc.

Treatment

1. <u>Chinese herbs</u>

    a. Concoction prepared from

Honeysuckle flowers	6 ch'ien
Forsythia suspensa	5 ch'ien
Niu pang-tzu (<u>Arctium lappa</u>)	2 ch'ien
T'ien-pien chu (<u>Aster</u> sp.)	4 ch'ien
Pai-t'ou weng (anemone)	4 ch'ien
Ch'ih-shao (water chestnut)	3 ch'ien
Tan-p'i	3 ch'ien
T'ieh ma-pien (<u>Verbena</u> sp.)	5 ch'ien
Licorice	1 ch'ien

    (This prescription is suited for use in presence of high fever, flushed face, thirst, red tongue, yellow coated fur on tongue, and rapid forceful pulse in patients.)

- 332 -

b. Concoction of ya-chih ts'ao (spider wort).

c. Shelled pumpkin seeds, pulverized. Take 80 gm each time, three times a day, for 7 to 14 days in succession.

2. Western medicines

a. Furfuryl prophylamine. Dosage: 60 mg/kg/day in four divided doses, for 14 days. This drug has side effects such as vomiting, abdominal pain, diarrhea, muscular spasms in calf of leg etc., so during the first two days, the dosage is cut in half to gradually build up drug tolerance. It is prohibited for use by patients with liver and/or kidney diseases. Where it produces emotional disturbances such as quarrelsomeness and crying in some patients, the drug should be discontinued.

b. Pao-t'ai-sung, 0.1-0.2 gm is given by mouth, three times a day. If the fever is still not controlled after a week of medication, change over to hormones.

c. Hydrocortisone, 100 to 300 mg daily, given in a 5-10 percent dextrose intravenous drip. Or, take cortisone 5-10 mg, three to four times daily.

It is only after treatment with the drugs described, to control fever and other acute symptoms that treatment by antimonials is considered. If the patient's condition is good and the fever is kept below 100°C, long-range treatment using antimonials in small doses may be considered.

B. Chronic Schistosomiasis

Some cases of repeated infection with the schistosomiasis cercariae and those cases of acute schistomiasis that were not basically cured usually develop into chronic schistosomiasis. These patients are usually emaciated and weak, beset by diarrhea, abdominal distension and hepatosplenomegaly. Young persons so afflicted are small and may show stunted growth and some effect on the appearance of secondary sexual characteristics. Generally, diagnosis is determined by the patient's history, physical examination and stool culture or stool collection to examine for larvae and eggs.

Treatment

Tartar emetic 20-day course. The total dose is figured on the basis of 25 mg/kg body weight. The daily dose is given by intravenous injection. For distribution of the dose to be given each day, see Table 6-5-1.

- 333 -

Table 6-5-1. Dosage Chart for 20-Day Treatment Using Tartar Emetic (25 gm 1 kg body weight)

(1) 针次 / (3) Injection sequence \ (2) 体重 Body weight	20	21	22	23	24	25	26	27	28	29	30	31	32	33	34	35	36	37	38	39	40	41	42	43	44	45	46	47	48	49	50	51	52	53	54	55	56	57	58	59	60
总剂量 Total dosage	50	53	55	58	60	63	65	68	70	73	75	78	80	83	85	88	90	93	95	98	100	103	105	108	110	113	115	118	120	123	125	128	130	133	135	136	140	143	145	148	150
1	2	3	3	2	3	3	3	3	3	3	3	3	3	4	4	4	4	4	5	5	5	5	5	5	5	5	5	5	5	6	6	6	6	6	6	6	6	6	6	7	7
2	3	3	3	4	4	4	4	4	4	5	5	5	5	5	6	6	6	6	6	6	6	7	7	7	7	7	7	7	7	7	7	7	8	8	8	8	8	8	8	7	7
3	3	3	3	3	3	4	4	4	4	4	4	4	5	5	5	6	6	6	6	6	6	6	6	7	7	7	7	7	7	7	7	8	8	8	8	8	8	8	8	8	8
4	3	3	3	4	4	4	4	4	4	4	4	4	4	5	5	6	6	6	6	6	6	6	6	7	7	7	7	7	7	8	8	8	8	8	8	8	8	8	8	8	8
5	3	3	3	3	3	4	4	4	4	4	4	4	4	5	5	5	6	6	6	6	5	6	6	6	6	7	7	7	7	8	8	8	8	7	8	8	8	8	8	8	8
6	2	3	3	3	3	3	3	3	3	3	4	4	4	4	4	4	5	5	5	6	5	5	6	6	6	6	6	6	6	6	6	6	7	7	7	7	7	7	7	7	8
7	3	3	2	3	3	3	3	3	3	3	4	4	4	4	5	4	5	5	5	6	5	5	6	6	6	6	6	6	6	6	6	6	7	7	7	7	7	7	7	7	8
8	2	2	2	3	3	3	3	3	3	3	3	4	4	4	4	4	4	5	5	5	5	5	6	6	5	5	5	6	6	6	6	6	7	7	7	7	7	7	8	8	8
9	2	2	2	3	3	3	3	3	3	3	3	3	4	4	4	4	4	4	5	5	5	5	6	6	6	6	5	6	6	6	6	6	6	6	6	7	6	7	8	8	8
10	2	3	2	2	2	3	3	3	3	3	3	3	3	4	4	4	4	4	4	4	5	5	6	6	5	5	5	6	6	6	5	6	6	6	6	6	6	6	8	8	8
11	2	3	2	2	2	3	3	3	3	3	3	3	3	3	4	4	4	4	4	4	5	5	6	6	5	5	5	6	6	6	5	6	6	7	5	7	6	7	7	7	7
12	2	3	2	2	2	3	3	3	3	3	3	3	3	4	4	4	4	4	4	4	5	5	6	6	5	5	5	6	6	6	5	6	6	7	6	7	6	7	7	7	7
13	2	3	2	2	2	3	3	2	3	3	3	3	3	3	3	3	3	4	4	4	5	5	4	5	5	5	5	6	6	6	5	6	6	7	6	7	6	7	6	6	6
14	2	3	2	2	2	3	3	3	3	3	3	3	3	3	4	4	4	4	4	5	5	5	4	5	5	5	5	6	6	6	5	6	6	6	6	7	6	7	6	6	6
15	2	3	2	2	3	3	3	3	3	3	3	3	3	4	4	4	4	4	4	5	5	5	4	5	5	5	5	6	6	6	5	6	6	6	6	7	6	7	7	6	6
16	2	3	2	3	3	3	3	3	3	3	4	4	4	4	4	5	4	5	5	5	5	5	5	5	5	6	6	6	6	6	6	6	6	6	6	7	6	7	7	7	7
17	2	3	2	3	3	3	3	3	3	4	4	4	4	4	5	5	5	5	5	5	5	5	5	5	6	6	6	6	6	6	7	7	7	7	7	7	7	7	7	8	7
18	3	3	3	4	4	4	4	4	4	4	4	4	5	5	5	5	5	5	5	5	5	5	5	5	6	6	6	6	6	7	7	7	7	7	7	7	7	7	8	8	8
19	3	3	3	4	4	4	4	4	4	5	5	5	5	5	5	5	5	5	5	5	6	6	6	6	6	6	6	6	7	7	7	7	7	7	7	8	8	8	8	8	8
20	3	3	3	4	4	4	4	4	5	5	5	5	5	5	5	5	5	5	5	5	6	6	6	6	6	6	6	7	7	7	7	7	7	7	7	8	8	8	8	8	8

Note: Body weight in chart is based on kg, total dosage and each individual dose is the amount of 1 percent tartar emetic in ml.

Key:
(1) Injection sequence
(2) Body weight
(3) Total dosage
(4) Amount for each dose

For males, the total dosage should not exceed 1.5 gm; for females and males in less fit condition, it should not exceed 1.3 gm. Patients in serious condition and not very good physical shape can have their total dosage figured on the basis of 22-24 mg/kg body weight. To each tartar emetic intravenous injection, add 20-40 ml of 25-50 percent dextrose solution, after which give injection slowly.

Indications and contraindications of antimonial therapy. Antimonials are definitely toxic, and a short-term or long-term course of treatment must be selected in the very beginning, in conjunction with the patient's condition. This is done to curtail any reaction and prevent any untoward accidents.

1. Short-term therapy is best suited for those cases of chronic schistosomiasis in reasonably good health, with no complications. Males over 55 years old, females over 50 years, and children less than 6 years old should use long-term therapy.

2. Long-term therapy is suited for those cases of chronic schistosomiasis in poorer physical condition, or cases of acute schistomiasis whose fever has subsided, or those cases of late schistosomiasis uncomplicated by jaundice and ascites.

3. Contra-indications. Antimonial therapy should not be given those patients who show the following conditions:

a. Acute infectious diseases or chronic fevers.

b. Cases with disturbances in cardiovascular compensation function, or those with serious arrhythmias.

c. Hypertension with readings over 160/100 mm, or patients with lower readings accompanied by heart, brain, or kidney complications.

d. Acute or chronic hepatitis, or suspected hepatitis (long range therapy may be considered for cured cases of hepatitis in whom liver function has been restored to normal for more than a year).

e. Acute or chronic hepatitis, or active tuberculosis.

f. Late stage schistosomiasis complicated by jaundice or ascites.

g. Pregnant women and nursing mothers.

h. Patients previously treated with antimonials less than 6 months ago.

<u>Precautions in antimonial therapy and treatment of reactions</u>.
Be familiar with the indications and contra-indications for such treatment. Observe the patient from start to finish. Take a careful and
detailed history, give patient a thorough physical examination, and write
up a brief but concise record, and depending on the patient's condition,
examine the blood and urine, if necessary.

Before initiating treatment, accurately check the patient's weight,
and twice a day, record his temperature and listen to his heart, check his
liver and sclera. Treat reactions in time, and determine whether to stop
injections and observe patient, or to terminate treatment.

After course of therapy has been completed, continue to observe patient
for 2 days. In those with severe reactions, extend period of observation.
Have necessary first aid items ready when such courses of therapy are being
given.

Some reactions frequently associated with antimonial therapy are listed
below:

1. <u>Extravasation of injection</u>. Be careful when giving the injection
that leakage outside the vein (extravasation) does not occur. If the patient
feels pain, withdraw needle and search for another vein. If an extravasation
has already occurred, immediately inject into site 5-10 ml physiological saline
or 1 percent procaine (given subcutaneously) to dilute the antimonial.

2. <u>Fever</u>. If the patient's temperature goes up beyond 37.5°C following an injection, stop injections, and observe patient to discover cause and
treat accordingly. If systemic symptoms such as high fever and hepatic tenderness appear, take antipyretic measures immediately -- terminate antimonial
therapy and treat with acupuncture, hormones and parenteral fluids.

3. <u>Nausea and vomiting</u>. Needle-puncture the "nei-kuan," "tsu-san-li"
points. Give atropine 0.3-0.6 mg, or phenothiazine 25 mg, by mouth or by
intramuscular injection. Mild cases do not need therapy discontinued. But
those patients who continue to be bothered by nausea and vomiting, and those
mentally deteriorated, stop injections immediately and observe, and give supplementary fluids to see if problem was caused by antimonial therapy.

4. <u>Coughing</u>. Slow down injection speed.

5. <u>Skin rash</u>. Give benadryl or phenergan 25 mg. Generally, it is
not necessary to stop injection treatment.

6. __Toxic hepatitis__. Before the condition sets in, there frequently is continued nausea and vomiting, hepatomegaly and tenderness, jaundice etc. In such cases, discontinue antimonial therapy immediately. Give intravenous injections of dimercapto-succinate dissolved in 10 ml of injection -- use water, 2 to 4 times daily. Also give 10 percent dextrose solution, 1000 -- 2000 ml daily, by intravenous drip. Support with large doses of vitamins B and C. If necessary, add hydro cortisone or cortisone.

7. __Arrhythmia__. During treatment, the heart rate may be lower than 60 beats per minute, or exceed 100 beats per minute (120 in children). Or where extra-systole exceeds three per minute, discontinue injections, prescribe bed rest, and observe patient closely for further developments. In presence of excessive bradycardia or extrasystole, administer 0.5-1 gm atropine intramuscularly or intravenously, 2 to 3 times a day.

8. __Cardiac intoxication__ (Adams-Stokes syndrome). This is one of the most serious reactions to antimonial intoxication, where emergency treatment given in a matter of seconds makes the difference between life and death. This syndrome usually appears in the final stage of treatment, though it can also occur within 2 to 3 days following a course of short-term therapy. This syndrome can cause paroxysmal ventricular tachycardia or ventricular fibrillation. The clinical manifestations are sudden fainting, convulsions, cyanosis and disappearance of heart sounds. Frequently before an attack, the patient experiences changing emotions, mental apathy, fever, continued vomiting, frequent extrasystoles etc. However, the condition may set in suddenly without marked forewarning. It is important to be on guard at all times.

__Emergency measures for cardiac intoxication.__

a. Immediately give intravenous injection of atropine 1-2 mg, repeating dose every one-half to one hour for 3 to 4 times in succession. Watch the patient's condition. If there is no recurrence, give atropine 0.5 - 1 mg by hypodermic injection, repeated every 4 to 6 hours until a pink coloring has returned to the patient's cheeks, and his heart rate is stable around 100 beats a minute. If the heart rate drops below 90 per minute, his face becomes pale and symptoms are heightened, change to intravenous instead of hypodermic injection. If, after 48 hours, there are no further attacks, discontinue atropine.

Large doses of atropine can also cause an intoxication reaction. It is manifested as rosy cheeks, ischidrosis, dilated pupils, excitability, mania etc. At this time the atropine dosage must be reduced or discontinued. Instead, isopropyl-epinephrine 0.5 - 1 mg added to 5 percent dextrose 500 ml given by slow intravenous drip is used to regulate the heart rate until it reaches about 100 beats a minute.

b. Keep patient quiet. Give luminal 0.1 gm or sodium amytal 0.2 gm intramuscularly, once every 4 to 8 hours to help patient sleep.

c. Neutralize acidosis. Frequently, acidosis appears after the Adams-Strokes syndrome sets in. Give soda bicarbonate 2 gm by mouth every 2 hours for 3 to 4 times. It is best to give an intravenous drip of 5 percent sodium bicarbonate, 100-250 ml.

d. Detoxify. Use dimercaprol.

Besides the measures described above, give oxygen when necessary. To keep the environment quiet, a nursing attendant must stay with patient, observing him closely until he comes out of critical condition.

C. Late-Stage Schistosomiasis

Late-stage schistosomiasis may be defined as chronic schistosomiasis accompanied by the following conditions:

(1) Liver cirrhosis. Ascites, distention, pronounced abdominal veins, hepatomegaly are all indications of portal hypertension present.

(2) Splenomegaly. Enlargement of spleen goes beyond line across from navel, and which may be accompanied by splenic hyperfunction (splenomegaly, thrombopenia or cytopenia, petechiae).

Treatment

The course of illness in late-stage schistosomiasis is quite complicated. Since many of the victims are in poor health, improvement of their health is a prime consideration, before any long-range antimonial therapy is contemplated.

In principle, treatment of liver cirrhosis patients is the same as that for portal hypertension cirrhosis (See section on "Liver Cirrhosis). With respect to splenomegaly, if treatment with Chinese herbs does not show marked improvement, splenectomy should be considered.

Chinese herbs

Clean roots or stems of niu-nai-chiang, also called kan-jui (Euphorbia sieboldiana), and sun dry or oven-dry. Pulverized and sieve out lumpy residue. Prepare into a powder medication, a honeyed pill (half powder half honey), or capsule.

Give one a day in doses of .04 - 1.5 fen, the dosage used determined by the severity of illness and the patient's condition. Give early in the morning, on an empty stomach, and down with some warm boiled water.

Do not give to pregnant women and those prone to vomiting. Generally, the side effects of this medication are slight nausea and vomiting, and abdominal pain. If reaction is severe, proper treatment should be given. Avoid the use of salt during period of treatment.

This prescription is usually effective for acute, chronic, or late stage schistosomiasis.

Other prescriptions used in the differential treatment of symptoms include the following:

1. <u>To resolve clots and clear the "lo" passageways</u>. This is suited for use in schistosomiasis where hepatosplenomegaly, ascites, and wasting away of the four extremities are predominant, and characterized by a thready pulse, white-coated fur on a purplish tongue.

Clean three large live turtles (or 5 small ones) in cold water. Extract juice, mix with a little sweet wine, and take with warm boiled water. Take once a day for 1 to 2 months.

2. <u>To promote diuresis</u>. Suited for patients with mild, moderate, and severe ascites, and who are still active and in fairly good physical condition. Niu-nai-chiang (<u>Euphorbia sieboldiana</u>) with its pronounced effect along these lines has already been cited. Others include the following:

    a. Shih-ts'ao-yuan ["ten-date pill], 1 ch'ien, 2 to 3 times a day.

    If dizziness, nausea, and abdominal pain appear after medication, needle puncture the "nei-kuan" and "tsu-san-li."

    If patient feels exhausted from sudden release of excess water, give half bowl of cold rice gruel.

    If patient becomes clammy and sweaty around brow and forehead, feels palpitation, and pulse becomes rapid and thready, give concoction prepared from 5 ch'ien of tang-shen (<u>Campanumea</u> sp) immediately.

    b. After ascites has subsided, maintain improvement with a combination shen-ling-pai-shu powder (prepared from tang-shen, fu-ling, pai-shu, dried tangerine peel, shan-yao, burnt licorice, chieh-keng, toasted pien-tou (Doliehos lablab), toasted lotus, sha-jen, (Job's tears), or a hsiang-sha six-element concoction (containing tang-shen, fu-ling, pai-shu, licorice, tangerine peel, pan-hsia, mu-hsiang, and sha-jen).

3. To <u>strengthen the spleen and resolve moisture</u>. Suited for use in cases of schistosomiasis showing hepatosplenomegaly, facial pallor, abdominal distension, and diarrhea, characterized by a thready pulse, and a white and oily fur on tongue.

Concoction of	
Ts'ang-shu	3 ch'ien
Pu-ku-chih	3 ch'ien
Hou-pu	3 ch'ien
Pai-shu	3 ch'ien
Chu-ling	3 ch'ien
Tse-hsieh	3 ch'ien
Mu-hsiang	1.5 ch'ien
Sha-jen	1.5 ch'ien

If abdominal cramps and loose stools (like duck droppings) are also present, add mild fu-p'ien (aconite), 3 ch'ien pre-concocted, and 1 ch'ien of dry ginger.

4. To <u>promote diuresis and resolve moisture</u>. Suited for cases of late-stage schistosomiasis complicated by ascites, a scanty and burning urination, a red tongue hardly fur-coated at all.

Concoction of	
Pan-pien-lien	4 liang
Pai-shu (potional)	3 ch'ien

Generally, the urinary function improves after 1 or 2 weeks with more urine passed, the ascites subsides, and patient feels better.

5. To <u>warm the yang and promote diuresis</u>. Suited for cases of schistosomiasis characterized by facial pallor, chills, loose thin stools, abdominal bloatiness, scanty urine, a white tongue fur, and a pale tongue.

Concoction of	
Pai-shu (Atractylis ovata)	4 ch'ien
Ts'ang-shu (Atractylis japonica)	1.5 ch'ien
Fu-ling (Poria cocos)	4 ch'ien
Roots of cottonwood	1 liang
Tzu-shih (nut of lindera)	4 ch'ien
Hsu-chang-hsing	1 ch'ien
Garlic	3 cloves

If energy is deficient, add tang-shen 4 ch'ien; if blood is deficient, add tang-kuei 3 ch'ien; if extremities are cold, add slices of aconite (fu-p'ien), 1.5 to 3 ch'ien.

6. To <u>strengthen the yang and nourish the body</u>. Suited for schistosomiasis dwarfism, where the size of adults are like that of children with a absence of puberty hair growth and menses. Characterized by extreme weakness

and emaciation, sallow complexion, falling hairs, and thready pulse. Generally, powdered placenta, Ho-che ta-ts'ao-yuan, shih-ch'uan ta-pu yuan are prescribed, 1-3 ch'ien, 3 times a day.

The herbal prescriptions just described are certainly effective towards treating ascites, and improving the patient's physical condition before further treatment with antimonials or splenectomy are contemplated.

Filariasis

Filariasis is caused by parasitism of the filaria in the lymph nodes and lymphatics in the human body. The larvae produced by the Filaria is called microfilariae. When mosquitoes feed on the blood of filariasis patients, they suck the microfilariae into their systems where they continue to develop. When these mosquitoes bite a new host, these microfilariae are introduced into the lymphatic system of another victim where they develop into mature filariae. Their continued growth can cause redness, pain and obstruction in the lymphatic system. Sometimes, this lymphangitis is seen as a red line running up and down an extremity (called "flowing fire" or "liu-huo" by the native populace). Sometimes the patient experiences periodic bouts of fever, shows lymphadenopathy or elephantiasis. Sometimes chyluria (when urine is milky white) is present. If blood from an early case is taken at night for examination, the infective microfilariae are often seen (Figure 6-5-1).

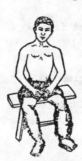

Figure 6-5-1. Elephantiasis of lower extremities.

Prevention

1. Promoting the Patriotic Health Movement on a wide scale, and carry out mosquito eradication measures properly.

2. Treating patients affected with disease in its early stages thoroughly.

Treatment

1. New acupuncture technique. Insert "seven-star" needles into the following points until bleeding ensues: the "tsu-san-li," "yin-ling-ch'uan," "san-yin chiao." Follow with cupping technique or hot compresses.

2. Chinese herbs. Treatment should clear and facilitate moisture-heat [removal] from the hsia-chiao, using remedies such as the following:

a. Concoction of
   Fang-chi   3 ch'ien
   Niu-hsi   3 ch'ien
   Huang-pai (phellodendron sp.)   3 ch'ien
   Cinnamon sticks   1 ch'ien
   Gypsum   8 ch'ien

   This prescription is good for early stages of elephantiasis when patient feels much localized pain.

b. Concoction of fresh eucalyptus leaves (chopped), 3 liang, cooked for 2 hours until the fluid, after removal of residues, is reduced to 60 ml. Take in one dose. (This prescription is effective as a microfilaricide.)

c. Roots of glutinous rice plants, 2 liang, in concoction. Take for a month.

d. Concoction prepared from

   P'i-hsieh   5 ch'ien
   Chu-liang   3-5 ch'ien
   Tse-hsieh (Eupatorium sp.)   3-5 ch'ien
   Hua-shih (talc)   3-5 ch'ien
   Che-ch'ien-tzu (plantago)   3-5 ch'ien
   Ch'ih-ling   3-5 ch'ien
   Phellodendron   1-3 ch'ien
   Chih-mu   1-3 ch'ien
   Mu-t'ung   1-3 ch'ien

   (The two prescriptions mentioned above are effective for treating chyluria.)

e. Concoction of

   Wei-ling hsien   3 ch'ien
   Wu-I   3 ch'ien
   Tzu-ts'ao   3 ch'ien
   Tang-kuei ends   3 ch'ien
   Fang-chi (coccolus sp.)   4 ch'ien
   Hung-hua (caramus)   1.5 ch'ien
   Ch'uan-shan-chia (crocodile)   2 ch'ien

(This prescription is effective for treating elephantiasis.)

3. Western medicines

Hetrazan therapy:

a. For adults, 200 mg each dose, 3 times a day, for 7 days in a row.

b. When given in mass treatment, adult dose is 400 mg each time, 3 times a day, for 3 days in a row.

Dosage for children is reduced according to calculations. For patients who show reaction to hetrazan, change to carbasone, given twice a day, 0.5 gm each time, for a total of 10 days.

During the course of treatment, because of large amounts of micro-filariae being killed, reactions such as chills, fever, headache, vomiting etc., may appear. In such instances, given aspirin compound 1 to 2 tablets, or needle-puncture the "t'ai-yang," "ho-ku," "nei-kuan" and other points. If dyspnea is present, give hypodermic injection of 0.1 percent epinephrine 0.1 percent, and stop all other medication.

Ankylostomiasis

Ankylostomiasis or hookworm disease, is commonly called "sang-hsieh-huang" [mulberry-leaves yellow], "lai-huang ping" and "huang-pan ping" by the local populace. The ova produced by the hookworms that are parasitical in the human body are expelled in the stools and they hatch in dirt fertilized with human manure where they develop into threadlike larvae. When people are working barefoot in fields so fertilized, the larvae penetrate the skin and enter the body of a new host. Carried by the circulation through the heart and lungs, they reach the pharynx, are swallowed and enter into the small intestines where they develop into adult hookworms, feed on the host's blood, and produce ova. Examination of stool specimen taken at this time will show the presence of hookworm ova.

When the hookworm larvae penetrate the skin, the victim discovers a characteristic itching sensation in the local area, followed by appearance of a rash. When he scratches, the wheal gradually swells and forms a small blister that can become purulent. Following this, the throat feels itchy, the patient coughs and spits up, the sputum frequently blood-streaked. After 5 or 6 weeks, the patient experience some epigastric discomfort, or even pain. The bowels are constipated and loose alternately, the stools sometimes blood-streaked or containing undigested food. Other signs are anemia, facial pallor, a sickly yellowing of skin, purplish spots on whites of the eyes, generalized edema, general weakness, palpitation at the slightest physical exertion. In a few patients, there is an inclination to eat rice grains uncooked, dirt, charcoal, leaves and other substances. In children this affects further growth and development. In pregnant women, such a disease can cause abortions or premature delivery.

Prevention

1. Centralized management of excreta. Store feces in special crook and keep covered for 1 to 2 months until all ova have perished before using as fertilizer. Do not defecate anywhere.

2. Preventing further infection. Rub squeezed garlic juice, or crushed leaves from ch'ou mao-tan (Clerodendron bungei), or tobacco tar scraped from smoking pipes, on hands and feet. After working in the fields, wash or soak hands and feet in solution of tea-seed residues or soapy water.

3. Active treatment of all patients suffering from disease.

Treatment

1. New acupuncture therapy technique

Needle-puncture the "ta-chui," "ch'u-ch'ih," "tsu-san-li," and "p'i-yu" points, using moderate stimulation, once a day. Apply moxibustion after needling.

2. Treatment of early skin rash.

    a. Apply hot compresses to itchy areas, changing compresses every half a minute (keeping temperature of water as hot as bearable) for about 10 minutes each treatment. For patients with numerous wheals, the affected hand or foot may be soaked in very hot water instead, for several seconds repeatedly for about half an hour. While this serves to allay the itching, it also exerts a larvicidal effect on the larvae already penetrated into the skin.

    b. Dissolve wei-sheng yuan (camphor ball) in cold boiled water and apply to affected parts.

3. Chinese herbs

Treatments should emphasize purging the worms, with additional benefit of supplementing energy and blood.

    a. Concoction of

Ephedra	1 ch'ien
Su-tzu	3 ch'ien
Almonds	3 ch'ien
Licorice	1.5 ch'ien

b. Concoction of

Pai-pu (<u>Stemona japonica</u>)   3 ch'ien
Almonds   3 ch'ien
Licorice   1 ch'ien

The prescriptions given above are both suited for coughing
and dyspnea.

c. Pill prepared from pulverized mixture of the following:

Lei-yuan (<u>Omphalia lapidecens</u>)   3 liang
Fei-tzu (<u>Torreya nucifera</u>)   3 liang
Betelnut   4 liang

Mix with some water and wine and roll pills the size of soybean. For adults, take 2 ch'ien each time, 3 times a day, on
an empty stomach. One course of therapy takes 5 days.

d. Concoction of

Fei-tzu   1 liang
Betelnut   1 liang
Hung-t'eng (<u>Sargentodoxa cuneata</u>)   1 liang
Kuan-tsung (<u>Crytomium fortunei</u>)   5 ch'ien

Take concoction with 2 to 3 cloves of garlic, for 3 days in
a row.

4. <u>Western medicines</u>

a. <u>Hexylresorcinol</u> 1 gm taken in early morning on an empty stomach.
Do not bite into capsule. Wait 5 hours before taking any food.
If there is no bowel movement within 24 hours, give patient 30
ml of 25 percent magnesium sulfate. Side effects of this drug
are few, and suited for patients in poor health or those who
show reaction to other drugs.

b. For <u>treatment of anemia</u>. Give ferrous sulfate, 0.3 to 0.6 ml
each time, 3 times a day.

Ascariasis

The ascaris, or roundworm, shaped like an earthworm is a parasite living
in the small intestines of the human body. It continues to produce large numbers of ova which are expelled with the stools, and become attached to leaves
of vegetables or dirt [when the excreta is used as fertilizer]. Under suitable

temperature and humidity conditions, the ova matures in about 2 weeks, and become sources of infection via food taken by mouth. In the small intestines, the larvae are hatched from the eggs and penetrate the intestinal wall where they enter the blood stream and be transported to the lungs. From the bronchi, they enter into the pharynx, are swallowed and gain access to the esophagus and back into the small intestines where they develop and mature.

Ascariasis is a frequently seen disease that often recurs. It is even more common among small children. Some of its characteristics are the following: coin-size white blotches on the face called "worm spots"; bluish or purplish specks on the sclera of the eye; granular and papilla-like red specks half hidden on the mucous membrane behind the lower lip and the surface of the tongue. These are all signs of diagnostic value. If there is abdominal pain, it is generally felt in area around the navel, sporadic, varying in intensity, and occurring usually in early morning or when the stomach is empty. The patient usually likes to eat sweets and dried foods, and grinds his teeth in his sleep. Small children with heavy infestations usually show a big abdomen, have an enormous appetite, and do not put on any weight. In some cases, the worms will even bunch up and cause intestinal obstruction. If the ascaris enters into the bile duct, it can cause bile duct ascariasis. Examination of stool specimen taken from patient will show the presence of ascaris ova.

Prevention

Strengthen program of health and hygiene education, and stress the importance of washing hands before meals and after defecation, and not defecating any place. Strengthen the management of excreta disposal. Staples such as fresh yams and fresh turnips should be washed and peeled before eaten raw. Small children in particular, must develop the habit of washing hands and keeping nails trimmed.

Treatment

1. _New acupuncture therapy_. When there is abdominal pain, needle-puncture the "jen-chung" and "tsu-san-li" points, using moderate stimulation. Ordinarily, needle the "szu-feng" and squeeze out some yellow fluid, once a week.

2. _Chinese herbs_. Treatment should kill the worms and strengthen the stomach, using medications such as the following:

   a. Concoction of root bark from k'u-chien (Melia azedarach), well-scraped of its outer red covering, 5 ch'ien to 1 liang decocted for 3 to 4 hours down to 60 to 80 ml. Take on empty stomach in early morning, two mornings in a row.

   b. Shih-chun-tzu (Quisqualis indica), roasted and shelled, 1 liang. Take 3 ch'ien each time, on empty stomach in the morning, chewing well before swallowing. Take for three mornings in a row. Rest for 3 days. Repeat treatment again.

c. Pai-ying (<u>Solanum lyratum</u>) fruit or roots, 1 liang, in concoction. Take once in the morning, and once in the evening.

d. Concoction of

Shen-ch'u (roasted)	3 ch'ien
Wheat sprouts (roasted)	3 ch'ien
Shan-cha (hawthorne)	3 ch'ien
Pai-shu (<u>Atractylis ovata</u>)	3 ch'ien

This prescription is used for its restorative effect after
the worms have been expelled.

3. <u>Western medicine</u>

Piperazine citrate tablets (Ch'u-hui ling): Dosage based on 160
mg/kg body weight/day, in two doses. The maximum dose for adults each day
should not exceed 3 gm (not to exceed 2.4 gm/day for children), given two days
in a row.

Besides this, pagoda confection (a vermifuge and vermicide) can also
be given to children, one piece for each year in age, in one dose. Repeat
after a lapse of 7 days.

<u>Note</u>: For ascaris-caused intestinal obstruction: Give 1 cup (about
50-60 ml) of vegetable oil or sesame oil to patient by mouth. The oil can
loosen up the knotted clump of worms, alleviate pain, and aid expulsion of
worms in the stool. Or, squeeze juice from bulbs of 10 stalks of green onions,
mix with 1 to 3 tablespoonsful of sesame oil, and give to patient. If this
treatment is still ineffective, immediately refer patient for other treatment.

Fasciolopsiasis

The trematode which causes fasciolopsiasis is shaped like a slice of
ginger. It is a parasite frequently found in the small intestines of man and
hog, where it produces ova that are expelled with the stool. In water, these
ova hatch into larvae which penetrate the body of the snail, a "pien-chuan+
lei." Inside the intermediate snail host, these larvae develop into cercariae
which are liberated and become attached and encysted on aquatic plants such
as red-water caltrops and water chestnuts. When people eat the red caltrops
and water chestnuts raw, the encysted cercariae is introduced into the human
small intestines where they break out and develop into mature trematodes.

Frequently seen signs of this disease are abdominal distention and
pain, peristaltic noises, a foul-smelling stool containing much undigested
food, an avaracious appetite, weakness, facial pallor, emaciation, and
puffiness. Examination of stool specimen will show presence of fasciolopsis
ova. When the trematodes are numerous, they are often passed in the stool,
and seen as slices of ginger.

Prevention

1. Strengthening health and hygiene education. Aquatic plants such as red caltrops and water chestnuts should best be cooked before eating. When eaten raw, they should be scalded first and skins should be pulled off by hand (instead of biting and tearing into them with teeth).

2. Proper measures to manage excreta disposal. Treat infected humans and infected hogs accordingly.

Treatment

1. **Chinese herbs**. Treatment should emphasize warm expulsion supported by spleen and stomach-restoring action.

   a. Betelnut 1 to 2 liang (half the dose for children) decocted to a concentrate. Take once in morning on empty stomach, 2 to 3 times in succession. This prescription is quite effective as a vermifuge, and it is not necessary to take another purgative.

   b. Concoction of

Betelnut	5 ch'ien
Black prunes	2 ch'ien
Licorice	1 ch'ien

   Take one preparation a day, for 3 to 5 days in succession.

   c. To promote restoration of spleen and stomach function following trematode expulsion, use hsiang-sha lu-chun-tzu yuan (a patent medicine), 3 times a day, 3 ch'ien each time. To be taken after meals with a little boiled water.

2. **Western medicine**

   (Use hexylresorcinol (See section "Ankylostomiasis").

Enterobiasis

The pinworms which cause enterobiasis are quite small, resembling white threads about 1 cm in length. These pinworms are found parasitic within the human large intestine. Because of careless personal hygiene, the eggs are frequently introduced by mouth from ova-contaminated fingers or food. Once inside the human intestines, the ova are hatched and the larvae develop into adults.

A characteristic of this disease is anal itching, particularly severe at night. Sometimes, an examination of the anus in the middle of the night will show small white worms crawling out. Examination of stool specimen will show presence of ova. Infants infested with this disease are frequently fretful during the night, but happy and normal in the daytime. Some children are fitful in their sleep frequently crying out in nightmares. In others, the scratching leads to ulcerations around the anus. In young females, the trematodes may crawl into the vulva to cause vulvar itching or vaginitis.

Prevention

1. Good personal hygiene and cleanliness. Stress the importance of washing hands, taking baths, and changing clothes frequently. In families or kindergartens with heavy infestations, have undergarments and underpants especially, boiled to kill any ova attached.

2. Treatment of patients accordingly.

Treatment

1. __Chinese herbs__. Treatment should concentrate on killing the worms, taking two approaches: internal treatment and external treatment.

    a. __Internal treatment__

        (1) Powder of shih-chun-tzu (<u>Quisqualis indica</u>), 3 fen for each year in age of child, to a maximum of 1 ch'ien 2 fen. Take 3 times a day with decoction of pai pu (<u>Stemona sessifolia</u>) 3 ch'ien. Take for 6 days in a row to complete a course of therapy.

        (2) Concoction of

Betelnut	3 ch'ien
Nut meats of <u>Torreya nucifera</u>	3 ch'ien
Black prunes	3 ch'ien

    b. __External treatment__

        (1) __Garlic retention enema__. Crush 3 liang of ta-suan (garlic), and soak in cold boiled water for 24 hours. Filter and save fluid. Use 20-30 ml each evening, given as retention enema at bedtime. Continue for 7 nights, to complete one course of treatment.

        (2) __Stemona-black prune retention enema__. Take 1 liang of pai-pu (Stemona sessifolia), 5 ch'ien of black prunes, and add 2 bowls of water. Decoct and reduce fluid to 1 bowl. Use as retention enema, as described before, for 10 days in succession.

2. __Western medicine__

Use piperazine citrate (ch'u-hui ling), 50 mg/kg body weight/day, to be given in early morning on an empty stomach, 10 days in a row. As a prophylactic measure after cure, take medication for 2 days every week, for 4 weeks, to prevent re-infection.

Taeniasis

The tapeworm (or taenia) which causes taeniasis or hookworm disease is also called "ts'un-pai ch'ung" [inch white-worm]. It is parasitic in the human small intestine, a flat, long and segmented worm, its segments joined together to resemble a long piece of white tape.

The term "ts'un-pai ch'ung" derives from the segments expelled by the worm. After the ova contained in these segments are eaten by swine or cattle, the eggs hatch and larvae are liberated. These larvaes in turn, penetrate the intestinal wall and enter into the blood or lymphatic circulation to be transported to the muscle and become encysted in the muscle of swine and cattle. If humans eat less than thoroughly cooked infested pork and beef, the larvae will develop into adult worms in side the human intestine, and the human victims will have acquired port (or beef) tapeworm disease. Mild cases generally show few symptoms, but in the more severe cases such signs as vague abdominal pain, alternation between constipated and loose stools, nausea and vomiting at times, abdominal distension after meals, poor digestion, and dizziness will be noted. Over a period of time, emaciation, a withered yellow complexion and general weakness will appear. Examination of stool specimen will uncover ova. Patients infested with pork tapeworm disease can often re-infect themselves and produce cysticercosis.

Prevention

1. Avoiding consumption of beef or pork not thoroughly cooked.

2. Proper treatment of patients in time. Strengthen management of excreta disposal measures. Do not let excreta contaminate grassy pastures and water sources, in a move to prevent infection of man and animal.

Treatment

1. Chinese herbs. Treatment should emphasize purging the worms supplemented by regulating action to restore the stomach and spleen.

    a. Concoction of betelnut 1 to 4 liang. Take concoction cold.

    b. Powdered pumpkin seeds, 4 liang, taken at one time. Follow 3 hours later with dose of Glauher's salt 3 ch'ien.

    c. Powdered lei-yuan (Omphalia lapidecens), 2 liang, pulverized, divided into 3 doses.

2. Western medicine

Atebrine 0.8 gm on empty stomach in early morning (0.6 gm for children under 12 years of age, and 0.4 gm for those under 6 years of age). Take with an equal amount of soda bicarbonate. Two hours later, take 40 ml of 50 percent magnesium.

SECTION 6. Medical Illnesses

Upper Respiratory Tract Infections

Upper respiratory tract infections is a blanket term covering viral
or bacterial infection of the nasal cavity, larynx, trachea and bronchus.
It is also called "cold" or "flu." Persons whose physique is not the
strongest are the most susceptible to colds when the weather alternates
suddenly between hot and cold, especially when they perspire profusely after
working hard.

Upon catching cold, the symptoms are dryness and itchiness of throat,
sneezing, running nose, nasal stuffiness, followed by general myalgia, chills,
fever (some patients have no fever), headache, coughing, etc. Most patients
will recover in 3 to 7 days.

Prevention

1. Attention to changes of weather, and dress accordingly.

2. Chinese herbs

   a. After exposure to cold, immediately take some ginger tea
      prepared by steeping fresh ginger in boiling water, with
      brown sugar added. It will cause some slight perspiring.

   b. Concoction of
      Leaves of huang-ching   2 liang
      Lu-pien ching   2 liang
      T'ien-pien-chu   2 liang
      Mint leaves   1 liang
      (This preparation is enough for 10 persons for
      one day)

Treatment

1. New acupuncture therapy. Same as that for epidemic influenza.

2. Chinese herbs. Same as that for epidemic influenza.

Acute Bronchitis

Acute bronchitis is an acute inflammation due to bacterial or viral
infection, or physical and chemical irritation of the trachea and bronchi.
It can also develop from upper respiratory tract infection. Generally, the
onset is acute, accompanied by chills, fever, headache, sore throat and general aches and pains all over the body. In the beginning stage, it is generally manifested as a sporadic dry cough that loosens up one and two days
later with some mucus or thin sputum coughed up. The sputum becomes more

profuse and thickens to a purulent yellow or white mucus gradually. Most frequently seen are the wind-chill (feng-han) and wind-heat (feng-je) types of bronchitis.

Wind-chill bronchitis. Characterized by much coughing and expectorating of thin mucus or white and thick sputum, accompanied by slight fever, a thin and white fur on tongue, and a floating tense pulse.

Wind-heat bronchitis. Characterized usually by fever, a dry cough, difficulty in bringing up sputum, or a thick sputum when coughed up. Fur on tongue is a thin yellow, and the pulse is slippery and rapid.

Prevention

Same measures as those taken for upper respiratory infection.

Treatment

1. New acupuncture therapy. Use medium stimulation on needles inserted into "t'ien-tu," "feng-lung" points, once a day. Also use cupping technique over the "fei-yu" point.

2. Chinese herbs.

    a. For wind-chill bronchitis. Treatment should dissipate wind-chill, and stop the coughing, and resolve the sputum using remedies such as the following:

        (1) Concoction of

Ching-chieh	2 ch'ien
Tzu-wan [Aster tataricus]	2 ch'ien
Pai-pu [Stemona sp.]	3 ch'ien
Chieh-keng [Platycodon sp.]	3 ch'ien
Pai-ch'ien	3 ch'ien
Dried tangerine peel	2 ch'ien
Licorice	1 ch'ien

        (2) Concoction of

Su-hsieh	4 ch'ien
Almonds	3 ch'ien

    b. For wind-heat bronchitis. Treatment should clear the lungs and reduce the fever, using remedies such as:

        (1) Concoction of

Fresh ephedra	2 ch'ien
almonds	3 ch'ien

Unprocessed gypsum	1 liang
Kou-lou peel	3 ch'ien
Huang-lien [Coptis chinensis]	1 ch'ien
Fa-hsia	1.5 ch'ien
Licorice	1 ch'ien

(2) Concoction of

Pai-pu [Stemona sessifolia]	4 ch'ien
Almonds	3 ch'ien
Sang pai-p'i [white bark of mulberry]	3 ch'ien
Sha-shen	4 ch'ien
Loquat leaves	5 ch'ien

(3) Concoction of 5 ch'ien of che-ch'ien-tzu (Plantago sp.)

3. Western medicines

Pencillin 400,000 units given intramuscularly once or twice daily. Or terramycin (also called tetracylene), 0.25 gm, is to be taken by mouth, 4 times a day.

Chronic Bronchitis

Chronic bronchitis is also called "chronic cough" by the local populace. It is due mostly to changes caused by repeated bouts of acute bronchitis. Smoking over a long period of time or long-term irritation by dust and harmful gases can also cause chronic bronchitis.

The important clinical manifestations are a chronic, paraxysmal cough that brings up mucoid sputum. Frequently, it becomes worse in cold weather, particularly severe at early morning or at night, coughing continuously until sputum is raised before experiencing a sense of relief. Because the nature and causes of coughing vary, the three commonly seen types are cold cough (han-ke), feverish cough (jeh-ke), and dyspneic cough (ch'i-hi).

Cold cough, characterized by chills, coughing, a productive white and foamy sputum, shortness of breath, and sometimes inability to lie down flat on back. Coat on tongue is white and moist, pulse is tight and slippery.

Feverish cough, characterized by fever, coughing, and a yellow purulent sputum. Coat on tongue is slightly yellow, and pulse is slippery and rapid.

Dyspneic cough, characterized by nausea and tachycardia, dyspnea on the slightest exertion, accompanied by cyanosis and difficulty in lying down flat because of the dyspnea. Tongue is red and hardly coated. Pulse is rapid.

Prevention

1. Attention to keeping warm to avoid taking chill.

2. No smoking. Treat acute bronchitis radically.

Treatment

1. New acupuncture therapy. Use medium stimulation on needles applied to the "t'ien-tu," "feng-lung," "nei-kuan," and "fei-yu," once a day. Moxibustion may be used in conjunction with treatment.

2. Chinese herbs.

    a. For cold cough. Treatment should warm the lungs and resolve sputum, using remedies such as the following:

        (1) Concoction of

Ephedra	2 ch'ien
Cinnamon sticks	1.5 ch'ien
Pai-shao	3 ch'ien
Hsi-hsin	1 ch'ien
Dried ginger	1 ch'ien
Pan-hsia [Pinella sp.]	3 ch'ien
Wu-wei	1 ch'ien
Licorice	1 ch'ien

        (2) Almond cough syrup (patent medicine)

        (3) Plaster [poultice] for soles of both feet prepared by crushing the following, and mix with egg:

Almond	7 ch'ien
White pepper	7 ch'ien
Glutinous rice	7 ch'ien
Chih tzu (gardenia)	6 ch'ien
Peach kernel	6 ch'ien

    b. For feverish cough. Treatment should clear the lungs and resolve sputum using remedies as the following:

        (1) Concoction of

Wa-wei	1 liang
Loquat leaves	1 liang
Fresh ginger	2 ch'ien

(2) Mixture of

Powdered oyster shell	3 ch'ien
Ch'ing-tai	1 ch'ien

Dissolve in rice water, to be taken 3 times daily.

(3) Concoction of

Honeysuckle	4 ch'ien
Forsythia	4 ch'ien
Fritillaria sp.	2 ch'ien
Niu-pang-tzu	3 ch'ien
Kuo-lou-p'i	3 ch'ien
Almonds	3 ch'ien
Coptis chinensis	1.5 ch'ien
Fa-hsia	1.5 ch'ien
Licorice	1 ch'ien

c. For dyspneic cough. Treatment should consolidate the lungs, and lower the energy activity, using the following concoction:

K'uan-tung hua	3 ch'ien
Pai-ch'ien	3 ch'ien
Yuan-chih	3 ch'ien
Wu-wei tzu (gall)	1.5 ch'ien
Ginkgo seeds	5 ch'ien

For patients with a kidney deficiency, add processed ti-huang (Rehmannia sp.) 4 ch'ien and huai shan 5 ch'ien; for those with anemia, add tang-kuei 4 ch'ien.

3. Western medicines

a. Control of infection, using penicillin or in combination with intramuscular injection of streptomycin.

B. Caffeine by mouth for nausea and dyspnea symptoms, 0.1 gm each time. Intravenous injections of 50 percent glucose 20 ml added to 25 percent caffeine 10 ml, once or twice daily.

Asthma

Asthma here covers both bronchial asthma and asthmatic brionchitis, the result of bronchial spasm and mucus obstruction of the air passageway. It is characterized by a repeatedly occurring expiratory difficult that does not permit lying flat during an attack, and the patient is forced to sit up to breathe (Fig 6-6-1) with a noisy mucus rasp in his throat. This ailment must be differentiated from the asthma caused by cardiac failure.

Types

On the basis of different clinical manifestations, asthma is generally classified as cold asthma (han-ch'uan), feverish asthma (jeh-ch'uan), mucus asthma (t'an-ch'uan), and deficiency asthma (hsu-ch'uan).

Cold asthma. Accompanied frequently by coughing and the raising of white sputum, headache and aches all over body, cold and clammy extremities, and aversion to cold. Coat on tongue slightly white, and pulse is tight.

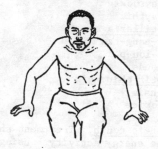

Figure 6-6-1. Sitting up to breathe

Feverish asthma. Accompanied by fever, restlessness, parched mouth, a preference for cold food, thick yellow mucus, scanty sputum that is difficult to cough up, dry stools and yellow urine. Furthermore, some burning is felt by urethra during passage of water, tongue is red with yellow coating, and pulse is rapid and smooth.

Mucus asthma. Characterized by a wheezing cough and much mucus present, the mucus in throat sounding like a buzz saw. The chest feels tight or the sides are painful, the mouth wide open and the shoulders are raised during respiration. The patient cannot lie down. Coating on tongue is thick, white and oily, but the pulse is tight and slippery.

Deficiency asthma. Unwise to let asthma become chronic and lower the body's resistance to disease. Usually, the breaths are short, the throat sound is low, and the asthma becomes more severe on slightest body exertion. At night, the pillow has to be raised considerably before patient can be comfortable and fall asleep. Facial pallor without any sparkle is also characteristic. The tongue is pink and uncoated, and the pulse is deficient.

Prevention

Abstinence from smoking and avoiding inspiration of irritable dust or gases. Attention to keeping warm and avoidance to "taking chill."

Treatment

1. New acupuncture technique. Apply medium stimulation to needles inserted in "ting-ch'uan," "t'an-chung," "t'ien-tu," "nei-kuan" points, once daily. Include moxibustion.

2. Chinese herbs

    a. For cold asthma. Treatment should dispel cold and quiet the wheezing, using remedies such as the following:

        (1) Pulverized mixture in equal parts of:

            Ephedra
            Almonds
            Pai-pu (Stemona sessifolia)
            K'uan-tung-hua

            Moisten with water to form pill. Take 2-3 ch'ien each time, 3 times a day.

        (2) Concoction of

Ephedra	2 ch'ien
Loquat leaves	6 ch'ien
Hu-t'o tzu	6 ch'ien

        (3) Toasted grasshoppers (those with pointed heads and long legs the best), 10, pulverized. Take all, with sweet wine. Repeat several times.

    b. For feverish asthma. Treatment should clear fever, resolve sputum and quiet the asthma. Using remedies such as the following:

        (1) Toasted and pulverized, 4 liang of white-necked earthworms, 1-2 ch'ien to be taken each time with granulated and boiled water, for 3 times daily, using granulated sugar.

        (2) A concoction of

Fresh goat's bile	4 liang
Honey	0.5 chin

        Steam for 1-2 hours until it reaches proper consistency. Take 1 tablespoon morning and evening until well.

c. **For mucus asthma.** Treatment should resolve the mucus and relieve the wheezing, using remedies such as the following:

(1) Pills prepared by mixing honey with a pulverized mixture consisting of the following:

Roots of fen-t'iao-erh ts'ai	2 chin
Dried orange peel	2 chin
Ginkgo nut meats	2 liang

Take 3 ch'ien each time, 3 times a day.

(2) Concoction of

Shih hou tzu	1 ch'ien
Pei-mu [Fritillaria sp.]	1 ch'ien
Chieh-keng	1 ch'ien

d. **For deficiency asthma.** Treatment should restore the deficiency and relieve the wheezing, using remedies such as the following:

(1) Powdered placenta, 1-2 ch'ien each time, 3 times a day.

(2) Concoction of

Walnut meats	2 liang
Pu-ku-chih (Psorales sp.)	4 ch'ien
Wu-wei-tzu (gall)	1 ch'ien

(3) Lu-wei Ti-huang yuan (patent medicine containing Rehmannia glutinosa) take 3 ch'ien each time with concoction of:

Cinnamon	5 fen
Wu-wei-tzu	1 ch'ien

(Suitable for asthma due to kidney deficiency)

3. **Western medicines**

(1) Caffeine 0.1 gm 3 times daily. For children reduce dosage, and base according to 4-6 mg/kg/time, 3 times a day.

(2) Ephedrine 25 mg, 3 times daily. For children, reduce dosage, and base according to 0.5-1 mg/kg/time, 3 times daily.

Lobar Pneumonia

Lobar pneumonia is an acute ailment caused by bacterial (usually the pneumonia diplococcus) infection. It frequently invades one large lobe of the lung. The onset is acute, frequently accompanied by chills, high fever, coughing and chest pain. The sputum coughed up is rusty -- a characteristic of this illness. The lips become blistered, and percussion of chest over the affected area reveals a dullness, while stethoscopic examination will uncover moist rales or lowered respiratory sounds. In serious cases such as toxic pneumonia, other symptoms, besides those just described, are clammy sweating, cold extremities, blood pressure drop, shallow respirations, rapid thready pulse, and even stupor.

Types

Clinically, lobar pneumonia may be considered generally as lung-heated (feverish or fei-jeh) or lung-closed (congestive or fei-pu) types.

Feverish lobar pneumonia, characterized by coughing, fever, and aversion to cold. Fur on tongue is white and thin or yellow, and pulse is rapid.

Congestive lobar pneumonia, characterized by coughing, dyspnea, high fever, hidrosis and thirst. Fur on tongue is yellow.

Prevention. Same as that for upper respiratory tract infections.

Treatment

1. **New acupuncture therapy**. Apply medium stimulation to needles inserted in the "ta-chui," "fei-yu," "nei-kuan," points. Give treatment once a day.

2. **Ear acupuncture**, using "hao" needle inserted into the pulmonary region designated on the pinna of the ear. Use a twirling movement, allowing the needle to be retained for 30 minutes. Treat in this manner once a day for 3 to 5 times in succession.

3. **Chinese herbs**

    a. **For feverish lobar pneumonia**. Treatment should clear fever in the lungs, using medications such as the following:

        (1) Concoction of

Ju-hsing ts'ao	1-3 liang
Pan-lan-ken	0.5-1 liang

        (2) Concoction of

Dandelions	5 ch'ien
Ta-ch'ing hsieh	5 ch'ien

(3) Concoction of

Honeysuckle	1 liang
Forsythia	1 liang
Fresh lu-wei [Phragmites communis]	2 liang
Seeds of tung-kua [Chinese waxgourd]	2 liang
Seeds [Job's tears]	5 ch'ien
Ju-hsing ts'ao	1 liang
Chieh-kong	2 ch'ien
Walnut meats	1.5 ch'ien

b. **For congestive lobar pneumonia.** Treatment should lower fever and clear the lungs, using remedies such as the following:

(1) Concoction of

Ephedra	2 ch'ien
Almonds	3 ch'ien
Gypsum powder	2 liang
Fresh licorice	1.5 ch'ien
Honeysuckle	5 ch'ien
Chieh-keng	3 ch'ien
Ju-hsing ts'ao	1 liang

(2) Concoction of

Pai-mao-ken (white congongrass)	1 liang
Ju-hsing ts'ao	1 liang
Honeysuckle	5 ch'ien
Forsythia	3 ch'ien

4. Western medicine

Depending on the patient's condition, selective use (singl or in combination) of sulfapyrimidine or sulfathiazole, penicillin, streptomycin (should be used in conjunction with penicillin, for old or weak patients, or serious cases), and/or tetracycline (to be used in addition to aforementioned drugs, if latter prove ineffective or if patient is seriously ill).

Lung Abscess

Lung abscess is a localized purulent infection in the lung tissue. Its onset is rather sudden accompanied by chills, fever, coughing, chest pain, and on excessive amount of purulent sputum that has a characteristically unpleasant or fishy odor. If this sputum is collected in a glass jar, it will separate into three layers: the upper, consisting of bubblyfroth; the second,

mucus; and the lower layer, purulent residues. This disease occurs frequently
as a complication to lobar pneumonia, and is generally placed in the lung-heated
(feverish or fei-jeh) category. Fur on tongue is mostly thin and white, or
slightly yellow, and the pulse is slippery and rapid.

Prevention

The same measures like those taken as precautions against upper respiratory tract infections are to be taken.

Treatment

1. _Postural drainage._ For patients with upper lobe lesions, have patient
sit or stand, to allow the purulent mucus to be expelled; for patient with mid-
lobe lesions, have patient lie down in recumbent position, and elevate foot of
bed about 1.5 feet; for patients with lower-lobe lesions, have patient lie down
in prone position and raise foot of bed about 1.5 feet. Repeat procedure 3 to
4 times daily for about 15 minutes each time.

2. _Acupuncture therapy._ Same as that given for lobar pneumonia.

3. _Chinese herbs._ Treatment should clear the fever and eliminate pus,
using remedies such as the following:

    a. Concoction of

Ju-hsing ts'ao	1-3 liang
Chieh-keng	3 ch'ien

        Take with additional water

    b. Concoction of

Ta-suan [garlic]	2 liang
Dandelions	1 liang
Honeysuckle	1 liang
Lu-pien ching	1 liang

    c. Concoction of

Barley	1 liang
Lu-ken [rushes]	1 liang
Lai-fu tzu	1 liang
Seeds of tung-kua [Chinese wax gourd]	1 liang
Nai-shen	3 liang

d. Concoction of

Wei-ching [stems of rushes]	5 ch'ien
Job's tears	5 ch'ien
Seeds of Chinese wax gourd	5 ch'ien
Peach kernels	3 ch'ien

4. Western medicines

Generally, penicillin 1,200,000 to 2,000,000 units/day is given in divided doses. Depending on the patient's condition, streptomycin 1-2 gm/day or tetracycline 1-2 gm/day may be added.

Acute Gastroenteritis

Acute gastroenteritis results from eating bacteria-contaminated or spoilt and toxic food. It usually occurs during the summer and winter months. Overheating or exposure to cold are frequently predisposing factors. Those eating together frequently come down together with the ailment. The onset is generally acute accompanied by nausea and vomiting, epigastric pain, diarrhea with thin or watery stools, (though without blood in stools nor tenesmus).

Types

According to difference in symptoms, acute gastroenteritis is generally classified as cold-damp (han-shih) and damp-feverish (shih-jeh) types.

Cold-damp gastroenteritis. Characterized by chills and fever, nausea and vomiting, mild epigastric pain, diarrhea with watery stools, stream of urination clear, and absence of thirst. Fur on tongue is white and thin, and the pulse is sunken and rapid.

Damp-feverish gastroenteritis. Characterized by vomiting and diarrhea, the vomitus bitter and acid, and the stools smelly, accompanied by headache and fever, apprehension, parchness and thirst, no appetite, yellow and scanty urine, and high fever. Fur on tongue is yellow and oily, and the pulse is slippery and rapid.

Prevention

1. Attention to food sanitation. Do not eat food or fruit that are spoilt. Do not drink untreated [or boiled] water. In summer, make sure that vegetables consumed are fresh. Cover food after being cooked. Be sure to cover leftovers before storing away.

2. All-out effort to eliminate flies together with measures strengthening excreta management, environmental sanitation and the disinfection [and purification] of drinking water.

Treatment

1. New acupuncture therapy. Apply medium stimulation to needles inserted in the "t'ien-shu," "nei-kuan," and "tsu-san-li" points in once or twice daily treatments. For those cases showing cold-damp symptoms, add moxibustion to "ch'i-hai" and "ch'i-chung" points.

2. Chinese herbs.

    a. For cold-damp gastroenteritis. Treatment should warm the center and dispel cold, using remedies such as the following:

        (1) Concoction of

Huo-hsiang	3 ch'ien
Hou-pu [Magnolia sp.]	1.5 ch'ien
Dried orange peel	2 ch'ien
Fu-ling	3 ch'ien
Wu-chu-yu	1.5 ch'ien
Dried ginger	2 ch'ien
Tzu-ssu leaves	1.5 ch'ien
Pan-hsia	2 ch'ien

        (2) Concoction of

Smart weed	1 liang
Camphor bark	1 liang
Fresh ginger	3 slices

        (3) Huo-hsiang chen-ch'i yuan (patent medicine), 3 ch'ien each dose, 2 to 3 times a day.

    b. For damp-feverish gastroenteritis. Treatment should clear fever and promote moisture removal, using remedies such as the following:

        (1) Concoction of

Lu-pien ching, roots	1.5 liang
Yeh nan-kua, roots	1 liang
Tieh sao-chou [bushclover], roots	5 liang

        (2) Concoction of

Ko-ken [Pueraria sp.]	5 ch'ien
Huang-ch'ing	2 ch'ien
Huang-lien [Coptis chinensis]	1.5 ch'ien
Licorice	1 ch'ien

(3) Concoction of

Lu-tou (mung bean)	2 liang
Che-ch'ien ts'ao	1 liang

If the patient cannot take his medications because of vomiting, apply some fresh ginger juice to the tip of his tongue beforehand, then give medicated concoction.

3. Western medicines.

a. For cases with severe abdominal pain, give atropine by mouth or intramuscularly.

b. For severely dehydrated patients as the result of prolonged diarrhea, encourage patient to drink more fluids and give 1500 ml 5 percent dextrose by I.V.

c. Give sulfaguanidine to relieve inflammation.

Ulcers

Ulcers, commonly called "stomach trouble" by the local populace embraces both gastric ulcers and duodenal ulcers. Epigastric pain is the chief indicator of this ailment. The pain of gastric ulcer usually occurs a half hour or hour after a meal, while that of duodenal ulcer generally takes place before meals when the stomach is empty. Exposure to cold, lack of moderation in eating, and nervous tension are all predisposing factors. The history of illness is a long one, with a record of repeated attacks, particularly frequent during fall and winter. The pain is frequently related to food, and the attack may be accompanied by belching and heartburn. In some cases secondary complications such as gastric bleeding, ulcer perforation, or obstruction, may occur.

Types

Because of differences in the predisposing factors of pain and the nature of the pain itself, this ailment may be typed clinically as cold-pain (han-t'ung), fever-pain (jeh-t'ung), energy-pain (ch'i-t'ung), blood-pain (hsueh-t'ung) types.

Cold-pain ulcers. Characterized by pain following exposure to cold and consumption of cold and raw foods. During the painful spell, chills, abdominal distension, non-dryness of mouth, and nausea are felt. However, pain is relieved after a hot compress has been applied.

Fever-pain ulcers. Seen frequently in individuals prone to alcoholic beverages and peppery foods. Since heat (fever) is already in the stomach, a burning sensation is felt during gastric pain attack. Other characteristics are parchness and a thick coating of fur on the tongue.

Energy-pain ulcers. Characterized by onset of pain when the energy collects in a mass, and relief or lessening of pain when the energy is dispelled. The stomach is generally distended. Hiccups and release of flatus by rectum are common.

Blood-pain ulcers. Characterized by a characteristic sharp and cyclic pain occurring in a definite location, the result of stagnant blood retention. If the hemorrhage is not stopped, massive hematemesis may occur, or the stools passed may be tar-black.

Treatment

1. New acupuncture therapy technique. Apply medium stimulation to needles inserted in the "chung-wan," "nei-kuan," and "tsu-san-li" points.

2. Chinese herbs.

   a. For cold-pain [cold exposure pain] ulcers. Treatment should warm the centers and dispel the chill, using remedies such as the following:

      (1) Mixture of wei-ling hsien, toasted dry and pulverized. Take 1-2 ch'ien for each dose, with boiled water.

      (2) Mixture prepared from the following, baked dry and pulverized:

Tu-hsing	3 ch'ien
Ch'ing-mu hsiang	3 ch'ien
Hsu chang-hsing	2 ch'ien

      Take 1 ch'ien each time, 3 times a day.

      (3) Liang-fu yuan (patent medicine). Take 2 chien each time, 3 times daily.

   b. For fever-pain ulcers. Treatment should clear fever and alleviate pain, using remedies such as the following:

      (1) Concoction of

Kuo-lou p'i	4 ch'ien
Coptis chinensis	1 ch'ien
Pan-hsia [Pinellia sp.], processed	1.5 ch'ien
Szechwan melia	3 ch'ien
Yen-hu-so	1.5 ch'ien

      (2) Powdered niu-p'i hsiao crushed fine, 1 ch'ien taken with boiled water.

(3) Concoction of

Ko-hua [flowers of _Pueraria_ sp.]	3 ch'ien
Chi-chu [buckthorn]	3 ch'ien

This prescription is suited for gastric pain arising
from alcohol indulgence.

c. <u>For energy-pain ulcers</u>. Treatment should break up liver congestion and correct energy circulation, using remedies such as
the following:

(1) Concoction of

Hsiang-fu	3 ch'ien
Ssu-hsieh [leaves]	1.5 ch'ien
Chi-he [trifoliate orange]	2 ch'ien

(2) Pulverized mixture of

Ch'ing-p'i	1.5 ch'ien
Wu yao	1.5 ch'ien

Divide into 2 doses, and take with warm boiled water.

d. <u>For bleeding [blood-pain] ulcers</u>. Treatment should stop bleeding and absorb clots, using remedies such as follows.

(1) Pulverized mixture of

Wu-ling-chi [bat droppings]	2 ch'ien
P'u-huang	1 ch'ien

Take with some boiled water.

(2) Yen-hu-so [<u>Corydalis ternata</u>] 3 ch'ien, roasted with wine
and finely crushed. Take with boiled water.

(3) Crushed mixture of

Cuttlefish bones	8 ch'ien
Chekiang fritillaria	2 ch'ien

Take 2 ch'ien each time, twice a day. For cases with
hematemesis and bloody stools, add pai-chi (pulverized)
8 ch'ien to prescription.

(4) Concoction of

Pai-mao-ken	1 liang
Nelumbo root sections	5

Mix in a little chiu-tsai juice before the whole concoction is taken. This prescription is suited for continuous hematemesis.)

3. Western medicine

   a. Antispasmodics. Beladonna compound, 1-2 tablets taken 3-4 times daily; atropine 0.3-0.6 mg 3 times daily, and for severe pain, 0.5 mgm given hypodermically.

   b. Antacids. "Wei-shu-p'ing" 2-3 tablets 3 times a day. Soda bicarbonate or aluminum hydroxide can also be used.

Liver Cirrhosis

Liver cirrhosis during its distended abdomen phase is also called "tympanum." This condition is due mostly to migrating hepatitis or chronic hepatitis, or the final stage of schistosomiasis that causes liver tissue damage.

Early stage liver cirrhosis is characterized by dizziness and fatigue, poor appetite, diarrhea, abdominal distension and flatus, possibly epistaxis of unknown origin, fine red streaks (capillary dilation) on face, and a black and dark, dull complexion, particularly of both cheeks. Liver is enlarged and hard.

Late-stage liver cirrhosis is characterized by a poor appetite, distended abdomen, epistaxis, swelling of legs, anorexia, scanty and yellow urine, dry and lusterless skin, dark complexion, "red spiders" on face, neck and chest, reddening palms similar to the cinnabar palms (chu-sha chang) described by the local populace which calls it "liver palm," and some jaundice. Splenomegaly may be prominent in others and the liver cannot be felt. In some cases, where the hard liver is palpable, its surface contours are felt to be irregular and bumpy. In other cases with abdominal enlargement, ascites may be present, and migrating dullness are detected upon percussion.

Complications may be upper digestive tract bleeding, hepatic coma etc.

Types

Liver cirrhosis is generally seen as energy deficient (ch'i-hsu), abnormal-solid (hsieh-shih), and combination balance-deficient abnormal-solid (cheng-hsu hsieh-shih) types.

The energy deficient type is characterized mostly by dizziness, weakness, fatigue, poor appetite and abdominal distension. Fur on tongue is thin, and pulse is deficient.

The abnormal-solid type, generally seen in young patients in reasonably good health, is first seen with symptoms such as ascites, abdominal distension, scanty and yellow urine, and edema of foot. Pulse is usually rapid and "wet."

The balance-deficient and abnormal-solid type, seen mostly in late-stage liver cirrhosis is characterized by anorexia, abdomen tympanum, bluish markings on abdominal wall, scanty urine, and poor appetite. Pulse is usually deficient and rapid.

Prevention

1. Revolutionary determination on part of liver cirrhosis patients to fight disease, armed with Mao Tse-tung thought.

2. Early and timely treatment of infectious hepatitis, chronic hepatitis, schistosomiasis etc.

Treatment

1. General

   a. Low salt or salt-free diet for late-stage patients with ascites. Abstention from alcohol to be enforced. Give soybean products, fruits and fresh vegetables in diet, and include suitable amounts of sugar, lean meat, eggs, and fresh fish. Cut down on animal fats.

   b. Dry Yeast or vitamin B complex, vitamin C etc.

2. New acupuncture therapy. Apply medium stimulation to needles inserted in "nei-kuan," "tsu-san-li," "yin-ling-ch'uan," "san-yin-chiao" points, with that in "nei-kuan" penetrating the "chih-k'ou" and the "yang-ling-ch'uan" penetrating the "yin-ling-ch'uan." Apply needle puncture once daily.

3. Chinese herbs

   a. For energy-deficient cirrhosis. Treatment should concentrate on restoration and nourishment, using drugs such as the following concoction of

Tang-shen	3 ch'ien
Pai-shu	3 ch'ien
Fu-ling	3 ch'ien
Tang-kuli	4 ch'ien
Dried ginger	3 slices
Licorice	1 ch'ien

   b. For abnormal-solid cirrhosis. Treatment should resolve the abnormal "solidity" of the cirrhosis, using remedies such as the following:

   (1) Concoction of

Fang-chi [Cocculus ps.]	3 ch'ien
Fu-ling	3 ch'ien

Pai-shu	3 ch'ien
Processed fu-tzu	3 ch'ien
Ta fu-p'i	3 ch'ien
Hou-pu [Magnolia sp.]	2 ch'ien
Dried ginger	2 ch'ien
Licorice	1 ch'ien

(This concoction is suitable for abdominal distension, fatigue, watery stools, and a thick and oily tongue in the hydrated patient.

(2) Concoction of

Cinnamon sticks	3 ch'ien
Tse-lan	3 ch'ien
Ch'ih-shao	3 ch'ien
Red dates	5

(This concoction is suited for blood-clot type cases with presence of abdominal mass, vascular "spiders," a "liver" palm, cyanosed tongue, and facial pallor.)

c. For the balance-deficient and abnormal solid type of cirrhosis, Treatment should emphasize restoration and diuresis, using preparation such as the following concoction of:

Tang-shen	5 ch'ien
Tse-hsieh	5 ch'ien
Flaming pieh-chia	5 ch'ien
Mu-t'ung	4 ch'ien
Mu-hsiang	4 ch'ien
Almonds	4 ch'ien
Shih-hu (pre-cooked)	6 ch'ien
Che-ch'ien-tzu	2 liang
Toasted oyster (pre-cooked)	2 liang
Dried gourd	2 liang

To be taken for several weeks.

Other effective prescriptions

(1) Concoction of

Pan-pien-lien (fresh)	2 liang
Huang-tan ts'ao	1 liang

Take 3 to 5 brew-doses in succession.

(2) Concoction of

- 369 -

Tzu-wei roots	0.5 - 1 chin
Huang ching, roots	6 ch'ien
Che-ch'ien-ts'ao	3 stalks
Hawthorne, roots	2 liang
Suan-p'an-tzu, roots	4 liang
Lu-pien-ching	1 liang
Shui-teng-hsin	3
Yellowed gardenia, roots	1 liang

For the first concoction dose, add a small amount of sweet wine, for the second, add two pieces of bean curd; for the third, add 1-2 feet of hog intestines; for the fourth, add some lean pork. This concoction requires considerable brewing before the wine, bean curd, hog intestines, or lean pork is added. Generally, 10 bowls of water is needed to brew the concoction down to one bowlful. One dose to be taken daily on empty stomach in early morning or late evening.

(3) Concoction of

Yellow gardenia roots	.05 - 1 liang
Mao-ken	1 liang
Chi-chu (roots)	1 liang
Sophora japonica blossoms	5 ch'ien
T'u-fu-ling	0.5-1 liang
Huang-t'an (roots)	3 ch'ien
Date palm, roots	0.5-1 liang
Liu-hsieh pai-ch'ien	3 ch'ien
Hu-chang	4 ch'ien
Pai-chu shu, roots	5 ch'ien
Wu-pao shu, roots	5 ch'ien
Mei-hsieh tung-ch'ing, roots	3 ch'ien

One dose (a concoction) to be taken daily for 2-3 consecutive doses. After this, steam-cook pig's feet in subsequent concoctions.

4. Western medicines

a. For ascites and edema. A diuretic shuang-ch'ing ke-niao-se [a hydrochlorothiazide?] 25 mg, 3 times a day, together with potassium chloride 0.9 gm 3 times a day. However, do not use during the pre-hepatic coma stage in case it invokes hepatic coma.

b. For ruptured esophageal varices and bleeding. Agrimonine or vitamin K_3.

- 370 -

c. For hepatic coma

    (1) Low protein and low salt diet. Do not give patient any
         drugs containing ammonium, e.g., ammonium chloride.

    (2) Daily intravenous drip of 28.8 percent sodium glutamate
         80 ml added to 1000 ml of 5 percent dextrose, given slowly.

    (3) Solution of 10 percent dextrose, 1000-2000 ml with 1-2 gm
         vitamin C added, given daily. Keep ratio of dextrose and
         physiologic saline at 4 = 1.

    (4) Hydrocortisone 100-200 mg added to 500 ml of 10 percent
         dextrose given by I.V., once a day.

    (5) Antibiotics given, if infection is present.

Prolapse of Rectum

In prolapse of the anus, the rectum is protruding outside the anus.
Prolific child-bearing, excessive bearing down during the parturition process,
chronic diarrhea and dysentery, hemorrhoids, and chronic coughing are all predisposing factors. Frequently seen in small children and older persons with
constitutional deficiencies, this condition must be differentiated from internal hemorrhoids, prolapse (Table 6-6-1).

Table 6-6-1. Differentiation of Anal Prolapse from Internal Hemorrhoids

Disease	Form	Color	Bleeding
Anal prolapse	Circular or spiral	Pink or fresh red	Does not bleed easily
Internal hemor-rhoid prolapse	Hemorrhoid nucleus obvious	Dull red or bluish purple	Bleeds easily

Treatment

1. New acupuncture therapy. Apply medium amount of stimulation to the
"pai-hui," "ch'ang ch'iang," "cheng-shan," points, once daily. At "pai-hui"
point, give additional moxibustion.

2. Chinese medicines

    a. Concoction of

        Huang-chi   5 ch'ien
        Tang-shen   5 ch'ien
        Sheng-ma   3 ch'ien
        Licorice   2 ch'ien

(This concoction is used chiefly to restore energy.)

b. Concoction of following for bathing affected area:

Dry alum	2 ch'ien
Wu-p'ei-tzu (gall)	5 ch'ien

c. Castor bean (shelled) 5 ch'ien, crushed, for compress applied over the pai-hui point. Keep in place with gauze dressing. Change dressing daily, for 3 days in succession.

Glomerulonephritis

Glomerulonephritis is commonly referred to as "kidney disease." It is an allergic reaction to infection by hemolytic streptococci or other bacteria. It frequently occurs as a secondary complication following upper respiratory tract infection, scarlet fever or some purulent skin disease. It is seen in two forms: as acute or chronic glomerulonephritis.

Acute Glomerulonephritis

Edema is frequently seen in the beginning, generally starting around the head and face. Or sometimes the edema starts from the feet. In severe cases, the edema is generalized. The urine turns reddish or brown, scanty in quantity accompanied sometimes by polyuria and dysuria, and edema (generally not too severe). Red cells, albumin, and casts in the urine are characteristic of this disease.

Types

According to differences in clinical symptoms, it is frequently seen as wind-damaging (shang-feng) and moisture-damaging (shang-shih) types.

Wind-damaging glomerulonephritis is characterized by an acute onset resulting mostly from exposure to wind and cold after perspiring. The edema first appears on the eyelids, then the face, accompanied by fever, chills, aversion to wind, and by anhidrosis. Fur on tongue is white and moist, and pulse is floating.

Moisture-damaging glomerulonephritis is characterized by fluid retention in the body, the edema usually first noticed in the feet. The breathing is coarse and the patient cannot lie down flat. Fur on tongue is white, and the pulse is sunken and fine.

Prevention

1. Attention to avoiding skin infections and exposure to dampness and cold.

2. Early and timely treatment of hemolytic streptococcal infection affecting the upper respiratory tract (including the tonsils) or the skin.

Treatment

1. Bed rest and warmth, and a low salt diet (no sodium-containing condiments such as salt, soy sauce, etc.) Restriction of fluid intake during acute phase. Low-salt diet permitted (salt intake limited to 1-1.5 gm/day) after edema has basically subsided.

2. New acupuncture therapy. Apply medium amount of stimulation to "kuan-yuan" point penetrating the "chung-chi," and other points such as the "yin-ling ch'uan" and the "san-yin chiao." Repeat treatment daily.

3. Ear acupuncture therapy. Apply needle puncture to areas designated for the kidneys and the bladder.

4. Chinese herbs

    a. For wind-damaging glomerulonephritis, treatment should clear the lungs and promote moisture removal, with remedies such as the following:

        (1) Concoction of

Tzu-su	3 ch'ien
Chinese waxgourd pellings (tung-kua p'i)	2 liang

        (2) Concoction of

Ephedra	1.5 ch'ien
Almonds	3 ch'ien
Tzu-pei fou-p'ing [duckweed sp.]	2 ch'ien

        (3) Concoction of

Ma-huang (ephedra)	2 ch'ien
Almonds	3 ch'ien
Dried orange peel	1.5 ch'ien
Fu-ling peelings	4 ch'ien
Ta-fu-p'i	2 ch'ien
Ginger peelings	1.5 ch'ien
Sang-pai p'i	3 ch'ien

    b. For moisture-damaging glomerulonephritis, treatment should channel out excess moisture and promote diuresis, with remedies such as the following:

(1) Concoction of

    Che-ch'ien ts'ao (fresh)   4 liang
    Corn silk (fresh)   4 liang
    (If dried, use only 2 liang of each.)

(2) Concoction of

    Ch'ih hsiao-tou [Phaseolus angularis] 1 liang
    Ma-pien ts'ao [verbena]   5 ch'ien
    Che-ch'ien ts'ao   5 ch'ien
    Han-lien ts'ao   1 liang
    Pai mao-ken   1 liang
    Tse-lan hsieh   3 ch'ien

(3) Concoction of

    Tan-fu p'i   3 ch'ien
    Wu-chia p'i   3 ch'ien
    Fang-chi   3 ch'ien
    Barley   8 ch'ien

(4) Concoction of

    Black soybean   1 liang
    I-mu ts'ao (motherwort)   1 liang

(5) Concoction of chin-ying tzu (stem peelings?) steamed with
lean meat and eaten.

5. Western medicines

    a. If streptococcal infection is still present, give penicillin
       or other antibiotic, but no sulfa drugs since they may crystal-
       lize in the glomeruli and complicate the patient's condition.

    b. If the blood pressure is high, consider using reserpine, shuang-
       ch'ing ke-niao-se [hydrochloro thiazide?] or other tension
       lowering compound.

Chronic Nephritis

    Chronic nephritis usually develops after acute nephritis. A gradual
puffiness frequently affects the face and lower extremities (edema may be
absent in other cases). The patient gradually feels tired, back aches,
appetite is poor, and nausea, facial pallor or sallowness may be present.
Generally, there is no fever. In some cases, infection and overwork may
invoke edema, hematuria, albuminuria, and other acute nephritis symptom,
flaring up repeatedly sometimes.

Types

This illness is seen chiefly as kidney-deficient and spleen-deficient types.

Kidney-deficient chronic nephritis is characterized by scanty urine, thin water stools, facial pallor, dyspnea on the slightest exertion, headache, and backache. Tongue is thin, coating is white and slippery, and pulse is sunken and fine.

Spleen-deficient chronic nephritis is characterized by scanty urine, general fatigue, distended upper abdomen, and poor appetite. Tongue quality is pink, fur is white, and pulse is fine and weak.

If the yang is deficient and the cloudy yin rises, symptoms of uremia such as nausea, vomiting, a rise in blood pressure, itchy skin, dyspnea, palpitation, and even restlessness, coma, and convulsions may appear, indicating the critical nature of this ailment.

Prevention

1. All-out effort in war against chronic illnesses by allowing development of body resistance to overcome illness.

2. Thorough treatment of acute nephritis cases in time. Avoid exposure to cold and extreme exhaustion.

Treatment

1. New acupuncture therapy. Apple needles to "kuan-yuan," "shen-yu," "yin-ling-ch'uan," "san-yin-chiao" points once daily for a total of 15 times for one course of treatment.

2. Chinese herbs

    a. For kidney-deficient type. Treatment should warm the kidneys and promote diuresis, using remedies such as the following:

        (1) Concoction of

Cinnamon	1 ch'ien
Fu-ling	5 ch'ien

        (2) Chi-seng shen-ch'i yuan (patent medicine), 3 ch'ien each dose, 3 times a day.

(3) Concoction of

Processed aconite	3 ch'ien
Dry ginger	1-2 ch'ien
Pai-shu [Atractylis ovata]	3-5 ch'ien
Pai-shao [Paenia albiflora]	3 ch'ien
Fu-ling bark	5 ch'ien
Hu-lu-pa (gourd)	3 ch'ien

b. For spleen-deficient type. Treatment should strengthen the spleen and promote diuresis; with remedies such as the following:

(1) Concoction of

Fu-ling bark	1 liang
Large dates	1 liang
Ch'ih hsiao-tou	1 liang

(2) Cooked in one pot

Barley	4 liang
Huai-shan	1 liang

When done, eat residue ingredients.

(3) Concoction of

Huang-ch'i	5 ch'ien
Fang-chi	5 ch'ien
Pai-shu	3 ch'ien
Fu-ling, bark	5 ch'ien
Chu-ling	5 ch'ien
Tse-hsieh	5 ch'ien
Dried orange peel	5 ch'ien
Ta-fu-p'i	4 ch'ien
Che-ch'ien-tzu	5 ch'ien

If the yang is deficient and the unclear yin rises [to dominance], and the stomach feels full and distended after a eating, treatment should support the yang to resolve the yin "cloudiness," using the following concoction of

Tang-shen	5 ch'ien
Processed fu-tzu [aconite]	3 ch'ien
Dried orange peel	2 ch'ien
Fu-ling	5 ch'ien
Hou-pu	1.5 ch'ien
Fresh pan-hsia [Pinellia sp.]	2 ch'ien
Fresh ginger	3 slices

3. Western medicine

    Use shuang-ch'ing ke-niao-se [hydrochlorothiazide?] to promote
diuresis. If edema is absent but albuminuria is strongly positive, give
cortisone dehydrocortisone 5-10 mg, 3-4 times a day, by mouth. This type
of hormone should not be used over a lengthy period. Note the indications
for their use.

    If uremia occurs, correct the acidosis in time and give symptomatic
treatment.

Pyelonoephritis

    Pyelonephritis is usually caused by ascending bacterial infection intro-
duced via the urinary passageway (urethra, bladder, ureters, and the renal
pelvis). It is seen mostly in women and among children.

    This ailment is generally due to moist heat descending, characterized
chiefly by polyuria, urinary urgency, and dysuria. The urine is cloudy with
an unpleasant odor. Low-grade fever and percussion pain over the kidney region
may also be present.

Types

    Clinically, the disease may be classified as acute and chronic. Acute
pyelonephritis is usually a "solid" illness, chronic pyelonephritis, a "deficient"
one.

    Solid-type pyelonephritis is characterized by fever, chills, and backache.
Thirst, urinary urgency, dysuria, cloudy urine, a thin and yellow coating on
tongue, and a rapid forceful pulse may be present.

    Deficient-type pyelonephritis is characterized by its long duration,
patient's poor health, poor appetite, a low-grade fever, backache, slight
edema, a thin and white coating on tongue, and a sunken and slow pulse.

Prevention

    1. Attention to perineal cleanliness and menstrual hygiene in women.
For infants, frequent diaper change to assure cleanliness.

    2. Timely treatment of pinworm disease and purulent infections in
small children.

Treatment

    1. New acupuncture therapy techniques. Apply medium stimulation to
"kuan-yuan," "chung-chi," and "san-yin-chiao" points, once daily.

2. __Chinese herbs__

   a. For __solid-type pyelonephritis__. Treatment should clear fever
      and promote diuresis, using remedies such as the following:

      (1) Concoction of

Wild chrysanthemum	0.5-1 liang
Honeysuckle	0.5-1 liang
T'u fu-ling (smilax)	0.5-1 liang
Dandelion	0.5-1 liang

      (2) Concoction of

Che-ch'ien ts'ao [plantago], fresh	2 liang
Ta-suan [leeks], fresh	1 liang

      (3) Concoction of

Honeysuckle	5 ch'ien
Forsythia	3 ch'ien
Crude ti-huang	5 ch'ien
Chih-mu	3 ch'ien
Huang-pai [phellodendron]	3 ch'ien
Niu-hsi	3 ch'ien
P'i-hsieh	4 ch'ien
Mu-t'ung	3 ch'ien
Licorice	1.5 ch'ien
Chieh-keng	1.5 ch'ien

   b. For __deficient-type pyelonephritis__. Treatment should restore
      the yin and clear fever, with remedies such as the following
      concoction of

Lu-wei ti-huang yuan (patent medicine)	3 ch'ien
Honeysuckle	5 ch'ien
Nu-chen-tzu [Ligustrum sp.]	5 ch'ien
Han-lien-ts'ao	5 ch'ien

      To be taken twice daily.

3. __Western medicine__

   a. Furantoin 100 gm, 4 times a day, by mouth.

   b. Chloromycetin or tetracycline 0.25 gm, 4 times a day.

Calculi in the Urinary System

Calculi formed in the urinary system, and usually called "shih lin," include those stones formed in the kidney, ureters, and bladder. Clinically, the symptoms are hematuria, and dysuria, frequently accompanied by renal colic (which radiates from the kidney region in back toward the bladder and genitals in front) of such severity that the patient oftentimes pales, breaks out into a cold sweat, becomes nauseous and vomits. In cases of vesical calculi, polyuria and urinary urgency and other signs of bladder irritation appear. Sometimes small stones are expelled in the urine. The cause of this disease is generally recognized as the descent of an accumulation of moist heat, accompanied by a rapid and tense pulse and a normal looking tongue.

Prevention

1. More boiled water to be taken regularly.

2. A brew of chin-ch'ien ts'ao (5 ch'ien each time) every other day, to be taken over a long period of time in cases of stones in the urinary system, following stone expulsion or surgery.

Treatment

1. New acupuncture therapy. Apply strong stimulation to the "shen-yu," "chung-chi" and "san-yin-chiao" points, once every day.

2. Chinese herbs. Treatment should clear fever, resolve [eliminate] stones, and promote diuresis, using remedies such as the following:

   a. Extract of ch'ing-mu-hsiang [Aristolochia sp.] prepared by soaking 40 gm in 100 ml of 40 percent alcohol for a week. Given by mouth, 3 times a day, 10 ml each time.

   b. Concoction of

Chi-hsueh ts'ao, fresh	4 liang
Chin-ch'ien ts'ao	4 liang

   c. Concoction of

Chin-ch'ien ts'ao	2 liang
Che-ch'ien ts'ao	1 liang
Pai-mao-ken	1 liang
Yen-hu-so	3 ch'ien
Chi-nei-chin	3 ch'ien
Ya-hsiao [tooth fragments] pulverized	3 fen

   d. Concoction of

Shih-wei	5 ch'ien
Tung kuei-tzu	3 ch'ien
Mai	3 ch'ien

Talc	1 liang
Che-ch'ien [plantago]	4 ch'ien

e. Concoction of

Pien-hsu	5 ch'ien - 1 liang
Hai-chin sha	5 ch'ien - 1 liang
Ch'u-mai	5 ch'ien - 1 liang
Chin-ch'ien ts'ao	1 - 2 liang
Yen-hu-so	3 ch'ien
Licorice (sticks)	2 ch'ien

Dosage modification: For hematuria, add

Ta-suan	5 ch'ien
Hsiao-suan	5 ch'ien
Crude ti-huang	5 ch'ien

For fever, add 5 ch'ien each of honeysuckle and forsythia.

3. Western medicine

During attacks of acute pain, give intramuscular injection of atropine 0.5 mg.

Retention of Urine

Retention of urine is sometimes called "lung-pi" [torpor]. It is due mostly to urinary passage obstruction, inflammatory irritation of the urinary tract, certain nervous conditions, or surgery or trauma to the back or abdomen. The patient frequently feels the urge to pass urine, but cannot do so. Distress from the distension is quite severe, and dullness is heard upon percussion of lower abdomen. This disease may be due to a deficiency/weakness in kidney energy or to the presence of moist heat in the bladder.

Kidney-deficiency type of urine retention is characterized by a slow onset, usually appearing after a serious bout of illness. The urge to urinate is present, but it is impossible to pass any urine. The area below the umbilicus is cold, as are the feet. The mouth is not dry, but fur on the tongue is thin and white, and the pulse is thready and weak.

Moist-heat type of urine retention is characterized by the rapid onset, anuria or the passage of urine in scanty drops, severe distention of sub-umbilical area, fever, feverish delirium accompanied by bladder distension and anuria. Coating on tongue is yellow and thick, and the pulse is rapid and forceful.

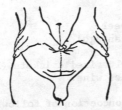

Figure 6-6-2. Compression method.

Treatment

1. __New acupuncture therapy__. Apply a medium amount of stimulation to needles placed in the "kuan-yuan," "yin-ling-ch'uan" and "san-yin-chiao" points, once or twice daily. Coordinate with hot compresses given to lower abdominal area.

2. __Digital pressure method__ (performed by barefoot doctor). Have patient lie on his back. Place both thumbs, overlapping each other, over the "li-niao" (diuretic) point (at midpoint of imaginary line joining the navel and the pubis symphysis, near the "kuan-yuan" point), other fingers resting on ridge of hipbone, and apply pressure, first lightly, then heavier. After the urine starts to flow, it is not necessary to repeat pressure, but keep hands in compressing position until urination is finished. Do not release hands while the urine is being passed. (Figure 6-6-2).

3. __Chinese herbs__

    a. For __kidney-deficient retention of urine__. Treatment should warm the kidneys to circulate the urine, using remedies such as the following:

        (1) Concoction of

Cinnamon	2 ch'ien
Bark of fu-ling [__Poria cocos__]	4 ch'ien

        (2) Concoction of

Sheng-ma [__Cimifuga__ sp.]	3 ch'ien
Che-ch'ien ts'ao (plantago)	5 ch'ien

        (3) Concoction of

Huang-ch'i [__Astragalus__ sp.]	3 ch'ien
Tang-shen [__Campanumaea__ sp.]	3 ch'ien
Pai-shu [__Atractylis ovata__]	3 ch'ien
Tang-kuei	3 ch'ien

Sheng-ma	1.5 ch'ien
Ch'ai-hu	1.5 ch'ien
Dried orange peel	2 ch'ien
Che-ch'ien (plantago)	4 ch'ien

(4) Toasted and pulverized crickets (3) and mole crickets (3) taken with sweet wine.

(5) Concentrated concoction of following for foot soak

Tzu-su [Perilla frutescens]
Tsung-pai [white part of leeks]
Shih-ch'ang-p'u [Acorus grammineus]

Use herb residues for frequent massaging of suprapubic area.

b. For moist-heat type retention of urine. Treatment should resolve [excess] energy, clear fever, and demoisturize, using remedies such as the following:

(1) Concoction of

Crude ti-huang	4 ch'ien
Mu-t'ung [Akebia sp.]	3 ch'ien
Bamboo leaves	3 ch'ien
Licorice (sticks)	3 ch'ien

(2) Concoction of

Che-ch'ien ts'ao [plantago]	5 ch'ien
Hsien-he ts'ao [Agrimonia pilosa]	3 ch'ien
Bark of fu-ling [Poria cocos]	3 ch'ien
Almond kernel	1 ch'ien
Rush	1 ch'ien

(3) White-necked earthworms (several) melted in sugar and taken with boiled water.

(4) Concoction of

Hai-chin-sha [Lygodium japonicum]	1 liang
Che-ch'ien-ts'ao [plantago]	1 liang
Chi-hsueh ts'ao	1 liang
Chrysanthemums	1 liang
Chieh-keng [Platycodon grandiflorum]	3 ch'ien
Tzu-wan [Aster sp.]	3 ch'ien
Dried orange peel	2 ch'ien

4. Catheterization, when necessary.

Rheumatic Arthritis

Rheumatic arthritis is also called "pi-cheng" [numbness disease]. It is related to a systemic allergic reaction produced after streptococcal infection of the human body. It frequently is induced by exposure to wind, cold, and dampness. In many patients, a migrating type of redness, swelling, heat, and limited movement are noted in large joints such as the knees, ankle, elbow, and wrist. This may be accompanied by fever, a pink circular type of skin rash, and bean-size nodules under the skin that do not hurt nor itch. This disease must be differentiated from rheumatoid arthritis (mostly symmetrical involvement of small joints with joint deformity).

Types

Generally seen are the following two types:

Wind-chill-dampness type of numbness, characterized by a slow and gradual onset usually involving the hands, feet, arms, legs, waist, and back which become painful. However, this pain is not fixed — sometimes it is here, and sometimes it is there. Sometimes the joints become quite swollen and numb, though the skin coloring shows no change. Generally, the swollen joint will feel better after application of hot compresses. Sometimes the condition is accompanied by an aversion to cold, by fever and hidrosis. Fur on tongue is thin and white or white and oily. Pulse is floating and tight.

Feverish and numb type of rheumatic arthritis is characterized by a more rapid onset accompanied by fever or a continuous low-grade fever, red and swollen joints, hot and extremely sensitive to touch. Mouth is dry, patient is restless, urine is yellow and scanty, tongue is red, its coating yellow and oily or yellow and dry, and pulse is slippery and rapid.

Prevention

1. Prevention of upper respiratory tract infections, and timely surgical removal of inflamed tonsils.

2. Active and thorough treatment of patients suffering from rheumatism, to prevent further development into rheumatic heart disease.

Treatment

1. New acupuncture therapy. Apply medium stimulation to needles placed in the following points, once a day:

    a. Upper extremities: "ch'u-ch'ih," "chien-yu," "wai-kuan," and "hou-ch'i' points.

b. Lower extremities: "huan-t'iao," "chueh-ku," "hsi-yen," "yang-ling-ch'uan," "tsu-san-li."

For wind-chill moist type numbness inoxibustion can be used; for severe redness and swelling in joints, perform shallow puncture of local area, using "hao-chen" until slight bleeding ensues.

2. Chinese herbs

a. For <u>wind-chill moist-type numbness</u> treatment should control wind, dispel cold, and promote moisture elimination to open up "lo" passageways, using remedies such as the following:

(1) Extract of

Chih-chu p'ao-tan [<u>Aspidistra elatior</u>]	0.5 chin
White wine	1 chin

Let mixture steep for 1-2 days. To be given 3 times a day, 15 ml each dose.

(2) Concoction of

Red lotus seeds	0.5 chin
San-pai ts'ao	4 liang

To be taken with a little white wine.

(3) Concoction of

Chi-hsueh t'eng	1 liang
Yin-yang-huo, roots	1 liang
Shen-chin ts'ao	3 ch'ien
Ch'uan ti-feng	3 ch'ien
Mulberry twigs (roasted)	5 ch'ien

(4) Hsiao-huo-lo tan (patent medicine), 1 pill to be taken twice a day, with some white wine or boiled water.

(5) Dried and pulverized crude pan-hsia (<u>Pinella</u> sp) mixed with 75 percent alcohol for local application.

b. For <u>feverish type of rheumatic arthritis</u>, treatment should clear fever, control "wind" and open up the "lo" passageways, using remedies such as the following:

(1) Concoction of

Wu-chia-p'i	3 ch'ien
Jen-tung t'eng	1 liang
Mulberry twigs	1 liang

(2)   Concoction of

Wei-mao ken	1 liang
Chu-ku, roots	1 liang
Chin-ying-tzu	1 liang
Mao-ken	1 liang

(3)   Concoction of

Jen-tung t'eng	2 liang
Crude li-huang [Rehmania glutinosa]	1 liang
Niu-pang tzu (toasted)	5 ch'ien
Feng-feng	3 ch'ien
Fang-chi	3 ch'ien

(4)   Hsi-tung yuan (patent medicine). To be taken twice a
day, 3-4 ch'ien each time, with some warm boiled water.

3. Western medicines

a. Aspirin 1 gm four times a day, by mouth. Or, sodium salicylate
1-2 gm four times daily, by mouth.

b. Cortisone 5-10 mg four times a day, by mouth. Suitable for those
cases of rheumatic carditis and rheumatic arthritis who do not
respond, or who are allergic to sodium salicylate. Reduce dosage
gradually after symptoms have receded, until dosage is finally
5-10 mg daily. The complete course of therapy lasts 1-2 months.

c. Sulfadiazine or penicillin for those rheumatism cases accompanied
by high fever, streptococcal infection of the tonsils or throat.

Note: Generally, after the rheumatism is temporarily controlled,
other body parts or function affected by the rheumatic condition
can also recover. However the heart valves and valvular folds
frequently incur permanent scar damage because of the inflammation, causing a varying degree of functional disturbance. Such
a condition is called chronic rheumatic heart valve disease.

Rheumatoid Arthritis

Rheumatoid arthritis is also called "li-chieh feng," [literally rheumatism in joints]. It is a chronic systemic ailment due mostly to invasion by
wind, cold and dampness. Generally, onset is slow, though fever may be present
during the acute stage. Distribution of joint pathology is frequently symmetrical, beginning with small joints, especially proximal joints of the fingers, and
later involving the wrist, elbow and kneejoints. These joints frequently swell
up spindle-shaped. In the later stages, the joints are mostly deformed, stiff,
and inflexible (Figure 6-6-3).

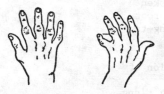

Figure 6-6-3. Rheumatoid arthritis

Prevention

Measures same as those for rheumatism.

Treatment

1. New acupuncture therapy. Apply needle puncture, using strong stimulation, to the following points, once a day. For digital and wrist joints, the "yang-ch'ih" and "ta-ling" points; for the elbow joint, the "ch'u-ch'ih" and "ch'ih-tse" points; for the shoulder joint, the "chien-yu" point, for the hip joint, the "feng-shih" and the "huan-t'iao" points; for the knee joint, the "hsi-yen" and "yang-ling-ch'uan" points; for ankle joint and joints of the toe, the "k'un-lun" and "ch'iu-hsu" points; for the spinal column, the "ta-chui" point.

2. Chinese herbs. Treatment should suppress the wind and dispel the cold, activate the blood and clear the "lo" passageways, using remedies such as the following:

    a. Concoction of

Hsun-ku-feng	1 liang
Hsu-chang-hsing	5 ch'ien
Processed szechuan aconite	1.5 ch'ien
Processed ts'ao-wu [Aconitum chinense]	1.5 ch'ien
Large dates	5

    b. Concoction of

Hsi-ch'ien ts'ao	1 liang
Mulberry sticks	1 liang
Mu-tse	1 liang
Mugwort leaves	1 liang
Shan-chi-chiao	1 liang

One concoction to be taken every day, for a period of half a month.

c. Concoction of

Lo-shih t'eng	5 ch'ien
T'u-niu-hse	5 ch'ien
Mu-tse	5 ch'ien
Ti-yu	1 liang
Mulberry sticks	1 liang
Pine branches [knots]	1 liang
White wine	1 liang

One concoction/dose per day for a period of half a month.

d. Concoction of

Mulberry sticks	1 liang
Su chi-chieh [logwood sticks?]	3 ch'ien
Pine knots	3
Bamboo joints	5
Fir tree knots	5
Camphor tips	1.5 ch'ien
<u>Sophora japonica</u> joints	3 ch'ien

(This concoction/prescription is suited for painful swelling
of small joints.)

e. <u>Poultice/compresses</u>. Used for painful swelling of extremity
joints where joint activity is restricted. Poultice is prepared from the following materials, crushed fine.

Mulberry sticks	3 ch'ien
Cinnamon sticks	1.5 ch'ien
Niu-hsi	4 ch'ien
T'ou-ku ts'ao	5 ch'ien
Fang-feng	3 ch'ien
Pi-hsieh	5 ch'ien
Ju-hsiang	1.5 ch'ien
Mu-hsiang	1.5 ch'ien
Myrrh	1.5 ch'ien
Chiang-huo	4 ch'ien
Tu-huo	4 ch'ien
Hung-hua	3 ch'ien
Tang-kuei [Angela smensis]	3 ch'ien

Add white wine and water to the pulverized material to form
consistency of a thick paste. Apply paste to affected joint.
Change compress two times a day.

3. <u>Western medicine</u>

Salicylate acid or aspirin, as well as dehydrocortisone may be
given by mouth.

Heart Failure

Heart failure is a frequently seen complication of heart disease. The most common etiological factors are rheumatic, hypertensive, atherosclerotic or pulmonary heart disease. Because of certain etiological factors, Myocardial function is inadequate, blood is not completely pumped out with each heart contraction, and a circulatory disturbance results. Clinically, this is seen as signs and symptoms of cardiac failure. Heart failure is generally classified as left heart failure and right heart failure.

Left heart failure is manifested chiefly as stagnation of the pulmonary circulation. The first sign is dyspnea, which first appears during working exertion, becoming increasingly severe as the lips and tips of body extremities become cyanosed. The left side of heart is enlarged, the heart beat is increased, and murmurs are heard over apex of heart, while moist rales are heard over the lungs.

Right heart failure is manifested chiefly as stagnation of the systemic circulation, accompanied by dyspnea, palpitation, coughing, epigastric distension and slight pain, cyanosed lips and fingertips. The edema is first seen in the lower extremities, progressing later to involve the whole body. At the same time, pleural effusion, ascites or noticeable protrusion of jugular veins may be seen. The heart is enlarged, murmurs are heard. Rales are heard over the lungs, and enlargement and pressure pain are noticed.

Prevention

1. Possession of a faith and determination to overcome illness. Female patients with a cardiac condition are best advised to avoid any pregnancy, to reduce the load on the heart.

2. Attention to prevention and timely treatment of any upper respiratory tract infection in cardiac cases. Set up an orderly schedule for work and rest.

Treatment

1. General

   a. Absolute bed rest for serious cases in semi-recumbent position. Activity may be increased after condition improves.

   b. Saltfree diet for patients suffering from cardiac failure. After condition improves, a low-salt diet is allowed, with daily salt intake limited to 2-3 gm.

   c. Antibiotics to be given immediately in presence of acute infection. For those with rheumatic involvement, give anti-rheumatic medication. For those with hypertension, give blood pressure lowering drugs.

2. **Chinese herbs**

   a. Concoction of fresh roots of wan-nien ch'ing [Rohdea japonica],
      5 ch'ien - 1 liang

      One concoction dose is taken daily. (This prescription is
      suited for chronic heart failure.)

   b. Concoction of

Tan-shen	0.5 - 1 liang
Tang-kuei	3 - 5 ch'ien
Ch'ih-shao	3 - 5 ch'ien
Peach kernel	2 - 4 ch'ien

   (This prescription is suited for rheumatic heart diseases)

   c. Concoction of

Fu-ling	5 ch'ien
Cinnamon sticks	3 ch'ien
Pai-shu	3 ch'ien
Licorice	1 ch'ien
Tan-shen	5 ch'ien
Huang-ch'i [Astragalus henryi]	3 ch'ien
Mu-fang-chi	3 ch'ien

   (This prescription is suited for those cardiac cases with
   generalized edema, asthma, hard and painful stomach, a
   blackish complexion, and a sunken pulse)

3. **Western medicine**

   Judicious use of cardiac stimulants such as digitalis or cedilanid.
Watch for accumulative dose intoxication.

   Aminophylline, hydrochlorothiazide [?] or hypertonic dextrose may
be given to promote diuresis.

   For restlessness, give luminal 0.1 gm or sodium amytal 0.2 gm to
keep patient quiet.

Hypertension

   The causes of primary hypertension are still not understood, though
the condition is generally considered to be related to nervous tension over
a long period of time or to heredity. Secondary hypertension is due mostly
to kidney disease and intracranial tumors. The patient may present with
symptoms of headache, dizziness, cranial pressure, tinnitus, palpitation,

numbness of extremities, neck rigidity, restlessness, insomnia etc. The blood pressure is frequently above 140/90 mm. In serious cases, the head also feels heavy, the lower limbs are weak, and the patient feels he is floating on water -- hence the feeling of "head heavy and feet light."

Types

Clinically, the liver-yang [energy] dominant type and the kidney-yin deficient type are more commonly seen.

Liver-yang dominant hypertension is characterized by dizziness, head-ache, ruddy complexion and bloodshot eyes, constipation, a reddish tongue coated by a yellow and oil fur, a tense or tense and slippery, but forceful pulse.

Kidney-yin deficient hypertension is characterized by dizziness, head-ache, tinnitus, palpitation, insomnia, "spots before eyes," to reddish tongue or a bright red "fur-less" tongue, and a tense and rapid pulse.

Prevention

1. Establishment of an optimistic attitude and a strong deter-mination toward fighting the disease. According to the severity of the condition, coordinate all living, working, and mild physical culture activities.

2. Light diet high on vegetables but low in fat content.

Treatment

1. New acupuncture therapy. Needle using a medium amount of stimula-tion, needle the following points, once a day: the "ch'u-ch'ih," "pai-hui," "fend-ch'ih," "tsu-san-li."

2. Chinese herbs

    a. For liver-yang dominant hypertension treatment should quiet and stabilize the liver and clear it of heat [excess], using remedies such as the following:

        (1) Concoction of

            Ch'ou wu-'tung leaves (tender)   1 liang.

        (2) Concoction of

            Wild chrysanthemums   3 ch'ien
            Hsia k'u-ts'ao   3 ch'ien

(3) Concoction of

K'ou t'eng	3 ch'ien
Ch'ung-wei tzu	3 ch'ien
Chi-ts'ai (Shepherd's purse)	1 liang
Ch'ueh-ming-tzu	5 ch'ien
Hsi-ch'ien ts'ao	5 ch'ien

b. <u>For kidney-yin deficient hypertension</u>, treatment should nourish and restore the kidneys and stabilize the liver, using remedies such as the following:

(1) Lu-wei Ti-huang wan (patent medicine) 3 ch'ien, and Tzu-chu wan (patent medicine), 0.5 - 1 ch'ien, both taken simultaneously, twice a day.

(2) Concoction of

Nu-chen-tzu [<u>Ligustrum</u> sp.]	1 liang
Han lien ts'ao	5 ch'ien
Moutan, bark	3 ch'ien

(3) Concoctions of

Lung-ku (refined)	3 ch'ien
Oyster shell (refined)	3 ch'ien
Magnetite	3 ch'ien
Che-shih [hematite]	3 ch'ien
Tu-chung	3 ch'ien
Sheng-tieh lo [cast iron droppings?]	1 liang

3. <u>Western medicines</u>

Use reserpine or other hypotensive drug selectively, with a tran-quillizer such as phenobarbital. To reduce vascular brittleness, "Lu-t'ung" [channel-opening] tablets could be used.

Stroke

The condition referred to as stroke includes cerebral hemorrhage, cerebral thrombosis, cerebral embolism, cerebrovascular spasm, and subarachnoid hemorrhage in what are called cerebrovascular accidents. This section will concentrate mainly on the prevention and treatment of cerebral hemorrhage.

Cerebral hemorrhage usually develops from hypertensive disease, and may be described in two phases: the apoplexy phase and the "p'ien-ku" or after-effects phase.

- 391 -

The _apoplexy phase_ refers to the immediate conditions surrounding a stroke attack. It is characterized by its acute onset, the sudden fall, coma, incontinence, stertorous breathing, accompanied by hemiplegia. Clinically, apoplexy is further classified as "closed" or "detached." In "closed" apoplexy, both hands of the patient are clenched, the jaw is locked, the face is red, breathing is coarse, fur on tongue is yellow and oily, and the pulse is tense and rapid. In "detached" apoplexy, the eyes are closed but the mouth is open, the patient shares, respirations are weak, hands are limp, the bladder is incontinent, the tongue is parched, and the pulse is weak or slow.

The _side effects phase_ refers to post-apoplectic complications. This is chiefly hemiplegia, where the patient wishes to move and cannot, the eyes and mouth are distorted, saliva and even food drools from corner of patient's mouth, the fur on tongue is white and oily, and the pulse is usually tense and rapid.

Prevention

1. _General treatment_. Prescribe absolute bed rest, with avoidance of routine moves and raising the head somewhat higher. Comatosed patients should be catheterized, fed nasally, and given oxygen, when necessary. After patient's condition has stabilized, change his position frequently, to avoid bedsores.

2. New _acupuncture therapy_. For "closed" apoplexy, needle the "pai-hui," "jen-chung," and "yung-ch'uan" points; for "detached" apoplexy, acupuncture (moxibustion added) the "ch'i-hai," "kuan-yuan."

For post-apoplectic _side effects_, needle the "chien-yu," "ch'u-ch'ih," "wai-kuan," "ho-ku," "feng-shih," and "huan-t'iao" points for extremity paralysis. For speech difficulties, needle the "shang-lien-ch'uan" (one finger's width over the lower jaw). For nystagmus, needle the "ti-ts'ang" point penetration the "chia-che" point.

3. _Chinese herbs_.

   a. For "closed" apoplexy, treatment should open the innards, quell the wind and resolve sputum with remedies such as the following:

   (1) T'ung-kuan san [a powder] blown into the nose to cause sneezing.

   (2) Mixture of

   Nan-hsing   1.5 ch'ien
   Rock sugar, crushed   .25 ch'ien

   Used to rub distal aspect of molars alongside buccal surface to cause jaw to unlock. Or, fleshy fruit of black prunes may be used to rub teeth along gumline for the same purpose.

(3) Niu-huang ch'ing hsin wan, 1-2 pills crushed and taken
with water (for fever-based "closed" symptoms); or su-ho-
hsiang wan, 1 pill, crushed and taken with water (for
cold-based "cold" symptoms).

b. For "detached" apoplexy, treatment should supplement energy
and restore yang vigor, using remedies such as the following:

(1) Concoction of

Ginseng	3 ch'ien
Tu-tzu [aconite]	2 ch'ien

(2) Concoction of

Fresh nan-hsing	3 ch'ien
Fresh Szechuan aconite, peeled	1.5 ch'ien
Fresh fu-tzu [aconite]	1.5 ch'ien
Mu-hsiang	1 ch'ien

Crush above ingredients, and use 2-3 ch'ien each time for
concoction brewing with 5 ch'ien of ginseng (if ginseng is
not available, substitute with tang-shen, using twice the
amount called for).

c. For after-effect complications

(1) For hemiplegia, concoction of

Tang-kuei ends	3 ch'ien
Szechuan Conioselinum unvittatum	1.5 ch'ien
Huang-ch'i [Astragalus henryi]	5 ch'ien
Peach kernel	2 ch'ien
Ti-lung	3 ch'ien
Ch'ih-shao	3 ch'ien
Hung-hua	1 ch'ien

(2) For strabismus: pulverized mixture of

Pai fu-tzu [white aconite]	3 ch'ien
Mummied silkworms	2 ch'ien
Whole centipede	1 ch'ien

To be taken twice daily, 1 ch'ien each time.

For external application, make ointment from

Castor seeds	2 ch'ien
Ju-hsiang	1 ch'ien

Spread on gauze and apply on healthy side.

Epilepsy

Epilepsy is called "yang-tien-feng" by the local populace. It is due mostly to an imbalance of wind, mucus, and energy. The onset is frequently sudden with the patient first emitting a loud cry that is followed by a loss of consciousness, generalized convulsions, lockjaw, cyanosis, foaming at the mouth (sometimes bloody if tongue or lips have been bitten), bloodshot eyes, dilated pupils, and incontinence. After these symptoms have persisted for a few minutes, the patient enters into a stuporous sleep. In some cases, the victim sleeps for at least half an hour before he slowly regains consciousness. Upon awakening, the patient has a headache and experiences mental fatigue, generalized pain and discomfort, and does not remember anything about the epileptic episode. The severity of the epileptic attack may be mild or severe. In mild attacks, the patient only takes on a fixed stare and stand or sit, as if in a trance, and drops anything held in his hands at this time without knowing, and becomes quite pale. Such an episode is called a "small epileptic attack." In some cases, this phenomenon is a daily recurrence, or one that takes place every few days, or every few months. In some cases, attacks occur several times a day.

Treatment

1. **New acupuncture therapy**

   a. During attack, needle the "jen-chung," "shao-shang," and "yung-ch'uan" points.

   b. At other times (no attack), use medium stimulation on needles inserted into "ta-chui," "yao-ch'i," and "shen-men" points, once daily. For the "yao-ch'i" point, use needles 2.5-3 ts'un [inches] long, and insert at point 2 inches upward from the coccyx

2. **Chinese herbs.** Treatment should dispel sputum formation, quell the wind, open up the innards, and stabilize the convulsions [the convulsive mechanism], using remedies such as the following:

   a. Concoction of

K'ou t'eng	1 liang
Oyster	2 liang

   b. Mixture of

Alum	8 liang
Cinnabar	1 liang
Magnetite	1 liang

   Crush into fine powder. For each dose allow 6 fen. Adult dosage the first month, 3 times daily; the second month, 2 times daily; and the third month, once daily.

c. Pulverized mixture of

Szechuan pei-mu [Fritillaria roylei]	5 ch'ien
Tan nan-hsing	3 ch'ien
Pan-hsia	3 ch'ien
Shih ch'ang-p'u	3 ch'ien
T'ien-ma	3 ch'ien
Ku-fan	2 ch'ien

To be taken twice daily, 3 ch'ien each time.

d. Concoction of

Ch'ing meng-shih	2-4 ch'ien
Ch'eng-hsiang	1-3 fen
Crude ta-huang [rhubarb] to be added later	1.5 ch'ien
Huang-ch'in [Scutellaria baicalensis]	3 ch'ien

3. Western medicines

   a. Phenytoin sodium 0.1 gm (adult dose), 3 times a day, the total
       daily dose not to exceed 0.6 gm.

   b. "Li-min-ning" [sedative] 10 mg (adult dose), 3 times a day.

Neurasthenia

Neurasthenia generally occurs after excessive tension caused by higher
nervous system activity when mental activity reaches a relative state of exhaustion. The patient may complain of dizziness, headache, cranial pressure,
tinnitus, spots before eyes, poor memory, inability to concentrate, bad temper,
poor sleeping habits or insomnia, daytime fatigue, backache and weakness in
legs. Additional signs and symptoms in still other cases are palpitation,
dyspnea, hidrosis and other circulatory symptoms. Poor appetite and gastric
distension and pain and other digestive tract symptoms may be seen in still
others. In some, genito-urinary tract symptoms such as impotency, premature
ejaculation, and "wet dreams" predominate. This disease is a functional ailment. However, it must be differentiated from several organic-type diseases,
to prevent misdiagnosis.

Prevention and Treatment

Analyze the nature of disease and its causes for explanation to
patient. This explanation will remove the patient's fears and point out
the items worthy of our daily attention, such as the proper scheduling of
work and rest activities. Everyday living must be orderly and provide
challenging opportunities.

2. <u>New acupuncture therapy</u>. Apply medium stimulation to needles inserted in the "yin-t'ang," "nei-kuan," "shen-men," and "san-yin-chiao" points. For poor appetite and gastric bloatiness, add the "chung-wan" and "tsu-san-li" points. For nocturnal emissions and impotency, add the "kuan-yuan" and "shen-yu" points.

3. <u>Chinese herbs</u>. Treatment should cultivate the heart and quiet the nerves, using remedies such as the following:

   a. T'ien-tzu ts'ao, heat-dried and crushed. Mold into honeyed pills the size of sterculia nuts. To be taken twice daily, 3 ch'ien each dose.

   b. Concoction of

Fresh pai-ho [lily]	2-4 liang
Seeds of <u>Zizyphus vulgaris</u> (toasted)	5 ch'ien

   c. Concoction of

Yeh-chiao t'eng	1 liang
Wu-wei-tzu (gall)	1.5 ch'ien

   d. Extract of yin-yang-huo prepared by soaking 1 liang of herb in 3 liang of white urine, for 7 days. Throw away residue. To be taken twice daily, 2-5 ml each time.

   e. <u>Patent medicines</u>.

      (1) For bad temper and difficult control of emotions, "Hsiao-yao Wan," 3 times daily, 3 ch'ien each time.

      (2) For poor appetite, when the heart and spleen are deficient, "Kuei-p'i Wan" or "yang-hsin Wan," twice a day, 3 ch'ien each time.

      (3) For dry mouth with little salivation, where the yin is deficient and body "fire" is dominant, "Chu-sha-an-shen Wan," 1-2 ch'ien at bedtime or "Pu-hsin Wan" 3 ch'ien twice a day.

      (4) For impotency, premature ejaculation or nocturnal emission, "chin-so ku-ching Wan," 3 ch'ien twice a day.

Trigeminal Neuralgia

The trigeminal nerve is located on the face (Figure 6-6-4). Sudden, short, and periodic jabs of acute pain (sensation is like needle jab, knife cut, or a burning pain) are felt on the face, in the upper or lower jaws, or around the region of tongue may indicate trigeminal neuralgia. Etiology of the condition is unclear. It may be due to cold exposure, face washing, talking, brushing teeth, or swallowing. The sudden onset of pain is generally written all over the face. The more commonly seen types are wind-chill (feng-han) related, or liver-wind (kan-feng) related.

Wind-chill trigeminal neuralgia is generally characterized by an aversion to wind, running nose, a floating pulse and a white fur on tongue.

Liver-wind trigeminal neuralgia is characterized by presence of sharp stabbing pain, a burning sensation over affected area, a rapid pulse and a red tongue.

Treatment

1. New acupuncture therapy. Apply stong stimulation to needles inserted in the "hsia-kuan" through to the "chia-che" (puncture here is shallow, just under the skin between these two points), "ho-ku," "lieh-ch'ueh," and "t'ai-yang" points.

2. Ear acupuncture therapy. Needle puncture or bury needles in those areas of the ear lobe that correspond to the upper jaw, lower jaw, and cheeks.

3. Seal-closure of acupuncture points. To 0.5 ml of 95 percent alcohol, add 1 ml of 1 percent procaine, and inject (seal-closure) into the "hsia-kuan" point. This approach is quite effective for treating resistant trigeminal neuralgia. After the point has been sealed, a burning sensation is felt for 2-3 days before it dissipates.

4. Chinese herbs

a. For wind-chill trigeminal neuralgia. Treatment should channel the wind and dispel the cold, using remedies such as the following concoction of

Ching-chieh	3 ch'ien
Feng-feng	3 ch'ien
Chiang-huo	1.5 ch'ien
Hsi-hsin	1 ch'ien
Mint	1.5 ch'ien
Pai-ch'i	3 ch'ien
Mummied silkworms	3 ch'ien
Licorice	1 ch'ien

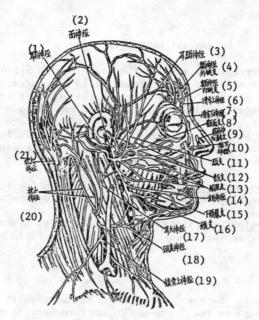

Figure 6-6-4. Distribution of the trigeminal nerve

Legend:
(1)	Posterior auricular nerve	(11)	Temporal nerve, branch
(2)	Facial nerve	(12)	Zygomatic nerve, branch
(3)	Auriculo-temporal nerve	(13)	Buccinator nerve
(4)	Frontal nerve, lateral	(14)	Mental nerve
(5)	Frontal nerve, medial	(15)	Inferior alveolar nerve
(6)	Supretrochlear nerve	(16)	Cervical nerve, branch
(7)	Infratrochlear nerve	(17)	Great auricular nerve
(8)	Zygomatic nerve	(18)	Cutaneous colli nerve
(9)	Anterior ethmoid nerve, external nasal branch	(19)	Supraclavicular nerve
(10)	Infraorbital nerve	(20)	Smaller occipital nerve
		(21)	Greater occipital nerve

b. For <u>liver-wind trigeminal neuralgia</u>, treatment should quiet the liver and quell the wind, with remedy such as the following concoction of

Mulberry leaves	3 ch'ien
Chrysanthemums	1.5 ch'ien
K'ou-t'eng	3 ch'ien
Hsia-ku ts'ao	3 ch'ien
Pai chi-li	3 ch'ien
Ligustrum	3 ch'ien
Han-lien ts'ao	3 ch'ien
Ts'ao ch'ueh-ming	3 ch'ien

5. **Western medicines**

Various analgesic or tranquillizing agents such as aspirin compound, analgesin phenytoin sodium etc. are used.

Migraine Headache

Migraine headache, commonly referred to as "pien t'ou-feng" (migraine rheumatism) by the native population, is a periodic one-sided headache. During an attack the eyes see nothing but a blackness in front, broken up by flashes of stars and light, and nausea and vomiting become overwhelming when the headache is excruciating. This ailment is seen mostly in women given to ill temper and insomnia, who usually experience a bitter taste in the month and dryness of throat, and present a tense pulse and fur-less tongue.

Treatment

1. **New acupuncture therapy.** Apply strong stimulation to needles inserted in the "t'ai-yang," "lu-ku" penetrating the "chiao-sun," and "tsu-lin-li," once or twice daily.

2. **Chinese herbs.**

Treatment should channel [open up] the wind and clear fever; restore the blood and stabilize the liver, with remedies such as the following:

a. Mei-hsieh tung-ch'ing (roots), peeled, 3-5 liang, cooked with 3 eggs and eaten.

b. Ta-ch'ing, roots, 4 liang, cooked with 4 liang of lean pork and eaten.

c. Concoction of

Ta-ch'ing [roots]	1 liang
Gypsum	5 ch'ien
Mildly salted black soybeans	3 ch'ien
Conioselinum unvittatum	3 ch'ien

d. Concoction of

Hsia-ku-ts'ao [Brunella vulgaris]	3 ch'ien
Kou-t'eng [Uncaria sp.]	4 ch'ien
T'ien-pien chu [Aster trinervius]	5 ch'ien
Lu-pien-ching [Serissa sp.]	5 ch'ien
Shui chin-ts'ai	4 liang

To be taken 3 days in a row.

e. Crushed radish juice mixed with a little camphor to be used as nose drops. Technique: Have patient lie on back and place nose drops in nostril of affected side. If both sides affected, drop both nostrils.

f. Concoction of

Crude ti-huang	3 ch'ien
Tang-kuei	3 ch'ien
Crude pai-shao	3 ch'ien
Conioselinum unvittatum	1.5 ch'ien
Chrysanthemum	1.5 ch'ien
Mother-of-pearl	5 ch'ien

Sciatica

Sciatica is commonly associated with rheumatic sciatic neuritis and slipped lumbar disc. When the sciatic nerve is invaded by different etiological factors, pain and tactile pain are felt in area over the nerve.

The onset of illness is frequently acute, and there is a history of cold exposure or trauma. It usually occurs on one side with a burning sensation, the pain felt like needle jabs, and becoming increasingly severe. It starts from the buttocks or the lower lumbar region and radiates downward along the posterior aspect of the thigh to the foot. During a painful attack, the victim cannot cough too hard, nor can he strain at stool. When he is standing up, the waist curves over to the painful side. In severe cases, he may not be able to walk or turn over. In such situations, the patient prefers lying on his side and flexes the lower extremity on the painful side upward, in a move to lessen the pull on the nerve and cut down on the pain. Testing patient's knee-bend reflex [Kernig's sign] will show that patient experiences pain when the knee of affected side is extended.

Treatment

1. New acupuncture therapy. Apply strong stimulation to needles inserted into the "huan-t'iao," "wei-chung," "yang-ling-ch'uan," "k'un-lun" points, once daily. Apply moxibustion after needles have been removed.

2. Chinese herbs

a. Concoction of

Tan-shen	4 ch'ien
Niu-hsi	4 ch'ien
Hsu-tuan	3 ch'ien
Papaya	3 ch'ien

b. Root bark from jui-hsiang, 3 ch'ien, roasted dry and pulverized. To be taken with boiled water, 3 times a day.

3. Western medicines

   Sodium salicylate, 1 gm 3 times a day may be given patients suffering from rheumatic sciatic neuritis. Other drugs such as aminopyrine, analygine etc. may be used selectively.

Anemia

   Anemia is a lower than normal reading of red blood cells and hemoglobin in the blood of the human body caused mostly by a lack of iron, overly great loss of blood, or hemolysis.

   Generally, symptoms of this disease include dizziness, poor appetite, fatigue, tinnitus, a sallow complexion, paleness in coloring of conjunctiva and nailbeds, pale lips and tongue, shortness of breath following exertion, palpitation, a reduced red cell count and a particularly low hemoglobin index. According to the manifestation of symptoms, anemia is seen more frequently in two forms: anemia due spleen-stomach weakness, and anemia due to energy and blood insufficiency.

   Anemia resulting from spleen-stomach weakness is characterized by a poor appetite, facial pallor, thin coating of fur on a pale tongue, and a slow and fine pulse.

   Anemia due to energy and blood insufficiency is characterized mostly by shortness of breath, palpitation, dizziness, tinnitus, fatigue and weakness, thin-coated fur on pale tongue, and a fine and weak pulse.

Prevention

   Active measures to prevent and treat the primary cause of anemia: use of anthelmintics to purge hookworms, radical treatment of hemorrhoids, active measures to stop bleeding, and proper feeding of infants.

Treatment

   1. New acupuncture therapy. Apply medium stimulation to needles inserted in the 'ta-chui," "ch'u-ch'ih," "tsu-san-li," "p'i-yu" points once daily. Needle puncture may be followed by moxibustion on points.

   2. Chinese herbs

      a. For anemia due to spleen-stomach weakness, treatment should supplement and restore energy and blood, with remedies such as the following:

      (1) Concoction of

                    Huang-ch'i [Astragalus henryi]   3-5 ch'ien
                    Tang-kuei   3 ch'ien
                    Hsien-t'ao ts'ao   2 ch'ien

          (2)   Burnt huang-ch'i   5 ch'ien
                    Tang-shen   3 ch'ien
                    Toasted pai-shu   3 ch'ien
                    Tang-kuei   3 ch'ien
                    Purple tan-shen   4 ch'ien

          One concoction/dose to be taken daily.

          (3)   Concoction of

                    Processed ho-shou-wu   5 ch'ien
                    Tang-kuei   4 ch'ien
                    Large dates   5 ch'ien
                    Black soybeans   1 cup

3.   Western medicines

     a.   Ferrous sulfate taken after meals. Continue medication for a
          month after condition shows improvement. During course of
          treatment, also take vitamin C 100-200 mg, 3 times a day.

     b.   Ferric ammonium citrate. Used chiefly to treat children, the
          dosage is 5-10 ml of 10 percent ferric ammonium citrate given
          3 times a day, after meals. Avoid using in conjunction with
          antipurine. Discontinue ferric ammonium citrate when anti-
          pyretics and analgesics are needed to treat colds and influenza.

     c.   Vitamin B, folic acid, and vitamin C used selectively.

                              Hemorrhagic Diseases

     Any condition which shows a marked tendency to bleed, such as the spon-
taneous appearance of petechiae on the skin and mucous membrane, or bleeding
that will not stop, is considered a hemorrhagic disease or "purpura." Clinically, thrombopenic purpura and anaphylactic purpura are more commonly seen.

                         1. Thrombopenic Purpura

     This disease is further classified as primary or secondary, with second-
ary thrombopenic purpura seen associated with other ailments (such as infections, anemia etc.) This disease falls within the scope of "blood-heated"
(hsueh-jeh) ailments that may be further distinguished as acute or gradual.
The acute cases are generally blood-heated, while the gradual cases are mostly
blood-deficient with heat present. The main symptom is bleeding under the

                                   - 402 -

skin seen as pin points, petechial or blue-black spots distributed unevenly, more on extremities than on the trunk. Mucous membrane bleeding is seen most often as epistaxis, bleeding from the gums, and rarely internal-organ bleeding manifested as hematemesis or bloody stools. Tongue quality is pink, pulse is fine and rapid, or deficient and rapid. If bleeding continues over a long period of time, or if the bleeding amount is rather large, symptoms of anemia will appear.

Prevention

1. Attention at all times, to any bleeding tendency. Protect against trauma.

2. Consumption of red dates [hung tsao] which has some effect on the prevention and treatment of this ailment.

Treatment

1. <u>New acupuncture therapy</u>. Apply light stimulation to needles inserted in the "ta-chui," "ch'u-ch'ih," "hsueh-hai," and "tsu-san-li" points, once daily. Treatment may also be combined with some moxibustion.

2. <u>Chinese herbs</u>

    a. For <u>blood-heated thrombopenic purpura</u>, treatment should clear the heat [fever] and stop the bleeding, using remedies such as the following:

        (1) Concoction of

T'ien-pien chu	2 liang
Han-lien ts'ao	2 liang
Pan-pien-lien	2 liang

        (2) Concentrated concoction of

Fresh hsiao-suan	1 liang
Fresh mao-ken	1 liang
Fresh crude ti-huang	1 liang
Fresh leave of <u>Thuja orientalis</u>	5 ch'ien

One concentrate to be prepared per day, divided into 2 doses.

        (3) Concoction of

Tzu-ts'ao	3 ch'ien to 1 liang
Ti-ting [clover]	3-5 ch'ien
Crude ti-huang coals	3-5 ch'ien
Ch'ih shao	2-4 ch'ien
Tan-p'i	1.5-3 ch'ien
Leaves of <u>Thuja orientalis</u>	5 ch'ien - 1 liang

- 403 -

Nelumbo root sections	5 ch'ien - 1 liang
Pig's feet (fatty oil removed)	3 ch'ien

b. For blood-deficient thrombopenic purpura, treatment should restore the blood and stop bleeding, using remedies such as the following:

(1) Eat fresh longana meats, 5 ch'ien twice a day. Prepare 2 chin of longana.

(2) Concoction of

Hsien-he ts'ao	1-2 liang
Pai-chi	3 ch'ien
Red dates	5 - 10

If anemia is also present, add

Tang-shen	3 ch'ien
Tang-kuei	3 ch'ien
Processed rehmannia [shu-ti]	3 ch'ien

(3) Beef thighbone (fresh), simmered in soup, without salt or oil added.

3. Western medicines

Vitamin C 100 gm, 3 times daily given by mouth.

Hsien-he-ts'ao liquid, 10 ml each time, 3 times daily.

Cotton ball pressure compress soaked in 1:1000 adrenalin used to treat local bleeding in mucous membrane.

Cortisone, 10 mg, three times a day by mouth, in acute cases. Drug dosage is reduced gradually and discontinued upon easing of symptoms.

2. Anaphylactic Purpura

Anaphylactic purpura is caused by an increase in vascular wall permeability and brittleness as the result of an allergic reaction. The onset is acute, and distribution of the purpura is generally symmetrical. This is seen mostly involving the lower extremities and may involve urticaria (hives). It may also appear as serious disseminating abdominal pain, arthralgia, bloody stools, or hematuria. Because of differences in individual makeup in clinical manifestations, most cases of anaphylactic purpura are seen as energy and blood insufficient and liver-dominant spleen-deficient types.

The energy and blood insufficient type of anaphylactic purpura is characterized by facial pallor, scattered distribution of petechiae, a fine [thready] pulse, pink tongue covered with thin fur coating.

The liver-dominant and spleen-deficient type of anaphylactic purpura is susceptible to flares of temper and complains of dizziness, fatigue, poor appetite, purpura of lower extremities, abdominal pain, a tense and fine pulse and thin coating of fur.

Prevention

1. Use extreme caution in prescribing drugs for patients with allergic tendencies. Do not give the same medication or food if patient has shown earlier sensitivity to them.

2. Consider stopping medication when patient shows abnormal reaction during course of treatment.

Treatment

1. New acupuncture therapy. Use medium stimulation on needles inserted into "hsueh-hai," "tsu-san-li," and "ch'u-ch'ih" points, once daily.

2. Chinese herbs

    a. For energy and blood deficient type, treatment should restore energy and blood, using remedies such as the following:

        (1) Concoction of

Huang-ch'i [Astragalus henryi]	5 ch'ien
Tang-shen [Campanumaea pilosula]	3 ch'ien
Tang-kuei [Augelica sp.]	3 ch'ien
Processed ti-huang [Rehmannia sp.]	5 ch'ien
Burnt licorice	1.5 ch'ien
Hsien-he ts'ao	1 liang
Red dates	10

For bleeding which may accompany defecation, add coals of ti yu 3 ch'ien; for hematuria, add hsiao-su 3 ch'ien and pai mao-ken 1 liang; for bleeding from gums and nose, add hsuan-shen 3 chien, for hematemesis add/substitute hematite 8 ch'ien, 3 nelumbo root sections, and "shih-hui-san" (patent medicine), 3 ch'ien.

        (2) Pa-chen wan (patent medicine), 3 ch'ien 3 times a day. Concoction of hsien-he ts'ao (Agrimonia sp.) may be used to help down the medication.

b. For <u>liver-dominant and spleen-deficient</u> anaphylactic purpura, treatment should calm the liver and support the spleen, using remedies such as the following:

(1) Concoction of

Ching-chieh [Nepeta japonica] spikelets, (toasted black)	2 ch'ien
Pai-shao	3 ch'ien
Dried orange peel	1.5 ch'ien
Pai-shu, roasted	3 ch'ien
Huai-shan-yao	8 ch'ien

One concoction per day, divided into two doses.

(2) Concoction of

Pai-shao	4 ch'ien
Licorice	2 ch'ien
Crude ti-huang	3-5 ch'ien
Black prunes	1 ch'ien
Fang-feng	1.5 ch'ien
Hsiao chi [Cirsium sp.]	1 liang
Huai-hua [Sophora sp.]	3-5 ch'ien
Red dates	10

3. <u>Western medicines</u>

a. Benadryl or Phenergan prescribed to counteract allergy, 25 mg given 3 times daily.

b. Cortisone tablets, 10 mg, 3-4 times daily for severe cases. Once symptoms ease up, reduce dosage gradually until drug is finally discontinued.

Leukemia

Leukemia results from a malignant change in the body's blood formation process, manifested chiefly as an unusual proliferation of white cells in the blood-forming tissues, and the appearance of immature white cells in the peripheral blood stream. On the basis of its severity, leukemia is generally seen as acute or chronic leukemia.

<u>Acute Leukemia</u>

Usually seen in children and young adults, acute leukemia sets in rapidly accompanied by sudden high fever, headache, and generalized aches and pains. Very rapidly, anemia and bleeding appear, with enlargement of the liver, spleen and lymphatic nodes. The patient is pale and weak and afflicted with ulcerative necrotic stomatitis and faucitis. The white cell count of blood is markedly increased, with large numbers of abnormal and immature red blood cells, and a decreased number of platelets present.

Treatment

1. **Chinese herbs** (tested formula)

   a. Concoction prepared from white blossom she-she ts'ao, 2-3 liang. One concoction/prescription is to be taken daily until the blood picture is normal again before taking the second prescription [given in (b)?]

   b. Concoction of

Tang-shen [Campanumaea sp.]	5 ch'ien
Pai-chiang ts'ao	5 ch'ien
Pai-shu	3 ch'ien

2. **Other treatment**

   a. **Supportive therapy**, in form of high-calorie diet, blood transfusions etc.

   b. **Prevention of infection** through selective use of penicillin.

This ailment must be treated by a combination Chinese and western medicine approach, an unending search for herbal remedies and continual evaluation of new experiences in treatment and control of the disease.

Chronic Leukemia

Of slower onset and longer duration (average 2-5 years), chronic leukemia presents a less acute set of symptoms. Early symptoms are generally facial pallor, generalized weakness, dizziness, fever, hidrosis, weight loss, epistaxis and bleeding at gum line and under the skin. Frequently, abdominal distension and pain and diarrhea are present. The sternum is subject to pressure pain. Hepatomegaly, splenomegaly and lymphadenopathy are also present.

Treatment

1. **General**. Suitable rest and nourishment.

2. Kuei-p'i wan (patent medicine) given when symptoms ease up, 3 ch'ien twice a day.

During an acute attack in chronic leukemia, the spleen will suddenly become enlarged, and there is hemorrhaging, high fever, and a marked increase of immature white cells in the peripheral blood and bone marrow. Treatment at this time should be like that for acute leukemia.

Endemic Goiter

Goiter is called "ta po-tzu ping" [big-neck disease] by the local populace. It is a compensating hyperthyroidism due to a lack of iodine in the
food. Generally, this condition is seen in plateau and upland regions as an
endemic occurrence, hence the term endemic goiter. In external appearance,
the neck, (Figure 6-6-5), as well as the thyroid glands on both sides of neck
are enlarged, the enlarged tissues soft to the touch. Upon further progression of the disease, some nodes of inequal size are felt over the thyroid
region. When this enlargement takes on critical proportions, respiratory difficulties will appear, as will a dry cough, hoarseness, and swallowing difficulties. These complications are generally related to respiration.

Prevention

1. In areas of higher incidence, provide children and pregnant women
with foods such as laminaria and seaweed that are rich in iodine content.

2. Use iodized salt. Preparation: To one kilogram of salt, add 1 gm
of potassium iodide or sodium iodide, and use for daily table salt, allowing
1.2 gm per person. Since iodine is highly volatile, pay attention to proper
storage.

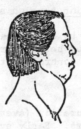

Figure 6-6-5 Endemic goiter

Treatment

1. New acupuncture therapy. Apply medium stimulation to needles inserted once a day in the "t'ien-tu," "a-chih-hsueh," and "ch'u-ch'ih" points.
To locate the "a-shih hsueh," lift up the enlarged thyroid mass and insert
the fine hao needle through the center, giving full attention to avoiding the
carotid artery below.

2. Chinese herbs

Treatment should open up the liver and relieve stagnation, and resolve the edema, using prescriptions such as the following:

a. Infusion of roots of huang tu, half a chin in 5 chin of white wine, steeping for 7 days. One small cup is to be taken each time, once in the morning and once in evening.

b. Concoction of

Ho-shou-wu	5 ch'ien - 1 liang
Algae	5 ch'ien - 1 liang

c. Concoction of

Algae	1 liang
Seaweed	1 liang
Laminaria	1 liang
Oyster	4 ch'ien
Cuttlefish bone	3 ch'ien
Hsiang-fu (sedgegrass)	3 ch'ien
Hsia-ku ts'ao	3 ch'ien

d. Concoction of

Hsia-ku ts'ao	4 ch'ien
Processed pan-hsia [Pinellia sp.]	3 ch'ien
Szechwan fritillaria	3 ch'ien
Oyster	1-2 liang
Seaweed	5 ch'ien
Laminaria	5 ch'ien

3. Western medicines

a. Potassium iodide 10-15 mg by mouth, once daily for 20 days (one course of treatment). Treat intermittently over a year's time. Note that iodine preparations should not be used over a long period of time as this may lead to hyperthyroidism.

b. Dessicated thyroid preparation, 60 mg 3 times a day given over a half-year period can cause the enlarged thyroid to dissipate. Best suited for pregnant women.

Beriberi

Beriberi is called "jan-chiao ping" [soft (weak) leg's disease] by the local populace. It is caused by a vitamin B_1 deficiency which results in a weakness in the lower extremities and difficulty of movement.

Symptoms seen in the early stage are poor appetite, indigestion, weight loss, insomnia, general weakness, muscular pains, and a weighted feeling in the legs. Among infants, the signs are regurgitation of milk, night fretfulness, weak efforts at nursing, weak crying, scanty urine etc. Clinically,

- 409 -

when accompanied by edema of lower foot, the condition is damp (shih) beriberi; without edema, the condition is dry (kan) beriberi. During the course of illness, when symptoms such as palpitation, dyspnea, nausea, and thirst appear, it it said that beriberi has involved the heart (chiao-ch'i ch'ung hsin).

Prevention

1. An improved diet for the patient or wet nurse, to include food stuffs high in vitamin B_1, such as unpolished rice, rice gruel, red beans, soybeans, peanuts, fresh vegetables etc. Do not eat highly polished white rice.

2. Active measures taken to prevent and treat other ailments, among which diarrhea is the most important. During course of illness, give patient a supplement of several vitamins.

Treatment

1. New acupuncture therapy. Apply medium stimulation to needles inserted once daily into the "tsu-san-li," "yang-ling ch'uan," and "chieh-hsi" points.

2. Chinese herbs

a. For damp beriberi, treatment should open up the "lo" passageways and promote moisture removal, with remedies such as the following:

(1) Concoction of

Betelnut	3 ch'ien
Dried orange peel	2 ch'ien
Papaya	4 ch'ien
Wu-chu-yu [Cornus officinalis]	1.5 ch'ien
Leaves of tzu-su	2 ch'ien
Chieh-keng	3 ch'ien
Fresh ginger	3 slices

(2) Concoction of

Tsang-shu [Atractylis ovata]	3 ch'ien
Huo-hsiang [Agastache sp]	1.5 ch'ien
Knots on fir branches	3

(3) Concoction of

Ch'ou-mu-tan [Clerodendron bungei] (roots)	1 liang
Tangerine leaves	2 liang
Knots of fir branches	8 liang

Use concoction for bathing affected areas.

b. For dry beriberi, treatment should neutralize the blood, clear
fever, and promote moisture removal, using prescription such
as the following concoction of

Crude ti-huang [Rehmannia sp.]	3 ch'ien
Tang-kuei	3 ch'ien
Pai shao [Palnia albiflora]	3 ch'ien
Ch'uan kung [Conioselinum unvittatum]	1.5 ch'ien
Niu-hsi	3 ch'ien
Mu-kua [papaya]	3 ch'ien
Huang-pai [Phellodendron sp.]	2 ch'ien
Chih-mu	2 ch'ien
Barley	4 ch'ien

3. Western medicines

a. Vitamin B_1, 5 - 10 mg each time, by mouth, 3 times a day.
For seriously ill patients, intramuscular injections may be
given.

b. Yeast tablets, 1-3 gm by mouth each time, 3 times a day.

Section 7   Surgical Conditions

Fractures

Damage to the continuity of bone, whether due to trauma or certain
diseases, is called a fracture.

Fractures usually affect surrounding tissue. Depending on whether
or not the fracture damages muscle sufficiently to cause a break in the skin,
fractures are further classified as open (compound) or closed (simple). Depending on the extent of the fracture, fractures are also classified as complete fractures,   complete fractures, and crushing fractures.

Clinical Manifestations

The local signs are swelling, bruises, pain or tenderness, and deformity.
Crepitus is also heard when the bone moves. Function is frequently partially
or completely lost. If there is vascular and nerve damage, hemorrhage and a
feeling of numbness will be noticed on distal side of fracture.

The most important systemic reaction may be shock, as the result of excruciating pain, excessive blood loss and serious organic damage. This reaction is most prone to appear in physically weak patients. For this reason, before local examination of patient, his overall condition must be checked first.

Treatment

Successful treatment calls for proper mastery of reduction technique, good fixation of fracture, and effective functional training [physical therapy].

1. Reduction

Proper reduction is the key to good union in a fracture. Generally, manual reduction involves four steps -- traction, separation, opposition and fixation -- maneuvered in sequence to correct early the angle, overlapping, rotation, and deformity caused by the fracture. Commonly used manipulation first calls for manual examination by touch and feel to determine the type of fracture and the amount of displacement in order to ascertain a reduction technique. Then traction is applied by a grasp of both ends of the fracture which separates the overlapping ends. While traction is thus applied, the distal end of fracture is rotated or extended as necessary to align the two sections on the same axis -- protruding bone sections pushed back and depressed sections elevated. In case of a double fracture, separate the fractured section using clamp manipulation. Generally, traction can be applied in direction in line with bone, the force increasing from light to heavy, until the fractured ends are separate from each other. After this, manipulate from a posterior to anterior direction or support fracture from inside to outside direction to align the distal section of bone with the proximal end. At the same time, correct any rotational abnormalities and restore fractured bone to its original position. Besides this, a massage-pinch technique can also be used to correct positioning of the displaced end, and massaging will soothe and open up the meridian passageways to allow good blood circulation and reduction of swelling.

2. Fixation

After a fracture has been reduced and it is given a local dressing, the part is placed on pressure padding and splinting and finally bandaged. This technique exerts a certain amount of pressure and maintains the correct positioning of part.

a. Splints. Depending on the nature and site of fracture, splints of different shapes, lengths, and thicknesses are used. Most commonly used are splints made of willow or fir, or even thick carboard, or bamboo strippings. Because of differences in fracture sites, local fixation, which is superior to joint fixation or digital (toe or finger) fixation, is used.

b. <u>Pressure padding</u>. Absorbent and soft "mao-pien" paper of definite shape and strength or soft cloth may be used for padding. Thickness size and shape of padding must be suited to the fractured extremity for fixation to be most effective.

c. <u>Bandaging</u>. Four double-layered cloth bandages of a fingers' width are needed. Tightness of the bandage should be just right. If too tight, the constriction may injure the fractured limb; if too loose, fixation is ineffective. After bandages have been tied, inspect part for good circulation, movement, and sensory feeling.

3. <u>Chinese herbs</u>

Treatment of fractures calls for a coordination of the local part to the whole, and of external treatment with internal treatment. Experience has shown that a reasonable use of drugs plays an important role in hastening the process of bone union.

a. Belt braided from the root bark of yuan-hua (Daphne sp.) and roots of wei-ling-hsien (<u>Clematis chinensis</u>) to be worn at all times, the longer the better. When injury is sustained, scrape/rub off 1 ch'ien of belt with white wine (or boy's urine), and take internally. This can alleviate the pain from external or internal injury and stimulate blood circulation to resolve bruises.

b. Concoction of

Ku-sui-pu   1 liang
Feng-wei ts'ao   1 liang

To be taken after reduction. Suitable for all kinds of fractures.

c. Extract obtained by grating equal parts of feng-ya-hsueh (roots), hsi-ts'ao (roots), and chu-sha-ken (<u>Ardisia crenata</u>) in wine, and used for external application over fracture. Or, a crab-shell extract (pulverized dried crab shells soaked in wine) is taken by mouth, one small cup 3 to 5 times daily, before meals.

Caution: Not for pregnant women.

d. Concoction of honeysuckle, acorns, and mugwort for bathing affected part. After reduction of fracture has been accomplished, the part may be given a compress prepared from a crushed mixture of violets, chi-hsueh ts'ao, plantago, verbena, brunella, shui su, p'u-pai chin, and fu-shui ts'ao.

- 413 -

If bark of fir is used for fixation [as splint?], drop a few drops of the above mixture into dressing, and change dressings weekly. This prescription is suited for open and closed fractures.

4. Functional training [physical therapy]

From a very early stage, reasonable and planned functional training must be carried out to realize the principle of "movement and inactivity co-ordination." Not only do functional training exercises stimulate local and general blood circulation, they are also beneficial to the union of fractures. The course of training follows a gradual pattern of little to big, light to heavy in the practice of handshakes, extension and flexion, internal rotation, standing, climbing, carrying light loads etc.

During the final stages of fracture mending, joint adhesions, muscular atrophy, swelling of extremities, and pain which are frequently noted may be treated with an intensified program of physical therapy coordinated with acupuncture, massage, and drug therapy using the following prescriptions:

a. Concoction of

Shen-ching ts'ao	3 ch'ien
T'ou-ku ts'ao	3 ch'ien
Liu-chi-nu	3 ch'ien
Mulberry sticks	3 ch'ien
Pine branches	3 ch'ien
Artemesia	3 ch'ien
Hu-chang	3 ch'ien

Use for bathing affected part. For internal consumption, add roots of wu-chia-p'i 1 liang, mix with half and half water and wine. Decoct.

b. Concoction prepared from 3 ch'ien each of tang-kuei, pai-shao, ch'uan-tuan, kou-chi, Szechuan conioselinum, mulberry sticks, and niu-hsi.

Besides these treatment approaches, analgesics, dolantin (demerol) or procaine could be used to relieve pain, depending on individual circumstances. In the following paragraphs, the treatment of several commonly seen fractures will be described.

Double Fracture of Forearm

In the forearm are the radius and ulna, and between them is an inter-osseous membrane. Double fracture involving both the radius and ulna are commonly seen in infants and young adults, the result of a direct blow or fall when hand hits ground with great impact. Most commonly seen are green-stick fractures, horizontal fractures, spiral fractures, or comminuted frac-tures.

Local examination frequently shows swelling, cyanosis, pain, tenderness, deformity, crepitus, pseudo-joint action, and loss of function in affected limb.

Treatment

1. For greenstick fracture only slight traction to correct deformity, and application of splint to fix the fracture are all that is necessary.

2. For a horizontal fracture or a spiral fracture with displacement, reduce fracture while using herbs prescribed above for alleviating pain. Have assistants first apply traction, then correct deformity according to direction of displacement. Manipulation is same as that for a single fracture. For more serious open fracture, consider consultation after carrying out proper first aid treatment.

3. Fixation. While traction is being applied, apply anti-swelling ointment, place semicircular bone-separating cellulose cotton padding between ulna and radius, and fix reduction with two fir splints or a fore-and-aft plaster-of-paris cast. Bandage and support arm in sling suspended from neck. Generally, the period of fixation lasts from 6 to 8 weeks. When patient goes to bed, elevate the affected limb. Also, pay attention to the color, warmth and feeling of the back of hand and fingers.

4. Chinese herb treatment. Consult information listed under "Frac-tures."

5. Functional training. For the first two weeks, concentrate on hand-shake exercises and extension-flexion activity of the wrist-joint. During the 3rd week, add internal rotation of shoulder, forward extension, and posterior extension movements. During the 4th week, the activity range is increased, including rotating activity of the forearm.

Distal Fracture of Radius

Fracture of the radius 2-3 cm for its distal end is commonly seen in the middle-aged and aged population. It is due mostly to a sudden fall in-curred by the victim forward or backward, when he tries to break it and hits the ground with the palm. Because various postures of the fall differ, so the type of fracture seen also varies. Among them, an over-extension fracture of the radius at its distal end is the most commonly seen (Figure 6-7-1).

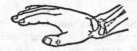

Figure 6-7-1. Displacement in distal fracture of the radius

The symptoms following injury usually are noted as local swelling and pain, tenderness, shifting of distal end of fracture backward and displacement of radius forming a fork-like deformity, accompanied by loss of wrist function.

Treatment

1. <u>Manual reduction</u>. The patient is usually placed in a sitting position. <u>Perform reduction</u> under anesthesia using traction to extend the limb, align the ends and correct with feel and touch. Finally, massage the fracture area to resolve bruises and relax muscles.

2. <u>Fixation by splinting</u>. While the patient's forearm is in traction apply a dressing, then place a cushion across the lateral and posterior aspects of the radius at its distal end, cover anterior aspect with a long piece of fir bark that extends from the palm up to lower wrist and support the posterior aspect with a short piece of fir bark to immobilize the wrist. Make sure splinting for the radius and ulna is narrower than ordinary. Complete fixation of the splint with bandaging. Keep splint on for about 4 weeks.

3. <u>Chinese herbs</u> (same as those listed in previous section)

4. <u>Functional training</u> (physical therapy). Same as that described in previous section.

Fracture of Femur

A break in that part of the thighbone between the acetabulum and the patella is called a fracture of the femur. It results mostly as the result of some forceful impact such as a blow or a collision, and is seen frequently in children under 10 years of age. Its next greatest incidence is among healthy young adults.

The fracture usually occurs at junction of lower third and mid-third of bone. Next would be somewhere on the upper or lower third of bone. Signs of fracture are local swelling, marked pain and tenderness, excruciating pain felt in fracture area when sole of foot or knee are tapped, a noticeable shortening of affected limb, external rotation and angular deformity, possibly crepitus and pseudo-joint movement of thigh, and shock in presence of severe pain.

Treatment

Deformed knitting of bone in cases of fracture of the femur occurs quite easily, leading to more serious complications. Therefore, it is important during the course of treatment, to prevent overlapping of fractured ends, angular union and rotational movement of these segments, "frozen" knee joint, etc.

1. Reduction

Fractures that were not displaced do not need any reduction and need only dressings and splint fixation. Cases with marked displacement should have reduction done under analgesia. The patient is usually lying down, and one assistant helps to stabilize the pelvis before various manipulation techniques, depending on the site of the frature, are used:

a. For fracture in upper third of thighbone, exert traction in a slightly external rotatory direction to correct the shortened deformity, with another assistant supporting the affected limb extended slightly outward. The physician feels and massages over the fracture site to correct the displacement.

b. For fracture in mid-third of thighbone. Because of tendency of part to form an external angular deformity, the physician uses the "top-shaving" technique to further correct the deformity, after traction has been applied to correct the "shortening."

c. For fracture in lower third of thighbone. After the assistant has bent the patient's knee and applied traction to the lower end of the femur, the physician uses the "end-holding" technique to correct depression in the distal segment of the fracture by aligning opposing ends of the fracture.

2. Fixation

Use four pieces of wood splint and 3-4 section of pressure cushioning. Concentrate on dressings of anti-inflammatory medications after reduction has been done. Placement of pressure cushioning and splints must be accurate.

3. Chinese herbs (Same as those described for previous sections).

4. Functional training. After the first week, institute extension and flexion exercises for the ankle and knee joints. After the third week, start on similar exercises to maintain agility of the hip joint, and encourage patient to walk with assistance of cane. After two months, the patient may try walking unaided.

Compression Fracture of Thoraco-lumbar Spine

Compression fracture of the thoraco-lumbar spine generally occurs on vertebral column between the 12th thoracic vertebra and the 1st lumbar vertebra. Causes of this type of fracture are numerous, e.g., the compression that occurs at juncture of the thoracic vertebrae with the lumbar vertebrae after the feet and pelvis both hit the ground after a high fall. The clinical manifestations are excruciating pain in back around lumbar region, restricted movement of spinal column, difficulty in assuming a standing or sitting position, and even difficulty in turning over. In serious cases, injury to the spinal nerve may result in paraplegia, incontinence of feces, retention of urine etc. Examination will reveal the following findings:

    a. Protruding abnormality in fracture site, accompanied by marked tenderness.

    b. Pain over injury when tapped; a throbbing ache felt in head.

    c. Neck-bending test, positive. Have patient lie in recumbent position and bend his neck forward (for chin to touch chest) and patient feels pain over the fracture site.

Treatment

Transporting a patient with a compression fracture of the thoraco-lumbar spine, all care must be taken to prevent antiflexion of the vertebrae to avoid aggravating the injury. For unstable fractures accompanied by dislocations or spinal cord damage, consider transfer. Stable fractures may be treated as follows:

    1. **Reduction**

        a. **Suspension reduction**. Before any reduction measure is taken, give Chinese herbs or dolantin to relieve pain. Then, have patient lie on bed in prone position and suspend his lower limbs with his trunk tilted slightly forward for about 15 minutes. This procedure utilizes the patient's own weight to exert traction on the compressed vertebrae, while the physician can check the affected area with his palm, (dusted with talc) massaging lightly to accomplish reduction.

        b. **Back-carry reduction method**. After an analgesic has been given the patient, the physician slowly maneuvers the patient on to his back, with the patient's fracture resting on his (the physician's) sacrum [in back-to-back positioning]. While an assistant pulls the patient's legs in a downward direction, the physician slowly bends over to make the patient overextend. After about 2-3 minutes, reduction is accomplished.

2. _Fixation_. After reduction has been completed, apply compress over injury, and immobilize patient in a special anterior and posterior movement-controlling cast or splint for 2-3 months.

3. _Chinese herbs_. Effective for internal consumption are certain herbs that open up the meridians and activate the lo passageways, and stimulate the circulation and resolve bruises, in concoctions such as the following:

a. Concoction of

Fu-shui ts'ao	2 ch'ien
Tao-tou he	2 ch'ien
Mu-tse ts'ao	2 ch'ien
Hung-hua [carthamus]	2 ch'ien
Tang-kuei ends	3 ch'ien
Nan wu-wei-tzu	3 ch'ien
Wu-chia-p'i	3 ch'ien
Tzu-wei	3 ch'ien
Niu-wei ts'ai	5 ch'ien

b. Concoction of

Ch'ih-shao	5 ch'ien
Tang-kuei	4 ch'ien
Hsu-tuan	4 ch'ien
Pu-ku-chih	4 ch'ien
Ku-sui-pu	4 ch'ien
Wu-ling-chih	3 ch'ien
T'u-p'i [tortoise]	3 ch'ien
Ti-lung	3 ch'ien

One prescription/dose to be taken daily.

4. _Functional training_. Beginning the day after fracture has been reduced, encourage patient to practice hyper-extension of back exercises in bed. He can wear cast and try some light exercises out of bed. However, patient must not engage in any anteflexion movement for 2-3 weeks.

Dislocations

If the articular surface of a joint becomes dislocated from its normal position, the condition is called a dislocation. It is frequently caused by trauma sustained in a fall. Its symptoms are manifested chiefly as joint swelling, pain, disturbance in joint function, deformity and elastic fixation (where muscles and tendons around the joint cause the dislocated part to assume a special elastic and fixed position). The most common types of dislocations will be described in sections that follow.

A. Dislocated Mandible

Mandibular dislocations are seen mostly in the aged or persons of weak constitution. The dislocation frequently results when the mouth is open and the jaw sustains a blow, or when it is stretched in a yawn, or when the mouth is opened wide in a burst of laughter. Such dislocations could become habitual. After the jaw becomes dislocated, the mouth cannot close properly, saliva drools from the corners of the mouth, chewing food is difficult, speech becomes unclear, and a depression may be felt on side of head just anterior to the ear.

Manual reduction. Generally no anesthesia is needed. Sit patient so his head and back are lined close up to the wall. The manipulator covers both thumbs with gauze or clean rag, and inserts them into the patient's mouth, resting over molars in lower jaw. The other fingers hold onto the jaw externally at the left and right mandibular angles. Then the two thumbs slowly exert pressure on jaw downward, then push gently backward for jaw to snap back into place. (Figure 6-7-2). At this time, quickly slide the two thumbs out

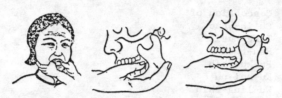

Figure 6-7-2. Dislocation of mandible.

of oral cavity. After reduction has been accomplished, use a broad bandage to support the jaw for a day or two. Make sure that patient refrains from opening mouth too wide or eating hard foods or snacks for at least 3 weeks.

B. Dislocated Elbow

When the body falls backward with the elbow in a slightly bent position, it is very easy for the elbow to become dislocated when the palm hits the floor first in the fall. After the dislocation has occurred, the affected elbow becomes swollen and painful, held in a semiflexed position. The arm cannot straighten out, a depression is seen in front of the elbow, and a protruding backward deformity caused by the ulnar notch is seen in back of the elbow. (Figure 6-7-3).

Treatment

1. Reduction technique. Before starting on the manipulation, inject 10-15 ml of procaine into the affected joint cavity, then manipulate dislocation. Have patient in sitting position. The manipulator grasps the patient's wrist and supports the elbow space with his knee. Then, while traction is applied, the forearm is bent gradually to snap joint back into place (Figure 6-7-4).

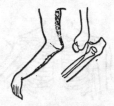

Figure 6-7-3. External appearance of dislocated elbow.

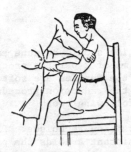

Figure 6-7-4. Reduction of dislocated elbow.

2. <u>Fixation of joint at 90°</u> after successful reduction. Support limb with triangular bandage for two weeks.

3. <u>Chinese herbs</u>. Crush and use as poultice for application over affected joint the following:

> Tangerine leaves
> Loquat leaves
> Plum leaves
> Leaves and pollen of hibiscus

C. Dislocated Shoulder

The range of joint movement of the shoulder is extensive, though un-stable. It is a joint that frequently becomes dislocated. The cause is mostly a fall during which the forearm extension and uplift allows the palms to hit the ground first. After the joint is dislocated, the affected shoulder loses its normal shape and becomes a square shoulder (Figure 6-7-5), local pain is present, and the joint is not mobile. When the elbow of the affected limb is placed against the chest wall, the hand cannot touch the shoulder on the opposite side.

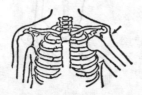

Figure 6-7-5.   Dislocated shoulder joint

Treatment

1. <u>Reduction</u>. Reduction should be done early. Before the procedure is carried out, inject 15-20 ml of 2 percent procaine into the joint cavity to anesthetize the part. If the muscles are soft, inject 0.005-0.01 gm morphine subcutaneously to facilitate the reduction procedures. Commonly used manipulation techniques include the following two:

   a. The <u>sitting-position technique</u>. Place the patient in a sitting position. Assistant A holds the patient firmly around his chest. Assistant B grasps the wrist and elbow of arm on the injured side and exerts traction downward and laterally. The manipulator places both hands under the axilla to support and push the humerus superiorly and laterally to accomplish reduction.

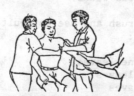

Figure 6-7-6.   Reduction of dislocated shoulder joint
          by the sitting-position technique.

   b. The <u>lying-down technique</u>. With the patient lying down, the manipulator grasps the wrist of the affected arm with both hands and places one foot up against the patient's axilla (for a dislocated right shoulder joint, use the right foot, and a left foot for a left joint). Exert traction slowly by pulling the arm and use foot to push the humerus in an outward direction. When a sound like the head of humerus snapping back in joint socket is heard, reduction is accomplished. (Figure 6-7-7).

- 422 -

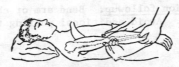

Figure 6-7-7. Reduction of dislocated shoulder joint in
the lying-down position.

2. Post-reduction followup. Immediately after the dislocation is corrected, turn the forearm inward toward the body, the elbow angled against the
chest. Bandage and support in triangular arm sling. Immobilize for 2-3 weeks,
(Figure 6-7-8). Spontaneous and natural movement of the affected limb should
be started slowly after 6 weeks.

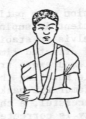

Figure 6-7-8. Immobilization of dislocated shoulder joint
after reduction.

3. Chinese herbs. Herbs used are the same as those recommended for
treating a dislocated elbow.

Note: Semi-dislocation of Head of Radius
in Small Children

This dislocation is seen usually in children between the ages of two
and six years. It usually results from a pull on the forearm by a parent when
the child is being dressed or when he is falling. When seen, elbow movement
is restricted or weak, the arm cannot be raised, and there is pain though swelling and deformity are lacking.

Treatment

1. Reduction technique. Sit child on lap of adult, with manipulator
facing the youngster. With one hand grasping the child's wrist, the other hand
grasping the humerus at head, the manipulator extends the child's forearm and
exerts some slight force to overextend and rotate limb anteriorly and posteriorly
to correct dislocation. Following this, the pain immediately dissipates, and
shoulder activity becomes spontaneous.

2. <u>Post-reduction followup</u>. Bend arm of child 90° and support arm in sling for several days. Avoid additional pulling to avoid habitual semidislocation.

Dislocated Hip Joint

A dislocated hip is usually caused by a blow on knee causing it to deflect posteriorly when the hip joint is flexed and adducted. After the dislocation has occurred, great pain is felt locally, the joint cannot move, the lower extremity is shortened and assumes a position of adduction and inversion. The buttocks on the affected side also exhibits a protrusion.

Reduction technique

a. Perform reduction with patient under spinal or general anesthesia. Then place patient in supine position. Have assistant hold and support the pelvis to stabilize it. Then the manipulator slowly flexes knee of affected limb, bending it to form 90° angle with the hip joint, and exert traction on the femur in a longitudinal direction while rotating the femur internally and externally to help head of femur fit back into the acetabulum. When the reduction is successful, a characteristic snap is heard and the joint deformity is corrected. (Figure 6-7-9)

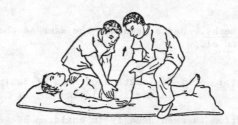

Figure 6-7-9. Reduction of dislocated hip joint.

b. Order post-reduction bed rest for at least 3 weeks, during which time the patient cannot get out of bed to carry anything heavy.

Sprains

When joint movement exceeds normal limits the damage inflicted on muscle, tendon, ligaments and joint capsules by heavy blows, twists or pulls is generally called a sprain or soft tissue damage. Colloquially, it is called "shang-chin" [meaning sinew injury]. Commonly seen sprains are described below in brief.

1. Wry Neck

Wry neck is also called "lo-chen" [meaning dropped occiput]. It is due mostly to an improper position assumed by neck in sleep, or to exposure to wind and cold, or to a slight degree of sprain. Following injury, the head is deflected to one side, the neck is painful, uncomfortable, and all spontaneous movement of the neck is gone.

Prevention and Treatment

1. Sleep with flat pillow, not letting it be too high or too low, to avoid the neck catching cold.

2. Slap-hit technique: Have patient sit down facing the operator. The operator uses the side of his right palm to slap the "chien-ching" point on the patient's affected side 20 to 30 times. The sprain will usually ease up after this treatment.

3. New acupuncture therapy. Needle the "chieh-hsi" point first, using strong stimulation. Then needle the "t'ien-ch'u," using medium stimulation. If the patient does not recover completely, repeat needling technique the following day.

Crushing Knee Injury

The kneejoint is the largest joint in the human body, and damage is easily incurred after the knee has sustained crushing injury. Its clinical manifestations frequently are tears of the lateral collateral ligament, rupture of the meniscus, hematoma of the patellor bursa etc. Following injury, local pain is severe, movement is restricted, and redness and swelling are frequently noted.

Treatment

1. New acupuncture therapy. Medium stimulation is applied to needles inserted into "tou-pi," "yang-ling-ch'uan," "a-shih," points, once daily. This can also be coordinated with hot compress applications.

2. Chinese herbs. Treatment should stimulate blood circulation and resolve bruises, reduce swelling and alleviate pain, using

    a. Compresses of
       (1) Equal amounts of fresh sprouts of chiu-ts'ai and gardenia, crushed and mixed with a little flour and wine.

       (2) One liang of tsa-chiang-ts'ao [sorrel], crushed for poultice.

       (3) O-pu-shih ts'ao, crushed and mixed with wine.

       (4) Fresh pan-hsia [Pinella sp.], pulverized and mixed with white wine, for poultice use.

b. Medications taken by mouth
(1) Concoction of t'ieh-ma-pien, 1 liang, mixed with a little white wine.

(2) Concoction of

Roots of wan-nien-ch'ing	5 fen
Roots of date palm	2 ch'ien

Taken with a little rock sugar and rice wine.

(3) Concoction of

Kuei-wei	4 ch'ien
Ch'ih-shao	4 ch'ien
Su-mu	4 ch'ien
Leaves of tse-lan	3 ch'ien
Peach kernel	3 ch'ien
Mulberry sticks	3 ch'ien

(4) T'ieh-ta wan (patent medicine), 1 tablet to be taken each time, twice a day.

Sprained Ankle

Excessive rotation of the ankle medially or laterally during work or exercise may cause a sprain in the ankle. Following the sprain, the ankle is swollen and painful, and walking is difficult.

Treatment

1. <u>New acupuncture therapy</u>. Apply medium stimulation to needles inserted in the "k'un-lun," "chueh-ku," "ch'iu-hsu," points once daily. Use cupping technique after needles have been withdrawn. If local swelling and redness are severe, point-puncture (enough to cause a little bleeding) first, then apply cupping technique or apply hot compress.

2. <u>Chinese herbs</u>. Same as those used for crushing knee injury.

Acute Back Strain

Acute back-strain is called "hsien-yao" by the local populace. It is usually the result of stress under a heavy load on the shoulder or forceful exertion in extending the lower extremity or in bending over. Following injury, movement of the lumbar spine is restricted, and motions such as bending over, leaning backward, turning sideways, walking etc. are impossible. Furthermore, the injured area shows marked tenderness. If this condition is not treated in time and allowed to become chronic, the backache will remain -- sometimes severe and sometimes slight. The amount of pain will be related to the weather quite often, becoming more severe in rainy and cold weather.

Prevention

Back-strain frequently results from a careless distribution of force while working. For example, keeping the legs straight and bending over to pick up a load can easily cause the condition. To avoid damage, bending the knees while keeping the back straight is the posture to assume. Pay attention to working-mode postures.

Treatment

1. _Acupuncture therapy_. Use strong stimulation on needles inserted to "chih-shih," "o-shih," and "wei-chung" points, once daily. Use cupping technique after needle treatment.

2. _Chinese herbs_.

    a. _Compresses_ [poultices]

        (1) Dry and pulverize whole plants of mao-kao ts'ai [Drosera sp.] and mix desired amount with cold boiled water to form a soybean-size pill. Place over the "chih-shih" point and keep in place with adhesive tape. Remove after 24 hours.

        (2) Wan-ying kao, kou-p'i kao (both patent medicines) applied over affected area.

    b. _Medications to be taken internally_.

        (1) Concoction of hsu chang-hsing, 3-5 ch'ien, mixed with little white wine.

        (2) Scrapings from "golden belt," 5 fen to 1 ch'ien, taken with white wine (golden belt made from a braiding of yuan-hua [daphne] roots and wei-ling-hsien [clematis] roots that is worn on human body -- the longer worn and the more perspiration soaked, the better.)

        (3) Concoction of

Tang-kuei	4 ch'ien
Ch'ih-shao	2 ch'ien
Tse-lan	2 ch'ien
Szechwan melia	2 ch'ien
Yen-hu-so	2 ch'ien
Kou-chih	4 ch'ien
Processed Szechwan aconite	1.5 ch'ien

3. _Western medicines_

    a. Yu-san-t'ung [patent medicine?], 1-2 tables, twice daily.

    b. Local procaine (1 percent) block.

Boil

A boil is an acute purulent inflammation of a hair follicle or a sebaceous gland, caused by bacterial infection. Occurring mostly in the summer, boils are generally located on sites such as the face, back of neck, groin, axilla, etc., where the hair follicles are more numerous. A boil first appears as a soybean size bump, erythematous and painful, shallow-based, and topped by a small yellowish white pustule. Once the pus comes to a head and the pustule erupts, the pus is allowed to drain out and recovery is on the way. Generally, large boils or furuncles may be accompanied by some slight constitutional symptoms, such as a low-grade fever, headache, general malaise, poor appetite etc. If squeezed or injured otherwise by trauma, boils pose some danger, particularly those around the nose and mouth. These boils should not be squeezed.

Prevention

Attention to personal hygiene and skin cleanliness. Do not squeeze boils or injure in any other manner, in case the infection spreads.

Treatment

1. Chinese herbs, used to clear fever and detoxify.

   a. Concoction of
Honeysuckle	5 ch'ien
Wild asters	5 ch'ien
Forsythia [blossoms]	3 ch'ien

   b. Concoction prepared from 4 liang of fresh portulaca, thoroughly washed, for taking by mouth. At the same time, also crush a suitable amount of portulaca with a small amount of salt. Use as dressing over boils. Change daily.

   c. Concoction prepared from 4 liang of fresh dandelions thoroughly cleaned. Also crush a suitable amount of fresh dandelions, and use for dressing over boils. Change daily.

   d. Leaves of hibiscus, dried and pulverized. To be taken with cool boiled water.

2. Western medicine

   Large amounts of antibiotics or sulfathiazole etc., given when the boils and furuncles become serious threats and liable to cause a generalized infection.

Felon

A felon is a purulent inflammation that can occur anywhere on the body, though the more common sites are the head and face, fingers, toes, etc. If results from bacterial invasion through an open wound (puncture wound, abrasion, scratch, bruise, insect bite etc.)

At onset, its size is about that of a kernel of corn (usually located on head and face), or eyes of the snake (usually on finger tips or distal part of toes), firmly rooted, numb yet itchy. Very quickly, erythema edema, pus formation and sloughing take place. Very painful, such felons or whitlows may be classified as mild cases or severe cases.

Mild felon is characterized by a hard red local swelling that is hot to the touch. It is first numb then painful. Accompanying symptoms are chills, fever, parchness, a dry hard stool, a dark concentrated urine, etc. If the core (root) of the felon is eliminated with the pus, the swelling and pain ease up immediately.

A severe felon is characterized by "brown spread of felon toxin." The crown of the felon becomes black and depressed suddenly without any pus present, the surrounding skin area turns purple, and the patient's temperature shoots up, accompanied by retching, restlessness, parchness, great thirst, constipation or diarrhea, delirium and respiratory difficulty. The pulse is generally solid, tongue dry, fur yellow or black. These signs all indicate the critical nature of the felon involvement, and emergency measures combining traditional Chinese and western medicine must be taken.

Prevention

1. Attention to personal hygiene and skin cleanliness. When the skin suffers any injury, treat it in time.

2. No pressing or squeezing of felons with fingers. Avoid such handling to prevent dangerous spread of toxins.

Treatment

1. New acupuncture therapy. Use triple-edged needle to prick-puncture the "ling-t'ai" and "wei-chung" points until they begin to bleed.

2. Chinese herbs

   a. For mild cases treatment should clear fever and detoxify, using remedies such as the following:

      (1) Concoction of
Honeysuckle	1 liang
Wild aster	1 liang
Dandelion	1 liang
Violet	1 liang
Tzu-pei t'ien-kuei	1 liang

(2) Concoction of

Violet	1 liang
Honeysuckle	1 liang
Ginkgo nuts [fruit]	10
Chieh-keng	3 ch'ien
Chih-mu	1 ch'ien

(3) Burweed bug (taken from stem of burweed <u>Xanthium</u>
    strumarium before season of the white dew [first part of
    September] soaked in sesame oil. Place bug over crown of
    ulcer and fix with a black plaster patch.

(4) She-mei, a suitable amount crushed, for use as poultice.

(5) Flowers and tender leaves of the hibiscus, 4 liang, crushed,
    for use as poultice. (This prescription is suitable for
    use in the early stage of felon development or in the
    later purulent stage. Before [felon] ripening, it can
    resolve the inflammation. After the felon has ripened
    and started draining, it is astringent.)

(6) Pulverized mixture of the following:

Cantharis	7
(Roasted to glutinous rice, rice removed)	
Scorpions	3
(blanched and dry-roasted in soil)	
Hsuan-shen (roasted)	3 ch'ien
Hsueh-chieh	3 ch'ien
Pistachio	1 ch'ien
Myrrh	1 ch'ien
Rock sugar	6 fen

Place in jar and seal. Break felon with a sterile needle
and apply an amount of this medicated mixture about the
size of a mung bean. Cover with gauze. Change in a day.
This medicated powder can alleviate swelling, promote pus
drainage, and extract the purulent core and all.

b. For severe felon. Treatment should cool the blood, clear fever
    and detoxify, using remedies such as the following:

(1) Concoction of

Rhinoceros horn	1 ch'ien
(buffalo horn 1.5 ch'ien may be used as substitute)	
Crude ti-huang	6 ch'ien
Tan-p'i	3 ch'ien
Ch'ih shao	3 ch'ien
Honeysuckle	1 liang
Dandelion	1 liang
Wild chrysanthemum	1 liang

Violet	5 ch'ien
Tzu-pei t'ien-kuei [buttercup]	5 ch'ien
Pan-chih-lien	5 ch'ien
Ch'i-hsieh I-chih-hua	3 ch'ien

For excessive thirst, add bamboo leaves and gypsum. For constipation, add ta-huang [rhubarb], hsuan-ming-fen. For delirium, add "An-kung niu-huang wan" or "tzu-hsueh tan" 1 tablet [both patent medicines].

(2) Pill to purge felon toxin, consisting of pulverized

[separately] Realgar	5 ch'ien
Fresh ta-huang [rhubarb]	1 liang
Pa-tou shuang [essence of croton?]	2 ch'ien

Add 3 ch'ien flour and mix; add vinegar to moisten and form pills the size of radish seeds. For each dose, give 5-9 pills (not to exceed 9 pills) with some warm boiled water. After one or two bowel movements, give patient 1 bowl of cold mung bean juice to stop loose stools. (This prescription is suited for those with infected felons on face and who are constipated. DO NOT GIVE TO PREGNANT WOMEN AND THOSE IN POOR HEALTH.

3. Western medicines

Penicillin 200,000 units, four times a day by intramuscular injection.

Tetracyclene 250 mgm by mouth each time, 4 times a day.

If necessary, administer parenteral fluids.

Carbuncle

A carbuncle is an acute purulent infection caused by bacterial (such as the Staphylococcus aurens) invasion of several hair follicles or sebaceous glands. Occurring anywhere on the body, it is characterized by local swelling, fever, excruciating pain, pus formation, and sloughing. Its involvement is more extensive. The lesion presents a diameter between 2 and 3 inches across, and contains several pustulas, resembling a beehive. The extent of carbuncle development may be considered in the early stage, suppuration stage, and the sloughing-off stage.

The early stage of carbuncle development presents a local swelling between skin and muscle tissue -- shiny, smooth, hot, red and painful accompanied by chills, fever, headache and other systemic symptoms. Fur on tongue is a little yellow, and the pulse is rapid.

The <u>suppuration stage</u> shows an elevation of local swelling topped by a yellow peak, and the pain is even more severe. If pressed, the swelling shows a marked induration that bounces back upon release of pressure -- a sign that suppuration has already taken place. Accompanying symptoms may be high fever, thirst, constipation etc. The fur on tongue is dry and yellow, and the pulse is tight and rapid.

In the <u>sloughing-off stage</u>, pus drainage follows a break, sometimes accompanied by purplish-black clots. If drainage is good, swelling and pain will both subside, and healing takes place gradually. However, if drainage is poor, and the exudate is clear and thin, then necrotic tissue is not being removed properly for granulation to occur. Healing occurs more slowly then. The tongue is red and shows no fur, and the pulse is deficient and weak.

Prevention

Attention to personal hygiene. Maintain cleanliness of the skin, and treat all boils in time.

Treatment

1. Chinese herbs

a. During early stage, treatment should clear fever, detoxify, and reduce swelling, using remedies such as the following:

(1) Concoction of

Tang-kuei bits and pieces	3 ch'ien
Ch'ih-shao	3 ch'ien
Wild chrysanthemum	5 ch'ien
Dandelion	1 liang
Honeysuckle	1 liang
Pistachio	3 ch'ien
Myrrh	3 ch'ien
Fang-feng	2 ch'ien
Chekiang fritillaria	3 ch'ien
Pai-chi	3 ch'ien
Dried orange peel	1.5 ch'ien
Licorice	1.5 ch'ien

(2) Grated ch'i-hsieh I-chi-hua [<u>Paris polyphylla</u>] mixed with water as concentrate, for frequent local application.

(3) Blossoms and leaves of fresh hibiscus, 4 liang, crushed for poultice application.

b. During suppuration stage, treatment should clear fever, detoxify, and promote thorough suppuration, using remedies such as the following:

    (1)   Concoction of

Tang-kuei bits and pieces	3 ch'ien
Tsao tz'u [locust thorns?]	2 ch'ien
Honeysuckle	8 ch'ien
Dandelion	8 ch'ien
Forsythia	5 ch'ien
Crocodile (roasted)	3 ch'ien
Pai-chi	3 ch'ien
Licorice	1.5 ch'ien

    (2)   T'ien-hsien-tzu [Scopolia japonica], 1 liang, mixed with
        water, for dressing.

    (3)   Leaves and flowers of hibiscus, 4 liang, crushed, for
        dressing.

  c. During sloughing-off stage, treatment should detoxify, support
      tissues, and promote drainage, using remedies such as the
      following:

    (1)   Concoction of

Fresh huang-ch'i [Astragalus sp.]	5 ch'ien
Honeysuckle	5 ch'ien
Tang-shen [Campanamueae sp.]	3 ch'ien
Pai-shu	3 ch'ien
Pai-chi	3 ch'ien
Fu-ling	3 ch'ien
Licorice	1.5 ch'ien

    (2)   Crushed mixture of following for dressing:

Leaves and flowers of hibiscus	4 liang
Castor beans	3 ch'ien

        (This medication is suitable for already erupted carbuncles
        still containing pus)

    (3)   Granulation powder prepared as follows:

Lu-kan-shih [zinc]	5 ch'ien
Ti-ju shih	3 ch'ien
Talc	1 liang
Hsueh-chieh [Calamus sp.]	3 ch'ien
Cinnabar	1 ch'ien

        Pulverize. Sprinkle with water. Dry, then add camphor
        5 fen (pulverized). Apply over wound and cover with
        gauze.

2. **Western medicine**

    Sulfonamides and antibiotics, used selectively.

Cellulitis

Cellulitis is a necrotic infection of the subcutaneous tissues, as the result of bacterial invasion. It usually occurs along the four extremities and/or the neck. It may be caused by trauma to the skin, or by diffusion of a local focus of infection. The local part is red, edematous, and painful, with no delineation of infection boundaries. The edema is worse than that seen in erysipelas (Table 6-7-1).

When the cellulitis is severe, systemic symptoms such as chills, fever, headache, poor appetite, thirst, and constipation are present. Frequently, lymphadenopathy accompanies the condition. Fur on tongue is thin and yellow. Pulse is rapid.

Prevention

Attention to cleanliness of the skin. Treat various wound infections in time. Increase general resistance to disease and infection.

Treatment

1. _Chinese herbs_. Treatment should be directed toward clearing fever and purifying body of toxins.

    a. External [local] treatment

        (1) Wild chrysanthemums in suitable amount, crushed and used for poultice and dressing.

        (2) Hibiscus flowers and leaves in suitable amounts, crushed and used for dressing.

        (3) Ch'i-hsieh I-chih-hua [Paris polyphylla], grated, steeped in wine, and used for local application.

    b. Internal treatment, by medications [taken by mouth] such as the following concoction of

Honeysuckle	5 ch'ien
Wild chrysanthemum	5 ch'ien
Violet	5 ch'ien
Tzu-pei t'ien-kuei [buttercup]	5 ch'ien
Dandelion	5 ch'ien

Prescription modifications

        (1) For yet to "ripen" suppuration, add tsao-tz'u [locust thorns), 2 ch'ien,

        (2) For constipation, add fresh rhubarb 3 ch'ien; hsuan-ming-fen 1.5 ch'ien [in a separate package to be taken with boiled water].

(3) For yellowish-red urine, add che-ch'ien ts'ao [plantago].

(4) For conditions where focus of infection is on head and face, add huang-ch'ing [Scutellaria baicalensis] 3 ch'ien.

(5) For conditions where focus of infection is along lower extremities, add huang-pai [phellodendron] 3 ch'ien.

(6) For sloughing-out, add huang-ch'i [Astragalus sp.] pai-ch'i 3 ch'ien each.

2. Western medicines

a. Sulfathiazole 1 gm four times daily. Double the initial dose and add an equal amount of soda bicarbonate to be taken at the same time. Stay on medication for the usual time of 3-4 days.

b. Terramycin or tetracyline 400,000 units given by intramuscular injection, once or twice daily (Be sure to conduct a skin test beforehand, to rule out any allergies.)

Table 6-7-1. Differentiation of Cellulitis from Erysipulas

Item Disease	Cellulitis	Erysipelas
Invaded tissue	Subcutaneous tissue	Reticular lymphatic vessels within the mucous membrane and/or under the skin.
Predisposed sites	Four extremities, neck	Legs, face
Redness	Dull red, central area marked, peripheral areas lighter	Bright red, lighter at center -- a brownish yellow -- bright red at edges
Swelling	Severe, marked at center, less severe around edges	Slight, edges raised slightly
Boundaries	Unclear	Clear
Pain	Continuous, accompanied sometimes by a pecking sound	Pain in lower extremities not great; more severe in head and face
Suppuration	Frequent	Rare
History of recurrence	None	Frequent
Complications	None	Repeated attacks affecting the lower extremities may lead to hypertrophy and thickening of skin

- 435 -

Erysipelas

Erysipelas is an acute pyoderma caused by streptococcal infection of the skin or the reticular lymphatics of the mucous membrane. Disease onset is sudden, and accompanied by chills, fever, local erythema, and a burning sensation over the slightly elevated lesion noted by its well-delineated boundaries. The lesion progresses rapidly, the redness frequently developing into a yellow vesicle. The ailment is often accompanied by nausea, vomiting and stupor, and delirium in serious cases. Fur on tongue is thin and yellow, and pulse is generally slippery and rapid. Erysipelas occurring on the head is called "p'ao-t'ou huo-tan" [head-embracing fiery erisipelas]; that below the waist is referred to by the local population as "nei-fa tan-tu" [internally-caused erysipelas poisoning]; that along the legs is called [liu-huo" [running fire]; and that idsseminated over the whole body is called "ch'ih yu-tan" [wandering red erysipelas].

Prevention

Timely treatment of breaks in the skin and dermaphytosis.

Treatment

Using Chinese herbs, treatment should clear fever, detoxify, cool the blood and resolve bruises, with remedies such as the following:

(1)   Concoction of
      Pan-lan-ken   1 liang
      Wild chrysanthemum   5 ch'ien
      Huang-pai [phellodendrom]   4 ch'ien
      Ts'ang-shu   3 ch'ien
      Niu-hsi   3 ch'ien

(2)   Crushed mixture, 3-5 ch'ien each, of she-mei [Indian strawberry], pan-chih-lien, and kuo-lu-huang. To be taken with rice water in equal amounts.

(3)   Juice of crushed she-mei, for external application and dressing.

(4)   Crushed mixture of
      Rape seed   5 ch'ien
      She-han   5 ch'ien
      T'ieh-ma-pien   5 ch'ien
      She-mei   5 ch'ien
      Kao-ts'ai   1 liang

      Mix with half bowl of rice rinse water. First take 1 c [by mouth]. Then mix remaining brew with half-cup rapeseed oil for application on affected parts, about 10 times daily.

Tuberculosis of the Cervical Nodes

Tuberculous nodes of the neck is also called "li-tzu" [scrofula]. It is caused by tuberculosis bacilli infection via the oral cavity, dental caries, nose and throat. It is seen mostly in young adults. In the early stage, general discomfort is lacking, and the node about the size of a bean is only hard, though movable. Skin color does not change and no pain is felt. In the intermediate stage, the lymphatic nodes become more enlarged, chronic inflammation and adhesions are noted, and the chain of nodes formed becomes immovable. In the final stage, the swelling softens, the local skin coloring turns into a dull red, and a white puslike fluid is discharged. Frequently, when one node heals, another breaks, to result in a chronic tuberculous ulcer. Serious cases may be accompanied by recurring afternoon fever, coughing, hidrosis, facial pallor, dizziness, mental exhaustion, poor appetite etc.

Prevention

Attention to oral hygiene, and early treatment of dental caries, to prevent invasion by the tuberculosis bacilli.

Treatment

1. New acupuncture therapy. Apply medium stimulation to needles inserted in the "a-shih" (direct puncture into the enlarged lymph node), "kan-yu," "t'ai-ch'ung" points, once every day. However, do not puncture the "a-shih" point if suppuration has set in in the node.

2. Chinese herbs

   a. During the early stage, treatment should "loosen" the liver and restore the blood, relieve congestion and resolve sputum, using remedies such as the following:

      (1) Concoction of
          P'ao-shih-lien   1 liang
          Hsia-ku ts'ao   8 ch'ien

      (2) Special pill compounded from
          Hsuan-shen   }   8 liang
          Tu-li (oyster)   } pulverized   8 liang
          Szechwan fritillaria }   8 liang
               to which is added
          Hsia-ku ts'ao   2 chin
          Concoct into cream, then add honey to form pills the
          size of sterculia nut. For each dose, give 3 ch'ien,
          twice daily.

b. During the intermediate stage, treatment should "consolidate" the toxin and help suppuration "ripen," with remedy such as the following:

Tsao-tzu [locust thorns]	4 liang
K'un-pu [laminaria]	4 liang
Seaweed	4 liang
Hsia-ku ch'iu	4 liang

Add 5 chin of water, and concoct so that concentration measures only 2.5 chin after cooking. Strain and add 2 chin of hung ts'ao [red dates]. After concentrate is dried, the red dates may be eaten, once in the morning, and once in the evening, 10 dates each time.

c. During the final phase, treatment should restore the kidneys and lungs, with remedies such as the following:

(1) "Hsiao chin-tan" (patent medicine), one tablet each time, twice daily (may be taken during the early and post-sloughing phases. If deficiency symptoms appear, add the following concoction.

Tang-shen	3 ch'ien
Huang-ch'i (Astragalus sp.)	3 ch'ien
Tang-kuei	3 ch'ien
Hsuan-shen	3 ch'ien
Crude ti-huang	5 ch'ien
Ti-ku p'i	5 ch'ien
Red dates	10 ch'ien

(2) "Ch'ung-ho kao" (patented ointment) for local application. After all pus has drained from the lesion, "sheng-chi san" (patent medicine) may be sprinkled over surface of scrofula.

3. Western medicines

a. Streptomycin 0.5 gm given by intramuscular injection, twice in one day. Depending on the patient's condition, injections may be given daily or twice a week.

b. Isoniazid 0.1 gm, three times daily.

c. PAS (p-amino salicylate) 2 gm, four times daily, by mouth. Both drugs could be used while disease is progressing. Once absorption has been stabilized, continue with either isoniazid or PAS. However, remember that prolonged drug use can bring on drug tolerance or drug resistance.

- 438 -

Acute Appendicitis

Acute appendicitis is also called "ch'ang-yung" [abscessed intestine] or cecitis. Its causative factors may be 1) obstruction of the cecal cavity due to stool impaction, twisting of the cecum, parasites etc.; and 2) bacterial infection, the chief culprits being the B. coli and streptococci.

Abdominal pain felt at onset usually begins in the upper middle abdomen around the navel. After several hours, it shifts to the lower right abdomen as a continuous pain accentuated by periods of greater severity.

The cecal point [McBurney's point] in the right lower abdomen (located on laterial 1/3 of imaginary line joining the iliac spine of hipbone and the navel) exhibits tenderness, rebound tenderness, and muscular tension.

This ailment is due mostly to congestion of energy and blood in the internal organs which becomes heated, and becomes abscessed after a long period of time. It is generally accompanied by symptoms such as chills, fever, nausea, vomiting, no appetite, yellow stools etc. Fur on tongue is usually thin and oily, or slightly yellow. The pulse is generally solid and rapid.

Treatment

1. <u>New acupuncture therapy</u>. Puncture the "tsu-san-li" and "lan-wei" points, 2-4 times daily, retaining needles for 30 minutes to 2 hours each time. If high fever is present, include the "ch'u-ch'ih" and "ho-ku" points; if vomiting is present, include the "nei-kuan" point.

2. <u>Chinese herbs</u>

    a. Concoction of

Hung-t'eng	1 liang
Violets	1 liang

    b. Concoction of

Ta-huang [rhubarb]	1.5 ch'ien
Mu-tan p'i [bark of peony root]	3 ch'ien
Seeds of tung-kua [chinese wax gourd]	5 ch'ien
Peach kernel	3 ch'ien
Glauber's salt	1.5 ch'ien
Pai-chiang ts'ao	1 liang
Ya-tsao [teeth grindings?]	2 ch'ien

(This prescription is suitable for use in early stage of illness when constipation is present.)

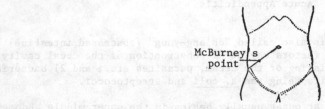

Figure 6-7-10. The cecal point [McBurney's point] illustrated.

    c. Concoction of

Barley	5 ch'ien
Seeds of tung-kua (Chinese waxgourd)	5 ch'ien
Honeysuckle	5 ch'ien
Tan-p'i (bark of peony root)	3 ch'ien
Ten-hu-so [Corydalis sp.]	2 ch'ien
Forsythia	3 ch'ien
Peach kernel	2 ch'ien
Pai-chiang ts'ao	3 ch'ien
Ch'ing-p'i	2 ch'ien
Violet	3 ch'ien

    d. Concoction of

Pai-chiang ts'ao [Patrinia sp.]	1 liang
Pan-lan ken	1 liang
Coix lacryma	5 ch'ien
Fu-tzu [aconite]	2 ch'ien
Honeysuckle	5 ch'ien
Tang-kuei	3 ch'ien

(This prescription is suitable for use in the final stage
when suppuration has already occurred.)

    e. Concoction of

Hsuan-shen	3 ch'ien
Mai-tung	2 ch'ien
Licorice	1 ch'ien
Seeds of Chinese waxgound	1 liang
Fresh ti-yu	3 ch'ien
Tang-kuei	3 ch'ien
Huang-ch'ing [Scutellaria baicalensis]	3 ch'ien
Coix lacryma	1 liang

(This prescription is suitable for chronic appendicitis).

3. Western medicine

    Penicillin 200,000 units every 6 hours given by intramuscular in-
jection. Streptomycin 0.5 gm twice daily, given by intramuscular injection.

Acute Cholicystitis and Cholelithiasis

Most cases of acute cholecystitis and cholelithiasis occur concurrently, due chiefly to gallstone obstruction, bile backup, and bacterial infection (Figure 6-7-11). Abdominal pain is frequently located in the right side between the ribs and the upper right abdomen, continuous and increasing in severity.

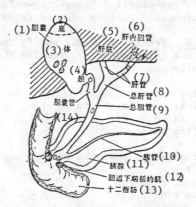

Figure 6-7-11. Diagram illustrating cholecystitis and cholelithiasis.

Key: (1) Gallbladder (5) Liver (9) Common bile duct
(2) Base (6) Interlobular ducts (10) Pancreatic duct
(3) Body (7) Hepatic duct (11) Pancreas
(4) Neck (8) Common hepatic duct (12) Oddi's sphincter
(13) Duodenum
(14) Cyctic duct

When the gallbladder is obstructed, the pain presents as a periodic twisting pain that often radiates to the back of the left shoulder. Upon examination, the gallbladder region of the upper abdomen shows marked tenderness and rebound tenderness. At the same time, symptoms such as fever, nausea, vomiting, or jaundiced whites of the eyes are noted. This ailment is due mostly to a congestion and release of moisture and heat [fever]. Fur on tongue is thin and white or slightly yellow. The pulse is usually tight and rapid.

Prevention

Patients who incur painful attacks regularly should cut down on greasy foods, and eat food that is more easily digested, to prevent attacks from occurring too frequently.

Treatment

1. Keep patient in a <u>semi-recumbent position</u>. Allow some liquid nourishment, but avoid greasy rich foods. For those in more serious condition, do not give food by mouth, but give parenteral fluids.

2. <u>New acupuncture therapy</u>. Apply strong stimulation to needles inserted into "nei-kuan," "tsu-san-li," "yang-ling-ch'uan," "t'ai-ch'ung" points. Retain needles for 30 minutes. Perform once or twice daily.

3. <u>Chinese herbs</u>. Treatment should purify the liver and relieve congestions and stimulate the gallbladder and resolve the gallstone(s) by using remedies such as the following:

    a. Concoction of

White-blossomed she-she ts'ao	5 ch'ien
Feng-wei ts'ao	5 ch'ien
Chin-ch'ien ts'ao	1 liang

    b. "Stone-resolving" powdered mixture consisting of

Yu-chin fen	2 fen
White alum, powdered	1.6 fen
Huo-hsiao fen	3.5 fen
Talc	6 fen
Powdered licorice	1 fen

Take the above dose 2 to 3 times daily. DO NOT give to pregnant women. For children, reduce dosage accordingly.

    c. Concoction of

Chin-ch'ien ts'ao	1 liang
Crocodile (roasted)	3 ch'ien
Po-ch'i (fresh)	1 liang
Yu-chin	4 ch'ien
Chi-nei-chen	3 ch'ien
Hsiang-fu	3 ch'ien
Niu-hsi	3 ch'ien
Talc	5 ch'ien
Seaweed	5 ch'ien

Prescription modification

    (1) For energy congestion, omit seaweed, and add

Ch'ai-hu	3 ch'ien
Tangerine leaves	1.5 ch'ien
Fresh orange peel	2 ch'ien
Dried orange peel	2 ch'ien
Ch'un-hsiang	8 fen

(pulverize and take by mouth.)

        (2) In case of nausea and vomiting, add
             Pan-hsia (Pinella sp.)   3 ch'ien
             Grain sprouts   4 ch'ien
             Tso-chin wan (patent drug)   1 ch'ien

        (3) In case blood clots, add
             Pistachio   1.5 ch'ien
             Myrrh   1.5 ch'ien
             Yen-hu-so (Corydalis sp.)   3 ch'ien
             Wu-ling chih   3 ch'ien
             P'u-huang   1.5 ch'ien

        (4) In case of moisture-heat (fever), add
             Huang-ch'ing [Scutellaria sp.]   3 ch'ien
             Gentiana   3 ch'ien
             In case of jaundice, add artemesia, 1 liang.

4. Western medicines

    a. Antispasmodics and analgesics. Give 50 percent magnesium
        sulfate solution 10 ml by mouth, 3 times daily. Or give
        atropine 0.5 mg, subcutaneously. In presence of severe pain,
        inject dolantin 50 mg and atropine 0.5 mg together. However,
        avoid using morphine independently, since Oddi's sphincter at
        the lower part of the common bile duct and the cystic duct can
        become spasmodic and increase the pressure within the gallbladder
        and the common bile duct to cause pathological changes. If there
        is jaundice, injections of vitamin K may be used.

    b. Antibacterials. Penicillin and streptomycin are used. For
        those patients more seriously ill, add tetracycline or chloro-
        mycetin 1.0 gm to 1000 ml parenteral fluid and give to patient
        by intravenous drip. For patients less seriously ill, give
        tetracyline, terramycin or coptin by mouth to hasten reduction
        of inflammation.

5. Surgical treatment

        If after the procedures described above have been tried to no avail,
and the gallbladder continues to show marked enlargement, the symptoms are
heightened. The temperature continues to rise and when a gallbladder abscess
or acute obstructive and suppurative inflammation of the cystic duct is suspected,
early and timely surgical intervention should be done.

- 443 -

Bile Duct Ascariasis

Bile duct ascariasis is called "hui-ch'ueh" by many Chinese medicine practitioners. It is seen usually among children and young adults, as the result of fever, achlorhydria, diarrhea etc., whereby ascaris inside the intestines move around haphazardly as the result of environmental changes. At this time, if Oddi's sphincter at the lower end of the common bile duct lose its elasticity, the ascaris will penetrate the bile duct (Figure 6-7-12). It is for this reason that the ailment is called bile duct ascariasis.

Characteristics of this condition are location of abdominal pain in the right lower part of the sternum, a sudden periodic fulgurant pain that sometimes radiate toward the right shoulder blade, imparting a special piercing sensation. During the attack, the patient hunches over on his side, his hands holding his abdomen, and breaks out in a cold sweat. His hands and feet are cold, and frequently there is nausea and vomiting. Sometimes ascaris are brought up in the vomitus. The fur on tongue is thin and white, and the patient pulse is thready and sunken. After an attack, the pain may be dissipated completely and the patient feels tired and sleepy.

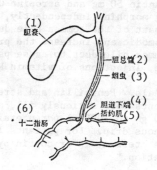

Figure 6-7-12. Diagram illustrating bile duct ascariasis.

Key: (1) Gallbladder   (4) Lower part of bile duct
     (2) Common bile duct   (5) Sphincter
     (3) Ascaris   (6) Duodenum

Prevention

Attention to personal hygiene to prevent ascaris infection, and to provide timely treatment. When a vermifuge is given, make sure the dosage is adequate. Otherwise such stimulation can cause the ascaris to panic and penetrate the bile duct.

<u>Treatment</u>

1. <u>Absolute bed rest</u>. Give rice gruel and thin congee. For those who cannot eat, administer parenteral fluids. After the attack has eased, give vermifuge in time, to prevent recurrences.

2. <u>New acupuncture therapy</u>. Apply medium stimulation to "chung-wan," "tsu-san-li," "yang-ling-ch'uan" points, retaining needles for 3 minutes, 2 to 3 times daily.

3. <u>Chinese herbs</u>

    a. "Wu-mei (black prune) wan" (patent medicine), 3 ch'ien, twice daily. Or, take with concoction prepared from chien [<u>Melia</u> sp.] 1 liang. For constipation, add hsuan-ming-fen to medication.

    b. Concoction of

Ch'ai-hu	3 ch'ien
Pai-shao	4 ch'ien
Acorn	3 ch'ien
Licorice	1.5 ch'ien
Szechwan pepper	2 ch'ien
Black prune	5 ch'ien
K'u-chien-tzu	5 ch'ien

    c. Rice vinegar 1 liang mixed with warm boiled water 1 liang, 3-4 times daily.

4. <u>Western medicine</u>

    a. To relieve spasms and alleviate pain: atropine 0.5 mg and phenergan 25 mg given by intramuscular injection. If necessary, repeat in 4-6 hours.

    b. To prevent against infection: chloromycetin or terramycin. If necessary, include streptomycin.

If signs and symptoms become more severe accompanied by chills, fever, jaundice etc., in spite of treatment given as prescribed above, then surgical treatment should be considered.

Acute Peritonitis

Acute peritonitis is usually caused by secondary infection, the result of perforation in an inflamed appendix, stomach or duodenum.

At onset, the abdomen feels intense generalized pain in the abdominal region. The severity is such that the patient dares not move, cough or turn -- movements which would increase the pain, particularly in area over original focus of infection. The skin over the abdomen is taut and hard, like a board.

There is marked tenderness and rebound tenderness, accompanied by symptoms such as fever, nausea, vomiting, abdominal distension, constipation, etc. Other signs are facial pallor, and a tired and worried expression. Fur on the tongue usually changes from white to yellow, and the pulse is thready and rapid.

Prevention

Early diagnosis and timely treatment of patients complaining of acute abdominal pain, to avoid the occurrence of acute peritonitis.

Treatment

1. **Basic.** Follow the procedures listed below, once diagnosis has been confirmed, since acute peritonitis usually requires early surgical intervention.

    a. Place patient in semi-recumbent position. This localizes the drainage of purulent fluid from the abdominal cavity into the pelvic cavity, and reduces the amount of toxin absorbed. In case an abscess is formed, this measure facilitates insertion of drain.

    b. Withhold food, connect suction apparatus to aspirate gas and fluid from stomach and intestine. This will reduce abdominal distention, restore peristalsis, and also help avoid or reduce the amount of gastrointestinal secretions draining into the abdominal cavity via the perforation.

    c. Control infection. Administer large doses of penicillin and streptomycin intramuscularly. Broad-spectrum antibiotics can also be given by intravenous drip.

    d. Provide fluid supplements, such as dextrose and physiologic saline, to prevent shock, correct the dehydration, and stimulate excretion of toxins in body. If necessary, give blood transfusion.

2. **New acupuncture therapy.** Such therapy can alleviate abdominal pain, relieve abdominal distension and stimulate peristaltic movement of intestines. The most often used acupuncture points are the "chung-wan," "t'ien-shu," "tsu-san-li," "nei-kuan," "ch'u-ch'in," "ho-ku" etc. For abdominal distention, include also the "kuan-yuan" and "ch'i-hai." For severe pain, include also the "chang-men."

3. **Chinese herbs.** Treatment should clear fever and detoxify, stimulate energy circulation and stop bleeding, and purge the moisture and open the bowels, using remedies such as the following:

- 446 -

a. Concoction of

Honeysuckle	1 liang
Forsythia	1 liang
Tan-p'i	5 ch'ien
Seeds of tung-kua [Chinese waxgourd]	5 ch'ien
Barley	4 ch'ien
Ta-huang [rhubarb], to be added later	3 ch'ien
Szechwan chien-tzu [Melia sp.]	3 ch'ien
Mu-t'ung	3 ch'ien
Licorice	3 ch'ien
Peach kernel	2 ch'ien
Pistachio	2 ch'ien
Myrrh	2 ch'ien
Mu-hsiang	2 ch'ien

(This concoction is suitable for use with cases of peritonitis, lowgrade fever, recurring afternoon fever, and local swellings.)

b. Concoction of

Honeysuckle	1 liang
Dandelion	1 liang
Chinese waxgourd seeds	1 liang
Forsythia	5 ch'ien
Violet	5 ch'ien
Tan-p'i	5 ch'ien
Ta-huang [rhubarb], added later	5 ch'ien
Huang-lien [Coptis chinensis]	3 ch'ien
Huang-ch'ing [Scutellaria sp.]	3 ch'ien
Mu-hsiang	3 ch'ien
Szechwan chien-tzu [Melia sp.]	3 ch'ien
Fresh licorice	3 ch'ien
Pistachio	3 ch'ien
Myrrh	3 ch'ien
Peach kernel	3 ch'ien
Bamboo leaves	1 ch'ien

(This concoction is suitable for cases of peritonitis presenting high fever and great prostration, fever, chills, thirst, flushed face and blood-shot eyes, dry mouth and parched lips, constipation, and bloody urine, and for patients with a slippery and rapid pulse, or a tense and rapid pulse.)

Intestinal Obstruction

The causes of intestinal obstruction most frequently are incarcerating hernia, post-operative intestinal adhesions (Figure 6-7-13), ascaris obstruction, intestinal intussusception (Figure 6-7-14), intestinal volvulus (Figure 6-7-15), tumor etc. In all these conditions, the intestinal contents cannot pass through the intestinal tube without interference. The onset is sudden and critical, and the chief clinical manifestations are pain, vomiting, distension, and obstruction. The abdomen experiences recurring bouts of crampy pain that is accompanied by local tenderness, rebound tenderness, nausea, vomiting, sweating, thirst, scanty urine, abdominal distension, no bowel movements nor expulsion of flatus. In some patients, fecal matter may even be noticed in their vomitus. This condition which involves the large intestine and the small intestine, is considered an internal ailment mostly of the "solid" variety. A few cases may be of the "deficient" variety with overtones of "solidness." Fever cases outweigh chill [han] cases. The pulse is tense, tight, slippery, and rapid. Fur on the tongue is usually white, yellow or oily.

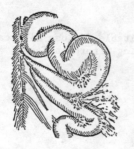 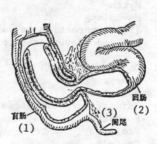

Figure 6-7-13. Intestinal obstruction due to acute angle formed by adhesions.

Figure 6-7-14. Intestinal intussuscep tion (where the ileum is prolapsed into the cecum).
Key: (1) Cecum (3) Vermiforme
(2) Ielum appendix

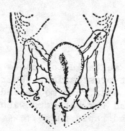

Figure 6-7-15. Volvulus involving the sigmoid colon.

1. General treatment

When a diagnosis of intestinal obstruction has been made, observe the following procedures immediately:

a. Withhold water and food from patient. Use suction apparatus on stomach and intestine to reduce abdominal distension.

b. Correct dehydration. Administer intravenous fluids. Besides normal daily requirements of 5-10 percent dextrose solution 1500-2000 ml, and 500-1000 ml of 5 percent dextrose in saline, fluid loss through repeated vomiting should also be replaced. In small children, this may be based on a requirement of 50-100 ml/kg, of which one-third to one-half should be normal saline.

c. Prescribe antibiotics. This is particularly urgent where strangulating obstruction is suspected, as the antibiotics may reduce the severity of bacterial infection and the production of toxins. Penicillin and streptomycin are most commonly used.

2. New acupuncture therapy. Apply strong stimulation to the "chung-wan," "t'ien-shu," "ch'i-hai," and "tsu-san-li" points, once or twice every day.

3. Chinese herbs. Treatment should open up the internal channels [stimulate circulation] to offset ill effects, and to stop the bleeding, using remedies such as the following:

a. Concoction of

Hou-pu [Magnolia officinalis]	1 liang
Chi-shih [Poncirus trifoliata]	3 ch'ien
Ta-huang [rhubarb], to be added later	5 ch'ien
Glauber's salt, steeped	1 liang

[This prescription is suited for all types of obstruction.]

b. Concoction of

Lai-fu tzu (roasted)	1 liang
Glauber's salt, steeped	5 ch'ien
Fan-hsieh hsieh [senna leaves]	4 ch'ien
Hsien-niu [morning glory]	5 ch'ien
Kan jui powder (steeped)	2 fen

(This concoction suited for those patients with a greater volume of fluid in the intestinal cavity.)

c. Concoction of

Wu-yao	2 ch'ien
Kuang-mu-hsiang	3 ch'ien
Hou-pu	3 ch'ien
Chi-he [covering of trifoliate orange]	2 ch'ien
Fresh orange peel	2 ch'ien
Dried orange peel	2 ch'ien
Peach kernel	2 ch'ien
Kuo-wei jan	3 ch'ien
Kernel of yu-li	3 ch'ien
Sesame seeds	3 ch'ien
Tang-kuei	5 ch'ien

(This concoction suited for cases with partial obstruction.)

d. Tested and tried procedure. Give patient 60-200 ml seed oil (can be peanut, sesame or rape-seed oil) by mouth, or introduce via gastric tube, once a day. This approach is certainly effective in the treatment of ascaris, adhesion-caused, or fecal obstruction.

4. <u>Surgical intervention</u>. When symptoms do not improve but become worse after observation for 12-24 hours following the treatment procedures previously described, surgery is considered. When possiblity of strangulating obstruction is suspected from the beginning; or when the condition becomes a total mechanical obstruction, surgical intervention becomes necessary. If there is delay, the consequences may be quite critical.

Hernia

Hernia called "hsiao-ch'ang ch'i," is a general term for dislocation or obvious shift in position of an organ.

<u>Types</u>

The types most commonly seen are femoral hernia, inguinal hernia, and umbilical hernia.

<u>Inguinal hernia</u>. Seen mostly in small children or middle-aged males. In the early stages, the signs are not particularly unusual -- only a feeling of increased abdominal pressure, particularly after standing for too long a time, manifested by an oval lump that appears on the medial aspect of the inguinal canal when the patient begins to walk. Sometimes this lump may protrude partially or completely into the scrotum. Usually the protrusion disappears upon pressure or when patient lies down (Figure 6-7-16).

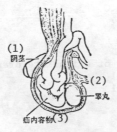

Figure 6-7-16. Inguinal hernia (hernia protruding into scrotum).

Key: (1) Penis   (3) Hernia contents
     (2) Testicle

Femoral hernia. Seen mostly in females, the hernia is hemispherical, located along the lower part of the femoral ligament and the upper medial aspect of the thigh. It can cause an incarcerated hernia very easily.

Infantile umbilical hernia. The protrusion is over the navel, seen mostly in females. It appears most prominently when the child is fretful and crying.

Hernia may be a deficiency type or solid-type ailment. In the deficiency condition, the energy is depressed and accompanied by pain. In the solid condition, the energy is congested and the blocked channels incur pain. Fur on the tongue is usually white and oily. The pulse is sunken and tense.

Prevention

1. Wrap diapers around the abdomen of infants securely but not too tight. Do not let infant stand at too early an age, nor let him cry nor cough too much.

2. Have patients participate in a program of regular exercise to strengthen the abdominal muscles, thereby exerting a protective reaction.

3. Provided active treatment to the aged for chronic diseases such as chronic bronchitis which may provoke a rise in intra-abdominal pressure.

Treatment

1. New acupuncture therapy. Apply medium stimulation to the "ch'i-hai," "san-yin-chiao," and "ta-tun" points, once a day. Moxa sticks can be further used in moxibustion over the "ta-tun."

2. <u>Chinese herbs</u>. Treatment should decongest the liver and correct energy flow, using remedies such as the following:

    a. Compress prepared from sorrel 5 ch'ien and coriander 3 ch'ien crushed with hot rice placed as poultice over the navel 3 to 4 hours each time for 2 to 3 times in succession.

    b. Pulverized mixture of

Ta-hui	2.5 ch'ien
Hsiao-hui	2.5 ch'ien
<u>Nephelium litchi</u> seeds	3 ch'ien
Tangerine seeds	3 ch'ien

To be taken with some brown sugar water, 3 ch'ien each time, twice daily.

c. Fresh pulp (fleshy fruit) of <u>Nephelium litchi</u>. To be taken twice daily, pulp from 15 fresh fruit each time, for several days in succession.

3. Western medicine

Injection of atropine when attack of inguinal hernia or femoral hernia becomes very painful.

4. Surgical treatment

Except for the very old, the weak, and those suffering at same time from serious illness, who cannot be treated by surgery, it is recommended that surgical treatment given in time be performed on all others. This is done to forestall cases of incarcerated hernia, and to strengthen and sustain the working manpower that is available.

Hemorrhoids

Hemorrhoids are small tumors (single or multiple) or piles formed by dilatations of the anorectal hemorrhoidal veins. This condition is seen mostly in young and mature individuals. It is caused chiefly by obstruction to the reflux action of the hemorrhoidal veins supplying the anus and the rectum (such as that seen in pregnancy or constipation where intra-abdominal pressure is increased or portal venous pressure is raised). Or they may be due to the ill effects of wind, dryness, moisture or heat, or overindulgence in hot and peppery foods. Based on their location, hemorrhoids may be classified further as internal or external hemorrhoids. Sometimes the hemorrhoids are mixed.

1. Internal Hemorrhoids

Varices occurring along the hemorrhoidal plexus inside the anus are called internal hemorrhoids (Figure 6-7-17). Their development is divided in three stages:

1. <u>Early stage hemorrhoids</u>. The core of the hemorrhoid is quite small at this time, and the chief symptom is bleeding. The blood which is a bright red covers, but does not mix with, the feces. The anus is not painful.

2. <u>Second stage internal hemorrhoids</u>. The core becomes bigger and frequently protrudes outside the anus. However, it retracts automatically after a bowel movement. The amount of bleeding is less than that seen with early-stage hemorrhoids.

3. <u>Third stage internal hemorrhoids</u>. The hemorrhoids become even larger now and protrude regularly during a bowel movement. They do not retract automatically, frequently requiring bed rest or digital manipulation

before retracting. When a hemorrhoid becomes strangulated, the pain becomes more severe. Such hemorrhoids can also cause peri-anal edema and even ulceration, gangrene or pus formation.

Treatment

1. <u>Keeping bowels open</u>. If bowels are constipated, have patient drink a cup of salt water every morning for mild cases, sometimes taken with some honey.

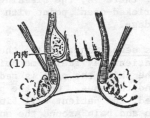

内痔
(1)

Figure 6-7-17. Internal hemorrhoids

Key: (1) Internal hemorrhoids

For more severe cases, prescribe some edible oil. For very severe cases, prescribe concoction of rhubarb roots (3 ch'ien), or a tea steeped from 2 ch'ien of senna leaves. Or order phenolphthalein, two tablets to be taken each time.

2. <u>New acupuncture therapy</u>. Apply medium stimulation to "ch'ang-ch'iang" and "ch'eng-shan" points, once a day.

3. <u>Prick-open therapy</u> (T'iao chih-liao fa)

a. <u>Locating the hemorrhoidal point</u>. Have patient expose his back, and sit him backwards on chair, his chest facing and leaning against the back of chair. Locate the hemorrhoid point below the 7th thoracic vertebra, but above the sacrum, and between a line drawn between the two axillas across the back. Characteristics of the hemorrhoid point: circular or oval in shape, protruding above the skin slightly, about size of the tip of a needle, slightly pigmented, usually grey, dull red, brown, or pink, the color not facing upon pressure. However, these points must be distinguished from freckles, keratoses, folliculitis, and small scratches. When the hemorrhoidal point is not noticeable, rub the patient's back with one hand, and watch for a change of the hemorrhoidal point to a fresh pink. If several similar points are found at the same time, they should be checked out according to the criteria just given. If they are all identical, select the point most inferior and closest to the hemorrhoids.

- 453 -

b. Technique. Sterlize skin over the hemorrhoidal joint, using iodine and alcohol. Use a large size suture needle to prick-open the skin of the hemorrhoidal point, after which direct the needle deeper and continue "pricking"until a glistening fibrous substance (shaped like fine flaxen) is picked up. Apply pressure [pull] to break. During the procedure, the placement of the needle must be parallel to the spine. The size of the "pricked-open" wound is about .05 cm in length and about 0.2-0.3 cm deep. If it is a true hemorrhoidal point, there is no bleeding. If there is, the bleeding is very slight. Finally, paint the "pricked-open" point with some iodine, and cover with adhesive bandage.

c. The patient's sensations. While the skin is being "pricked-open," the patient may feel some pain. Once the needle has penetrated the skin, the pain is reduced or some sensation may be felt around the anus. Once the prick-open procedure has been completed, the patient will find that the original feeling of congestion and pain around the anus has been dissipated or reduced.

d. Length of treatment. Generally one prick-open treatment will suffice. If not, repeat procedure after 10 days.

e. Conditions suited for. Internal hemorrhoids, external hemor-rhoids, mixed hemorrhoids, anal fissure, anal pruritus etc. The procedure is particularly effective for acute inflammations.

f. Precautions. Avoid heavy exertion for the rest of day after "prick-open" therapy. Also avoid highly stimulating foods. Patients who feel dizzy should be given bed rest immediately. This technique is ruled out for pregnant women.

4. Chinese herbs

a. Concoction of
Hei mu-erh [Auricularia auricula]   3 ch'ien
Pei-mu [Fritillaria sp.]   4 ch'ien
K'u-shen [Sophora flavescens]   5 ch'ien

b. Concoction of
K'u-shen (pan-roasted with vinegar)   5 ch'ien
     [Sophora flavescens]
Ti-yu [Sanguisorba sp.]   5 ch'ien
Sophora blossoms   3 ch'ien

The two prescriptions just described are used for treating bleeding from internal hemorrhoids.

c. Concoction for bathing local area, prepared from
   Wu-pei-tzu (gall)   5 ch'ien
   Glauber's salt   1 liang

   (This prescription is effective for treating painful everted
   internal hemorrhoids)

5. Injection therapy

   A sclerosing agent such as 5 percent oleum marrhuae stearate injected into the hemorrhoids is very effective for treating bleeding of first
and second stage hemorrhoids and rectal prolapse. Use about 0.5 ml of oleum
morrhuae stearate each time, once or twice a week. If the core of the hemorrhoids should protrude anytime, it should be returned [retracted] in time, to
avoid infection or strangulation.

2. External Hemorrhoids

   External hemorrhoids are located outside the anus, usually like grapes,
purplish-black, and symptomless. If the stool is dry or if there has been too
much straining at stool or too much strenuous exertion to cause rupture of
varices, rectal pain will ensue, heightened by sitting down and walking.

Treatment

1. New acupuncture therapy (same as that for internal hemorrhoids).

2. Chinese herbs

   a. Salve for local application following defecation, prepared from
      3 ch'ien of t'ien-kuei [Semiaquilegia adoxoides], freshly sliced,
      and steamed in a cup of pure tea oil over cooking rice.

   b. Mixture for local application, prepared from sprinkling 1 ch'ien
      of camphor (crushed fine) over 10 snails (shelled) and kept
      covered in crock for about half a day.

   c. Decoction for bathing local parts, prepared from
      Ju-hsing ts'ao [Houttuynia cordata]   1 liang
      Roots of k'u-lien [Melia sp]   1 liang
      Glauber's salt   1 liang
      Ma-ch'ih-hsien [portulaca]   1 liang

   d. Pill prepared from 1 liang each of honeysuckle and licorice
      finely crushed and mixed with water and wine to form ball.
      Prescribe 2-3 ch'ien each time, twice daily.

- 455 -

Leg Ulcers

Leg ulcers are also called "lien tsang." They occur on the medial and lateral aspects of the leg, frequently the result of trauma and infection. For example, if moisture and heat in the system bear down and clots obstruct the meridian and "lo" passageways, the ulcer becomes chronic and will not heal. The ulcer surface becomes depressed, cyanotic, painful and itchy, and discharges an oozing fluid, emitting a characteristically unpleasant odor. The margins of the ulcer are indurated, and the flesh turns black over a period of time. The skin surrounding the ulcer frequently presents a weeping rash. This is a rather resistant disease.

Prevention

For those patients suffering from varicosities of the lower extremities, protect the legs with elastic supports, [or elastic stockings], and make sure that treatment is given in time for any injury or infection sustained.

Treatment

1. __Electropuncture therapy__. Insert "hao" needles into skin about 1 fen from margin of ulcer toward the center, so that the needles can penetrate deeply into the base of the ulcer. Use 5-10 needles in each puncture application, after which hook them up with the electropuncture activator and turn the current on for 15 minutes (determined by the patient's tolerance). This treatment is given once a day, and continued for two to three courses of treatment (each course of treatment has 10 sessions).

2. __Chinese herbs__. Treatment should detoxify and promote moisture resolution, stimulate blood circulation and absorb clots, with remedies such as the following:

    a. Concoction of

Huang-ch'i [Astragalus sp.]	5 ch'ien
Honeysuckle flowers	5 ch'ien
Tang-kuei odds and ends	3 ch'ien
Phellodendron	3 ch'ien
Niu-hsi [Achyranthes Didentata]	3 ch'ien
Licorice	1.5 ch'ien

    b. Concoction for bathing the affected part twice a day, prepared from the following:

Dandelions	5 ch'ien
Chrysanthemums, wild	5 ch'ien
Leeks [bulbs]	3
Moxa leaves	3 ch'ien

c. Shan ts'ang-tzu oil for external application twice daily
    (prepared from dried shan ts'ang-tzu that is steeped in
    sesame oil).

d. Powdered toad for sprinkling over affected parts, twice daily.
    Prepared by skinning two toads that are then hearth-dried before
    crushing into powder.

e. Powdered pai-chih [Bletilla sp.] mixed with brown sugar con-
    centrate used as dressing, protected by covering of tea leaves
    or film and fixed in place by bandage. Dressing is changed
    every other day.

Frostbite

Frostbites are caused by circulation obstruction, as the result of cold.
They affect mostly the back of the hands, the fingers, ankles, toes, and the
ears. They occur most easily among those over-exposed to cold, those who engage in little physical activity in bitter cold weather, and in those with
poor circulation of blood and energy. Generally, they could be classified as
mild or severe.

Mild frostbite. In the beginning, the local area experiences a burning
prickly feeling which then is followed by numbness and a blanching of the skin.
Later on, the affected local areas become hard, congested, swollen and itchy.
The skin coloring has also changed, from a bright pink to a dull red.

Severe frostbite. The affected areas crack, the itching becomes more
severe, and the chilblain may ulcerate and discharge an infected ooze.

Prevention

1. Attention to keeping warm and dry. Step up physical activity.
Crushed bulbs of leeks may be applied, after heating in sunshine in the summer-
time, to those body areas most prone to frostbite, as a preventive against
recurrence.

2. Washing hands and feet in wintertime with a peppery concoction
which stimulates the local circulation.

Treatment

1. New acupuncture therapy. Tap local areas lightly with "mei-hua"
needles until some bleeding ensues. Repeat daily, but do not use this technique
on ulcerated areas.

2. **Chinese herbs**

   a. **For mild frostbite**

      (1) Concoction prepared from sproutings of leeks and eggplant, used for bathing hands and feet.

      (2) Radish (or piece of fresh ginger), warmed over open fire and sliced, for rubbing over affected areas.

      (3) Dried peppers, about a dozen or so, in concoction, for bathing affected areas. Or, 3 ch'ien of black pepper crushed, and dissolved in boiling water, used for bathing affected areas.

   b. **For severe frostbite**

      (1) Compress of a puffball ma-po [Lycoperdon gemmatum] over affected part, changed daily.

      (2) Oyster (or clam) shell burned and pulverized, for sprinkling over affected part.

      (3) Phellodendron 1 liang, pulverized, for sprinkling over affected area (This prescription is suited for frostbite accompanied by an inflammation).

      (4) Concoction for internal consumption, prepared from

Tang-kuei [Angelica polymorpha]	3 ch'ien
Cinnamon sticks	3 ch'ien
Pai-shao [Paenia albiflora]	3 ch'ien
Burnt licorice	1.5 ch'ien
Hsi-hsin [Asarum sieboldi]	1 ch'ien
Mu-t'ung [Akebia trifoliata]	2 ch'ien
Fresh ginger	2 slices
Red dates	3

Chapping

Chapping, called "ch'e ch'uan-k'ou" by the local populace, occurs chiefly on the hands and feet. It is commonly seen in the wintertime, since secretions from the sweat and sebaceous glands are reduced then, and the skin becomes dry, loses its usual elasticity and becomes chapped, that is cracked and slit open. Chapping occurs along the normal lines of the skin, though the length, depth, and width of the cracks vary. There may be bleeding and pain.

Prevention

1. Regular use of warm soaks before and after the winter season [to soften skin], followed by applications of chap-preventing ointment, clam oil or glycerine (do not use pure glycerine, but mix it half-and-half, with water).

2. Appropriate protection of hands while working, by wearing gloves etc.

Treatment

1. Chinese herbs

a. Special ointment prepared from

Sesame oil	2 liang
Crude ti-huang [Rehmannia sp]	5 ch'ien
Yellow wax	2 liang
Vaseline	1 liang

Preparation. The sesame oil is first heated in a pot, after which the crude ti-huang (sheng-ti) is added. After the mixture begins to thicken, strain to remove the ti-huang residue. Then add the wax and vaseline. Heat until the mixture is completely melted. Store in jars and use for application over affected skin areas.

b. Application prepared from mixture of

Mi-t'o-tseng [lead oxide] pulverized	1 liang
Tung oil	2 liang

c. Oily paste for local application prepared from equal parts of huang-pai [Phellodendron sp] and pai-lien [Ampelopsis sp.] pulverized, and mixed to the proper consistency with addition of peanut oil.

d. Ointment of pai-chih [Bletilla striata] prepared by steaming the pulverized plant over rice. Apply over cracks.

2. Western medicines

a. For small shallow fissures in skin, use adhesive tape method.

b. Ointment of benzoic acid compound (salicylic acid 6 gm, benzoic acid 12 gm, and vaseline to make 100 gm).

c. Sulfur ointment, boracic ointment, or salicylic ointment.

Corns and Calluses

Corns and calluses frequently occur on the toe margins and soles of the feet, caused by constant pressure, friction, the wearing of ill-fitting shoes, or long-distance walking. Locally, they appear as small and hard rounded areas of thickened skin, yellowish white, and yield to pain on pressure. Hardened areas with a mung-bean size core are corns; those without cores, but presenting only a thickened and hardened skin area are calluses.

Treatment

1. New acupuncture therapy

    a. Apply needle puncture to the center of the corn until patient feels pain. Retain needle for 20 minutes before removal. Then press and squeeze part until it bleeds a little.

    b. Apply 3-5 needles to area around the corn, followed by moxibustion, once a day.

2. Chinese herbs

    a. Compress prepared from the fruit of ya-tan-tzu [Brucea javanica] with shell removed applied locally. Fix with adhesive tape and bandage. After 7 days the corn or callus will fall off automatically. Mild cases require only one course of treatment. More severe cases may require several courses of treatment.

    b. Plaster prepared from fleshy part of wu-mei [black prune], crushed and mixed with salt and vinegar to form poultice.

    c. Mixture of pulverized toasted centipede and sesame oil for application over affected area. Remove application after one night. The corn or callus has turned black and will drop off in a week.

    d. Corn ointment (patent medicine) for application over affected area.

Impetigo

Impetigo called "huang-pao ts'ang" or "nung-ch'ao ts'ang" [terms describing the yellow vesicles or beehive appearance of the pustules], is a skin infection caused by the Staphylococcus aureus or Streptococcus hemolytica or a mix of the two organisms. It is usually seen in children, occurring most frequently on the face and the extremities. At onset, itchy red spots or a bloody-looking rash is seen on the skin, which very rapidly becomes purulent, changing into soybean size pustules. The skin surrounding the lesions becomes red, burning hot and painful. After the pustules erupt they dry up and form yellow scabs. However, the erupting pustular discharge will infect other skin areas and produce new pustules. The condition may be accompanied by lymphadenopathy, fever, thirst and other symptoms.

Prevention

1. Strengthened measures of hygiene and sanitation to be practiced in child care centers and elementary schools. Once a case is discovered, the patient must be placed in isolation treatment.

2. Attention to personal hygiene, with frequent bathing (no bathing upon appearance of disease, in order to prevent dissemination of infection) and frequent change of clothing. After the patient has recovered, boil and disinfect all towels, clothing and toys used by the patient.

Treatment

1. Chinese herbs. Treatment should clear fever, detoxify, and promote [excess] moisture removal, with remedies such as the following:

    a.   Suitable amounts of powdered ma-po [puffball Lycoperdon gemmatum] sprinkled over open sores.

    b.   Local preparation made from sesame oil or crushed portulaca juice mixed with the following ingredients, pulverized, for use on affected areas:

Ch'ing-tai [indigo flower]	2 liang
Gypsum	4 liang
Talc	4 liang
Huang-pai [Phellodendron sp.]	2 liang
Huang-tan [minimum]	1 liang

       Or, mix 2.5 liang of this pulverized mixture with 10 liang of vaseline, melt and cool. Use as ointment for local application.

    c.   Concoction for local bathing of affected parts once or twice daily, prepared from equal parts of tree bark of k'u-lien [Melia sp], eucalyptus leaves, and shui-lung [Jussiaea repens].

    d.   Salve prepared from suan-chiang [winter-cherry Physalis alkekengi], burnt and crushed fine with some camphor and mixed to right consistency with addition of sesame oil. The plant can also be concocted and the concoction used for bathing affected areas.

    e.   **Concoction for internal consumption, of**

Fresh sheng-ti [crude ti-huang]	5 ch'ien
Lien-ch'iao [forsythia]	5 ch'ien
Honeysuckle	5 ch'ien
T'u-fu-ling [Smilax glabra]	5 ch'ien
Mung-bean shells	5 ch'ien
Che-ch'ien-tzu [plantago]	4 ch'ien
Dandelion	1 liang

2. Western medicines

Gentian violet for external application. For cases with extensive skin damage, accompanied by fever and lymphadenopathy, injections of penicillin may be given.

Urticaria

Urticaria, also called "feng-chen k'uei" or "feng-t'uan" [wind rash or hives] by the local populace is a common allergic disease. The condition could be due to numerous factors such as the ingestion of certain foods and drugs, smell of certain odors, the presence of intestinal parasites, intolerance to temperature changes, or the onset of menstruation in women. In the beginning, the skin only shows pink or white wheals [hives] of various shapes and sizes. They may occur anywhere on the body and are very itchy. With scratching, the patches of hives increase even more, so that the skin becomes bumpy like k'u-kua [Momordica charantia]. Within a short time, the hives can subside automatically, though several breakouts could occur within a day's time. Serious cases are accompanied by symptoms such as nausea, dyspnea, abdominal pain, diarrhea or itchiness in the throat, respiratory difficulties etc. If after repeated attacks, the condition does not subside, the urticaria will become chronic.

Types

Generaly, the urticaria most commonly seen may be classified as the wind-chill (feng-han), wind-heat (feng-jeh), or anemic (hsueh-hsu) types.

Wind-chill urticaria. The hives are pale and itchy, easily breaking out when the weather is cold. Once the weather warms up, the urticaria will subside and not recur. Fur on tongue is thin and white, and the pulse is slow.

Wind-heat urticaria. The hives are a deep red, breaking out only in warm weather. The pruritus is very severe, and fever is present, accompanied by parchness, apprehension, constipation, and a concentrated yellow urine. Fur on tongue is yellow, the pulse rapid.

Anemic [blood-deficient] urticaria. The hives are reddish and light at the same time, and the itching is less pronounced, the urticaria usually appearing in the afternoon or evening. It is accompanied by apprehension, a low-grade fever, parchness and an aversion to drinking water. The tongue is pink and without fur, and the pulse is fine and rapid.

Prevention

The important consideration is removing the cause by tracking down any drug, food, or other substance or factor the patient may be allergic to. Once uncovered, the patient must avoid contact with these factors. If parasites are found, give appropriate treatment. Have patient stay away from strongly flavored foods or condiments.

Treatment

1. New acupuncture therapy (see section on "Pruritus")

2. Acupuncture point injection. Using 0.5 - 1 percent procaine, inject the "hsueh-hai," "san-yin-chiao" points, 0.5 - 1 ml to each point. Or dilute phenergan 25 mg with 10 ml of injection-use water, and inject 0.5 - 1 ml of dilution into each acupuncture point.

3. Chinese herbs

   a. For wind-chill urticaria. Treatment should loosen the wind and dispel the chill, using remedies such as the following:

      (1) Concoction of lu-lu-t'ung, taken internally.

      (2) Powdered ts'ang-erh tzu [the burweed Xanthium strumarium] (the whole plant), 2 ch'ien each time, three times a day.

      (3) Concoction of
          Tzu-p'ing [duckweed spirodela polyrhizd]   2 ch'ien
          Ephedra   1 ch'ien
          Ti-fu-tzu [Kochia scoparia]   3 ch'ien
          Fang-feng [Siler divaricatum]   1.5 ch'ien

      (4) Concoction of the following mixed with a suitable amount of brown sugar before consumption:
          Ching-chieh [Nepeta japonica]   5 ch'ien
          Prickly chi-li [Tribulus terrestris]   4 ch'ien
          Chi-he [Poncirus trifoliata]   3 ch'ien

      (5) Concoction of clematis (wei-ling-hsien) for bathing affected areas.

   b. For wind-heat urticaria. Treatment should dispel the wind and clear fever, using remedies such as the following:

(1) Concoction for internal consumption, of
Hsuan-shen [Scrophularia sp.]   3 ch'ien
Tzu ts'ao [Lithospernum sp.]   3 ch'ien
Chrysanthemum   3 ch'ien
Licorice   1 ch'ien

(2) Concoction of
Yin-ch'en [Artemesia capillaris]   1 liang
Tzu-p'ing [Spirodela sp.]   4 ch'ien
Fang-feng [Siler divaricatum]   1 liang
Leaves of ta-ch'ing [Clerodendron sp.]   3 ch'ien
Processed rhubarb   3 ch'ien
Lu-lu-t'ung   3 ch'ien

(3) Juice of shan k'u-kua [Momordica sp.?] mixed with water
for external application.

(4) Pai-pu [Stemona sessifolia] 5 ch'ien cooked in white wine,
2 liang, for application over affected part.

c. For anemic urticaria. Treatment should nourish the blood and
moisturize the body, using remedies such as the following:

(1) Concoction of the following for internal consumption

Crude ti-huang   5 ch'ien
Tang-kuei   3 ch'ien
Ch'ih-shao [water chestnut
            Heleocharis plantaginea]   3 ch'ien
Mummified silkworms   3 ch'ien
Cicada moltings   2 ch'ien

(2) Dried stems from the taro plant, 1-2 liang cooked with an
appropriate amount of pork spareribs.

4. Western medicines

a. Atropine for cases with noticeable gastrointestinal symptoms.

b. Adrenalin hydrochloride to be given immediately to cases with
edema of the throat. Also give cortisone by mouth.

c. Antihistamines such as benadryl for certain cases. For those
with more pronounced symptoms, give calcium gluconate by
intravenous injection.

Eczema

Eczema is a very common inflammatory skin condition, caused mostly by carelessness to skin hygiene or it may be due to some special body makeup. It can occur at any age and on any part of the body. Occurring on the head and face of infants, it is called milk eczema (nai hsien); on the ears, called encroaching boils (yueh-shih ts'ang); on the lower lip, goatee boils (yang hu-tzu ts'ang); on the elbow and knee spaces, bend's rash (szu-wan feng); and on the scrotum, genital pouch rash (shen-lang feng).

Types

Eczema maybe classified as acute or chronic.

Acute eczema. Manifested as a local redness and itching of the skin, the rash very rapidly presents as wheals and vesicles. After the vesicles have ruptured through scratching, they ooze a clear discharge. Finally scabs form and once the scabs are shed, the patient recovers.

Chronic eczema. Usually the result of repeated attacks of acute eczema, accompanied by skin changes -- thickening, increasing coarseness and fissuring, and a change in skin color to a dull red or grey. Oozing may follow scratching and rupture of lesions, though the involvement is more limited.

Acute eczema is associated mostly with moist heat (shih-jeh); chronic eczema, with anemia (hsueh-hsu).

Prevention

Attention to skin cleanliness, and avoidance of scratching and vigorous rubbing. During the acute stage, do not give prophylactic inoculations. This applies particularly to infants who should not be vaccinated when they have eczema.

Treatment

1. Acupuncture therapy. Use medium stimulation on needles inserted into the "ch'u-ch'ih," "hsueh-hai," and "san-yin-chiao" points, once a day.

2. Chinese herbs

a. For acute eczema. Treatment should clear fever and resolve moisture, using remedies such as the following:

(1) Concoction of the following for bathing affected areas:
Ts'ang-shu [Atractylis ovata]   3 ch'ien
Huang-pai [Phellodendron sp.]   3 ch'ien
K'u-shen [Sophora flavens]   5 ch'ien
T'u-fu-ling [Smilax glabra]   5 ch'ien

(2) Concoction prepared from 1-2 liang of leaves of ch'i-ta-ku [chickweed Sagina maxima]

(3) Powdered mixture for local application prepared from
K'u-fan [burnt alum]   2 parts
Dried orange peel   1 part

(4) Local use paste for applying over affected area, prepared from
Huang-tan [minimum]   5 ch'ien
Gypsum (refined)   1 liang
Camphor   6 fen

Mix with crushed rape seeds and concoct until right consistency is attained. Apply over affected parts twice daily.

b. **For chronic eczema**. Treatment should nourish the blood and moisturize [the skin], using remedies such as the following:

(1) Concoction of
Crude ti-huang   5 ch'ien
Shou-wu [Polygonum multiflorum]   5 ch'ien
La chi-li [thorny Tribulis terrestris]   5 ch'ien
Tan-p'i [bark of peony roots]   3 ch'ien

(2) Concoction of following for bathing affected parts
Yin-ch'en [Artemesia capillaris]   1-2 liang
K'u-shen [Sophora flavescens]   1-2 liang

(3) Mixed juices from the following for local application:
Ch'ing-tai [indigo flower]   3 ch'ien
Ma-ch'ih-hsien [portulaca]   appropriate amount

(4) Crushed dried silkworm cocoons for local application over affected parts, twice daily.

Dermatomycoses

Dermatomycoses are commonly seen fungus infections of the skin. Neglect of proper skin hygiene is usually the causative factor. Clinically, they are characterized by the appearance of eruptions, scab formation, encrustation, pruritus etc. The eruptions can appear anywhere on the body. Most frequently seen are tinea capitis, tinea corporis, tinea manuum, tinea pedis -- ringworms affecting the scalp, body, hand and foot.

1. Tinea Capitis

Tinea capitis or ringworm of the scalp, usually occurring among children between the ages of 6 and 15 years, is spread by primary infection through hair cutting equipment, pillows, hats, etc.

Types

According to morphological differences, ringworm of the scalp is further classified as tinea favosa (yellow ringworm) and tinea alba (white ringworm).

Tinea favosa is also called "fei ts'ang." At onset, light yellow pustules, the size of a pinhead, are seen at base of hair follicles. Later on they merge into itchy patches, oozing a yellow fluid. The hairs fall off and leave a permanent alopecia and scars.

Tinea alba is called "pai t'o ts'ang" [balding boils] or "lai t'ou" [scabies scalp] by the local populace. At onset, one or two small greyish-white specks are seen, followed by gradual proliferation into round or circular patches ranging in size as small as a bean or as large as a copper coin, with well delineated margins. The lesions are extremely itchy. Or they may present as vesicles that eventually form scabs, the scab shedding white dandruff. Generally the condition heals by itself when the patient reaches adulthood.

Prevention

1. Separation of haircutting equipment, hats, pillow cases etc., used by the patient. Boil after each use, to prevent transmission of infection to others.

2. Strengthening the enforcement of sanitary measures in public places such as barber shops, kindergartens, elementary schools etc. See that barbers understand basic facts related to the prevention and treatment of scalp ringworm. Barbering equipment and utensils should be sterilized before use on another patron.

Treatment

1. For tinea favosa. Treatment should dispel the moisture and kill the offending organism, using remedies such as the following:

    a. Roasted seeds of k'u-lien [Melia sp.] pulverized and mixed with equal amount of lard or vaseline, to be used as ointment for external application.

    b. Application prepared from pulverized mixture of the following combined with a suitable amount of tea oil.

Roots of wu-shui k'o [nettle Pouzolzia zeylanica]	1 liang
Leaves of liao-ko wang [Wickstroemia indica]	1 liang
Chiu-li kuang [Senecio scandens]	1 liang
Ta-fei-yang [Euphorbia hirta]	1 liang
Dried alum	5 ch'ien

2. For tinea alba. Treatment should dispel the wind and kill the offending organism, using remedies such as the following:

a. Crushed mixture of

Fresh disk of kuei-hua [Malua sp.], burnt	3-5 chin
Buffalo dung } in suitable amounts	
Dirt }	

Apply mixture overhead for 1-2 hours, once daily, for 3 days in succession.

b. Ointment prepared by pulverizing the following ingredients separately,

Realgar	3 ch'ien
Sulphur	3 ch'ien
Chaulmoogra	5 ch'ien

Then mix and add enough oil to form ointment. Before using, cut hair short or shave and shampoo hair. Cover with gauze or oiled paper. Repeat daily.

2. Tinea Corporis

Tinea corporis or body ringworm called "t'ung-ch'ien hsien" [copper-cash ringworm] by the local populace, is found mostly on the face, trunk, and the four extremities. At onset, dry erythematous plaques containing small macula form in annular layers, shaped like copper cash.

Treatment

1. Soaks prepared by mixing together

Hung-hua [Carthamus sp.]	5 ch'ien
Soda (laundry)	1 liang
Water	3 liang

2. Juice for local application, obtained by grinding 5 root tubers of Pinellia ternata (with outer covering removed) in a bowl to which a spoonful of vinegar has been added.

3. Tinea Manuum

Tinea manuum, or ringworm of the hands, is called "o-chang feng" [goose-foot rash] by the local populace. It usually occurs along the lateral aspects of the palm, on the palmar surface, or in the inter-digital spaces. In the beginning, the ringworm is seen as scattered or grouped vesicles or erythematous patches. Gradually, the skin thickens, and becomes hard, dry and scaly. In the winter when it is dry, the skin on the palm cracks easily.

Treatment

1. Solution for local application prepared by placing 4 ch'ien each of huang tan [minimum] and dry alum in one chin of boiling rice vinegar. Or, hands can be soaked in this solution for 50 minutes 3 times a day. Do not dry or wash hands after soaks, but let hands dry by themselves. In the winter, instead of rice vinegar, apply lard mixed with huang-tan solution over affected parts.

2. Leaves of castor plant, crushed, for application over affected areas.

3. Fermentation liquor obtained by steeping leaves of mu-lan [Indigofera tinctoria] in lime water for 3 days. Paint over affected parts.

4. Tinea Pedis

Tinea pedis or ringworm of the foot is called "Hongkong foot" by the local populace. In the beginning, small vesicles are noted between the toes. This is followed by erosion of the lesions and discharge of a smelly ooze. Pruritus and maceration of the skin alternate repeatedly and a permanent cure is not easily obtained.

Treatment

1. New acupuncture therapy. Apply medium stimulation to needles inserted in the "t'ai-ch'ung" and "t'ai hsi" points, once a day.

2. Chinese herbs

    a. Soaks of k'u-fan [burnt alum] 5 ch'ien dissolved in water for foot baths. Also sprinkle powdered burnt alum over affected parts.

    b. Pulverized mixture of the following for use on lesions

Camphor	2 fen
Ch'ing-fen	2 fen
K'u fan [burnt alum]	3 ch'ien

First soak foot in alum foot bath. Then roll alcohol sponges in pulverized mixture and place between toes. Bandage. Change dressing daily until lesions are healed. Do not stop or skip treatment any one day during course of treatment.

c. Tincture/paint prepared by steeping powdered t'u-chin-p'i [bark of Hibiscus sp] 200 gm in 350 ml of water and 75 percent alcohol added to make 1,000 ml, for one week. The contents are then pressed, extracted and filtered before use.

Rice Paddy Dermatitis

Rice paddy dermatitis, called "shui-tu" [water poison] by the native populace is also referred to as "fertilizer sores." This condition occurs between May and August, particularly frequent during the double cropping season. It is caused by fertilizer and insecticide irritation encountered by farmers laboring in the rice paddies. Or, it may be caused by cercariae carried in their snail hosts, the t'ui-lo [Oncomelania hupeiensis?]. These cercariae can penetrate the human skin and cause an allergic reaction, though they cannot mature into adults in the human body. Such skin (of arms and legs mostly) that has come in contact with water collected in the paddies frequently break out in erythematous patches of small vesicles that are very itchy, and burning hot in many instances. If scratching breaks the vesicles, pain, pustules, and erosion frequently ensue. This ailment is generally classified in the moist-heat [shih-jeh] category. Skin tissue damage is comparatively slight, as staying away from the paddies for 2-3 days will allow healing and return of skin to normal. Skin tissue with comparatively severe damage will drag on over a longer period of time, if no suitable treatment is found for it.

Prevention

1. Before going into paddies to work, rub arms and legs with la-liao [smartweed], leaves of ch'iu-ts'ai or tung oil. Wash skin with soap and water after coming off the fields.

2. In fields that contain the t'ui-lo [oncomelania snail?], sprinkle lime or tea seed powder, and wait 6-12 hours before working in treated paddies.

Treatment

With Chinese herbs, treatment should clear fever and detoxify, using measures such as the following:

1. Concoction for application on affected areas, prepared from

   she-kan [Belamcanda sp.]   0.5 chin
   Table salt   1.5 liang
   Water   8 chin

   Cook for 1 hour and strain. Warm before use over affected areas

2. Concoction for bathing affected areas, of

   Wu-p'ei-tzu [gall]   1 liang
   She-ch'ang-tzu [Cnidium sp.]   1 liang

3. Concoction prepared from cooking a bunch of huang-ching [Vitex negundo] leaves.

4. Crushed mixture for local application, consisting of

   Realgar (pulverized)   5 ch'ien
   Leeks   1 ch'ien

5. Concoction for internal consumption, prepared from

   Honeysuckle blossoms   1 liang
   Licorice   5 ch'ien

Neurodermatitis

Neurodermatitis, commonly called "niu-p'i hsien" [water buffalo-hide ringworm] by the local populace, usually occurs on the back and sides of the neck, followed by areas such as the elbow space, the chest, sacrum, thigh, legs and perineum. It is usually localized. At onset, the local skin area becomes itchy, and because of continuous scratching by the patient, small rounded or multi-angular flat wheals appear. Later, over the local skin area, the skin gradually thickens and hardens, very much like a piece of coarse cowhide. The patient feels that a stubborn pruritus is ever present, so that over a period of time a vicious cycle of more itching is followed by more scratching which is followed by more itching. This phenomenon is frequently related to nervous factors; sudden changes in the living environment or other local exciting factor may provoke an attack of pruritus. The ailment takes a slow gradual course, so that after a period of time complete recovery is difficult.

Prevention

No scratching. Wash area with soapy water. Also avoid alcoholic beverages and other highly seasoned foods. Do not starch the collars of clothing too stiff.

Treatment

1. <u>New acupuncture therapy</u>.

   a. Apply strong stimulation to needles inserted into the "nei-kuan," "ch'u-ch'ih," "hsueh-hai," and "san-yin-chiao" points, once a day.

   b. Use the pricking technique with mei-hua needles over the affected part until some bleeding ensues. Then use mild moxibustion over area. Treatment is given once a day.

2. <u>Chinese herbs</u>

   a. Pulverized mixture of the following ingredients, in equal parts

         T'u-ching-chieh [Chenopodium]
         Ma-ying-tan [Santana camaro]
         San-ya-k'u [<u>Evodia lepta</u>]
         Liang-mein chen [<u>Zanthoxylum</u> sp.]
         Sulfur

      Add a suitable amount of tea oil, to form paste for local application.

   b. Paste prepared for local application, from
         Pa-tou [croton bean] (shelled)   1 liang
         Realgar   5 ch'ien

      After blisters have formed and dried up, apply again over affected area. Be sure not to smear any of this paste on top of normal skin. Avoid ingesting by accident.

   c. For small areas of neurodermatitis, use the adhesive tape method [to cover fissures and open lesions], and change every two or three days.

Vegetable Dermatitis

Vegetable dermatitis is also called "hung-hua ts'ao ts'ang" [red-flower grass (<u>Astragalus sinicus</u>) sores]. It is due to a reaction between the moisture-heat collected in the body system, the result of eating or contact with plants such as <u>Astragalus sinicus</u>, mustard greens, rape, turnips etc., and exposure to sunlight to cause an accumulation of toxins that erupts into a dermatitis. Hence it is also called vegetable dermatitis or vegetable-sunlight dermatitis. This condition is seen most frequently in the months between March and August, affecting most often the face, the back of the hands, the neck, and the four extremities. The clinical symptoms are erythema (without noticeable depressions) mainly, accompanied by numbness, pain, tightness, and a feeling of "ants crawling all over." In severe cases, a feeling of stuffiness in the head, nausea, high fever, maculae, vesicles, erosion and ulceration are, furthermore, present.

Prevention

Avoidance [do not eat] of certain vegetables, while working outdoors, it is best to wear a broad-brimmed straw hat and long sleeved jackets and trousers.

Treatment

1. <u>Chinese herbs</u>. Treatment should clear fever and detoxify. Using remedies such as the following:

    a. Concoction of dandelion (2 liang) tea. Drink instead of tea.

    b. Concoction for internal consumption, of

Mummified silkworms	3 ch'ien
Mint (to be added later)	1 ch'ien
Huang-lien [coptis chinensis]	5 fen
Dandelion	4 ch'ien
Huang-ch'ing [Scutelearia sp]	3 ch'ien
Shan-yao [Gardenia sp.]	3 ch'ien
Che-ch'ien-tzu [Plantago sp.]	3 ch'ien
Licorice	1 ch'ien

    c. Concoction for bathing

Ch'i-ta ku [Sagina maxima]	1 liang
Kung-pan-kuei [Polygonum perfoliatum]	1 liang
Honeysuckle	5 ch'ien

Bathe affected areas once or twice daily.

2. <u>Western medicines</u>

Large amounts of vitamins such as vitamin B complex, for serious cases.

Contact Dermatitis

Contact dermatitis is an acute dermatitis caused by skin contact with certain substances (such as certain insecticides, plasters, iodine, sulfonamides etc.). Its onset is acute and most cases present a history of contact with the offending agent. At the site where contact had been made are frequently seen erythematous maculae, edema, a dense collection of wheals or vesicles, frequently accompanied by an itchy or burning sensation. In serious cases, there is local erythema. Recovery is spontaneous several days later, upon removal of offending agent.

Prevention

Isolating the offending substance wherever possible. Once done, tell patient not to repeat experience.

Treatment

1. New acupuncture therapy. Apply medium stimulation to needles inserted in the "hsueh-hai" and "san-yin-chiao" points, once a day.

2. Chinese herbs. Treatment should clear fever and detoxify, using remedies such as the following:

    a. Concoction of following for bathing affected parts

San-ya-k'u [Evodia lepta]	2 liang
Ta-feng ai [Artemesia sp.]	2 liang
Kung-pan-kuei [Polygonum perfoliatum]	2 liang
Ch'i-ta-ku [Sagina maxima]	2 liang

    b. Concoction prepared with new shoots of suan-p'an-tzu [Glochidion puberum] for bathing affected areas.

    c. Concoction for bathing affected areas, prepared from a suitable amount each of water lily leaves, Glauber's salt, and mint.

    d. Concoction of

Honeysuckle	5 ch'ien
Crude ti-huang	5 ch'ien
Chrysanthemum indicus	5 ch'ien
K'u-shen [Sophora sp.]	3 ch'ien
Tan-shen [Salvia multiorrhiza]	4 ch'ien
Pai-hsien-p'i	4 ch'ien
Licorice	2 ch'ien

Drug Dermatitis

Drug dermatitis is caused by sensitivity of patient to a drug, whether taken orally or parenterally. Drugs causing this reaction frequently are antibiotics (penicillin the most common), sulfonamides, antipyretics and analgesics, tranquillizers etc. The onset is very acute, and a bright red drug rash resembling urticaria, measles, etc. is seen. Its distribution may be generalized or symmetrical, and very itchy. Some patients may feel a generalized burning sensation. In others, the reaction may be accompanied by fever, headache, nausea, poor appetite etc. In serious cases, jaundice, nephritis, blood diseases etc. may be present. Treatment must be given in time.

This ailment must be differentiated from drug intoxication. (See Table 6-7-2)

Table 6-7-2. Differentiation of Drug Sensitivity from Drug Intoxication

Drug sensitivity	Drug intoxication
Has a definite incubation period*	No incubation period
Occurring in individual cases	Occurs in any individual, once the intoxication dosage has been reached.
Not related to drug dosage. Can occur even with a small amount of drug.	Due chiefly to drug dosage being excessive
Later use of offending drug will still generate allergic reaction	Later use of drug still possible, as long as dosage controlled within given range.

* The incubation period refers to the period covering time when the drug is first ingested to the time the skin rash first appears. If this is the first occurrence, the incubation period is generally 7-9 days. If it is a repeat, the incubation period may be shortened to several minutes, though the range is usually 1-2 days.

Prevention

1. Avoid abusive use of drugs. Do a skin test before using penicillin or procaine on a patient.

2. Do not use a drug a patient has been sensitive to again [on the same patient].

Treatment

1. Chinese herbs. Treatment should cool the blood, clear fever, and promote diuresis, with remedies such as the following:

> a. Concoction [for internal consumption] of
> Honeysuckle blossoms   1 liang
> Crude ti-huang   1 liang
> Chrysanthemum indicus   5 ch'ien
> Artemesia capillaris   5 ch'ien
> Violets   4 ch'ien
> Mu-t'ung [Akebia trifoliata]   2 ch'ien

   b. Concoction of
       Honeysuckle blossoms

b. Concoction of	
Honeysuckle blossoms	5 ch'ien
Yen-so-yao [Cyclea hypoglauca]	5 ch'ien
Licorice	1 liang
c. Concoction of following for bathing:	
Ch'i-ta-ku [Sagina maxima]	1 liang
Kung-pan-kuei [Polygonum perfoliatum]	1 liang
Honeysuckle blossoms	5 ch'ien

Bathe affected parts with concoction twice daily.

2. Western medicines

Give antihistamines such as benadryl and phenergan by mouth. For severe cases, give cortisone by mouth. Force fluids.

Miliaria [Prickly Heat]

Miliaria, or prickly heat, is a common skin ailment seen in the summer time, caused by inadequate elimination [evaporation] of perspiration in unduly hot weather. At onset, small papules or vesicles appear on an erythematous base, distinctly delineated, but merging gradually into a patch. The skin feels burning hot, and the pruritus is prickly. The rash generally subsides spontaneously following good skin hygiene or a cooling change in the weather.

Prevention

Keep residences well-ventilated. Do not wear clothing too tightly, nor wear ill-fitted garments. Bathe frequently and maintain skin cleanliness.

Treatment with Chinese Herbs

1. Tea prepared from steeping 5 ch'ien of Lu-I San (patent medicine) in boiling water.

2. Fresh cucumber slices lightly rubbed over the prickly heat, 3 or 4 times daily.

3. Juice from crushed leaves of ssu-kua [vegetable sponge] (or ku-kua Momordica charantia), for application over rash.

4. Heat rash powder sprinkled locally.

Tumors

A tumor is an abnormal new growth occurring in certain body tissues or organs. It is one of the diseases that most endanger human life. However, the broad mass of workers, peasants and soldiers, and revolutionary health workers have made certain progress in treating tumors with Chinese herbs, and some good news is appearing on the horizon.

Types

At present, though the causes of tumors are not too clear, tumors can generally be classified as benign or malignant, according to the amount of danger they pose to the human organism.

A benign tumor is one that grows slowly, shows definite lines of demarcation separating it from surrounding tissues, does not metastasize, and does not pose any great danger to the human body. Examples are myoma, lipoma, osteoma, cyst, fibroma, etc.

A malignant tumor is one that grows rapidly, penetrates nearby tissues without any delineation of limits, metastasizes rapidly and seriously affects the health of the afflicted. Examples are carcinomas and sarcomas.

The approach toward tumors should emphasize early discovery, diagnosis and timely and early treatment. Otherwise benign tumors can sometimes change into malignant tumors. The treatment of malignant tumors is more demanding.

Malignant tumors most commonly seen are cancer of the breast, cancer of the cervix, carcinoma of the nasopharynx, lung cancer, stomach cancer, liver cancer, cancer of the colon, Osteosarcoma etc.(Table 6-7-3). Diagnosis of some of these types may require x-ray examination, blood studies or biopsy for confirmation.

Treatment

In the treatment of tumors, besides surgery, chemotherapy or deep x-ray therapy, extensive use of Chinese herbs also has a great future.

- 477 -

Table 6-7-3. Diagnosis of Frequently Seen Malignant Tumors

Disease	Important diagnostic characteristics
Mammary cancer	1. Seen mostly in women over 40 years old 2. Breast is raised, or an immovable lump is felt in breast 3. Nipple usually retracted, skin showing an orange-peel appearance 4. No pain in early stage, followed by metastasis toward the axilla or deeper tissues
Cancer of the cervix	1. Seen mostly in women over 40 years old 2. Incidence may be related to chronic cervicitis 3. Menorrhagia may be present, as well as frequent bloody discharge from vagina 4. Easily metastasizes toward other pelvic organs. Lower abdominal pain and backache may be present.
Carcinoma of the nasopharynx	1. Sensation of a foreign body in the nasopharynx. Fresh blood frequently mixed with nasal discharge 2. Incidence greatest during the prime of life, accompanied by rapid weight loss 3. Enlargement of cervical nodes 4. Frequent headaches. Paralysis of cranial nerves may occur.
Lung cancer	1. Chronic cough that never gets better. Blood in sputum. Seen mostly in older males. 2. Chest pain and hemothorax noted in late stage 3. Enlargement of nodes in the hilum, sometimes metastasizing to distal organ via the blood stream.
Gastric cancer	1. A history of ulcers over a long period of time in most cases 2. Reduced appetite, indigestion, belching, weight loss, anemia, fatigue, tumor palpable locally. 3. Bleeding from upper digestive tract or presence of occult blood in tarry stools. 4. Symptoms of obstruction in the late stage 5. Metastasis to lymph nodes above left collar bone
Cancer of the liver	1. Development rapid, with obvious signs such as weight loss appearing in a few weeks' time. 2. A continuous pain noted over liver region in right upper abdomen in most cases. Seen mostly in middle-aged males. 3. Jaundice, fever, anemia, ascites appearing in the late stage. 4. Hepatomegaly, the liver hard and surface nodular to palpation.

Table 6-7-3 (Continued)

Disease	Important diagnostic characteristics
Cancer of the rectum	1. Progress of disease slow, with changes in bowel habits noted. Incidence greater in women above middle age. 2. Blood in stools. Mucus present. Bowel movements becoming smaller gradually. Abdominal distension and flatus frequently present. 3. Invasion of sacral nerve in late stage, accompanied by lower abdominal pain. 4. Tumor felt by digital examination via the anus.
Osteosarcoma	1. Localized pain, more severe at night, sleep disturbed, appetite poor. Weight loss rapid. 2. Atrophy of affected limb, enlargement of involvement. Skin over local area taut and shiny, and the veins distended. 3. Pain on pressure locally. 4. Low-grade fever. Seen mostly involving extremities of young people. 5. Possible metastasis to lungs.

1. Chinese herbs frequently tried in the treatment of tumors include the following: pai-hua she-she ts'ao [Olaenlandia diffusa], pai-ying [nightshade Solanum lyratum], hsu yang-ch'uan [ch'i-ku ts'ao Sagina maxima], ssu-hsieh lu [Galium gracile], feng-wei ts'ao [bracken Pteris multifada], pan-pien lien [Lobelia radicans], lai ha-mo [frog], pan-chi-lian [Scut ellaria barbata], huang yao-tzu [Dioscorea bulbifera], ts'ang-erh ts'ao [burweed Xanthium strumarium?], mi-hou t'ao [Actinidia chinensis], pi-hsieh [chinaroot Smilax china] ti-erh ts'ao [Hypericum japonicum], hsia-k'u ts'ao [Brunella vulgaris], yeh chu-hua ken [roots of Chrysanthemum indicus], lung-kuei [Solanum nigrum], t'ien-kuei [Semiaquilegia adoxoides], shao-tzu [Gardenia jasminoides], and tzu-ts'ao [Lithospermum erythrorhizon]

2. Prescriptions [samples for reference] frequently tried in the treatment of tumors:

   a. For stomach cancer, a concoction of
Olaenlandia diffusa	2 liang
Roots of lu [bulrush]	1 liang
Blackened ginger	1 ch'ien
Scutellaria barbata	5 ch'ien
Shao-tzu [Gardenia sp.]	3 ch'ien

   One concoction/dose daily. Follow with roots of bulrush tea.

b. For <u>lung cancer</u>. Concoction of

Pai-ying [<u>solanum lyratum</u>]   }   2 liang
Oaenlandia diffusa   }   of each,
Lobelia radicans   }   the fresh
Scutellaria barbata   }   plant*

* If dried, use only half the measurement. Drink as
would tea.

For severe pain, add ch'ing-mu-hsiang [<u>Aristolochia</u> sp.]
1 liang, and take with rice polishing water.

For hemoptysis, add 1 liang of chi-hsueh-t'eng [<u>Milletia
reticulata</u>]; if coughing becomes more severe, add yin-yang-
huo [<u>Epimedium sagittatum</u>] and ai-ti-ch'a [<u>Ardisia aponica</u>]
3 ch'ien of each.

(This prescription can also be used for treating cancer of the
liver, cervix and nasopharynx).

c. For <u>carcinoma of the esophagus</u>: powdered huang yao-tzu 3 ch'ien
3 times a day. The huang yao-tzu prepared as follows:

Take 12 liang of huang yao-tzu and steep in 3 chin of white
wine for 24 hours. Then place huang yao-tzu in cold water and
soak for another 7 days and 7 nights. Take out, dry and crush
into powder.

d. For <u>cancer of the rectum</u>:

(1) Concoction of pan-chi-lian [<u>Scutellaria barbata</u>] 3 ch'ien

(2) Concoction of following, to be drunk as tea
     Feng-wei ts'ao [<u>Pteris multifada</u>] 1 liang
     Po-ch'i [water chestnut]   2 liang

(3) Concoction of a suitable amount of ts'ang-erh ts'ao, for
     bathing affected area.

     The three prescriptions given above may be used simul-
     taneously.

e. For <u>cancer of the liver</u>: Pulverized t'ien chi-huang [<u>Hypericum
japonicum</u>] mixed with a suitable amount of rock sugar, taken
with boiled water, three times a day. This prescription is
also good for liver cirrhosis.

b. For cancer of the nasopharynx: Concoction prepared from 2 liang of she-kan [Belamcanda chinensis] to be taken internally. For external application over nasopharyngeal region, crush the herb (or mill with vinegar for painting over area).

g. For mammary cancer: Pulverized liao-ko-wang [Wickstroemia indica] 1-2 liang, mixed with cold boiled water or rice wine for local compress. (Can also be used to treat mastitis and mumps -- as local application).

h. For cancer of the cervix: Concoction of

Ssu-hsieh-lu [Galium gracile]	2-4 liang
Large dates	2-4 liang

To be taken daily.

i. For other cancers: Live frog wrapped in dirt, toasted [or baked over fire] until dirt is hardened and dry. Remove dirt and pulverize frog remains. Take 1 ch'ien of powdered frog, 3 times a day.

Section 8   Gynecological and Obstetrical Diseases

Menstrual Irregularities

Menstruation is a periodic manifestation of uterine bleeding. It is the result of follicular hormone action causing periodic changes in the endometrium lining the uterus, that is climaxed by its shedding and bleeding. The first menstrual period that ushers in the menarche occurs between the ages of 13 and 18 in females. After that, the cycle is repeated every 21-40 days, for a duration of 3-7 days each time. Around the age of 45 in females, menstruation will cease, in what is called the menopause.

Menstrual irregularities refer to the premature or tardy recurrence of subsequent menstrual periods, a prolonged period of menstrual flow, and heavy or scanty menses, all of which are caused by abnormal ovarian function. Because this condition may be due to certain gynocological ailments, infections or endocrine ailments, it is very important to track down the cause.

1. Premature Menstruation

When the recurring menstrual cycle is early by more than 8 or 9 days, it is called premature menstruation. It is generally considered as a solid condition (shih cheng) or a deficient [anemic] condition (hsu cheng).

A **solid condition** is characterized by a heavy flow, the menses colored red or purplish black, and containing clots. The abdomen is distended and crampy. Apprehension is present and patient is susceptible to bursts of ill temper. The stools are dry, the urine yellow, the pulse tight and rapid, and the coating on tongue yellow.

A **deficient or anemic condition** is characterized by scanty menses of light red coloring, a lack of pep and alertness, backache, weakness in legs, no energy, dizziness, palpitation, fine and weak pulse, and a pale and "furless" tongue.

2. Delayed Menstruation

When the recurring menstruating cycle is delayed by more than 8 or 9 days, it is called delayed menstruation. Frequently seen are three types: the uterine cold-moist (pao-chung han-shih) type, the blood-and-energy deficient (hsueh-ch'i liang hsu) type, and the energy stagnant blood clotting (ch'i-chi hsueh-yen) type.

The **uterine cold-moist type** is characterized by blackish scanty menses, abdominal [over uterine area] pain, relieved somewhat by hot compress, backache and weakness in legs, facial pallor, cold hands and feet. Chills, a sunken and slow pulse, and a thin and white coating on tongue.

The **blood-and-energy deficient type** is characterized by a small amount of light red menses, facial pallor, dizziness, palpitation, fragile health, poor appetite, a deficient pulse, and a pink and "fur-less" tongue.

The **energy-stagnant and blood-clotting type** is characterized by scanty purplish-black menses containing clots. Cramps felt over abdomen which is aversive to palpation and pressure. Apprehension, pain at the sides and a dry skin are also noted. The pulse is tight, accompanied by a dull red tongue.

Prevention

The resistance of women to disease over the menstrual period is poorer than it usually is, and they are more prone to become ill. For this reason, the following precautions should be observed during the menstrual period.

1. Avoidance of heavy work during this time. Production teams should pay further attention to safeguarding the health of women, and allow for their physiologic characteristics. Depending on local conditions observe the principle of "three assignments and three non-assignments" (that is assign dry work but not wet work during the menstrual period; assign light duty but not heavy duty during pregnancy; and assign nearby work detail, but not distant work detail during the lactation period).

2. Attention to adequate rest. Avoid cold, raw and highly seasoned foods and condiments (such as peppers, alcoholic beverages, etc.)

3. Attention to cleanliness of external genitals. Wash with warm water daily, but do not take tub baths. Abstain from sexual relations. Keep sanitary belt clean, to prevent bacterial contamination which may result in various menstruation connected ailments.

Treatment

1. New acupuncture therapy. Apply medium stimulation to needle inserted in the "kuan-yuan," "hsueh-hai," "san-yin-chiao" points before and after the menstrual period 5 to 7 times.

2. Chinese herbs

a. In premature menstruation

For a solid condition, treatment should regulate energy and blood circulation, using remedies such as the following:

(1) Concoction of
Tan-shen [Salvia multiorrhiza]   5 ch'ien
Tang-kuei   3 ch'ien
Ch'uan-kung [Conioselinum unvittatum]   3 ch'ien
Hsiang-fu [sedge Cyperus rotundus]   3 ch'ien

(2) Concoction of
Roots or flowers of yueh-yueh hung   5 ch'ien -
        [Rosa chinensis]   1 liang

(3) Concoction of
Ti-chin [Euphorbia sp.]   3 ch'ien
Tzu-chu ts'ao   3 ch'ien
Charred palm, aged   6 ch'ien

For an anemic condition, treatment should regulate and restore the blood and energy, using remedies such as the following:

(1) Concoction of
Huang-ch'i [Astragalus sp.]   5 ch'ien
Processed ti-huang   4 ch'ien
Tang-kuei   3 ch'ien

(2) Steamed brown hen (no salt) stuffed with following herbs
[after inner organs have been removed]

I-mu ts'ao [motherwort]   1.5 liang
Tang-kuei   1 liang
Wine   2 liang

Two hens to be eaten.

- 483 -

(3) Tang-kuei wan (patent medicine), 3 ch'ien each time, two times a day.

b. In delayed menstruation

For the uterine cold-moist type, treatment should be warm to dispel cold and moisture, with remedies such as the following:

(1) Concoction of
Tang-kuei   3 ch'ien
Fu-tzu   2 ch'ien
Moxa [Artemesia] leaves   1 ch'ien

(2) Concoction of
Ts'ang-shu [Atractylis ovata]   3 ch'ien
Hsiang-fu [sedge]   3 ch'ien
Tan-shen [Salvia multiorrhiza]   3 ch'ien

(3) Ai-fu ai-kung wan [an artemesia and fu-tzu compounded pill] (patent medicine), 2 ch'ien each dose, twice daily.

For the blood-and-energy deficient type, treatment should supplement the energy and nourish the blood, using remedies such as the following:

(1) Concoction of
Shu-ti [processed ti-huang]   4 ch'ien
Tang-shen [Campanumaea pilosula]   4 ch'ien
A-chiao [donkey hide glue]   3 ch'ien

(2) Pa-chen wan (patent medicine), 3 ch'ien each dose, three times a day.

(3) Fu-k'o shih-chen p'ien (patent medicine), 5 tablets each time, twice a day.

For the energy-stagnant and blood-clotting type, treatment should stimulate energy circulation and activate the blood, using remedies such as the following:

(1) Concoction of
Tan-shen [Salvia sp.]   4 ch'ien
Tang-kuei   3 ch'ien
Bat droppings   3 ch'ien
P'u-huang [Typha latifolia]   3 ch'ien
Hsiang-fu [sedge]   2 ch'ien
Kuang-p'i   1.5 ch'ien

(2) Concoction prepared with 3-5 ch'ien of chi-mu hua [Loropetalum chinense].

(3) I-mu kao (patent medicine) [ointment prepared from mother-
     wort], 1 teaspoonful each dose, twice daily.

Dysmenorrhea

Severe abdominal cramps felt before and after, or during the menstrual
period accompany the menstrual disorder called dysmenorrhea. It may also be
accompanied by backache, nausea, and vomiting. It may be due to tension because the patient does not understand the menstrual process fully, or due to
exposure to cold, an underdeveloped uterus, a narrowed cervix, abnormal positioning of uterus, or inflammation of a reproductive organ.

Types

According to the nature and manifestation of dysmenorrhea, it is commonly classified as cold [han], heated [jeh], deficient [hsu] and solid [shih]
types.

The cold type is characterized by scanty menses which is purplish-black,
by abdominal cramps that are eased by applications of heat, by a white and
oily fur on the tongue, and a sunken and slow pulse.

The heated type is characterized by a heavier menstrual flow which is
a brighter red, by abdominal cramps, an inclination for cold and an aversion
to heat, a flushed face, restlessness, parchness, and thirst, concentrated
brown urine, constipation, a yellow coated fur on tongue, and a rapid pulse.

The deficient type is characterized by scanty menses pale in color, dull
crampy pain, lassitude, backache, tired feet, facial pallor, pale uncoated
tongue, and a deficiently weak pulse.

The solid type is characterized by scanty menses containing purplish
black clots, backache and abdominal pain, distended and painful breasts, cyano-
tic-looking tongue, and a tight pulse.

Prevention

Educate young females on the facts of menstrual physiology, so that
understanding will remove those feelings of dread and tension. Make sure
that during the menstrual period, they keep from catching cold, have enough
rest, and forego strenuous activity.

Treatment

1. New acupuncture therapy. Apply strong stimulation to needles
inserted into "kuan-yuan" and "san-yin-chiao" points,   the "san-yin-chiao"

first when pain is present, and continue to twirl needle for 1-2 minutes. Then puncture the "kuan-yuan" and follow with moxibustion. If acupuncture is used about 3-5 days before onset of period, the therapeutic effectiveness is even more satisfactory.

2. Chinese herbs

    a. For cold type dysmenorrhea, treatment should dispel the cold and alleviate pain, using remedies such as the following:

        (1) Concoction of

Fresh ginger	3 slices
Brown sugar	2 liang

            Take with an equal amount of sweet wine.

        (2) Concoction of

Tang-kuei	1 liang
Hsiang-fu [sedge Cyperus sp.]	3 ch'ien
Roasted ginger	2 ch'ien

        (3) White pepper, 1 ch'ien mixed with some brown sugar, for internal consumption.

        (4) Concoction of

Leaves of tse-lan	3 ch'ien
Mugwort leaves	2 ch'ien

            Mix with 1 liang brown sugar for taking by mouth.

    b. For heat type dysmenorrhea, treatment should clear the fever and alleviate pain, using remedies such as the following:

        (1) Concoction of

Crude ti-huang	5 ch'ien
Tang-kuei	3 ch'ien
Tan-p'i	3 ch'ien
Shan-yao [Gardenia sp.] [stir-fried)	3 ch'ien
Hsiang-fu [Cyperus sp.]	3 ch'ien

        (2) Concoction of following:

Ti-ku-p'i	5 ch'ien
Hsuan-shen	5 ch'ien
Crude ti-huang	5 ch'ien
Phellodendron	2 ch'ien

    (3) Concoction of
          Tan-shen [Salvia multiorrhiza]   5 ch'ien
          Yen-hu-so [Corydalis sp.]   2 ch'ien

          Take about 4 or 5 days before onset of menstrual cycle,
          and discontinue

c. For deficient type dysmenorrhea, treatment should restore the
    deficiency, using remedies such as the following:

    (1) Concoction of
          Tang-shen [Campanumaea pilosula]   3 ch'ien
          Tang-kuei   3 ch'ien
          Hsiang-fu [sedge Cyperus rotundus] 2 ch'ien

    (2) Concoction of
          Tang-kuei   5 ch'ien
          Ch'uan-kung [Conioselinum unvittatum] 2 ch'ien
          Black soybean   1 liang

d. For solid-type dysmenorrhea, treatment should stimulate energy
    and blood circulation, using remedies such as the following:

    (1) Concoction prepared from 5 ch'ien of yang-t'i ts'ao
          [Emilia sonchifolia].

    (2) Concoction of
          Tse-lan   5 ch'ien
          Hsiang-fu [Cyperus sp.]   3 ch'ien

    (3) Concoction of
          Wu-ling-chih [bat droppings]   3 ch'ien
           P'u-huang [Typhus latifolia]   3 ch'ien
           Motherwort   3 ch'ien

3. Western medicines

    Analgesic tablets or atropine tablets.

Amenorrhea

    Absence of menstruation in females over 18 years of age who have never
menstruated, or absence of menstruation for periods longer than three months
(not related to pregnancy or lactation) in females who have begun to menstruate
is called amenorrhea. This condition may be caused by chronic illness, anemia,
malnutrition, under-developed uterus, tuberculosis of the genital organs, etc.

<u>Types</u>

Generally, amenorrhea may be classified into the deficient [anemic or hsu] type or the solid [shih] type. The solid type usually involves energy stagnation and formation of blood clots. The deficient type usually involve energy and blood inadequacy.

The <u>solid type of amenorrhea</u> is characterized by distension and pain in the lower abdomen which is also aversive to manual palpation, nausea, restlessness, ill humor, and a bitter taste in mouth. Coloring of tongue is purplish, the pulse is sunken, full, and uneven.

The <u>deficient type of amenorrhea</u> is characterized by a sallow or pale complexion, dizziness and spots before the eyes, palpitation and shortness of breath, poor appetite, delicate health, weakness of arms and legs, burning sensation in palms, rosy cheeks, apprehension, dry skin, recurring fever, cough symptoms in what is called "kan hsueh-lao" [dry tired blood]. The tongue tastes flat, non-coated. Pulse is usually deficient.

<u>Treatment</u>

1. <u>New acupuncture therapy</u>. Apply medium stimulation to needles inserted in the "kuan-yuan," "chung-chi," "hsueh-hai," and "san-yin-chiao" points, once daily or every other day. For deficient type amenorrhea, puncture the "kuan-yuan" point; for the solid type, the "chung-chi" point.

2. <u>Chinese herbs</u>

    a. For <u>solid type amenorrhea</u>, treatment should stimulate blood and energy circulation, using remedies such as the following:

        (1) Potion prepared from bringing 4 liang each water and rice wine with 4 liang of pan roasted silkworm droppings to a boil and strain. Take a cup, two times a day.

        (2) Concoction of
            Seeds of <u>Thuja orientalis</u>   5 ch'ien
              (pan roasted and pulverized)
            Niu-hsi   5 ch'ien
            Fresh chuan-pai [<u>Selaginella tamariscina</u>] 5 ch'ien
            Leaves of tse-lan [<u>Eupatorium</u> sp.]   1 liang

        (3) Medication prepared by pulverizing together
            Ta-huang [rhubarb]   3 ch'ien
              (pan-roasted with wine)
            Crude sheng-ti   3 ch'ien

        (This prescription is suitable for cases of amenorrhea, face flushing, epistaxis, and other patients with a solid pulse).

b. For deficient-type amenorrhea, treatment should regulate and restore energy and blood, using remedies such as the following:

    (1) Concoction of
I-mu ts'ao [motherwort] (dry)	5 ch'ien
Brown sugar	1 liang

        Take whole concoction at bedtime. Take for five nights in a row.

    (2) Pork liver, 3 liang, cooked with seeds of Thuja orientalis (pulverized) 3 ch'ien. Eat whole amount at once, for three days in a row.

    (3) Concoction of
Leaves of tse-lan [Eupatorium sp.]	3 ch'ien
Tang-kuei	3 ch'ien
Pai-shao	3 ch'ien
Moxibustion licorice	5 fen

3. Western medicine

For treating the cause of disease, consider using the following:

a. Vitamin E, 5 gm by mouth, 3 times a day (on average)

b. Progesterone 10 mg, given intramuscularly, once a day for a total of 5 days.

Pelvic Inflammation

Pelvic inflammation is an overall term embracing inflammation of the pelvic organs and tissues such as the uterus, fallopian tubes, ovaries, pelvic-peritoneum or pelvic connective tissue. It occurs mostly in married women due chiefly to bacterial invasion caused by careless sterile technique employed during delivery and abortion procedures and by not observing sanitary practices during the menstrual period. There are two types of pelvic inflammation acute and chronic.

1. Acute Pelvic Inflammation

The signs and symptoms are chills, fever, headache, lower abdominal pain and discomfort heightened by manual palpation, increased leukorrhea which may be pyogenic and has unpleasant odor, dry tongue and parched mouth, apprehension, brown concentrated urine, constipation, a furry yellow tongue, and a rapid and tight pulse.

Prevention

Promotion of modern child delivery technique and good sanitary practices for keeping the external genitals clean after childbirth and during the menstrual period. Make sure that sanitary belts, and paper pads are clean, and avoid sexual intercourse and tub baths during this time.

Treatment

1. <u>New acupuncture therapy</u>. Apply strong stimulation to needles inserted into the "t'ien-shu," "kuan-yuan," "hsueh-hai" and "san-yin-chiao" points, once daily.

2. <u>Chinese herbs</u>. Treatment should clear fever and detoxify, correct the energy and stimulate blood circulation, using remedies such as the following:

    a. Concoction of

Honeysuckle blossoms	1 liang
Forsythia blossoms	1 liang
Hung-t'eng [Sargentodoxa sp.]	1 liang
Pai-chiang ts'ao [Patrinia scabiosaefolia]	1 liang
Tan-p'i	1 ch'ien
Ch'ih-shao	1 ch'ien
Hsuan-hu	1 ch'ien
Peach kernel	2 ch'ien

    b. Concoction of

Lung-tan ts'ao [Gentiana]	3 ch'ien
Shan-yao [Gardenia sp.]	3 ch'ien
Huang-ch'ing	2 ch'ien
Ch'ai-hu [Bupleurum falcatum]	3 ch'ien
Crude ti-huang	5 ch'ien
Tse-hsieh [plantain species]	4 ch'ien
Tang-kuei	3 ch'ien
Che-ch'ien-tzu [Plantago sp.]	4 ch'ien
Mu-t'ung [Akebia trifoliata]	2 ch'ien
Licorice	2 ch'ien

    c. If accompanied by symptoms of a urinary infection, concoction of

Mu-t'ung	3 ch'ien
Chih-mu	3 ch'ien
Huang-pai [Phellodendron sp.]	3 ch'ien
Shan-yao [Gardenia sp.]	3 ch'ien
Pien-hsu [knotgrass Polygonum aviculare]	3 ch'ien
Chu-mai	3 ch'ien
Talc	4 ch'ien
Che-ch'ien tzu	4 ch'ien
Licorice sticks	2 ch'ien

3. Western medicines

   a. Penicillin 200,000 units given intramuscularly, every 6 hours.
      Streptomycin 0.5 gm two times a day. Both drugs can be used
      simultaneously. Or give tetracyline 0.25 gm by mouth, 4 times
      a day.

   b. In cases of post-partum or post-abortion bleeding, motherwort
      extract or ergot extract 3 ml, three times daily, to stop the
      bleeding.

2. Chronic Pelvic Inflammation

This condition is due mostly to inadequate or not soon enough treatment
of acute pelvic inflammation. Its chief clinical manifestations are a dull
ache in the lower abdomen, that is heightened before and after the menstrual
period. Menstrual irregularity may be present, and leukorrhea may be more
profuse. The patient may also be sterile. During an acute or subacute attack
of pelvic inflammation, the symptoms of acute pelvic inflammation may be
present.

Prevention

Timely treatment of acute pelvic inflammation.

Treatment

1. New acupuncture therapy. Apply medium stimulation to needles inserted in "kuan-yuan," "shen-yu," and "san-yin-chiao" points. Pucnture every
other day.

2. Chinese herbs

   a. Concoction of
      Tang-kuei   4 ch'ien
      Dandelion   4 ch'ien
      Ch'ih-shao [Paenia sp.]   4 ch'ien
      Fu-ling   4 ch'ien
      Tan-p'i [peony root bark]   3 ch'ien
      Shan-chih [Gardenia sp.]   3 ch'ien
      Ch'ai-hu [Bupleurum falcatum]   3 ch'ien
      Hsiang-fu [Cyperus rotundus]   3 ch'ien
      Hsuan-hu   3 ch'ien
      Che-ch'ien tzu   5 ch'ien

b. Concoction of

Cinnamon sticks	2 ch'ien
Fu-ling [Poria cocos]	5 ch'ien
Pai-shao [Paenia albiflora]	4 ch'ien
Hsiang-fu [Cyperus sp.]	3 ch'ien
Tang-kuei	3 ch'ien
Hsuan-hu	2 ch'ien

3. Treatment as acute pelvic inflammation for acute or subacute attacks.

Leukorrhea

A small amount of white or light yellow secretion is ordinarily found in the vaginal tract of women. An increase, such as that noted during puberty, before and after the menstrual period and during pregnancy is also normal. However, if there is a marked increase in the secretion ordinarily found, and it has a characteristic unpleasant odor, a change in color or shows a bloody tinge, and pruritus in the vagine is intense, this excessive secretion is termed leukorrhea. This condition is caused mostly by certain gynecological ailments, infections or careless hygiene.

Types

According to different manifestations, leukorrhea is frequently seen as the deficient (hsu cheng) type or the moist-heat (shih-jeh) type of luekorrhea.

The deficient type is characterized by a clear white discharge. Other signs are facial pallor, cool hands and feet, backache and weakness in legs, lassitude, flat taste in mouth, a clear long urinary flow, polyuria, pale uncoated tongue, and a deficient and weak pulse.

The moist-heat type of leukorrhea is characterized by a yellow or bloody discharge, foul-odored, pruritus, brown concentrated urine, constipation, a yellow furred tongue, and a tight or rapid pulse.

Prevention

Cultivation of good hygienic habits and keeping external genitals clean. Change underpants regularly.

Treatment

1. New acupuncture therapy. Apply medium stimulation to needles inserted in the "t'ien-shu," "ch'i-hai," and "san-yin-chiao" points, daily or every other day.

2. Chinese herbs

   a. For <u>deficient type leukorrhea</u>. Treatment should replenish the deficiency and stabilize the roughness, using remedies such as the following:

     (1) Crushed ginkgo nuts, 10, crushed and taken with soybean milk. Repeat for several days.

     (2) Concoction of

Chi-kuan hua [<u>Celosia cristata</u>]	5 ch'ien
Pai pien-tou ['white' white Doliches lablab]	1 liang

     (3) Concoction of

Base stalk of sunflower	4 ch'ien
Brown sugar	1 liang

     (4) Concoction prepared by steaming together

White-leafed wild tung (roots)	5 ch'ien
Cuttlefish bones	8 ch'ien
La hsien-ts'ao [Prickly amaranth]	1 liang
Local tang-shen	5 ch'ien

   b. For <u>moist-heat type of leukorrhea</u>. Treatment should clear fever and promote moisture, using remedies such as the following:

     (1) Concoction of

White root bark of ch'u [Ailanthus altissima]	4 ch'ien
Cuttlefish bones	4 ch'ien
Ts'ang-shu [<u>Atractylis ovata</u>]	3 ch'ien
Phellodendron	3 ch'ien
Tapioca	1 liang

     (2) Concoction prepared from a bunch of tallow tree leaves cooked in the second rinse of rice washings.

     (3) Concoction for bathing external genitals of

Tapioca	2 liang
Huai-shan-yan [<u>Dioscorea babatas</u>]	1 liang
Fu-ling	5 ch'ien
Chien-shih [seed of <u>Euryale ferox</u>]	5 ch'ien

If the discharge is white, add white granulated sugar. If the discharge is bloody, add an egg. If the patient is thin and weak, steam cook concoction with lean meat.

c. External treatment for leukorrhea and pruritus of the external genitals caused by various infections is described as follows:

(1) Concoction of
She-chuang-tzu [Cnidium monnieri]	2 liang
K'u-shen [Sophora flavenscens]	5 ch'ien
Phellodendron	5 ch'ien
Pai-chi [Heracleum lanatum]	5 ch'ien
Alum (heated and dried) (added later)	2 ch'ien

Bathe external genitals with concoction, twice a day.

(2) Pointed leaves from peach tree, 2 liang, washed and crushed by hand, then wrapped in gauze forming a long tube. Insert into vagina and retain for 20 minutes.

(3) Pulverized mixture of
Dry alum	1 ch'ien
She-chu'ang-tzu [Cnidium sp.]	2 ch'ien

Form into peanut-size pills by adding sufficient vinegar. Wrap in gauze and insert into vagina change daily.

(4) Pulverized alum (heated and dried) 1 liang, pulverized, for adding,in small amount, into water for bathing external genitals.

Uterine Bleeding

Sudden nonstop profuse bleeding from the vagina is termed "peng" or metorrhagia; nonstop flow of blood in dribbles and trickles from the vagina is termed "lou" or spotting. Together "peng-lou" refers to profuse and lesser amounts of uterine bleeding. The condition is due generally to certain gynecological diseases, blood diseases or tumor of the internal genital organs.

Types

Seen more frequently are two forms: the blood-energy deficient form and the blood-clot obstructing form, with the deficient (hsu) type occurring more frequently than the solid (shih) type.

The deficient type is characterized by intermittent nonstop bleeding over a long period in profuse amounts, pink or bright red, mental exhaustion, poor appetite, facial pallor, palpitation, dyspnea, lethargy, a pale fur-less tongue and a fine weak pulse.

The solid type is characterized by continuous discharge or bleeding in moderate amounts, purplish black clots, pain in lower abdomen, tenderness to touch, restlessness and apprehensions, petechial or red tongue, and a rapid or sunken and rough pulse.

Prevention

1. Abstention from sexual intercourse during the menstrual period. Avoid fatigue and highly seasoned foods and condiments.

2. Suitable amount of rest after childbirth. Make sure that the new mother has regained all her strength before going back to work in productive labor.

3. Timely treatment for premature menstruation once discovered that the amounts have become increasingly heavy.

Treatment

1. New acupuncture therapy

    a. Use medium stimulation on needles inserted into the "kuan-yuan," "hsueh-hai" and "san-yin-chiao" points, once daily.

    b. Moxibustion to the "yin-pai" (paired), each given a once-over flaming.

2. Chinese herbs

    a. For deficiency uterine bleeding. Treatment should restore the energy and stop bleeding, with remedies such as the following:

        (1) Concoction of following [for internal consumption]

Huang-ch'i [Astragalus hoantchy]	5 ch'ien
Tang-shen [Campanumaea pilosula]	4 ch'ien
Tang-kuei	3 ch'ien
Pai-shu [Atractylis ovata]	3 ch'ien
Meats of longana [fruit]	3 ch'ien
Dates	3 ch'ien
Mu-hsiang [Saussurea lappa]	1 ch'ien
Toasted yuan-chih [Polygala tenuifolia]	2 ch'ien
Sheng-ma [skunk bugbane]	2 ch'ien
Moxa	2 ch'ien

        (2) Concoction of

A-chiao [donkey-hide glue]	4 ch'ien
Ashes of moxa leaves	2 ch'ien
Tang-kuei	3 ch'ien
Processed ti-huang [Rehmannia glutinosa]	4 ch'ien
Pai-shao [Paenia albiflora]	3 ch'ien
Ashes of ti-yu [Sanguisorba sp.]	4 ch'ien
Hsueh-yu-t'an [burnt hairs]	3 ch'ien

(3) Pulverized lotus seed-case (burnt), taken with boiled water, twice daily.

(4) Mixture of
Hsueh-yu-t'an [burnt hairs]	2 ch'ien
Ch'en-tsung-tan	2 ch'ien
Pai-ts'ao hsiang	2 ch'ien

Added to half cup boy's urine, for taking by mouth.

b. For <u>solid-type uterine bleeding</u>. Treatment should clear fever and prevent the bleeding, using remedies such as the following:

(1) Concoction of
Chih-mu [<u>Anamarrhena asphodeloides</u>]	4 ch'ien
Huang-pai [<u>Phellodendron</u>] (pan fried with salt water	3 ch'ien
Tang-kuei	4 ch'ien
Hsiang-fu [<u>Cyperus</u> sp.]	3 ch'ien
Crude ti-huang	1 liang
Pai-shao [<u>Paenia</u> sp.]	4 ch'ien
Ch'uan-kung [<u>Conioselinum unvittatum</u>]	1 ch'ien
Leaves of tse-lan [<u>Lycopus lucidus</u>]	3 ch'ien
San-ch'i [<u>Gynura segetum</u>]	1 ch'ien

(2)
Tse-pai [<u>Thuja orientalis</u>]	3 ch'ien
Mugwort	3 ch'ien
I-mu ts'ao [motherwort]	3 ch'ien

(3) Concoction of
Tang-shen [<u>Campanumaca pilosula</u>]	3 ch'ien
Tan-shen [<u>Salvia multiorrhiza</u>]	3 ch'ien
Tang-kuei	3 ch'ien
Aster	3 ch'ien
Ashes of bat droppings	3 ch'ien
Ashes of p'u-huang [<u>Typha</u> sp.]	3 ch'ien
Ashes of ching-chieh [<u>Nepeta japonica</u>]	1.5 ch'ien
Ting-hsiang [<u>Carophyllus aromaticus</u>]	5 fen

3. Western medicines

If bleeding does not stop, immediately give I.M. injection of methyl testosterone 25 mg to help stop it. If bleeding persists, repeat 1-3 shots. This may induce a temporary hemostatic effect.

Other anti-coagulants may be used selectively, depending on the patient's condition.

Prolapse of Uterus

Prolapse of the uterus termed "yin-t'ing" or "yin-ch'ia" by the local populace refers to the uterus sagging or protruding outside the vagina. Depending on the extent of the prolapse, it may be considered as light, moderate or severe. This ailment occurs mostly among women working at physical labor. It is due chiefly to inadequate recuperation from childbirth whereby the central energy is depressed when the physical condition of the body is still weak, or due to invasion of moisture-heat (shih-jeh) under the circumstances.

Types

Clinically, prolapse of the uterus is seen as the energy-deficient (ch'i-hsu) type or the moisture-heat (shih-jeh) type.

The energy-deficient type of uterine prolapse is characterized by a sagging of the uterus into the vagina or a partial protrusion of it outside. The lower abdomen frequently experiences a distended and "pulling down" sensation, the organ very easily prolapsed upon bearing down or squatting. However, it retracts automatically when the patient lies down to rest. Also present may be mental apathy, palpitation, dyspnea, weakness, frequent urination, thin loose stools, increased leukorrhea, a lightly furred pale tongue, and a deficient and weak pulse.

The moist-heat type of uterine prolapse is characterized by an irreversible prolapse that cannot be retracted after a period of time. Other signs are painful swelling, ulceration, a watery yellow discharge, a weighted-down sagging feeling in the lower abdomen, backache, increased leukorrhea, a yellow concentrated urine, constipation, a yellow and oily fur on tongue, and a tight and rapid pulse.

Prevention

A good program of maternal health and birth control planning. Effect a system that protects women during the menstrual period, pregnancy, parturition, and lactation. Promote the new modern method of birth delivery. Repair perineal tears in time. Allow adequate rest during the post-partum period, and keep patient from engaging in heavy work for 6 weeks.

Treatment

1. New acupuncture therapy

   a. Apply medium stimulation to needles inserted in the "kuan-yuan," "san-yin-chiao," points, in treatment given once a day.

   b. Apply moxibustion to "pai-hui" point using wheat grain, about 5 to 7 flamings each time.

c. Shallow-puncture the "pai-hui" using hao-chen [fine needles] until skin begins to bleed. Cover with a suitable amount of crushed castor beans. Change dressing every 24 hours. If the uterus has retracted, then remove medication and wash off residue.

2. Chinese herbs

a. For energy-deficient type. Treatment should restore the central energy by supporting and elevating it, using remedies such as the following:

(1) Concoction of
Huang-ch'i [Astragalus hoantchy]   1 liang
Tang-shen [Campanameae sp.]   5 ch'ien
I-mu ts'ao [motherwort]   5 ch'ien
Sheng-ma [Cimicifuga foetida]   3 ch'ien

(2) Pu-chung I-ch'i wan (patent medicine) 3 ch'ien each time, two times a day.

(3) Steam-cooked hen in broth, prepared with the following herbs:
Roots of chin-ying-tzu [Rosa laevigata] 4 liang
Roots of p'i-ma [Castar plant]   4 liang
Roots of cotton plant   1 liang
I-mu ts'ao [motherwort]   1 liang

b. For the moist-heat type. Treatment should clear fever and promote [excess] moisture removal until symptoms show change for better. Then follow with medications to restore energy and raise [its level].

(1) Concoction of
Lung-tan ts'ao [gentiana]   2 ch'ien
Huang-ch'ing [Vitex negundo]   1.5 ch'ien
Hei-chih [Black gardenia?]   3 ch'ien
Tse-hsieh [Alisma plantago]   3 ch'ien
Ch'ai-hu [Bupleurum falcatum]   1 ch'ien
Tang-kuei   2 ch'ien
Mu-t'ung [Akebia trifoliata]   2 ch'ien
Ch'e-ch'ien-tzu [Plantago sp.]   3 ch'ien
Licorice   1 ch'ien

(2) Concoction of following for bathing affected organ
She-ch'uang-tzu [Cnidium monnieri]   1 liang
K'u-shen [Sophora sp.]   1 liang
Dried alum   3 ch'ien
Wu-p'ei-tzu [Chinese gall]   3 ch'ien

- 498 -

Vomiting of Pregnancy

The vomiting of pregnancy is also termed "wu-ts'ao" [bad obstruction].
It frequently begins after the 6th week of pregnancy and continues on for 4
to 6 weeks before dissipating. The severity of the vomiting varies with different individuals. In mild cases, there is only a feeling of nausea and some
vomiting the first thing in the morning upon awakening. In severe cases, the
vomiting is more pronounced, occurring possibly several times in a day. This
is one of the characteristic signs of pregnancy.

Types

Because of differences in signs and manifestations, the vomiting of
pregnancy is generally considered in three forms: the stomach/spleen deficient-
weak (p'i-wei hsu-yao) type, the excess mucus [sputum] obstructive (shih-t'an
ts'o-chi) type, and the gastric fever regurgitating (wei-jeh shang-I) type.

The stomach/spleen deficient-weak type is characterized by vomiting,
feeling of fullness in chest and mouth, aversion to eating and vomiting upon
ingestion of food, mental apathy, lethargy, pale white fur on tongue, and a
slippery and weak pulse.

The excess mucus obstructive type of vomiting is noted more often in
women of plump build. It is characterized by a mucus-type of vomitus, chest
discomfort, palpitation, dizziness, flat taste in mouth, a white and oily furred
tongue, and a slippery pulse.

The gastric fever regurgitating type is characterized by a "vomitus"
consisting mostly of bitter fluid [bile] and acid [HCl], restlessness and
apprehension, an affinity for cold food, a yellow-furred tongue, and a slippery
and rapid pulse.

Treatment

1. New acupuncture therapy. Apply medium stimulation to the "nei-kuan"
and retain needle for 30 minutes. Give treatment daily.

2. Chinese herbs

a. For stomach/spleen deficient-weak type, treatment should invigorate the stomach and stop the vomiting, using medications such
as the following:

(1) Pulverized mixture of
Processed hsiang-fu [Cyperus rotundus] 1 liang
Leaves of hua-hsiang [Agastache rugosa] 5 ch'ien
Sha-jen [Amomum xanthiodes]   2 ch'ien
Each dose, 2 ch'ien to be taken with some boiled water.

(2) Concoction of
    Tsao-hsin t'u [stove ashes] (wrapped)   2 liang
    Toasted ginger slices   3

(3) Concoction of
    Dried orange peel   2 ch'ien
    Processed pan-hsia [Pinellia ternata]   3 ch'ien
    Bamboo shoots   3 ch'ien
    Black prunes   2 ch'ien
    Stove ashes (wrapped)   1 liang
    Fresh ginger   3 slices

b. For the excess mucus obstructive type, treatment should resolve
the sputum and stop and vomiting, using drugs such as the
following:

(1) Concoction of
    Processed pan-hsia [Pinellia sp]   3 ch'ien
    Fu-ling [Poria cocos]   5 ch'ien
    Fresh ginger   3 slices

(2) Concoction of
    Processed pan-hsia [Pinellia sp.]   3 ch'ien
    Pan-roasted pai-shu [Atractylis ovata]   3 ch'ien
    Fu-ling [Poria cocos]   3 ch'ien
    Huang-ch'ing [Scutellaria baicalensis]   1.5 ch'ien
    Dried orange peel   1.5 ch'ien
    Chih-he [Poncirus trifoliata]   2 ch'ien
    Toasted licorice   1 ch'ien

c. For the gastric fever regurgitating type of vomiting, treatment
should clear fever to relieve the vomiting, using remedies such
as the following:

(1) Ssu hsieh   1.5 ch'ien
    Huang-lien [Coptis chinensis]   8 fen
    Steep in boiling water and drink as tea.

(2) Concoction of
    Fresh bamboo shoots   3 ch'ien
    Mai-tung [Liriope graminifolia]   3 ch'ien
    Lu-ken [roots of bulrush]   4 ch'ien
    Dried orange peel   1 ch'ien
    Coptis chinensis   8 fen

Mastitis

Mastitis, also called "ju-yung" [breast abscess] is an ailment frequently seen among women during lactation. It is caused by invasion of pyogenic bacteria through cracked and fissured nipples. At onset, the breast is red and painful, nodular and hard, the milk flow obstructed. At the same time chills, fever, headache, myalgia, and a heavy uncomfortable feeling in the chest are noted. The mouth is dry and nausea may be present. After several days, the swelling growns larger and a throbbing pain is felt. This proves that after an abscess has formed, it will break, and pus or fluid will be discharged. Fur on tongue is thin and white or yellow, and the pulse is usually rapid, taut and smooth.

Prevention

During the latter stage of pregnancy, rub the nipples once or twice daily with a hot towel. After childbirth, pay attention to nipple cleanliness, and adhere to a nursing schedule for feeding. Make sure that the breast is emptied at each feeding. Should the nipples become cracked, treat immediately. (May use cooked lard mixed with the powdered sheng-chi san for application over cracked nipples).

Treatment

1. **Local treatment**. In the beginning use warm and moist towels as compresses over affected area, for about 15 minutes, 3-5 times a day, to help relieve the local congestion.

2. **New acupuncture therapy**. Use moderate stimulation on needles inserted into the "chien-ching," "t'an-chung," and "ho-ku" points in acupuncture treatment given once daily. Use cupping technique locally (making sure that opening of the cup is larger than the swelling). This is very effective during the early stages of painful swelling.

3. **Chinese herbs**

   a. During early stage of infection, treatment should reduce swelling and detoxify body of poisons, using remedies such as the following:

   (1) Concoction of
   Dandelion   2 liang
   Honeysuckle flowers   2 liang

   (2) Concoction prepared from 2 ch'ien pulverized shan tzu-ku with 1 liang of roots of ch'u-ma [Bochmeria nivea]

- 501 -

(3) Poultice prepared from crushing the following:

Dandelion	3 liang
Fresh leeks [bulbs]	10
Fresh leaves of yeh-chu	1 liang
Chrysanthemum indicus	

(4) Suitable amount of violets, crushed, for external application.

b. During pus-drainage stage, treatment should promote drainage and neutralize toxins, using remedies such as following:

(1) Fresh huang-ch'i [Astragalus hoantchy]   5 ch'ien
Honeysuckle flowers   5 ch'ien
Tang-kuei   3 ch'ien
Licorice   1 ch'ien

(2) Suitable amounts of the following, cleaned and crushed, and added to a suitable amount of rice washings
Creeping violets
Lien-ch'ien ts'ao [ground ivy]
Ta chin-chi wei [Pteris multifada]
Shan-chi-chiao [Litsea cubeba]

(3) Application prepared from flowers and leaves of fu-jung [Hibiscus mutabilis] 4 liang and brown sugar, a suitable amount. Crush before use.

(4) Processed gypsum 1 liang, and camphor 2 fen, pulverized separately, and use for sprinkling over affected breast.

(This preparation is used in cases where the pus had already completed draining, but wound is hard to eat.

Puerperal Sepsis

Puerperal sepsis, termed "ch'an-yu jeh [puerperal fever] is also called "yueh-tze ping" [month-old disease]. Its occurrence is due largely to careless hygiene and inadequate sterilization of delivery instruments, which allows bacterial invasion to set in and cause infection of the reproduction organs. Its clinical symptoms are fever, chills, headache, general malaise, a profuse, brownish-red and muddy, and smelly lochia. Examination will show poor contraction of the uterus and marked tenderness of the lower abdomen.

Prevention

1. Absolute abstinence from sexual relations for two months before delivery. Pay strict attention to personal hygiene.

2. Use of modern delivery [midwifery] method with strict adherence to asepsis technique. Observe good nursing practice during the post-partum period, with particular attention to those patients with post-partum bleeding and damage to the birth canal, to prevent infection.

Treatment

1. _Elevating head of patient_. Place her in semirecumbent position to promote good drainage of lochia.

2. _Chinese herbs._ Treatment should clear fever and eliminate toxins, break up clots and promote new tissue growth, with remedies such as the following:

a. Concoction of

Ch'ai-hu [Bupleurum falcatum]	5 ch'ien
Huang-ch'ing	3 ch'ien
T'iao-shen [ginseng sticks?]	3 ch'ien
Tang-kuei	3 ch'ien
Crude ti-huang	3 ch'ien
Pai-chao [Paenia albiflora]	3 ch'ien
Ch'uan-tung [Conioselinum unvittatum]	1.5 ch'ien
Dandelion	1 liang

b. Concoction of

Tang-kuei	3 ch'ien
Ch'uan-kung	2 ch'ien
Roasted ginger	5 fen
I-mu ts'ao [Leonurus-sibirieus]	1 liang
Peach kernel	2 ch'ien
Pai-chiang ts'ao [Patrinia scabiosaefolia]	1 liang
Hung-t'eng	1 liang
Lien-ch'iao [forsythia]	1 liang
Yen-hua [honeysuckle]	5 ch'ien

3. Western medicines

Pencillin 200,000 units given intramuscularly, every 6-8 hours. When necessary, additional injections of streptomycin 0.5 gm intramuscularly may be given twice daily.

Post-Partum Hemorrhage

Post-partum, also termed "ch'an hou hsueh-peng" [post-partum metrorrhagia], is caused chiefly by poor contraction of the uterus, retention of placental, birth canal damage, or blood diseases. The patient's physical condition may affect clinical manifestations such as the amount and rate of bleeding. If a large volume of blood loss occurs within a short time, signs and symptoms of acute anemia and shock may set in -- facial pallor, cold extremities, rapid and thready pulse, blood pressure drop, etc.

Types

Clinically, post-partum hemorrhage is seen in three forms: the energy-deficient (ch'i-hsu) type, the blood-heated (hsueh-jeh) type, and the blood-clot (hsueh-yen) type.

The energy deficient type of post-partum hemorrhage is characterized mostly by absence of abdominal pain, profuse bleeding that is red or light in color.

The blood-heated type is characterized by profuse bleeding which is bright red, parched mouth, and apprension.

The blood-clot type is frequently characterized by abdominal pain and discharge of purplish-black blood containing numerous clots.

Prevention

1. Calcium preparations and vitamins C and K to be started a week before the estimated birth arrival date. Check placenta after its ejection at birth, to see if it is still intact. Also give uterus-contracting agents by injection.

2. Repair of birth canal damage and perineal tears.

3. New modern method of delivery to be used to prevent bacterial infection.

Treatment

1. General

   a. Have puerpera lie flat in bed. Elevate the foot of bed, give hot drinks of sugared water.

   b. Feel for the uterus over the abdomen. Apply pressure to force out blood clots. Continue until the uterus becomes hard.

2. New acupuncture therapy. Apply a medium amount of stimulation to needles inserted into the "san-yin chiao" and "hsueh-hai" points. Or use wheat grain in moxibustion over the "yin-pai" point, giving it 3-4 flamings.

3. Chinese herbs. Refer to section on "Metrorrhagia."

4. __Western medicines__

    a. __Uterine contraction agent__. Give oxytocin 5-10 units (or 5-10 units of pituitrin).

    b. __Hemostatic drugs__. Intramuscular injection of vitamin K_3 4 mg, vitamin C 500 mg or agrinomine 5 ml.

Retained Placenta

    If after the foetus has been delivered and the placenta cannot deliver itself spontaneously over a period of time, this is called a retained placenta. It is due chiefly to the weak physical condition of the puerpera, an overly long period of labor, or exposure to cold during labor, so that the energy and blood circulation is affected. As the result, the capacity for uterine activity is weakened, and it cannot force expulsion of the placenta.

__Types__

    Clinically energy-deficient (ch'i hsu) and cold condensing (han-ying) forms of retained placenta are seen most frequently. If not treated in time, the consequence is frequently post-partum metrorrhagia endangering the life of the puerpera. Care must be taken.

    The __energy-deficient form__ of retained placenta is characterized by placenta retention, distension of lower abdomen, profuse bleeding, facial pallor, palpitation, dyspnea, chills, dizziness and weakness, possibly coma, flat taste in tongue, and a deficient and weak pulse.

    The __cold-condensing form__ of retained placenta is characterized by placenta retention, a cold aching pain in the lower abdomen, tenderness in the area, a less than excessive amount of bleeding, facial pallor, nausea, a flat-taste to the tongue, and a tight and rough pulse.

__Treatment__

    1. __New acupuncture therapy__. Apply medium stimulation to needle inserted into the "chung-chi" point. Use wheat-grain moxibustion on the "chih-yin" point, giving it 1-3 flamings.

    2. __Chinese herbs__

        a. For the __energy-deficient type__, treatment should supplement the energy and restore the blood in order to expel clots, with remedies such as the following:

(1) Concoction of
     Huang-ch'i [Astragatus hoantchy]   4 ch'ien
     Tang-shen [Campanumeae pilosula]   3 ch'ien
     Tang Kuei   2 ch'ien
     Pai-shu [Atractylis ovata]   2 ch'ien
     I-mu ts'ao [Leonurus sibiricus]   5 ch'ien
     Licorice   1 ch'ien

(2) Concoction of
     Tang-kuei   5 ch'ien
     Ch'uan kung [Conioselinum unvittatum]   2 ch'ien
     Peach kernel   2 ch'ien
     Roasted ginger   1.5 ch'ien
     Tang-shen   3 ch'ien
     I-mu ts'ao   5 ch'ien
     Moxa   2 ch'ien

(3) Ointment prepared from 1 liang of pulverized castor bean,
     for application over "yung-ch'uan" point. Remove and wash
     after placenta has been expelled.

b. For the cold-condensing type, treatment should warm the meridians
    to dispel the chill, stimulate blood circulation to expel clots,
    using remedies such as the following:

(1) Concoction of
     Shu-ti [processed ti-huang]   3 ch'ien
     Tang-kuei end pieces   3 ch'ien
     Ch'ih-shao   2 ch'ien
     P'u-huang [Typha latifolia]   2 ch'ien
     Kuei-hsin [Cinnamon sticks]   1 ch'ien
     Roasted ginger   1.5 ch'ien
     Black soybean (pan roasted)   5 ch'ien
     Licorice   1 ch'ien

(2) Pulverized
     Pan-roasted p'u-huang   3 ch'ien
     Bat droppings   3 ch'ien

     Take with warmed wine.

(3) Pulverized burnt [semi-burnt] disk of sunflower to which
     is added 2 liang of sugar. Take with wine.

(4) Concoction of
     Tung-kuei tzu [Malva Verticillata]   1 liang
     Niu-hsi [Achyranthes bidentata]   8 ch'ien

     To be mixed with 1/2 cup boy's urine for internal consump-
     tion. Also tickle throat of puerpera with finger or feather
     to induce vomiting which will help expel the placenta.

Inadequate Lactation
[Insufficient Milk Secretion]

Inadequate lactation indicates a lack in the milk supply or a shortage of milk during the lactation period. It is usually seen in blood and energy deficient women not getting proper nourishment during the puerperium. In some instances, it is caused by a congestion of liver energy which disrupts the energy and blood balance. Consequently, the two forms of the energy and blood deficient type and the liver-energy congestion type are more commonly seen.

The energy and blood deficient type of inadequate lactation is characterized by a scanty milk supply or absence of milk noted during the puerperium. The breasts are soft and not painful, accompanied by signs of facial pallor, dry skin, some apathy, dizziness, dyspnea, poor appetite, loose stools, a pale furless tongue, and a fine and deficient pulse.

The liver-congestion type is characterized by a lack of milk during the puerperium, distended and painful breasts, nausea and discomfort, restlessness, bad temper, poor appetite, a yellow-furred tongue, and a tight pulse.

Treatment

1. New acupuncture therapy. Apply medium stimulation to needles inserted in the "t'an-chung," "shao-tse," and "tsu-san-li" points, and apply moxibustion to the "tan-chung" additionally, every other day.

2. Chinese herbs

    a. For the energy-blood deficient type, treatment should supplement the energy and blood, with remedies such as the following:

        (1) Well-cooked dish of food, prepared from

Fresh shrimp	4 liang
Sweet wine	1/2 chin
Sugar	2 liang

        (2) Special dish prepared from

Huang-ch'i [Astragalus hoantchy]	5 ch'ien
Tang-kuei	3 ch'ien
Hsuan ts'ao [Miscanthus sinensis]	1 liang
Wang-pu-liu-hsing [cow soapwort]	3 ch'ien
T'ung ts'ao [Tetrapanax papyrifera]	3 ch'ien
Pig's feet	1 foot

Steam until well done.

(3) Special dish, prepared from

Toasted huang-ch'i [Astragalus hoantchy]	3 ch'ien
Tang-kuei	3 ch'ien
Pan-roasted pai-shu [Atractylis ovata]	2 ch'ien
Huai-shan [Dioscorea batatas]	5 ch'ien
Red dates	1 liang
Meats of lotus seeds	1 liang
Hog's stomach	1 liang

Steam-cook until well done.

b. For liver-energy congestion type of inadequate milk lactation, treatment should loosen up the liver and open up "lo" passageways, using remedies such as the following concoction of

Kua-wei	4 ch'ien
Tangerine, fibrous "string"	2 ch'ien
Green tangerine peel	2 ch'ien
Vegetable sponge fibers	4 ch'ien
Fresh hsiang-fu [Cyperus rotundus]	2 ch'ien
T'ung ts'ao [Miscanthus sinensis]	3 ch'ien
Tang-kuei	2 ch'ien
Wang-pu-liu-hsing [cow soapwort]	3 ch'ien

3. Western medicines

Lactation-inducing pills, 3 times daily, 5 tablets each time.

Section 9   Common Pediatric Ailments

Infantile Convulsions

Infantile convulsions is a common ailment found among a variety of pediatric diseases. Its occurrence poses an urgent situation because of its symptoms -- sudden spasms encountered in the upper and lower extremities, tight clenching of teeth, a roll of the eyes upward, and coma. It is due mostly to certain acute infections, internal ailments, high fever, or sudden fright, vomiting and diarrhea, chronic illness etc. It is generally classified as acute convulsions and chronic convulsions.

1. Acute Convulsions

Acute convulsions are usually caused by high fever. The symptoms are sudden quirks in the hands and feet as if patient were trying to grasp at

something, possible cervical rigidity, clenched teeth, rolling of the eyes
upward, and coma. It is generally seen as the wind-heat (feng-jeh) and the
wind-mucus (feng-t'an) types.

Wind-heat convulsions are characterized by red lips, intense parchness
and thirst, constipation, and scanty reddish urine. Fur on tongue is yellow,
and pulse is rapid and weak.

Wind-mucus convulsions are characterized by the presence of an excessive
amount of saliva and mucus in the mouth, coarse loud breathing, and sound of
mucus stuck in throat. The pulse is slippery and rapid and fur on the tongue
is yellow and oily.

Treatment

1. New acupuncture therapy. Use strong stimulation on needles inserted
into the "yin-t'ang," "jen-chung," "ho-ku," "t'ai-ch'ung" points.

2. Chinese herbs

a. For wind-heat convulsions, treatment should clear fever and
quell the wind, using remedies such as the following:

(1) Concoction of

Chin-yen hua [honeysuckle]   4 ch'ien
Lien-ch'iao [forsythia]   4 ch'ien
Leaves of ta-ch'ing [Clerodendron sp.]   3 ch'ien
Chrysanthemums   3 ch'ien
Fu-ling [Poria cocos]   3 ch'ien
Kou t'eng [Uncaria rhynchophylla]   3 ch'ien

(2) Powdered mixture of
Scorpion, pan-roasted   1 ch'ien
Centipede, pan-roasted   1 ch'ien
One fen each time, twice daily, to be taken with
concoction prepared from 2 ch'ien of mint.

(3) Niu-huang ch'ing-hsin wan (patent medicine), 1 tablet,
taken in 2 doses with boiled water.

(4) Poultice prepared from 7-8 white-necked earthworms,
cleaned and crushed, and applied over navel. Or place
earthworms in sugar which dissolves the worms and ingest
the sugar solution.

b. For <u>wind-mucus convulsions</u>, treatment should clear fever and resolve mucus, using remedies such as the following

    (1) Concoction of
        Kuo-lu-huang, crushed   1-2 liang
        [<u>Lysimachia christinia</u>]
        Kou-t'eng [<u>Uncaria</u> sp.]   4 ch'ien
        Bamboo shoots   2 ch'ien
        Pai-chieh ch'a [a neutralizing tea]   3 ch'ien
        Shui teng-hsin [<u>Juncus effusus</u>]   2 ch'ien
        Take with 5 ch'ien of bamboo drippings.

    (2) Pulverized mixture of
        Tan-nan hsing [<u>Arisaema</u> sp.]   5 ch'ien
        Chih-shih [<u>Poncirus trifoliata</u>]   5 ch'ien
        Huang-lien [<u>Coptis chinensis</u>]   4 ch'ien
        Take 2 ch'ien each time, with some water.

3. <u>Western medicines</u>

    a. Antipyretic: Analgine 5-10 mg/kg/dose, given intramuscularly.

    b. Antispasmodic: chlorpromazine 1-2 mg/kgm/dose, given intra-muscularly.

2. Chronic Convulsions

Chronic convulsions usually occur following attacks of severe vomiting and diarrhea. Its clinical characteristics do not have the sudden urgency of the acute form. Noted are sporadic spasms, comatosed sleep, nonclosure of eyelids when asleep, mental apathy, low grade fever, or no fever. Because of differences in the infant's physical condition, the symptoms that appear also vary. Generally seen are the yang-deficient (yang-hsu) and yin-deficient (yin-hsu) forms, most of them yang-deficient.

<u>Yang-deficient chronic convulsions</u> are characterized by cyanosis, sallowness, or pallor or facial coloring, vomiting, diarrhea, cold hands and feet, and a perspiring head. Fingerprint lines are pink, and the pulse is rapid and thready.

<u>Yin-deficient chronic convulsions</u> are accompanied by low-grade fever, thirst, restlessness, a flushed face, and sometimes a raspy noise in throat caused by nucus. The tongue is red and furless. The pulse is rapid and thready.

Treatment

1. **New acupuncture therapy**

   a. For <u>yang-deficient chronic convulsions</u>, treatment should restore the stomach/spleen, strengthen the yang and supplement the yin, using remedies such as the following:

       (1) Concoction of

Tang shen	3 ch'ien
Pai shu [<u>Atractylis ovata</u>]	3 ch'ien
Fu-ling	3 ch'ien
Toasted licorice	1 ch'ien
Dried ginger	1 ch'ien
Cinnamon	5 fen
Ting-hsiang [<u>Carophyllus aromaticus</u>]	5 fen

       (2) Filtered concoction of

Hu-chiao [pepper]	1 ch'ien
Toasted ginger	1 ch'ien
Cinnamon	1 ch'ien
Ting-hsiang	10 grains
Stove ashes	3 liang

   Allow concoction to settle. Pour off the clear portion and cook again [the clear portion] before ingestion.

       (3) Toasted and pulverized mixture of

Centipede	1
Beehive	2 ch'ien

   Divide into 5 packets. Take 1 packet each time with sweet wine, twice a day.

   b. For <u>yin-deficient chronic convulsions</u>, treatment should nourish the yin and restore body balance, using remedies such as the following:

Preparation using	
Egg yolk	1
Roasted oyster	3 ch'ien
A-chiao [donkeyhide glue]	2 ch'ien
Tortoise shell	2 ch'ien
Boy's urine	1 cup

   To prepare: First cook the oyster, tortoise shell. Then melt donkeyhide glue. Add egg yolk and urine last. Take in one dose. Make sure medication is hot.

3. <u>Western medicines</u>. Tranquillizers and anticonvulsives may be used selectively.

Marasmus (Kan-chi)

Marasmus is a common infantile ailment, which is due to a nutritional imbalance following illness or some injury to the milk supply. There are two kinds of marasmus: parasite-caused marasmus (ch'ung-chi), and dietary marasmus, where food is not properly digested and absorbed. These factors can cause infantile malnutrition, and result in marasmus. This ailment mostly involves deficiency/damage in the stomach/spleen, and the manifest symptoms frequently are quite complex. Characteristics of this disease are a bloated abdomen and skinny arms and legs.

Types

Generally, the solid type (shih-cheng), the deficienvy type (hsu-cheng) and the ocular involving type (yen-kan) are the three forms more commonly seen.

The solid type of ailment is characterized by a flushed face, restlessness, fretfulness and crying, a hard dry stool, scanty brown urine, and cyanosed fingertips.

The deficiency-type of marasmus is characterized by rosy checks with facial pallor, dry lips, an aversion to water, emaciation, mental apathy, diarrhea, clear urinary flow, and pink fingertips.

The ocular-involving type is characterized by red and swollen eyelids, pupils covered by a film, whites of the eyes bloodshot, night blindness, excessive lacrimation and difficulty in opening eyes. The pulse is tight and weak.

Prevention

1. Additional powdered milk or other easily digested food to be given in time when the maternal milk supply is inadequate. Start infant on food supplements earlier. Generally, congee, egg yolk and pureed vegetables may be given by time the infant is 6 months old.

2. Additional vitamin supplements.

3. Active measures to prevents and treat parasitical and other diseases.

Treatment

1. New acupuncture therapy.

   a. At the "szu-feng" point, insert needle intradermally, to a depth of 0.5-1 fen, after which squeeze dry with cotton. Repeat treatment every other day.

- 512 -

b. At "p'i-yu," "chung-wan," and "tsu-san-li" points, apply strong stimulation. Needle once daily.

2. <u>Spinal pinch-pull therapy</u> (nieh-chi liao-fa)

Apply pinch-pull technique to patient's spine, once in early morning before patient has had any food for 6 days in a row which is one course of therapy (refer to Chapter IV, section on "Spinal Pinch-Pull")

3. <u>Incision therapy</u>

Make a straight incision on the "ju-chi" area of palm located between the 2nd and 3rd digits.

4. <u>Chinese herbs</u>

a. For the solid-type ailment, treatment should reduce the "accumulation" and kill the parasites, with remedies such as the following.

(1) Powdered chiao-chuang [<u>Justicia</u> sp.] (dried), 2 ch'ien each time, taken with brown sugar water.

(2) Pulverized mixture of the following taken in specified doses:

Shan-cha [Hawthorne]	2 liang
Shen-ch'u	2 liang
Egg shells	2 liang
Cicada molting	2 liang
Betelnut	2.5 liang
Grain sprouts, roasted	2.5 liang

Dosage: for 1-3 years, 3 fen; 3-9 years, 6 fen; 9-12 years, 1 ch'ien; and over 12 years of age, 2 ch'ien each time, taken with some warm boiled water, three times daily.

(3) Pulverized mixture of the following taken in specified doses:

Shih-chun-tzu [<u>Quisqualis indica</u>]	5 ch'ien
K'u lien bark [<u>Melia</u> sp.]	5 ch'ien
Chiang-t'i [ginger]	4 ch'ien
Lei-wan [<u>Omphalia lapidecens</u>]	5 ch'ien
Fresh licorice	1.5 ch'ien

Dosage: For 1-3 years, 2-5 fen each time; for 3-9 years, 4-8 fen; for 9-12 years, 8 fen to 1 ch'ien. To be taken twice daily with some cool boiled water. Discontinue medication after 3-day course. After one week, resume 3-day regimen again. This prescription is used chiefly as an anthelmintic.

b. For the deficiency type of marasmus, treatment should strengthen the stomach/spleen and eliminate marasmus, with remedies such as the following:

(1) Concoction of
Huan-shan-yao [Dioscorea batatas]   3 ch'ien
Shih-chun-tzu [Quisqualis indica]   2 ch'ien
Dried tangerine peel   1 ch'ien
Chi-nei-chin   8 fen
Sha-shen [Adenophora stricta]   2 ch'ien

(2) Concoction of
Hu-t'o-tzu [Elacagnus pungens] (roots) 1 liang
T'ieh sao-chou [Lespedeza sp.]
Preheat in honey before concocting.

c. For the ocular-involving type of marasmus, treatment should restore the liver to promote clear vision, with remedies such as the following:

(1) Pulverized mixture of the following given in specified doses:
Ti-erh ts'ao   3 ch'ien
Fen-t'iao erh ts'ai   5 ch'ien
Chi-nei-chin   5 ch'ien
Shih-ch'ueh-ming   3 ch'ien
Chi-chiu-ch'u [brewer's yeast?]   4 liang
Dosage: For children under 3 years of age, 1 ch'ien each time; and 3-10 years, 2 ch'ien, taken with brown sugar water. To be taken 3 times a day, for 3-5 days in succession. Or steam with pork liver and eggs, to be eaten.

(2) Pulverized mixture of
Yeh-ming-sha [Bat droppings]   4 liang
Mi-meng hua [Buddlea officinalis]
Pai-shao [Paenia albiflora]   3 liang
Divide in 3 doses, and steam with pork liver for eating.

(3) Pulverized mixture of following after preliminary processing:
Fei-tzu [Torreya nucifera],   3 ch'ien
Pan-fry until it emits aroma
Mu-pi [Momordica sp.]   3 ch'ien
Pan-fry until it emits aroma
Yeh-ming-sha [Bat droppings]   6 ch'ien
warm dry to evaporate moisture
Sift and mix thoroughly. To use: Take 1 ch'ien of powder each time, place with 1 unwashed chicken liver in an enamel cup without any seasoning or oil, and steam cook until done. Eat contents 1 hour before mealtime. Do not drink any liquids with it.

Rickets

Rickets is also called "jan-ku ping," meaning "soft-bone disease." It is caused by non-absorption of calcium in the body, the result of a calcium deficiency in the diet, inadequate exposure to sunshine, or lack of Vitamin D in the body. Traditional Chinese medicine regards the ailment as the result of spleen and kidney insufficiency, and energy and blood deficiency. It is seen mostly in infants under 3 years of age, in those whose anterior fontanels still have not closed by the age of two, who show delayed dental eruption, large articulations between ribs and cartilage, that resemble a string of beads, a protruding rib cage in front and a protruding spine in back resembling a turtle hump, and curved and deformed-looking extremities (particularly noticeable in the lower limbs, sometimes bowlegged). In others, the cranium is square-shaped. In mild cases, the only signs may be fretfulness, ill temper, disturbed slumber, hidrosis, anorexia, muscular weakness, slow physical develop-ment etc. The mild cases are easier to treat. In severe cases where deformi-ties have set in, treatment may restore skeletal growth function, but the deformities cannot be corrected spontaneously.

Prevention

1. Sunbathing in appropriate amounts for infants within a month after birth.

2. Promotion of nursing by mothers. Include food supplements such as egg yolks to infant's diet after 6 months. Bottle-fed babies should have vitamins and calcium added to make up for nutritional deficiencies.

3. Including large amounts of fresh vegetables in the everyday diet.

Treatment

1. Frequent sunbathing. Include foods rich in vitamin D (such as egg yolks, fish fry, etc.). Also give more fresh vegetables to add more calcium and phosphorus to the diet.

2. New acupuncture therapy. Use medium stimulation on needles inserted into the "ta-chui," "p'i-yu," "shen-yu," "kuan-yuan," and "tsu-san-li" points, once a day. Or use wheat-grain moxibustion to one or two points, giving each point 2 to 3 flamings each time.

3. Massage therapy (t'ui-na fa). Use spinal pinch-pull technique, 2 to 3 times each day.

4. Chinese herbs. Treatment should supplement the spleen and kidney, using remedies such as the following:

a. Crushed pan-fried egg shell, pulverized. Take with some boiled water, 5 fen each time, 3 times daily.

b. Pulverized mixture of

Shen-ch'u	3 liang
Wheat sprouts	2 liang
Yellow soybean	1 liang
(pan-stirred till done)	
Calcium lactate	2 liang
(eggshells, browned and pulverized, 2 liang, may be substitute)	

Dosage: For infants 1-3, 3 fen each time; from 3-9 years, 5 fen to 1 ch'ien each time; 9-12 years, 1-2 ch'ien each time. To be taken 3 times a day with a little boiled water.

c. Pu-shen ti-huang wan (patent medicine) or Kuei-p'i wan (patent medicine), 1-2 ch'ien each dose, twice a day.

5. Western medicines

Cod liver oil, 5-10 ml, 3 times a day, given by mouth. Or, cod liver oil pills and calcium lactate (or calcium gluconate) may be given instead.

Infantile Diarrhea

Infantile diarrhea is a serious ailment of infancy, most commonly seen in the summer and fall. It is due mostly to an inadequate milk supply, over-feeding, unclean [not sanitary] food, or climatic changes. Clinically, the most noticeable symptom is the diarrhea itself, the stool resembling egg drop [like curdled milk?]. It may also be accompanied by vomiting, intestinal gurgling sounds, and abdominal pain. In serious cases, high fever, thirst, respiratory difficulty, cyanosis, lethargy and coma, and even convulsions, may be present.

Types

Infantile diarrhea is frequently seen in three types: the moist-heat (shih-jeh) type, the appetite-losing (sh'ang-shih) type, and the spleen-deficient (p'i-hsu) type.

The moist-heat type of diarrhea is characterized by its rapid onset and severity, averaging over 10 stools daily, and accompanied by vomiting, scanty urination, high fever, thirst, and even coma, and cramps. Frequently, dehydration and acidosis set in because emergency treatment was not given soon enough.

The appetite-losing type of infantile diarrhea is characterized by diarrhea, abdominal distension, abdominal cramps and some relief felt after stool passage, foul-smelling stools, nausea and vomiting, belching, and no appetite. Fur on tongue is thick, yellow, and oily.

The spleen-deficient type of infantile diarrhea is characterized by poor appetite, mental apathy, presence of undigested food in stools, cold hands and feet, and facial pallor. Fur on tongue is white and smooth.

Prevention

Promotion of nursing by mothers. Do not give infant too much food supplement at any one time. Pay attention to sanitary food habits and climatic changes, to prevent exposure to cold or heat.

Treatment

1. Follow rules of strengthening nursing care [practices]:

   a. Clean anal area with warm water after every defecation, and sprinkle talcum powder over area. Change diapers frequently.

   b. Give feedings slowly, with emphasis on frequent small feedings.

   c. For mild cases, curtail the amount of food given. Avoid raw, cold, oily and not easily digested food. For severe cases, temporarily skip feedings for one-half to one day, and give boiled water with salt and/or sugar added. Resume normal diet gradually after the patient's diarrhea seem to improve.

2. New acupuncture therapy

   a. Apply medium stimulation to needles inserted in the "t'ien-shu," "kuan-yuan," and "tsu-san-li" points, once a day. In presence of fever, include the "ch'u-ch'ih" and "ho-ku" points for acupuncture. Also include the "nei-kuan" point when there is vomiting, the "jen-chung" when there is coma, and the "ho-ku" and "tai-ch'ung" when there are cramps.

   b. Prick-puncture the "szu-feng" point until it is possible to squeeze out a small amount of yellow serous fluid.

3. Massage therapy [t'ui-na fa]. Employ spinal-pinch -- pull technique 3-5 times, until the area over the spine becomes hot. Massage abdomen for 5 minutes, rub the navel another 5 minutes, and push the 7th vertebra [in upward direction] 50 times, rub the "kuei-wei" 30 times, the "tsu-san li" 10 times, this treatment being given once daily.

4. **Chinese herbs**

   a. For the <u>moist-heat type of infantile diarrhea</u>, treatment should clear fever and promote moisture removal, using drugs such as the following:

   (1) Concoction of
   Jen-hsien [the <u>hsien ts'ai</u> spinach?]   5 ch'ien
   Ma-ch'ih hsien [portulaca]   5 ch'ien

   (2) Concoction of
   Huo-hsiang [<u>Agastache</u> sp.]   2 ch'ien
   P'ei-lan [<u>Eupatorium</u> sp.]   2 ch'ien
   Hou-pu [<u>Magnolia officinalis</u>]   8 fen
   Dried tangerine peel   5 fen
   Fu-ling [<u>Poria cocos</u>]   3 ch'ien
   Lu-I San   3 ch'ien
   (This prescription is suitable for use at onset of
   diarrhea when fever is absent.)

   b. For the <u>appetite-losing type of infantile diarrhea</u>, treatment should clear up "stagnant collections," using remedies such as the following:

   (1) Pulverized burnt hawthorne and chi-nei-chin in equal parts, 1 ch'ien taken with boiled water, 4 times a day.

   (2) Pao-huo wan (patent medicine), 3 ch'ien, crushed and taken with some water.

   c. For the <u>spleen-deficient type of infantile diarrhea</u>, treatment should strengthen the spleen and restore the stomach, using remedies such as the following:

   (1) Concoction of
   Tang-shen [<u>Campanumeae</u> sp.]   2 ch'ien
   Pai-shu [<u>Atractylis ovata</u>]   1.5 ch'ien
   Fu-ling [<u>Poria cocos</u>]   3 ch'ien
   Licorice   1 ch'ien
   Huo-hsiang [<u>Agastache</u> sp.]   1.5 ch'ien
   Kuang-hsiang   8 fen
   Fen-ko [arrowroot]   2 ch'ien
   (This prescription is suitable for diarrhea, fever, thirst,
   poor appetite, weight loss, and lethargy.)

   (2) Concoction of
   Tangerine peel   1 ch'ien
   Lotus seeds   4 ch'ien
   Seeds of <u>Coix lachryma</u>   5 ch'ien
   Che-ch'ien tzu [<u>Plantago</u> sp.]   2 ch'ien

5. Western medicine

If dehydration of the infant is severe, intravenous supplements may be given. For mild cases, give supplementary fluids by mouth (consisting of sugar 6 ch'ien, table salt 1 ch'ien, and soda bicarbonate 1.5 fen, dissolved in warm boiled water 200 ml).

Thrush

Thrush is seen mostly among infants. It is caused by <u>Candida albicans</u> or other fungus infection of the oral mucous membrane. Malnutrition and careless oral hygiene are predisposing causes.

At onset, milky white spots are noticed on the buccal mucosa and the surface of the tongue. These spots merge later into a large membranous patch that is not easily wiped off. There is excessive salivation, and over a period of time, the infection will spread and affect the pharynx and the nasal cavity. The whole mouth is snowy white and this extensive involvement will affect breathing and swallowing. In serious cases, low-grade fever, restlessness, poor appetite may be noted.

Types

According to variations in symptoms presented, most commonly seen are the solid-heat (shih-jeh) type and the deficient-heat (hsu-jeh) type.

The solid-heat type of thrush is seen mostly in patients presenting flushed complexions, who show signs of restlessness, dry stools, dark scanty urine and cyanotic fingertips.

The deficient-heat type of thrush is seen mostly in patients of pale complexion with rosy cheeks and dry lips. They are aversive to drinking water and are emaciated. Other symptoms are diarrhea, a pale urine and pinkish fingertips.

Prevention

Attention to oral hygiene and active treatment of any systemic disease present to increase body resistance to disease.

Treatment

1. Chinese herbs

   a. For solid-heat type, treatment should clear fever and neutralize toxins, using remedies such as the following:

- 519 -

(1) Concoction of niu-hsi [Achyranthes bidentata], 5 ch'ien to 1 liang.

(2) Concoction of huang pai [Phellodendron sp.] 3 ch'ien. Or pulverize and dust over affected areas.

(3) Pulverized mixture of following for local application

Borax	1 ch'ien
Realgar	1 ch'ien
Camphor	4 fen
Licorice	5 fen

b. For deficient-heat type, treatment should supplement the "hsu," and clear fever, using remedies such as the following:

(1) Concoction of
Huang-ch'i [Astragalus hoantchy] ⎫
Tang-kuei   ⎬ 2 ch'ien of each
Honeysuckle flowers   ⎭
Forsythia

(2) Feng-huang-I (hatched egg shell) roasted dry and pulverized, for blowing into oral cavity, 3 times a day.

(3) Pulverized mixture of

Camphor	5 fen
Borax	6 fen
Chu-sha [cinnabar]	5 fen
Hsuan-ming-fen [Glauber's salt]	5 fen

Add 1 liang of honey and mix well. First rinse mouth. Then apply honeyed mixture over affected areas.

Enuresis

Enuresis, commonly called "niao-chuang" [bed of urine], refers to the unconscious elimination of urine during sleep. Among infants less than 2 years, this is not considered unusual. However, if it occurs among older children and adults, it is due mostly to a deficiency in kidney energy. At the same time, the facies are accompanied by facial pallor, mental apathy, chills, cold hands and feet, polyuria etc. The fur on tongue is white and the pulse is sunken and delayed.

Prevention

Awakening [from sleep] every night at a set time for trip to bathroom to urinate. Cultivate good health habits, and appropriately control fluid intake in the evening.

- 520 -

<u>Treatment</u>

1. <u>New acupuncture therapy</u>. Apply medium stimulation to needles inserted in the "shen-yu," "kuan-yuan," and "san-yin-chiao" points, in acpuncture treatment given once every afternoon. Subject the "shen-ya" and "kuan-yuan" to moxibustion.

2. <u>Chinese herbs</u>. Treatment should supplement the kidney and restore the energy, using remedies such as the following:

a. Steamed hog bladder [for eating] containing the following herbs
Chin-ying tzu	5 ch'ien
Red dates	5 ch'ien
Litchi fruit	5 ch'ien
Hsien-mao [<u>Curculigo</u> sp.]	5 ch'ien

b. Steamed hog's bladder [for eating] containing
Sang piao-hsiao [mantis cocoon]	5 ch'ien
Huai shan [<u>Dioscorea batatas</u>]	5 ch'ien
Wu-yao [<u>Lindera strychnifolia</u>]	2 ch'ien
I-chih kernel	4 ch'ien

c. Cooked preparation [for eating] of following:
Wu-kuei [turtle] meat	0.5 chin
Black soybean	2 liang

d. Chin-so ku-ching wan (patent medicine), 2 ch'ien each time, twice daily.

Nocturnal Fretfulness [Colic]

Intermittent crying done by infants from nightfall to early morning is termed infantile nocturnal fretfulness [colic]. Its ailment is frequently accompanied by colic and few tears in most instances. It is generally seen as heart-heating (hsin-jeh) and spleen-chilling (p'i-han) types.

In <u>heart-heating cases</u> of nocturnal infantile colic, the infant's complexion is ruddy and lips are red. Tears flow freely and generalized fever, restlessness and constipation may be present.

In spleen-chilling cases of nocturnal infantile colic, the outstanding characteristics are facial pallor and pale lips, cool hands and feet, and loose stools.

Prevention

Frequent change of diapers and clothing. Do not wrap blankets and swaddling clothes too tight.

Treatment

1. <u>Massage therapy</u>. Massage balls of thumbs and 3rd fingers 20-30 times and grasp-massage the "tsu-san-li" area 20 times. Technique must be light and gentle.

2. <u>Chinese herbs</u>.

    a. For the <u>heart-heating type of infantile colic</u>, treatment should calm the heart and settle the nerves, using remedies such as the following concoction of

Sheng-ti [crude ti-huang]	1 ch'ien
Mu-t'ung [Akebia trifoliata]	1 ch'ien
Licorice	5 fen
Bamboo leaves	1 ch'ien

    b. For the <u>spleen-chilling type of infantile colic</u>, treatment should warm the "center" and calm the nerves. Using remedies such as the following concoction of

Dried tangerine peel	1 ch'ien
Mu-hsiang [Inula]	5 fen
Roasted ginger	5 fen
Licorice	5 fen
Seed of I-chih [Zingiber nigrum]	5 fen
Fu-ling	1.5 ch'ien

Favisin (Ts'an-tou Huang)

Favisin is an acute hemolytic anemia, that is caused by an allergic reaction to horsebeans, through ingestion of inadequately cooked or uncooked horsebeans, or through direct contact with the fresh horsebean or its pollen. It generally occurs during the horsebean picking season among children 5 to 14 years of age. Its onset is acute, accompanied by fever, headache, nausea, aches in the four extremities, jaundice (due to the hemolysis), and reddish urine. In severe cases, convulsions and coma leading to death may also occur.

Prevention

Educational program directed toward children for them not to eat fresh young horsebeans, nor to pick the blossoms. Fresh horsebeans must be cooked until well done.

Treatment

1. **Chinese herbs.** Treatment should clear the fever and cool the blood using remedies such as the following concoction of

Rhinoceros horns	1.5 ch'ien
(or substitute with 5 ch'ien of buffalo horn tips)	
Tan shen	4 ch'ien
Crude ti-huang	5 ch'ien
Ch'ih-shao	3 ch'ien
Bark of peony root	1.5 ch'ien
P'u-huang [Typha latifolia]	2 ch'ien
Donkey-hide glue	2 ch'ien
Charred luan-t'ou-fa [Achillea sibirica]	1 ch'ien
(converted)	

Modifications of basic prescription:

For fever, add 3 ch'ien each of honeysuckle blossoms and forsythia blossoms.

For jaundice, add hin-ch'en [Artemesia capillaris] 5 ch'ien.

For parchness and constipation, add hsuan-shen [Scrophularia sp.] 4 ch'ien and mai-tung [Ophiopogon japonicus] 3 ch'ien.

For mental confusion, add ch'ien-ch'ang-p'u [Acorus calamus] 5 fen.

For convulsions, add 4 ch'ien each of fresh lung-ch'ih and fresh oysters.

For vomiting, replace the donkey hide glue in prescription with 1 liang of fu-lung-kan [stove ashes].

2. **Western medicine**

Vitamin C 100 mg three times a day. If a low blood sugar coma, the result of not eating, is noted, quickly give 40-60 ml of 50 percent glucose by intravenous injection. If dehydration is noted, treat accordingly and give fluid supplement.

Summer Fever [Heatstroke?]

Summer fever, also termed "shu-jeh cheng" is frequently seen among infants less than 3 years of age. The clinical manifestations are usually a continuous pyrexia that does not recede, with the body temperature hovering between 38° and 40° centigrade. If the weather is stifling hot, the body temperature also rises, accompanied by thirst, polyuria, anhidrosis or some perspiration. Over a period of time, emaciation, facial pallor, restlessness and anorexia will set in. Fur on tongue is thin, white and oily. The pulse is rapid, floating, and weak. Generally, the fever and corresponding symptoms will subside with the advent of cooler weather.

Prevention

1. Cool and well ventilated places of residence recommended for infants with delicate physiques in the summer.

2. Chinese herbs. Tea concocted from 2-3 ch'ien of fresh huo-hsiang [Agastache rugosa].

Treatment

1. New acupuncture therapy. Use light stimulation on needles inserted into the "ch'u-ch'ih," "ho-ku," "tsu-san-li," and "t'ai-ch'ung," points, in treatment given once a day.

2. Massage therapy

Push-massage the area between the "yin-t'ang" to the "t'ai-yang" (in outward direction) 24 times; grasp-massage the "feng-ch'ih" and "chien-ching" 20 times, knead-massage the "ta-chui" 20 times, and push-massage the spine 200 times.

3. Chinese herbs. Treatment should clear summer heat and moisturize dryness, using remedies such as the following:

a. Concoction of
    Chin-ssu ts'ao [Pogonatherum crinitum]   1 liang
    Mai-hu [Bulbophyllum inconspicuum]   5 ch'ien

b. Tea from concoction of silkworm cocoons, 20 of them, without
    breaking cocoons. Modifications: For fever, thirst, polyuria
    and anhidrosis, add mild salted black soybeans 5 ch'ien; for
    cases with hidrosis, add 10 red dates.

c. Concoction of
    Mai-tung [Ophiopogon japonicus]   3 ch'ien
    Shih-hsien-t'ao [Pholidota chinensis]   5 ch'ien
    Tan-chu-hsieh [Lophatherum gracile]   1 ch'ien

d. Concoction of
    Chu-hsieh [bamboo leaves]   2 ch'ien
    Gypsum   5 ch'ien
    T'iao-shen   2 ch'ien
    Processed pan-hsia [Pinellia ternata]   1 ch'ien
    Mai-tung [Ophiopogon japonicus]   3 ch'ien
    Licorice   2 ch'ien
    Rice   1 spoonful

- 524 -

e. Concoction of

Shu-ti [processed ti-huang]	3 ch'ien
Huai-shan [Dioscorea batatas]	3 ch'ien
Fu-ling [Poria cocos]	2 ch'ien
Tan-p'i [bark of peony root]	1.5 ch'ien
Shan-yu [Cornus officinalis]	1.5 ch'ien
Mai-tung [Ophiopogon sp.]	1.5 ch'ien
Mulberry leaves	1.5 ch'ien
Fen-ko [Pueraria pseudohirsuta]	1.5 ch'ien
Licorice	1

4. Western medicine

Antipyretics such as aspirin, antipyrine etc. for high fever. For
poor appetite, vitamin B complex and vitamin C can be given.

Section 10   Diseases of the Sense Organs

Rhinitis

Rhinitis is frequently classified as acute, chronic and allergic.

Acute rhinitis is, most commonly, acute inflammation of the mucous
membrane of the nasal cavity, as seen during bouts of "colds" and "influenza."

Chronic rhinitis is the result of repeated attacks of acute rhinitis
or the effect of exposure to irritating gases over a long period of time. The
chief clinical manifestations are an alternating type of nasal obstruction (right
nostril stopped up when lying on right side, and left nostril stopped up when
lying on left), nasal discharge that may be sticky or purulent, a reduced sense
of smell, and headache.

Allergic rhinitis is characterized by a history of other allergies
(such as asthma, urticaria), and a sudden reaction to certain allergic substances or climatic changes in form of a sudden stopped-up nose, itchy nose,
sneezing, and large amounts of a clear nasal discharge.

Prevention

Strengthened program of physical training to increase body resistance.
Attention to climatic changes, to prevent colds.

Treatment

1. New acupuncture therapy. Apply medium stimulation to needles inserted in the "ying-hsiang" and "ho-ku" points, until nasal passageways are
cleared.

2. **Chinese herbs**. Treatment should loosen up the wind and clear fever, using remedies such as the following:

a. Concoction of
   O-pu-sh'ih ts'ao [Centipeda minima], dried 1 ch'ien
   Hsin-I [Magnolia liliflora]   3 ch'ien
   Ts'ang erh [Xanthium strumarium]   3 ch'ien

b. Pulverized mixture of
   Mao ken [Imperata cylindrica], dry   1 chin
   Nelumbo root, dry [Xanthium strumarium]   1 chin
   Ts'ang-erh [Xanthium strumarium], dry   1 chin
   T'ien-pien-chu [Aster trinervius], dry   5 liang

c. Concoction of
   Ma-huang [Ephedra]   1.5 ch'ien
   Almond [kernel]   3 ch'ien
   Gypsum   5 ch'ien
   Licorice   1 ch'ien

d. Mixture of
   O-pu-sh'ih-tsao [Centipeda minima], pulverized 30 gm
   Glycerine   70 gm
   Use as nose drops.

e. Solution of 10 percent garlic used as nose drops. Drop enough to reach the larynx. Shows good results.

3. **Western medicine**

Nose drops of ephedrine 1 percent, 3-4 times a day.

Sinusitis

Sinusitis is an infection of the sinuses by bacteria introduced from the nasal cavity through blowing the nose or sneezing during the last stage of acute rhinitis or during swimming.

This ailment, also called "pi-yuan" [nasal drip] is characterized by a thick nasal discharge and loss of a sense of smell. Clinically, it may be classified into acute and chronic forms.

Acute sinusitis. Its milder symptoms resembling those for acute rhinitis, include a stopped up nose, nasal discharge, a reduction in the sense of smell. Its more severe symptoms include frontal headache and distension, fever, general malaise, poor appetite, and local tenderness.

Chronic sinusitis. The result of repeated recurrences of acute rhinitis, or its ineffective treatment, the important manifestations are a thick yellow-greenish and foul-smelling nasal discharge, a loss of the sense of smell, head-ache and dizziness, a heavy-headed feeling, inability to concentrate, and for-getfulness.

Prevention

Regular physical training sessions to improve body resistance to disease, to prevent colds, influenza and other respiratory tract infections.

Treatment

1. New acupuncture therapy. Apply medium stimulation to the "yin-t'ang," "ying-hsiang," and "ho-ku" in acupuncture treatments given once a day.

2. Chinese herbs. Treatment should dispel the wind and clear fever, using remedies such as the following:

a. Inhalation of sung-hua fen [pine cone pollen?]

b. Pulverized ts'ang-erh-tzu [Xanthium strumarium] inhaled through nostrils.

c. Tao-tou [Canavallia ensiformis] (mature), roasted and pulverized, mixed with white wine (a suitable amount). Each dose 3 ch'ien, to be taken twice daily.

d. Concoction of

P'u-kung-ying [dandelion]	5 ch'ien
O-pu-sh'ih ts'ao	5 ch'ien
Hsin-I	3 ch'ien
Ts'ang-erh-tzu	3 ch'ien
Pai-chih [Angelica anomala]	3 ch'ien
Hsi-hsin [Asarum sieboldi]	1 ch'ien
Mint	1.5 ch'ien

Modification: ;For foul-smelling nasal discharge, add 3 ch'ien each of huang-ch'ing [Scutellaria baicalensis] and huang-pai [Phellodendron sp.]; for headache, add ch'uan-kung [Conioselinum unvittatum] 1 ch'ien and chrysanthemums 1.5 ch'ien.

Nasal Polyp

Nasal polyp, also termed "pi-chih" [literally nasal hemorrhoid] is the result of a pedunculated growth arising from the nasal mucosa. According to traditional Chinese medicine theory, it is formed by the chronic effect of wind, moisture, and heat on the lungs. Its presence is characterized by an increasing severity to nasal obstruction. The extent of this obstruction may vary according to the size of the polyp. When extremely severe, the nasal cavity can be obstructed completely, so much so that the polyp extends to the nasal vestibule. Large polyps may cause the bridge of the nose to widen, its external appearance full and large, in what is called a "frog-shaped" nose. At the same time, some watery or mucus discharge, accompanied by headache or a dull ache between the eyebrows, may be present. From the outside, a greyish white or light pink semi-translucent pedunculated growth is seen in the nasal cavity, which does not bleed when pushed.

Prevention

Active treatment of all chronic ailments affecting the nasal cavity. This may lower its incidence.

Treatment

1. New acupuncture therapy. Apply medium stimulation to needles inserted in the "yin-t'ang," "ying-hsiang," and "ho-ku" points, in treatments given once daily. This is effective for relieving headache or the dull ache felt in the area between the eyebrows.

2. Chinese herbs. Treatment should clear the lungs and open up the air passageways, using remedies such as the following:

   a. Pulverized realgar in suitable amounts, mixed with water. Soak cloth pledgets in solution and insert into nose, change dressing daily. Maintain treatment for 10 days.

   b. Crush and extract juice from man-t'ien-hsing [Hydrocotyle rotundifolia] 2 liang and mix well with a small amount of sugar. Drop on nasal polyp, several times a day for several days in a row.

   c. Concoction of
   Hsin-I [Magnolia liliflora]   2 ch'ien
   Kao-pen [Nothosmyrniun japonicum]   2 ch'ien
   Chih-mu [Anemarrhena asphodeloides]   3 ch'ien
   Lien-ch'iao [forsythia]   3 ch'ien
   Gypsum   3 ch'ien
   P'u-kung-ying [dandelion]   5 ch'ien
   Po-ho [mint]   1 ch'ien
   Licorice   1 ch'ien

3. Western medicine

Use of 1-2 percent ephedrine solution nose drops on small polyp(s) may relieve symptoms temporarily. Severe cases require surgical treatment. Recurrence is common.

- 528 -

Acute Tonsillitis

Acute tonsillitis, referred to as "j'u-o" or "o-tzu" [both implying a moth] by the local people is a common throat ailment caused by hemolytic streptococci. Exposure to cold and fatigue are predisposing factors. In general, the onset is acute and the throat is sore, frequently accompanied by chills, fever, general malaise, myalia of the extremities etc. In infants, the high fever may produce convulsions.

Upon examination, the throat is red, the tonsils are congested and swollen, and covered by specks of yellow or greyish white exudate that sometimes merge to form a pseudomembrane. It must be differentiated from diphtheria at this time. If the tonsillitis keeps recurring, it may develop into chronic tonsillitis.

Prevention

Active participation in physical training activities to increase body resistance to disease. Pay attention to climatic changes. Since chronic tonsillitis is frequently a foci of infection, it is possible for it to cause chronic infections of the ear, nose and throat, arthritis, pyelitis and rheumatic heart disease. For this reason, infected tonsils must be removed by surgery when necessary.

Treatment

1. New acupuncture therapy. Prick-puncture the "ho-ku" and "shao-shang" points until bleeding ensues, in treatments given once or twice daily. When fever is present, include the "ta-chui" and "chu-ch'ih" points for prick-puncturing.

2. Grasp-massage therapy. Have patient sit in chair with both arms extended forward, the thumb in superior and the little finger in inferior positions. The physician stands to the side in front of the patient, and places his right thumb against the right ball of thumb of the patient and brings the index, 3rd and ring finger to press on the patient's "ho-ku" point [at interdigital space between thumb and index finger], while using his left hand to press on the patient's right shoulder (over the collarbone), after which use his right hand to pull [the patient's]outward, and maintain in this position for 1 or 2 minutes. This technique has an immediate effect on patients suffering from very sore throats in which they can hardly swallow water.

3. Chinese herbs. Treatment should clear fever and neutralize toxins, using remedies such as the following:

      a. Concoction of
        Leaves of ta-ch'ing [Clerodendron cyrtophyllum] 1 liang
        T'u niu-hsi [Achyranthes bidentata]   1 liang

b. Pulverized mixture of
   Chu-sha ken [Andesia crenata]   2 ch'ien
   Huang-lien [Coptis chinensis]   2 ch'ien

c. Concoction prepared from sliced roots of hu-mu [Aralia chinensis].
   Use half for gargle, the other half for drinking.

d. Concoction of
   Mei-hsieh tung-ch'ing [Ilex asprolla]   3 ch'ien
   Roots of wan-nien-ch'ing [Rohdea japonica]   1 ch'ien

e. Pulverized wu-p'ei-tzu [gall] or pin-pen [camphor-boric?] powder
   (patent medicine) for nasal insufflation.

f. Concoction of
   P'u-kung-ying [dandelion]   1 liang
   Root of pan-lan [Strobilanthes sp.]   5 ch'ien
   Leaves of ta-ch'ing [Clerodendron sp.]   5 ch'ien
   Honeysuckle blossoms   4 ch'ien
   Forsythia blossoms   3 ch'ien
   One concoction/dose to be taken daily.

4. **Western medicine**

Antipyretic-analgesics and penicillin, sulfonamides etc., may be
used selectively. For those patients who cannot eat, suitable supplements
should be considered.

Laryngitis

Laryngitis is caused mostly by upper respiratory tract infection. Sometimes it may be caused by excessive use of vocal cards, excessive smoking,
drinking or breathing by mouth etc.

It is characterized clinically by sore throat and hoarseness. It may
further be classified into acute laryngitis and chronic laryngitis. Repeated
attacks of acute laryngitis will cause it to become chronic. The acute form
is generally classified as wind-chill (feng-han) or wind-heat (feng-jeh), while
the chronic form is classified as yin-deficient (yin-hsu).

Wind-chill laryngitis is characterized by tickling and pain in throat, a
thin sputum brought up, and a clear nasal discharge. Fur on tongue is thin.

    Wind-heat laryngitis is characterized by more severe coughing, hoarseness, a burning sensation to the sore throat, parchness, and possibly fever. Fur on tongue is yellow.

    Yin-deficient laryngitis is characterized by hoarseness, a dry throat, slight pain on swallowing, and possibly flushed cheeks. Tongue is bright red with no fur. Salivation is also absent.

Prevention

    Measures same as those for sinusitis.

Treatment

    1. **New acupuncture therapy** apply strong stimulation to needles placed in the "ho-ku" and "shao-shang" points. Puncture the "shao-shang" once daily using the prick-puncture technique, pricking until blood is seen.

    2. **Chinese herbs**

    a. For **wind-chill laryngitis**, treatment should resolve the wind and dispel the chill, using remedies such as the following concoction of

Ching-chieh [Nepeta japonica]	3 ch'ien
Fang-feng [Siler divaricatum]	2 ch'ien
Chieh-keng [Platycodon grandiflorum]	3 ch'ien
Mint	1.5 ch'ien
Mummified silkworms	2 ch'ien
Licorice	1 ch'ien

    b. For **wind-heat laryngitis**, treatment should clear fever and neutralize toxins using remedies such as the following:

    (1) Pulverized mixture of

Roots of chu-sha [Ardesia crenata]	3 ch'ien
Huang-lien [Coptis chinensis]	1 ch'ien

    Take with some cold boiled water.

    (2) Concoction of

Honeysuckle flowers	3 ch'ien
Forsythia	3 ch'ien
Niu-pang-tzu [Arctium lappa]	3 ch'ien
Chieh-keng [Platycodon chinensis]	3 ch'ien
Mint	1.5 ch'ien
Cicada molting	1 ch'ien

(3) Pulverized ch'ing-yu ts'ao [Rohdea japonica?], roasted gall pulverized, or Pin-peng san (patent medicine) used to insufflate the throat.

c. For yin-deficient laryngitis, treatment should cultivate and restore the yin, using remedies such as the following:

(1) Huang-pai [Phellodendron] soaked and cut into strips, 1 ch'ien each time, for sucking as a lozenge, 3 times a day.

(2) Tea steeped with

Shen hsieh	1.5 ch'ien
Ho tzu [Terminatia chebula]	3 ch'ien
Pan-ta-hai	3-5

(3) Concoction of

Fresh shih-hu [Dendrobium nobile]	5 ch'ien
Sha-shen [Adenophora stricta]	3 ch'ien
Crude ti-huang	5 ch'ien
Pai-shao [Paenia albiflora]	3 ch'ien
Mu hu-tieh	1 ch'ien
Mai-tung [Ophiopogon japonicus]	3 ch'ien
Chieh-keng [Platycodon sp.]	2 ch'ien
Licorice	1 ch'ien

Toothache

Toothache is commonly seen among ailments of the oral cavity. The causes of toothache may be pulpitis, apical periodontitis periodontitis, and trigeminal neuralgia. Except for dental caries toothache, most toothaches are related to wind, fire and stomach heat.

Prevention

Attention to oral hygiene. Cultivate the habit of brushing teeth after meals.

Treatment

1. New acupuncture therapy. Use strong stimulation on needle inserted into the "ho-ku" penetrating the "hou-hsi." Retain needle for 20 minutes after pain has been relieved.

2. Chinese herbs

a. Pulverized mixture of white pepper 30 percent and gypsum 70 cent, mixed into paste with cold water. Use to rub base [at gumline] of aching tooth.

- 532 -

b. Concoction of following for mouth rinse [retain in mouth for
    a while]
    Honeysuckle vine
    Shin hu-sui
    Ch'ing mu-hsiang
    Use residue from concoction for compress.

c. Poultice prepared from fresh chiu-ts'ai [leeks] 5 ch'ien, soaked
    in vinegar and crushed into paste. For local application over
    affected area, several times a day.

d. Concoction of I-chih-huang-hua [Solidago virgo-aurea] 6 ch'ien,
    strained, and taken with two duck eggs.

e. Li-chi (Nephelium litchi) stuffed with alum [after stone is re-
    moved], steamed while cooking rice. Place the fruit pulp over
    the aching tooth. When saliva begins to flow, pain will have
    been relieved. (In absence of li-chi fruit, a piece of crude
    ti-huang [Rehmannia glutinosa] can be used instead.)

f. Concoction of
    Processed ti-huang   4 ch'ien
    Crude ti-huang   4 ch'ien
    Huai-shan [Dioscorea batatas]   4 ch'ien
    Shan yu [Cornus officinalis]   2 ch'ien
    Tan-p'i [bark of peony root]   2 ch'ien
    Pai-chi-li [Tribulis sp.]   3 ch'ien
    Ku-sui-pu [Drynaria fortunei]   3 ch'ien
    Niu-hsi   3 ch'ien
    Hsi-hsin   5 fen
    Ch'ing-yen [converted]   1 ch'ien
    (This prescription is suitable for cases of chronic toothaches,
    where tooth is loose and sensitive. Typed as yin-deficient
    and fire-light).

3. Western medicine

    Analgesic to relieve pain, and sulfonamides and penicillin to relieve
inflammation, in accordance with patient's condition.

Furuncle of the External Auditory Canal
and Otitis Externa

A localized infection of hair follicle or sebaceous gland along the
external auditory canal is a furuncle; and a generalized inflammation of the
skin or subcutaneous tissue of the same canal is called otitis externa. Both
conditions are caused by heat-toxins. Its clinical characteristic is an earache that is aggravated by chewing. Pressure on the tragus or a pull on the

- 533 -

pinna will evoke even greater pain. The ear canal may show a localized swollen furuncle or generalized redness and swelling, congestion which frequently evokes a preauricular or post-auricular swelling. If the furuncle ripens and erupts, then pus will be discharged.

Prevention

Avoidance of poking around the ear with ear-scoops and cotton applicators. After the ears have been in water, be sure to use a cotton applicator to soak up water remaining in the ear canal.

Treatment

1. New acupuncture therapy. Use medium stimulation on needles inserted into the "I-feng," "wai-kuan," and "ho-ku" points, in treatment given once every day.

2. Chinese herbs. Treatment should clear fever and neutralize toxins, using remedies such as the following:

   a. Concoction of
      Honeysuckle blossoms   8 ch'ien
      Forsythia   4 ch'ien
      Tan-p'i [bark of peony root]   3 ch'ien
      Licorice   2 ch'ien

   b. Concentrate prepared by concocting fresh leaves of wild chrysanthemum [C. indicus]. After concoction has settled, use clear portion as ear drops.

   c. Compress prepared by mixing a suitable amount of t'ien hsien-tzu with water.

3. Western medicine

   a. For furuncle in the external auditory canal, 10 percent glycerine ichthyol; for otitis externa, 1-2 percent of glycero-carbolic acid or 4 percent boric acid alcohol.

   b. If swelling is marked, penicillin and sulfonamides may now be used.

   c. If furuncle has burst, or if secretion is present from otitis externa, the canal should be cleaned frequently with a cotton applicator soaked in 3 percent hydrogen peroxide, after which anti-inflammation ear drops (e.g., 0.5 percent chloramphenicol solution, 1 percent neomycin solution, or 4 percent boric acid alcohol etc.) are instilled. Several medications listed under section "Diseases of the Eye" can also be used.

Purulent Otitis Media

Otitis media, also termed "t'ing-erh" "erh-nung" [purulent ear], is a purulent infection of the middle ear caused by entrance of bacteria through the eustachian tube (particularly after forceful blowing of nose] after trauma to the ear canal or spread from an existing nasal infection. Acute otitis media is manifested chiefly as a sudden earache, a throbbing needle puncturing pain that is particularly severe at night. Because infants cannot complain, they can only cry and show great restlessness. Other manifestations are chill, fever with temperature as high as 40° centigrade in serious cases, reduced sense of hearing, and a light yellow or greenish-yellow discharge occurring after 5-7 days. Once the discharge has been drained, the fever will be coming down and the pain will subside gradually. In some cases, before treatment was given in time, the otitis develops into a long-term chronic condition that flares up repeatedly, accompanied by a purulent yellow and foul-smelling discharge, and deafness in what is called chronic otitis media.

If dainage is poor, the pus will be diffused into the surrounding area and post-auricular edema, headache, pyrexia, chills, neck rigidity, or coma etc. will appear. These are danger signs of a complicating purulent meningitis. Emergency measures must be taken promptly or have patient sent to the hospital immediately.

Prevention

1. Active treatment of diseases affecting the nasal cavity, upper respiratory tract infections and other respiratory tract ailments.

2. Preventing dirty water from entrance into the ear canal. Once that happens, clean and soak up immediately.

3. Active treatment of otitis media, to prevent recurrence or progression into a chronic condition which may cause other serious complications.

Treatment

1. New acupuncture therapy. Use strong stimulation on needles inserted into the "I-feng" and "wai-kuan" points in treatment given once daily. If fever is present, include "ch'u-ch'ih" and "ho-ku" points for acupuncture.

2. Chinese herbs. Treatment should quell the liver fire and resolve moisture-heat, using remedies such as the following:

    a. Concoction of

Ch'ai-hu [Bupleurum falcatum]	3 ch'ien
Lung-tan ts'ao [gentian]	3 ch'ien
Ch'ih-shao [Paenia sp.]	3 ch'ien
Shan-chih [gardenia]	3 ch'ien
Huang-ch'ing [Scutellaria baicalensis]	3 ch'ien
Honeysuckle blossoms	4 ch'ien
Forsythia blossoms	4 ch'ien

If pus is profuse, add shent-ti [crude ti-huang] 5 ch'ien; if earache is severe, add tu-li [oyster] 1 liang, hsia-ku-ts'ao [Brunella vulgaris].

b. Concoction of

Honeysuckle blossoms	8 ch'ien
Forsythia	3 ch'ien
Tan-p'i	3 ch'ien
Licorice	1 ch'ien

If the purulent drainage has continued over a long period of time without healing, include in prescription, huang-ch'i [Astragalus hoantchy] 4 ch'ien, pai-chih [Angelica anomala] 3 ch'ien.

c. Juice of fresh hu-erh ts'ao [Saxifrage sarmentosa], crushed. Juice is used for ear drops, given three times a day.

d. Extract prepared from a suitable amount of Kunming chi-hsueh-t'eng [Milletia reticulata] chopped and steeped in 95 percent alcohol for 7 days. Extract is then used as ear drops, given 3 drops to each ear, twice daily.

e. Pulverized mixture of

Wu-p'ei-tzu [gall] (burnt)	1 ch'ien
Ku-fan [burnt alum]	3 fen

Blow powder into ear (This prescription is suitable for chronic otitis media.)

3. Western medicine

Ear drops of 2 percent glycerocarbolic acid and 4 percent boric acid alcohol may be given before eardrum is punctured. When ear is draining, clean and wash with 3 percent hydrogen peroxide, after which instill an antibiotic solution or a 3 percent coptis chinensis solution.

Deaf-Mutism

Deaf-mutism is frequently a complication of certain acute infections (such as measles, epidemic poliomyelitis, epidemic Japanese B encephalitis etc.) incurred during childhood which led to loss of hearing and subsequent inability to learn how to talk. A few cases may be attributed to congenital causes (such as closure of external meatus or incomplete development of the inner ear).

Prevention

    1. Active prevention and treatment of acute infections and otitis media.

    2. Abusive use of drugs and medications (such as streptomycin etc.) to be avoided. Master strict observance of drug dosages.

Treatment

    In deafness and mutism, deafness is the chief paradox. So deafness should be treated first, after which the problem of mutism will be resolved through training. A strategy must be planned and followed in treating deafness. There must be patience, indefatigability, and confidence in the effort to complete treatment successfully.

    1. Treatment of deafness -- using new acupuncture therapy

        a. Selection of points

            (1) "Erh-men" (open patients mouth while inserting needle, puncturing until a response is evoked before needle is retracted subcutaneously. Then puncture through to the "t'ing-kung" "t'ing-hui," retaining needle slightly with finger bracing the handle of needle for 1-2 minutes, before finally extracting needle), "t'ing-hui," "t'ing-kung," "lung-hsueh" (between the "t'ing-hui" and "t'ing-kung")

            (2) "I-lung," "I-feng," and "I-ming."

            (3) "Pai-hui," "ya-men," and "shang-tien-ch'uan."

            (4) "Ho-ku," "chung-chu," "wai-kuan," "chih-cheng."

            (5) "Tsu-san-li," "lung-chung" and "ling-hsia."

        b. Treatment technique: From the group of acupuncture points just listed, select one pair each day on a rotational basis, to undergo a 10-15 minute course of treatment (the "t'ing-kung" and "I-feng" points cannot be used, simultaneously). Once a course of treatment has been found effective after acupuncture, intensive

speech training should be followed up. Generally, a cure is
evident after two to four courses of treatment. After this,
certain points should still be selected for acupuncture to
reinforce the treatment with another one to three courses.

2. Treatment of mutism -- using speech training

    a. Reinforcing hearing ability is the basis of speech training.
Use the learning by memorization technique to strengthen hearing ability.

    b. Mastering enunciation is the key to speech training. Simple-
to-complex training may consist of vocal cord vibration, nasal
sound training, tongue exercises, breathing exercises, pitch
adjusting etc.

    c. Learning speech [language] is revolutionary practice. By
organizing Mao Tse-tung thought promotion teams to participate
in production activities and the great revolutionary criticism
to learn and enrich speech and the language.

Styes

A stye, called "t'ou-chen yen" [needle-stealing eye] by the native populace, is an acute inflammation of the sebaceous glands in the eyelid. It may
be due to a deficiency of blood and energy and subsequent infection and invasion
by wind-toxins [feng-tu]. This ailment is prone to recur. Appearing on the
upper or lower eyelid margins (that appearing on the conjunctival surface under
the lid is called an "inner-stye"). At onset, it is only a small hard nodule
that is slightly itchy and painful. However, after a few days it suppurates
and erupts. Following drainage of the pus, the symptoms rapidly subside. A
bad stye often involve the whole eyelid, forming an abscess. It frequently
is accompanied by swelling of lymph nodes in front of the ear.

Prevention

Attention to personal hygiene. Wash handkerchiefs frequently. Do not
rub eyes with dirty hands. Actively treat conjunctivitis and other eye diseases.

<u>Treatment</u>

     1. At onset, local applications of hot towel compresses. Repeat three times daily, 15 minutes each time.

     2. <u>New acupuncture therapy</u>. Apply medium stimulation to needles inserted in the "ching-ming," "t'ai-yang," and "ho-ku" points, once daily.

     3. <u>Chinese herbs</u>. Treatment should dispel wind, clear fever, and neutralize toxins, using remedies such as the following:

         a. Moist compresses prepared from t'ien-hsien-tzu [<u>Aristolochia debilis</u>] 1 liang mixed with warm boiled water.

         b. Concentrate/juice from pai-chi [<u>Bletilla striata</u>] 1 ch'ien grated in white wine.

         c. Concentrate of huang-lien [<u>Coptis chinensis</u>] obtained by grating herb in cold boiled water.

         d. Concoction of

Chiang-huo [<u>Angelica sylvestris</u>]	2 ch'ien
Fang-feng [<u>Siler divaricatum</u>]	2 ch'ien
Ch'ih-shao [<u>Paenia</u> sp.]	3 ch'ien
Pan-lan-ken [<u>Strobilanthes</u> sp.]	3 ch'ien
P'u-kung-ying [dandelion]	5 ch'ien
Tsao-chiao [Chinese locust]	1.5 ch'ien

         If constipation is present, add fresh ta-huang [rhubarb], 3 ch'ien, later.

     4. <u>Western medicine</u>

         a. Sulfonamide and antibiotic eye drops and ointment for external use. Cases of serious infection require systemic medication.

         b. If suppuration has set in, break open with a sterile injection needle, allow to drain, then apply ointment. Refrain from squeezing stye at onset, to prevent spread of infection.

Acute Conjunctivitis

     Acute conjunctivitis is also called "ch'ih-yen" [red eye] or "t'ien-hsing ch'ih-yen" [heaven's red eye]. Seen mostly during the spring and fall seasons, it is an acute inflammation of the eye caused by bacteria. Its onset is quite sudden. The eyes become swollen and red, painful and itchy, aversive

to heat and light, "hot" watery, and discharging so profusely that the eyes
are frequently "stuck" shut. This ailment is usually classified as wind-hot
[feng-jeh], and besides the local symptoms just described, it is frequently
accompanied by headache, fever, parchness, dark concentrated urine, constipation etc. The tip of tongue is pink, the fur is yellow, and the pulse is rapid.
If suitable treatment is not instigated and the symptoms are allowed to drag
out, it becomes a chronic conjunctivitis.

Prevention

Good health education programs for the masses. Explain that this disease is transmitted by contact with the discharging secretions from the eye.
For this reason, the patient's towels and handkerchiefs must be boiled and
kept separate from articles used by others, to prevent spread of the infection.

Treatment

1. Maintaining cleanliness of the eyes. The affected eye(s) must not
be bandaged.

2. New acupuncture therapy. Apply strong stimulation to needles inserted into the "ching-ming" and "t'ai-yang" points. The "t'ai-yang" point
and the post-auricular vein may be pricked with a triple-edged needle until
it begins to bleed a little. Satisfactory results are obtained this way.

3. Chinese herbs. Treatment should "loosen" the wind and clear fever,
using remedies such as the following:

a.	Concoction of	
	Ma-huang [ephedra]	3 ch'ien
	Ts'ang-shu [Atractylis ovata]	1.5 ch'ien
	Spikes of ching-chieh	2 ch'ien
	Cicada molting	1 ch'ien
	Bat droppings	1 ch'ien
	Burnt silkworm droppings	3 ch'ien
	Mulberry leaves	1.5 ch'ien
	Huang-lian [Coptis chinensis]	5 fen
b.	Concoction of	
	Fresh ju-hsing ts'ao [Houttuynia cordata]	1 liang
	Yeh-chu-hua [Chrysanthemum indicus]	5 ch'ien
c.	Eye drops prepared from	
	Huang-lien [Coptis chinensis]	1 ch'ien
	Camphor	2 fen
	Human milk	

Steam mixture over rice [when rice is being cooked] for 30
minutes, cool, and instill drops in eyes several times daily.

d. Eyewash concoction prepared from
    P'u-kung-yin [dandelion]
    Chin-yen-hua [suitable amount]
    P'o-ho [mint] small amount
    Water

    Bathe eyes twice daily.

e. Concoction of
    Ma-huang   1.5 ch'ien
    Kuei-p'i [cinnamon bark]   1.5 ch'ien
    Hsi-hsin [Asarum sieboldi]   1 ch'ien
    Fu-p'ien [Aconitum fischeri]   1.5 ch'ien
    Fresh ginger   3 slices
    Red dates   3
    (This prescription is suitable for treating chronic conjunc-
    tivitis.)

4. Western medicine

a. Tetracycline 0.5 percent eyedrops (or other antibiotic eyedrops),
    instilled every 2 hours.

b. Application of opthalmic aureomycin ointment at bedtime to
    prevent eyelids from cracking or from being stuck by secretions.

c. For phlyctenular conjunctivitis applications of ophthalmic
    tetracycline cortisone ointment 4 times a day can be used.

Trachoma

Trachoma, also called "chiao-ts'ang" [peppery sores] is a common chronic
inflammation of the conjunctiva that is caused by the trachoma virus. No unusual
sensations are noted at onset, or maybe just a little itching. Later on as the
trachoma progresses, symptoms such as pain, sensation of a foreign body present,
photophobia, lacrimation, itching, increased secretion, blurred vision, etc.,
will appear. Eversion of the eyelid will reveal numerous small granules on
the conjunctiva, the conjunctiva presenting a coarse cloudy appearance (Figure
6-10-1). In severe cases, the upper lid is swollen and hard, the granules
piling up in an uneven layer. Rubbing the eyes will cause inversion of the
eyelashes and pannus to result in reduced vision or even blindness.

Figure 6-10-1   Trachoma

Prevention

Active treatment of trachoma and practice of good hygiene. Do not share use of towels, handkerchiefs, face basins etc., with trachoma patients. Do not rub eyes with dirty hands or dirty clothing. Remember that trachoma is an infection spread by direct contact. Be aware that it is a dangerous threat that can cause reduced vision.

Treatment

1. Eyedrops prepared from
Coptin sulfate	0.5 gm
Hsi-kua hsiang [Watermelon frost?]	5 gm
Yueh-shih [moonstone?]	0.2 gm
Phenylmercuric nitrate	0.002 gm
Distilled water	100 ml

   Drop eyes three times a day.

2. Special eyedrops prepared from Cock's "hua-ku" (round and red part found inside cock abdomen that resembles the gallbladder, but it is not the gallbladder)   3
Black prunes	3
Almonds [or apricot kernels]	7
Ch'uan-chiao [Szechwan pepper], crushed	2 ch'ien
Sha-jen [Ammomum xanthoides, crushed]	1 ch'ien
Feng-hua-hsiao [Glauber's salt]	3 ch'ien
Old copper cash [a true copper-green one would be ideal]	1
New embroidery needles	3
Distilled water	1 chin

   Take the above ingredients and place in a jar for steeping. Seal mouth of jar with wax. Remove after 7 days and filter contents twice to purify. Use as eyedrops for instillation three times a day.

3. Eyedrops of 0.5 percent tetracyline or other antibiotic to be instilled 2-3 times daily.

4. Cuttlefish bone stick dipped in powdered coptin use to "sand" off the trachomatous granules on the conjunctiva. (The cuttlefish bone is whittled down to shape of a flat rounded stick, one end shaped like a pencil tip. It is then sterilized.) (This technique is called "kuo-sha-yen" [scraping the trachoma] by the local populace.)

5. To treat other complicating eye conditions, consult the pertinent sections.

Keratitis

Keratitis is a broad term covering all inflammations of the corneal layers, due to viral or bacterial infection. At onset, a small greyish-white spot appears over the pupil, the peripheral blood vessels become congested, the whites of the eyes become "bloodshot," and photophobia, pain, lacrimation, and blurred vision are evident in what is called superficial punctate keratitis. If treatment is given in time, the fine punctate infiltrations are usually absorbed and no scars remain. If the condition is allowed to persist, the corneal tissues undergo destruction, greyish white punctate, strip-like, and macular cloudy lesions are noted over the pupils (Figure 10-2), and the patient experiences photophobia, lacrimation and pain in what is called ulcerative keratitis. Scarring remains after recovery from primary infection, to become corneal nebulas and maculas.

Superficial punctate keratitis largely resembles what the traditional Chinese medicine practitioner calls "chu-hsing chiang" [nebular obstruction], white ulcerative keratitis is largely like "hua-I pai-hsien" [flowery film – white bumps and depressions]. Due mostly to invasion by maelovent toxins and excesses of wind-heat, keratitis is seen mostly in the excessive wind-heat [feng-jeh p'ien-sheng] form and the excessive fever toxins [jeh-tu chi-sheng]

1.点 状   2.片 状

Figure 6-10-2   Keratitis

Legend: (1) Punctate
          (2) Macular

Excessive wind-heat keratitis is characterized by appearance of a stellar pannus over the pupillary area in the beginning, accompanied by symptoms such as headache, stuffy nose, local pain, photophobia, and lacrimation. Fur on tongue is thin, and the pulse is rapid.

Excessive fever toxins keratitis is characterized by spread of the stellar pannus that is transformed into thready strip-like or macular lesions. The whites of the eye become very bloodshot, and lacrimation and pain become quite severe. Restlessness and thirst are also evident. The pulse is rapid and bounding, and fur on tongue is yellow.

Prevention

Active treatment of trachoma, conjunctivitis, dacryocystitis, and other eye diseases. Also avoid trauma to the cornea. The measures are all important in preventing the development of keratitis.

Treatment

1. New acupuncture therapy (same as that used for treating conjunctivitis).

2. Chinese herbs

    a. For excessive wind-heat keratitis, treatment should resolve the wind and clear the fever, using remedies such as the following:

    (1) Concoction of

Ching-chieh [Nepetajaponica]	3 ch'ien
Fang-feng [Siler divaricatum]	3 ch'ien
Chrysanthemums	2 ch'ien
Cicada molting	1 ch'ien
Shed snakeskin (toasted)	1 ch'ien
Ku-ching-chu [Eriocaulon sp.]	3 ch'ien
Pai chi-li [Tribulis terrestris]	3 ch'ien
K'ou-I [Eriocaulon sieboldianum]	5 fen
Huang-lien [Coptis chinensis]	5 fen
Licorice	1 ch'ien

    (2) Eyedrops prepared from a small amount of snake bile and one drop of cold boiled water. Apply locally with a goose feather, several times a day.

    b. For wind-heat dominant type of keratitis, treatment should clear fever and neutralize toxins, using remedies such as the following:

(1) Concoction of
     Lung-tan ts'ao [gentian]   1 ch'ien
     Ch'ai-hu [Bupleurum]   1 ch'ien
     Tang-kuei pieces   1 ch'ien
     Ch'ih-shao [Paenia sp.]   1 ch'ien
     Huang-lien   1.5 ch'ien
     T'ien-pien chu [Aster trinervius] 3 ch'ien
     Mu-tse ts'ao [Equisetum sp.]   3 ch'ien
     White mulberry bark   3 ch'ien
     Ts'ao-ch'ueh-ming   5 ch'ien
     Crude ti-huang   5 ch'ien
     Che-ch'ien-tzu [Plantago sp.]   4 ch'ien
     Ts'ang-shu [Atractylis ovata]   1.5 ch'ien

(2) Poultice prepared from 2-3 leaves of hsiao-mao-ken
[crowfoot sp.], crushed, or pulverized mao-kao ts'ai
[sundew species] (whole plant) mixed with water to form
a triangular patch the size of soybean, and apply over
patient's "yang-pai" and "t'a-yang hsueh" acupuncture
points. Keep in place with adhesive strip, and remove
after 24 hours.

3. Western medicine

Eyedrops of 0.5 percent etracyline (or other antibiotic ophthalmic
solution) for instillation into eyes every 2 hours. Or an antibiotic ophthalmic
ointment may be applied 3-4 times daily (cortisone eye ointments are to be
avoided during the acute phase of any corneal ulceration).

Trichiasis

Trichiasis is frequently caused by shrinkage of trachomatous scar tissue
during the cicatricial stage, that causes the eyelashes to be turned inward.
The chief clinical manifestations are a stabbing pain felt by the eyeball,
lacrimation, a continuous sensation of a foreign body present. Because of this
continuous cilial irritation of the eyeball, complications such as conjunctival
congestion, corneal cloudiness, or corneal ulceration, or even loss of vision,
may result.

Prevention

Active measures taken to prevent and treat trachoma may lower the incidence of this condition. Cases already incurred should be treated immediately.

Treatment

1. New acupuncture therapy. On the lid whose lashes are inverted
(comparable to the surgical treatment site), prick-puncture with a hao-needle

- 545 -

until some oozing ensues. Then puncture the ching-ming hsueh. Repeat this treatment once every day.

 2. <u>Chinese herbs</u>

   a. Concoction for eye bath, prepared from

Ch'ing-yen [salt?]	2 ch'ien
Honeysuckle	3 ch'ien
Chrysanthemum indicus [yeh chu-hua]	3 ch'ien
Mu-tse [<u>Equisetum hiemale</u>]	3 ch'ien
Crude ti-huang	3 ch'ien
Tang-kuei	3 ch'ien
Evening silkworm droppings	3 ch'ien

   b. Powdered poultice prepared from pulverized Wu-p'ei-tzu [gall], 5 ch'ien, thoroughly mixed with honey 5 ch'ien. Apply poultice on upper and lower eyelids.

   c. Pledget of cloth containing several seeds of mu-pi [<u>Momordica cochinchinensis</u>], shelled and crushed, about soybean size, for insertion into nostril on side of affected lid. Nasal discharge and tearing will become heavier. Change pledget every 12 hours.

 3. <u>Surgical treatment</u>. Good results are obtained.

Night Blindness

     Night blindness, called "chi-meng" [chicken blindness] by the native population is usually caused by a vitamin A deficiency resulting from chronic illness and run-down health. Its outstanding characteristic is blurred vision which sets in at nightfall, but disappears the following morning when every- thing looks normal again. It may be accompanied by dry itching of the eyes, dizziness, backache, and other symptoms.

<u>Prevention</u>

     Intensive physical training to increase body resistance to disease. Health must be built up after illness. Include animal organs and nourishing food such as pork liver and carrots in the diet.

<u>Treatment</u>

     1. <u>New acupuncture therapy</u>. Apply medium stimulation to needles in- serted in the "kan-yu," "ching-ming" and "tsu-san-li" points, once daily. Moxibustion can also be applied over the "kan-yu" and "tsu-san-li" points.

2. <u>Chinese herbs</u>. Treatment should emphasize regulation of energy
and restoration of blood, using remedies such as the following:

    a.   Pulverized mixture of
        Ts'ang-shu [<u>Atractylis ovata</u>]
        (pre-soaked in rice rinsing)   1 liang
        Ku-ching ts'ao [<u>Eriocaulon sieboldianum</u>]   5 ch'ien
        Use 5 ch'ien each time in concoction. After it comes to a boil,
        drop in 3-4 liang of pork liver. Bring to boil again and cook
        until liver is almost done. Take after meals, three times a
        day for several days in succession.

    b.   Flowers from ssu-kua [vegetable sponge], 30, steamed with
        2 liang of pork liver. To be eaten.

    c.   Crushed mixture consisting of
        Chu-chi [<u>Lycium chinense</u>]   3 ch'ien
        Chrysanthemums   3 ch'ien
        Bat droppings   3 ch'ien
        Divide into two doses. Steam with pork liver each time. To
        be eaten.

    d.   Ming-mu ti-huang wan (patent medicine) or yang-kan wan (patent
        medicine), 3 ch'ien each dose, three times a day.

Eye Injuries

1. Blunt Injuries

     Any injury sustained by eye through the impact of an external force trans-
mitted by brick, stone, club, or fist where the eyeball is not ruptured is a
"blunt injury." In this category are the commonly seen bruised eyelids [black-
eye], hemorrhage beneath the bulbar conjunctiva, corneal abrasions, hemorrhage
into the anterior chamber, traumatic mydriasis and miosis, cloudiness or luxa-
tion of the lens, and infrequently, hemorrhages in the eyeball. If the impact
of the external force is very great, serious sequela such as rupture of the
eyeball may occur with subsequent escape of contents.

<u>Treatment</u>

    1. For contusions of the eyelids and subconjunctival hemorrhages, apply
cold compresses in the early stage, followed by hot compresses 2-3 days later,
to hasten resorption of bruises.

2. For corneal abrasions, treat as would keratitis. Pay particular attention to preventing infection.

3. For hemorrhage into the anterior chamber, besides cold and hot compresses, bandage the affected eye and curtail activity wherever possible. Hemostatic agents may be used. Observe the bleeding pattern. If other symptoms appear, or the bleeding increases and no absorption takes place, take the patient to hospital for further study.

4. Chinese herbs. Treatment should clear fever and neutralize toxins, stimulate blood circulation and reduce swelling, by using remedies such as the following:

   a. Leaves and flowers of fu-jung [hibiscus] crushed, for use as poultice for external application.

   b. Pulverized mixture of following with cool boiled water added to make poultice:

Crude ti-huang	5 ch'ien
Fresh ta-huang [rhubarb]	3 ch'ien
Hung-hua [Carthamus tinctorius]	3 ch'ien
Ch'ing-mu-hsiang [Aristolochia debilis]	2 ch'ien

5. If eyeball is ruptured, take patient to hospital immediately for treatment.

2. Traumatic Detachment of the Corneal Epithelium

This condition is frequently seen during the busy harvest season, when threshing the grain, missiles of rice or wheat, straw etc., may hit the corneal epithelium. The injured experiences excruciating pain, photophobia, lacrimation and other symptoms of irritation. If a 1-2 percent mercurochromed solution is dropped into the eye, after which it is washed out with 3 percent boric acid solution, the injured area may show up as a stain.

Prevention and Treatment

Strengthen the promotion of occupational safety measures, especially during the busy harvest season. When threshing grain, it is best that workers wear broad-brimmed straw hats, and wear them lower whenever possible. Once the eye is injured, treat immediately. Generally, antibiotic eyedrops or a 0.5 percent aureomycin eye ointment is used. Instill eyedrops or apply ointment 2-3 times a day. Bandage the injured eye, and watch closely for any changes, in order to prevent ulceration to the cornea.

3. Corneal and Conjunctival Foreign Bodies

Any dust and grit particles that are bounced onto the eye and become attached to the conjunctival sac without intruding into the cornea are conjunctival foreign bodies. Metal fragments and sand particles that become attached to or lodged in the cornea are corneal foreign bodies. The important characteristic of both these conditions is the sensation of a foreign body present and lacrimation.

Prevention and Treatment

1. To prevent foreign body intrusion, protection of the eyes is a "must." If a foreign body should gain entrance into the eye, avoid agitated rubbing of eyes with fingers. Close the eyes and allow the tears to flow. Sometimes the foreign body is washed out with the tears.

2. Conjunctival foreign bodies are mostly located on the palpebral conjunctiva and the orbital aspect though they could be lodged in other sites too. The eyelids should be everted under good light to help locate the foreign body. A cotton swab-stick soaked in saline or a clean handkerchief may be used to wipe it off.

3. Some corneal foreign bodies are more deeply embedded. Use a solution of 1 percent pontocaine to anesthetize eye, then swab foreign body off with a saline-soaked cotton applicator. If that proves ineffective, use a foreign body needle or an injection needle to dislodge it. Take care not to injure the cornea or to leave any foreign body particle behind. After foreign body removal instill 0.5 percent terramycin eyedrops or other ophthalmic solution, to prevent secondary infection.

4. Penetrating Injuries

Flying splinters from chopping wood or puncture wounds from sharp instrument (knife, scissors, scalpel, metal fragment, nails, lead threads, pieces of crock or glass etc.) may all cause rupture of the eyeball. Depending on the state of the injury, give prompt emergency treatment. First must be prevention of infection. Give an injection of penicillin or sulfonamides by mouth, tetanus antitoxin, and apply antibiotic ophthalmic ointment on the injured eye. Cover with sterile dressing, bandage, and take patient to the hospital immediately.

5. Burns and Chemical Burns

Most commonly seen are acid or base corrosive burns caused by chemicals such as sulfuric acid, hydrochloric acid, nitric acid, lime, ammonia etc. The injured palpebral tissue may turn red, blister, become edematous, and ulcerate. The conjunctiva becomes congested, edematous, and necrotic. The corneal epithelium may become detached, and the cornea itself turns white and cloudy, even becoming soft and hole-ridden in some cases. Cloudy scars of varying severity, and palpebral-bulbar adhesions often remain after healing. This is particularly true with base-caused chemical burns which are more prone to evoke deep tissue damage and produce many serious complications.

Prevention and Treatment

Corrosive burns caused by acids should be flushed with copious amounts of clear [clean] water, normal saline, or 2 percent bicarbonate of soda solution. For corrosive burns caused by bases [alkalis], if the solid object is still retained in the eye, its removal should be the first order. After foreign body removal, flush with copious amounts of 2 percent acetic acid solution or 3 percent boric acid solution with water. Flushing the burn area is critical to its recovery, the sooner done, the better. At the same time, have patient roll his eyes around to make sure the flushing action is thorough and the irritant is completely washed out. Following the flushing, give antibiotics to prevent infection, and instill atropine eyedrops to dilate the pupils, and apply a cod liver oil ointment or an antibiotic aointment to prevent adhesion between the palpebral and bulbar surfaces. For corrosive base burns, 0.5-1 ml of vitamin C may be injected under the conjunctiva.

Photoelectric Opthalmia
(Radiation Injury)

Commonly seen radiation burns of the eye are a photoelectric ophalmia caused by ultraviolet rays. Ultraviolet rays are easily absorbed by the conjunctiva and the cornea. The symptoms appear 6-7 hours following radiation exposure, manifested as conjunctival congestion, lacrimation, photophobia, pain etc. It generally subsides after a day or two.

Prevention

Yellowish green or dark sunglass goggles should be worn for work.

Treatment

Acupuncture of "ching-ming," and "t'ai-yang" points will bring quick relief. Drop eyes with human milk or cow's milk which also alleviates symptoms quickly.

CHAPTER VII. CHINESE MEDICINAL PLANTS

Section 1   Introduction (General Facts)

Common Terminology

1. ### General Terms

   Tree. Large and tall plant, woody, with an obvious main stem (the
   trunk). Examples are the pines, firs, camphorwoods, and Sophora
   spp.

   Shrub. Smaller and shorter plant without an obvious main stem,
   its numerous main stems arising from the roots. Examples are the
   thorns (Vitex negundo), camellias and roses (Rosa chinensis).

   Herb. Small short plant with pliable and soft stems and leaves,
   high in moisture content. Examples are the smartweed (Polygonum
   hydropiper) and common verbena (Verbena officinalis).

   Annual herb. Plant that blooms the same year it is sown, dying
   after •t has borne fruit. Examples are St. John's-wort Hypericum
   japonica (t'ien-chi-huang) and Olaenlandia diffusa (pai-hua she-
   hsieh ts'ao).

   Biennial herb. Plant that grows roots, stem and leaves one year,
   and blooms and fruits the following year, after which it dies.
   Examples are the artemesias such as Artemesia apiacea and the
   verbenas.

   Perennial herb. Plant that lives for more than two years. Examples
   are Coptis chinensis and the Indian turnip, Arisaema consanguineum.

Vine. Plant with long woody stem that creeps or climbs during growth. Examples are the spindle tree Celastrus articulatus (nan-she t'eng), Pueraria pseudohirsuta (k'o-ken), and the blood vine Sargentodoxa cuneata (ta-hsueh t'eng).

Wild plant. Plant that depends on nature as the medium of propagation and growth.

Cultivated plant. Plant that depends on artificial means of seed selection, cutting, grafting etc. for propagation and growth. Examples are the Andrographis paniculata and the jasmine Jasminum sambac.

Symbiotic plant. Plant that grows by itself while attached to another. Examples are Dendrobium nobile and Lepidogrammitis drymoglossoides.

Parasitic plant. Plant that lives on another, its roots penetrating deeply into the host plant and deriving nutrients from it for growth. Examples are a 2 to 3-feet tall plant parasitic on mulberries called "sang-chi-sheng," and a "rootless vine" Cuscuta japonica.

2. General Technical Terms

a. Roots

(1) Root tuber. Thick fleshy roots like those seen in the knotweed Polygonum multiflorum and the yam.

(2) Fibrous roots. Several or numerous slender fibrous roots of about the same size that branch out from base of the stem. Examples are those of leeks, the "psi-ch'ien" Cynanchum atratum, and Pycnostelma pedniculatum.

(3) Perennial roots. Roots that live on below ground after leaves and stems have died off, to bring forth new stems and leaves the following year. Examples are those of Chrysanthemum indicum and Achyranthes bidentata.

(4) Aerial roots. Roots that branch out from the plant stem, living off the moisture it absorbs from the air. Examples are those of the Ficus wightiana and Dendrobium nobile.

(5) Woody roots. Roots that are more woody and hard. Examples are those of trees and shrubs.

(6) Flesh roots. Roots that are large, tender and high in moisture content. An example is seen in roots of the Curculigo orchoides.

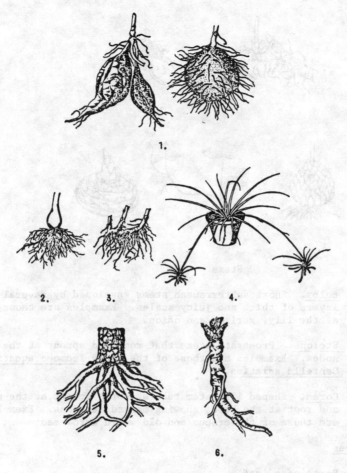

1.

2.   3.   4.

5.   6.

Roots

b. __Stems__

    (1) __Rhizomes__. Prostrate and subterranean root stems that
        look like roots and showing a markedly scaly leaf at
        each node. Examples are those of the __Imperata cylindrica__,
        __Huttuynia cordata__, __Polygonatum chinense__.

    (2) __Tuberous stems__. Short and fat subterranean stem tubers
        noticeably separated by a membraneous scale, each tuber
        crowned by a bud. Examples are those of potatoes, yams,
        and cassava.

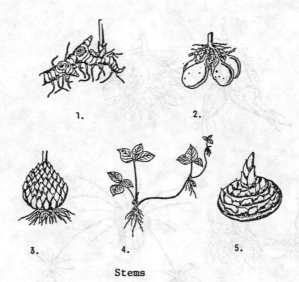

Stems

(3) <u>Bulbs</u>. Short subterranean stems enveloped by several layers of thick and juicy scales. Examples are those of the lily, garlic, and onion.

(4) <u>Stolons</u>. Prostrate stems that root and sprout at the nodes. Examples are those of the reedy <u>Ipomoea aquatica</u>, <u>Centella asiatica</u>.

(5) <u>Corms</u>. Shaped like stem tubers, corms sprout at the apex and root at the base, showing marked sections. Examples are those of the crocus and old world arrowhead.

c. <u>Leaves</u>

(1) <u>Parts of a leaf</u>

<u>Blade</u>: the expanded portion of the whole leaf.
<u>Petiole</u>: the part that attaches the leaf to the stem or tuberous stem.
<u>Stipule</u>: the small leaf at base of petiole, often paired (opposite).
<u>Apex</u>: tip of leaf.
<u>Base</u>: lower margin of leaf near the petiole.
<u>Axil</u>: the upper axillary space formed by attachment of petiole to the stem.
<u>Ochrea</u>: enlarged basal portion attached to stem like a sheath.

<u>Veins</u>: noticeable venation on leaf surface: (1) midrib,
(2) lateral veins, and (3) fine veins.
<u>Margin</u>: edges of blade.

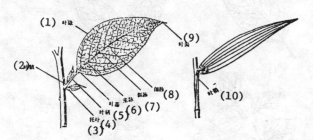

Parts of a leaf   The ochrea

Key: (1) Margin   (6) Midrib vein
      (2) Axil   (7) Lateral vein
      (3) Stipule   (8) Fine vein
      (4) Petiole   (9) Apex
      (5) Base   (10) Ochrea

(2) <u>Leaf classification</u>

<u>Simple leaf</u>: where only one blade grows from a petiole.

<u>Compound leaf</u>: where two or more leaflets grow from a
petiole.

<u>Pinnately compound leaf</u>: where the petiole extends into
a central axis from which leaflets grow from each side.

<u>Odd pinnately compound leaf</u>: where a single small leaflet
climaxes the tip of a pinnately compound leaf. Examples
are leaves of the horsebean and black locust.

<u>Even pinnately compound leaf</u>: where no small leaflet
climaxes tip of pinnately compound leaf. Example as seen
in leaves of the peanut.

<u>Trifoliately compound leaf</u>: where no central axis is
formed by the petiole; instead 3 small leaflets grow from
tip of petiole. Examples are leaves of the buttercup and
the arum <u>Pinellia ternata</u>.

<u>Palmately compound leaf</u>: where the petiole does not form a central axis; instead 5 or more leaflets grow from the tip. Examples are leaves of the ginseng and the <u>Gynura pinnatifida</u>.

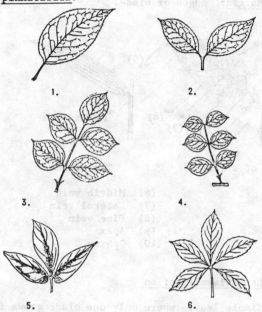

Key:
(1) Simple leaf	(4) Even pinnately compound leaf
(2) Compound leaf	(5) Trifoliately compound leaf
(3) Odd pinnately compound leaf	(6) Palmately compound leaf

(3) <u>Leaf arrangement</u>

<u>Alternate</u>: where leaves are arranged singly on stem, one to each node in an alternate left-right pattern, as in the mulberry, aconite, <u>Magnolia officinales</u>.

<u>Opposite</u>: where leaves are paired on the stem, two to each node, as in the Siberian motherwort.

<u>Whorled</u>: where three or several leaves grow from a node in a twirling radiating pattern, as in the oleander and Siberian yarrow (<u>Achillea sibirica</u>).

<u>Clustered</u>: where several leaves grow from a node, or where whorled leaves are grouped so close between nodes that pattern is not obvious, as in the ginkgo and larch.

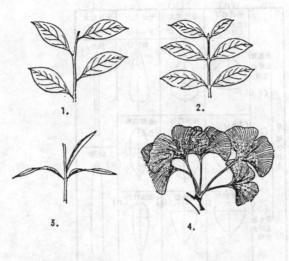

1.
2.
3.
4.

Key: (1) Alternate leaves   (3) Whorled leaves
      (2) Opposite leaves   (4) Clustered leaves

   (4) <u>Various leaf shapes</u>

    (a) <u>Leaf shape illustrations</u>

      i. The proportional length-width relationship in
       simple leaves

       Leaf shape classification based on its broadest
       part

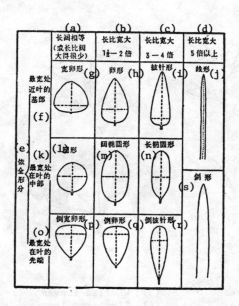

Key: (a) Length-width equal (or where length slightly longer than width)
(b) Length greater than width 1 1/2 to 2 times
(c) Length greater than width 3 to 4 times
(d) Length greater than width, more than 5 times
(e) On basis of whole leaf shape, divided into following categories
(f) Broadest part of leaf at base
(g) Broad ovate
(h) Ovate
(i) Lanceolate
(j) Linear
(k) Broadest part of leaf at center
(l) Round
(m) Broad oval
(n) Long oval
(o) Broadest part of leaf at tip
(p) Broad obovate
(q) Obovate
(r) Oblanceolate
(s) Ensiform

ii. <u>Common simple leaf shapes</u>

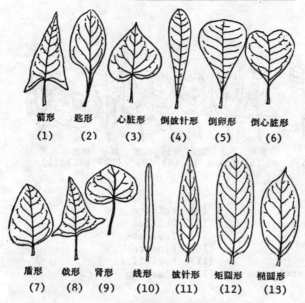

箭形	匙形	心脏形	倒披针形	倒卵形	倒心脏形
(1)	(2)	(3)	(4)	(5)	(6)

盾形	戟形	肾形	线形	披针形	矩圆形	椭圆形
(7)	(8)	(9)	(10)	(11)	(12)	(13)

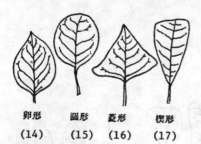

卵形	圆形	菱形	楔形
(14)	(15)	(16)	(17)

Key:
(1)	Sagittate	(10)	Linear
(2)	Spatulate	(11)	Lanceolate
(3)	Cordate	(12)	Oblong
(4)	Oblanceolate	(13)	Oval
(5)	Obovate	(14)	Ovate
(6)	Obcordate	(15)	Round
(7)	Peltate	(16)	Rhombic
(8)	Hastate	(17)	Cuneate
(9)	Reinform		

(b) Leaf bases

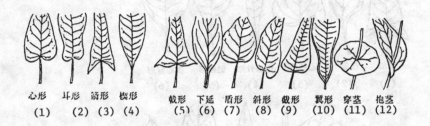

| 心形 | 耳形 | 箭形 | 楔形 | | 截形 | 下延 | 盾形 | 斜形 | 截形 | 翼形 | 穿茎 | 抱茎 |
| (1) | (2) | (3) | (4) | | (5) | (6) | (7) | (8) | (9) | (10) | (11) | (12) |

Key: (1)   Cordate   (7)   Peltate
        (2)   Auriculate   (8)   Oblique
        (3)   Sagittate   (9)   Truncate
        (4)   Cuneate   (10)   Pinnate
        (5)   Hastate   (11)   Perfoliate
        (6)   Extended, prolonged   (12)   Clasping

(c) Leaf apices

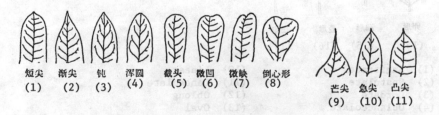

| 短尖 | 渐尖 | 钝 | 浑圆 | 截头 | 微凹 | 微缺 | 倒心形 | | 芒尖 | 急尖 | 凸尖 |
| (1) | (2) | (3) | (4) | (5) | (6) | (7) | (8) | | (9) | (10) | (11) |

Key: (1)   Obtuse   (7)   Emarginate
        (2)   Acuminate   (8)   Obcordate
        (3)   Acute   (9)   Aristate
        (4)   Rounded   (10)   Mucronate
        (5)   Truncate   (11)   Cuspidate
        (6)   Retuse

(d) <u>Leaf margins</u>

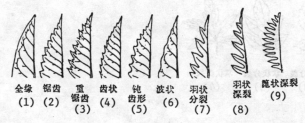

全缘 锯齿 重锯齿 齿状 钝齿形 波状 羽状分裂 羽状深裂 篦状深裂
(1) (2) (3) (4) (5) (6) (7) (8) (9)

Key: (1) Entire   (6) Undulate
      (2) Serrate   (7) Pinnate
      (3) Doubly serrate   (8) Parted pinnate
      (4) Dentate   (9) Pectinate

(e) Leaf venation

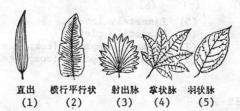

直出 横行平行状 射出脉 掌状脉 羽状脉
(1) (2) (3) (4) (5)

Key: (1) Parallel (nerved)   (4) Palmate
      (2) Parallel (pinnate)   (5) Pinnate
      (3) Radiate

- 561 -

(5) Leaf divisions

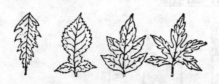

倒向羽裂　琴状分裂　掌状分裂　掌状深裂
(1)　　　　(2)　　　　(3)　　　　(4)

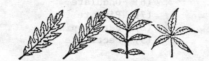

羽状浅裂　羽状深裂　羽状全裂　掌状全裂
(5)　　　　(6)　　　　(7)　　　　(8)

Key:　(1) Inverted pinnate　　　　(5) Pinnately lobed
　　　　(2) Salver-formed　　　　　(6) Pinnately cleft
　　　　(3) Palmately lobed　　　　(7) Pinnate compound (complete division)
　　　　(4) Palmately cleft　　　　(8) Palmate compound (complete division)

(6) Leaf texture

Membraneous: thin and soft, as in belladonna.
Fleshy: thick and juicy, as in sedum and bulrush.
Leathery: hard and tough, as in Osmanthus aquifolium,
　　　　　　　Berberis hepalensis.

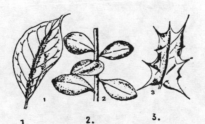

Key:　(1) membraneous
　　　　(2) Fleshy
　　　　(3) Leathery (coriaceous)

d. Flowers

Peduncle: the cylindrical part joining the flower and stem.
Floral receptacle: the expanded tip part of the peduncle.
Calyx: formed by several green leaf-like sepals growing from
the floral receptacle.
Petals: leaflike pieces in blue, white, red, or yellow colors
growing from the floral receptacle.
Corolla: formed by colored petals.
Inflorescence: form taken by many flowers in a patterned
arrangement on the flower stem.

Key: (1) Bracteal leaf
      (2) Bud
      (3) Corolla
      (4) Sepal
      (5) Pistil
      (6) Petal
      (7) Stamen
      (8) Pedicel
      (9) Peduncle

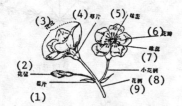

1. External view of a flower

Key: (1) Peduncle
      (2) Floral receptacle
      (3) Filament
      (4) Stamen
      (5) Pistil
      (6) Petal
      (7) Nectary
      (8) Sepal

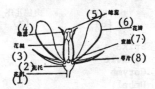

2. Anatomy of a flower

Some commonly seen inflorescences

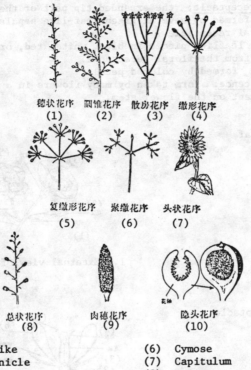

穗状花序
(1)　　　圆锥花序
(2)　　　散房花序
(3)　　　缴形花序
(4)

复缴形花序
(5)　　　聚缴花序
(6)　　　头状花序
(7)

总状花序
(8)　　　肉穗花序
(9)　　　隐头花序
(10)

Key: | | |
|---|---|
| (1) Spike | (6) Cymose |
| (2) Panicle | (7) Capitulum |
| (3) Corymb | (8) Racemose |
| (4) Umbel | (9) Spadix |
| (5) Compound umbel | (10) Hypanthodium |

e. <u>Fruits</u>

Some commonly seen fruits

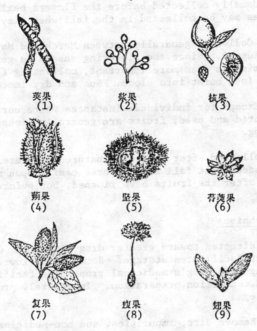

莢果
(1)

漿果
(2)

核果
(3)

蒴果
(4)

堅果
(5)

蓇葖果
(6)

復果
(7)

瘦果
(8)

翅果
(9)

Key: (1) legume   (6) Follicle
        (2) Berry   (7) Compound fruit
        (3) Drupe   (8) Akene
        (4) Capsule   (9) Samara
        (5) Glans (nut)

Collection, Processing and Storage

1. Season of collections

Different Chinese medicinal plants vary in their parts used for medicinal purposes. For some, the roots are used; in others, the stems, leaves, flowers, fruits or the whole plant. Since different parts of the plant mature at different seasons, collecting the medicinal part of the plant at the right time must be kept in mind.

        a. <u>Roots and rhizomes</u>. Generally collected in late fall or early spring. Plant nutrients at this time are generally stored in the roots or rhizomes. Their medicinal quality is better at this time.

b. __Barks__. Usually collected between February and May. Moisture content in the corium is high at this time, and facilitates easy bark stripping.

c. __Leaves__. Usually collected before the flowers begin to bloom. Some leaves may be collected in the fall when they begin to drop.

d. __Flowers.__ Collected generally between March and May, and during July and August. Since the flowering season is generally short, proper timing is even more important, collecting flowers still in bud or just burst into bloom. Sun and dry immediately.

e. __Fruits__. Except for individual instances where unripened fruits are collected and used, fruits are generally picked and collected on ripening.

f. __Seeds__. Collected after they have matured completely. Certain drug-use seeds that fall and disperse easily upon maturity are collected after the fruits have ripened, but before they split open.

2. __Processing technique__

Processing is directed toward greater drug efficacy. Cleaning and purifying the drug product facilitates storage. Removing or lowering drug toxicity to suitably change the drug's medicinal properties facilitates prescription compounding and concoction preparation. In general, processing consists of the following steps:

a. __Sorting__. Remove dirt, impurities, and non-medicinal use parts. Separate parts that have different medicinal uses.

b. __Washing__. Remove flowers and certain plants that should not be washed (such as __Plantago major__ var __asiatica__ and green bristlegrass). Most plants should be washed clean of dirt to meet drug requirements of relative cleanliness.

c. __Slicing__. For packaging and preparation convenience, slice all plants into different sizes, thicknesses, lengths and strips, in accordance with their shapes. Generally, thick and fat roots, rhizomes and woody vines are cut into thin slices; bark and leaves, into fine strips; whole plants, into sections. For external use, these slices may be crushed for the juicy component.

d. __Drying__. Drying in direct sunshine assures better storage. During rainy season or cloudy days, dry around a fire. Meats must be first seared by boiling water before drying, to help shorten drying process. Animal carcasses must first be steamed before drying, to prevent hatching of eggs. Aromatics must be dried in a well-ventilated shady place.

3. Storage and care

   a. Labeling. After cutting-sectioning and drying, be sure to
      label drug products to prevent misuse, particularly those
      plants that are hard to identify by just their external forms.

   b. Keeping dry. Store drug products in a dry and well-venti-
      lated area to prevent mildew and insect attack, oil loss and
      other property changes.

   c. Inspecting and sun-airing. Inspect stored drugs regularly,
      to check on boring bugs and mildew. Sun-air drugs regularly
      and frequently, particularly during the drizzly rainy season
      in May.

   d. Protecting medicinal plant resources. We must consider the
      long-range view in reasonable use of every herb and shrub picked,
      and avoid abuse and "over-picking" of this resource.

      (1) Planned collecting and use. Adopt a reasonable and thought-
          out plan that will meet present needs and consider future
          benefits at the same time.

      (2) Root retention and plant propagation. Pay attention to
          propagation of plants used for their roots or rhizomes.
          For many perennials, if the tops of root-use plants can
          substitute for roots, use the tops whenever possible, and
          leave roots in the soil. For annuals, leave the lower
          parts of plants whenever possible, to assure availability
          of seed stock for future propagation. For drugs used for
          their leaves, do not pick leaves all at once, or the plant
          will die. When collecting for bark, do not strip the whole
          bark. When collecting for roots, try not to damage the
          main tap root.

      (3) Comprehensive utilization. After plants have been collected,
          store parts of the plant that cannot be used for immediate
          medicinal purposes, for future reference. When clearing
          wild and unclaimed areas for environmental sanitation,
          pay attention to plants that can be used for medicinal
          purposes. Do not carelessly throw away or burn any plant
          material.

(4) Proper planting. On the basis of actual needs, reclaim
and use wild areas, the banks along streams, edges of
paddy fields and roadside for planting of those medicinal
plants used in greater amounts or needed for emergencies.

General Properties

"Properties" here refer to the drug's nature, taste and functional
action. In traditional Chinese medicine theory, the "four energies" (szu
ch'i) and "five tasks" (wu-wei) are used to describe drug properties.

The "four energies" are chill (han), heat or fever (jeh), warmth (wen)
and coolness (liang). Chill and coolness fall in the same category, but vary
in degree. A great deal of warmth (ta-wen) is comparable to heat or fever,
and a slight chill also amounts to coolness. Then there are balanced or
neutral (p'ing) drugs that do not tilt toward warmth nor coolness. Because
the "nature" of these drugs is not pronounced, they have not been classified
among drugs of the "four energies," though in actual practice they are included.
The "four energies" are seen from the body's reaction and the efficacy of drug
in treating the ailment. Generally speaking, drugs used to treat fever type
ailments fall into the chill or coldness category, while those used to treat
chill-type ailments fall into the heat or warmth category. For example, when
a person has taken cold, chills and headache appear. He drinks a bowl of fresh
ginger brew, perspires and recovers. This explains that fresh ginger is a warm-
nature drug. In another example, when one's throat is red and sore, accompanied
by thirst and fever, then after taking some dandelion tea, the fever will come
down and the illness is dispelled. This simply explains the cooling nature of
the dandelion. For this reason, after the different drug properties are understood, one can use drugs of different properties to treat different kinds of
illnesses. The phrase in traditional Chinese medicine that says "Chills --
treat with warmth; fevers -- treat with cold" is based on the principle of
using the "four energies" to treat disease.

The "five tastes" are the sour, bitter, sweet [pleasant], peppery
[acrid], and salty flavors, inherent in the drugs. Some bland and generally
tasteless drugs are, by practice, also included within the scope of the "five
tastes." Generally, sour-tasting drugs exert an astringent effect; bitter-
tasting ones, an antipyretic and moisture-drying effect; pleasant and sweet-
tasting ones, a soothing and tonic effect; peppery—tasting drugs, a dispersing
and stimulating effect; the salty drugs, a purgative effect; and the bland-
tasting drugs, a diuretic effect. These are general principles of disease
treatment based on the taste or flavor of drugs.

Energy and taste are inter-related. Different drugs may fall in the
same energy category, but taste differently. Or they may fall in the same
taste category, but act differently energywise. Or they may fall in one energy
category, but possessing several different flavors. These variations simply
explain the different properties and actions of different drugs. Besides a
grasp of common drug properties based on an understanding of principles posed
by the "four energies" and "five tastes," one must not be afraid to discover
any special drug properties or special drug action.

General Dosage and Usage

When drugs are given, one must take a scientific attitude and a creative approach at the same time. Information on the patient with respect to sex, age, general health, severity and duration of illness, climatic factors, etc., must be considered and analyzed.

Generally speaking, the amount of medication prescribed for a healthy individual may be greater than that for a weaker person; greater for a young adult than an aged person or child; also greater for a man than a woman. Smaller dosages are given for a milder disease, and larger doses for more severe illnesses. Chronic diseases should be treated slowly [prolonged] with smaller doses, and acute ailments should be given heavy dose(s) in an abrupt attempt to save the patient and dispel evil [effects of illness]. Dosage of drugs with strong or toxic properties should be strictly controlled -- from smaller to larger doses. Excessive use of bitter and cooling drugs are harmful to the stomach and spleen. Peppery and hot drugs should be given with care to patients with deficient and heat-dominating constitution. Purgative drugs that disrupt energy and blood should be avoided by pregnant women or used only with care. Few heat-type drugs should be used in the summer, and few cold-type drugs in the winter. Drugs containing light porous materials such as flowers and leaves should be used in small amounts, and those containing minerals and shells, in larger amounts. Aromatics to restore "breath" should be used sparingly, and juicy drugs to restore "taste" should be used more heavily. What has been described are only general principles prescribing drug use. In actual practice consider actual conditions and prescribe flexibly when needed.

As agents used for preventing and treating disease, Chinese herbs are most commonly given in the form of a concocted brew. That is, one or several medicinal herbs (dried or fresh) are cooked in water, after which the residue is discarded, but the brew is kept for drinking or for external use. The cooking time and cooking temperature [gauged by size of fire used] used are determined by the herb properties. Aromatics do not need cooking for any length of time. Minerals and mussel shells should be crushed before cooking. Plants containing hairs and much fine pollen should be wrapped in cloth before cooking.

If it is possible in the large rural areas to pick the herbs fresh, use the fresh product wherever possible. Besides being highly effective and convenient to use, fresh herbs can be brewed or squeezed for internal consumption medication, or crushed for external use.

In accordance with the continuing development of the mass movement stressing use of Chinese medicinal herbs to prevent and treat disease, the mass of workers, peasants and soldiers are cooperating with the barefoot physician to tear down superstitions, to experiment and create different dosage forms such as pills, tablets, powder, capsules, tinctures, syrups, ointments and injections from Chinese herbs, based on different plant properties and disease prevention and treatment needs. In this manner, they can effectively serve the new wave of industrial and agricultural production and national defense, while effectively stimulating the development of a combined practice of traditional Chinese and western medicine.

Section 2   Common Chinese Medicinal Herbs

1. I-tien-hsueh [Drop of blood]

Family: Menispermaceae

Scientific Name: Stephania, sp.

Synonyms: "Hsiung-huang-lien," "hsueh-mu shu' [blood root], "san-hsueh shu" [anticoagulant tuber].

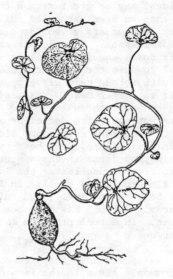

Morphology: Perennial herbaceous vine, found growing on hillsides, water's edge, and in forests, entwining tree trunks or prostrate. Tuberous root blackish-brown, covering coarse and scaly, greyish white in cross-section. Vine showing obvious longitudinal stripes. Break at leaf petiole releases purplish red juicy fluid. Leaves membraneous, peltate, venation purplish red, margins slightly undulated. Blooms in summer, flowers pale yellow. Fruits between September-November, similar to red legumes.

Properties and action: Cool and bitter, slightly poisonous. Stimulates blood circulation, dispels clots, detoxifies, and reduces swelling.

Conditions: (1) Poisonous snake bites, abscesses, mastitis; (2) manipulation (eg., fracture) injuries, post-partum (blood) clotting, abdominal pain etc.

Preparation: The tuberous roots is commonly used for medicinal purposes, mostly for external use. Oral dosage ranges from 1 to 3 ch'ien.

2. I-chi-kao [Siberian yarrow]

Family: Compositae

Scientific name: Achillea sibirica Ledeb.

Synonyms: "A stalk of artemisia," "fei-t'ien
wu-sung" [sky-flying centipede], "wu-sung
ts'ao" [centipede grass], "luan-t'ou-fa"
[unkempt hair].

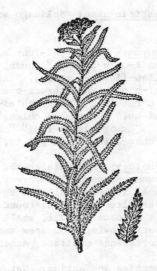

Morphology: Perennial herb. Wild or
cultivated. Stem erect, fusiform-striped,
branching above. Leaves alternate, lance-
linear, pectinate-pinnatifid into unevenly
denticulate fine lobes, half clasping stem,
silky-lanate especially dorsally. Blooms
in late summer, white flowers growing from
axil of apical leaf, inflorescence umbellate.
Achenes flat, long oval, winged.

Properties and action: Neutral, bitter and
sour tasting. Acts as carminative and
stomach tonic, clears meridian passages,
reduces inflammation and exerts bactericidal
effect.

Conditions most used for: (1) Stomach ulcers,
amenorrhea and abdominal cramps; (2) abscesses,
snakebites; (3) traumatic falls and bleeding.

Preparation: The whole plant is used, about
2-5 ch'ien each time, decocted in brew.

3. I-chi Huang-hua [Stalk of yellow flowers]

Family: Compositae

Scientific name: Solidago virgo-aurea
L.

Synonyms: "Hsiao pai-lung su" "ch'ao-
t'ien I-ch'u-hsiang," "huang-hua ts'ao,"
[yellow-flowered grass], "chien-tzu ts'ao,"
"k'ai-hou chien" [throat-opening arrow],
"tz'u tse-lan," "hsiao-ch'ai-hu," "hung
ch'ai-hu," "huang-hua chien," "chien-hsueh
fei," "huang-hua ma-lan," "chi-yu ts'ao,"
"wu-chao-chien," "ta-pai tu," "sheng-ma."

Morphology: Perennial herb. Wild grown
on sunny slopes. Stem erect, dark red.
Radical leaves, oval or long ovate; stem
leaves alternate, oval round to long
oval. Blooms in fall, small yellow
flowers growing from apex and axil,
inflorescence capitate, achene fruit.

Properties and action: Nature slightly
cooling; taste peppery [acrid] and bitter.
Aids digestion, relieves flatus, expels
worms, clears fevers and detoxifies.

Conditions used most for: (1) Influenza
headache, sore throat, malaria, and
measles; (2) gastric pain and vomiting,
and worms in small children.

Usage: The whole plant is used, from
5 ch'ien to one liang each time, prepared in decoction.

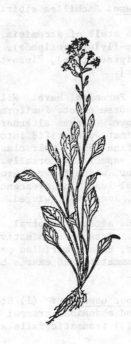

4. Ch'i-hsieh I-chi-hua [Seven leaves to a flower]

Family: Liliaceae

Scientific name: Paris polyphylla Sm.

Synonyms: "Tsao-hsiu," "Ts'ao-ho-che"
"Ch'i-yeh lien,""chung-lou," "tu-chiao
lien" [single-footed lotus], "yu-t'ou
san-ch'i" "t'ieh teng-t'ai."

Morphology: Perennial herb. Wildgrown on
fertile and shady alpine bogs. Rhizomes
sectioned. Stem single, 30-100 cm tall.
Leaves whorled at top of stem, apexes acute,
bases rounded, in arrangement of 6-10,
oval to extensive lanceolate, margins
intact, with short petioles. In summer,
single flower grows from whorled leaf.
Berry dark purple.

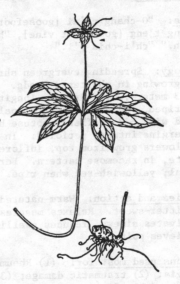

Properties and action: Bitter and slightly
"han" [cold-natured]. Clears fever and
detoxifies, resolves bruises and reduces
swelling.

Conditions most used for: (1) Poisonous
snakebites; (2) boils and ulcers; (3)
diphtheria; (4) epidemic Japanese B
encephalitis.

Preparation: Roots are used for medicine,
2-4 ch'ien each time, prepared as decoction.
Or roots may be crushed and pulverized for
insufflating on throat.

5. Ch'i-yeh Lien [7-leafed lotus]

Family: Araliaceae

Scientific name: Scheffera arboricola Hyata.

Synonyms: "0-chang ch'ai [goosefoot wood],
"0-ch'ang t'eng [goosefoot vine], "han-
t'ao yeh," "ch'i-chia p'i."

Morphology: Spreading evergreen shrub.
Mostly growing in sheltered woods. Stem
height 3 meters, cylindrical, longitudinally striped. Leaves alternate, palmate
compound with 5-7 leaflets, obtuse both
ends, margins intact, petioled. In spring,
white flowers grow from top, inflorescences
umbellate, in racemose pattern. Berries
spherical, yellowish-red when ripe.

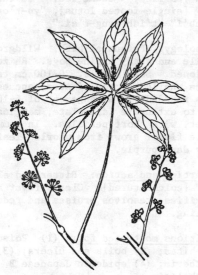

Properties and action: Warm-natured,
taste bitter-sweet. Relaxes muscles
and activates sinews, reduces swelling
and relieves pain.

Conditions used most for: (1) Rheumatoid
arthralgia; (2) traumatic damage; (3)
wound-caused bleeding.

Preparation: Stems and leaves for medicinal use, 5 ch'ien to 1 liang each time,
prepared as decoction. For external use,
crush fresh leaves for poultice to be
applied over affected parts.

6. Pa-chiao Feng [8-cornered maple]

Family: Marleaceae

Scientific name: Alangium chinense
(Lour.) Rehd.

Synonyms: San-chiao feng [3-cornered maple],
ch'i-chiao feng, "chieh-ku mu" "pai-chin-
t'iao," "shan-yao yu," "pa-chiao wu-t'ung,"
"pa-chiao chin p'an."

Morphology: Deciduous small shrub or tree.
Growing in upland hill thickets. Bark
light grey. Leaves alternate, varying
greatly into oblique-ovate, rounded,
truncate, or slightly cordate shapes;
apexes acuminate and bases slightly oblique;
margins 2-7 parted, into deltoid, deltoid-
ovate or crenate parts of various sizes;
branching reticulate veins on back of leaf
pubescent; petioled. Blooms in summer,
flowers white, cymose inflorescence
growing from axil. Berry oval shaped,
black when ripe.

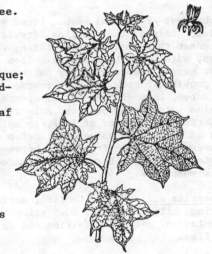

Properties and action: Neutral,
peppery to taste, toxic. Quells wind
[flatus], eliminates moisture, stimulates
circulation and keeps meridians open.
Also has contraceptive properties.

Conditions used most for: (1) Rheumatism,
numbness, traumatic injuries; (2) wound
injuries and bleeding; (3) snakebites.

Preparation: Roots and stems are used,
1-2 ch'ien each time, prepared in
decoction.

7. Pa-chiao Lien [Eight-cornered lotus]

Family: Berberidaceae

Scientific name: Dysosma auranticocaulis (H.M.) HU.

Synonyms: "Pa-chiao-p'an" [8-cornered platter], "lu-chiao lien" [6-corner lotus], "tu-yeh I-chih-hua" [one-flower-from-a-single-stalk], "tu-chiao lien" [single-footed lotus], "I-to yun" [a single cloud], "ho-yeh lien."

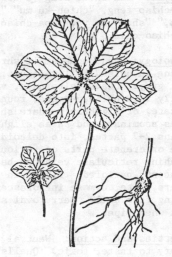

Morphology: Perennial herb. Found growing in damp shady spots in alpine forests. Sub-terranean rhizomes, knotted, thick, yellowish brown, with adventitious roots. Stem erect, light green, topped by fuzzy hairs. Leaves 1-2 growing at apex, peltate-rounded, margins 3-8 lobed, lobe deltoid-ovate, apexes acute, margins irregularly dentate, main rib radiating from center of leaf, to apical tips of lobes. In summer, yellowish white flowers growing 5-8 from joint between top of stem and leaf. Berry ovate-rounded, black when ripe.

Properties and action: Cooling, acrid-tasting, slightly toxic. Can stimulate circulation. Reduces swelling and de-toxifies.

Conditions used most for: (1) Snake and insect bites, bee stings; (2) abscesses, boils, tumors; (3) abdominal pain, non-descent of chorion when the fetus had died en utero; (4) traumatic injuries.

Preparation: Rhizomes are used medicinally, 1 to 3 ch'ien each time, prepared in de-coction. An appropriate amount can also be used externally.

Note: Similar to this species in form and function is the 8-corner lotus Dysosma chengii (chien) Kengf.

- 576 -

8. Pa-so Ma [Eight-spindled elder]

Family: Caprifoliaceae

Scientific name: Sambucus javanica Reinw.

Synonyms: "ch'ou ts'ao" [stink-weed],
"shuo-t'iao," "kung-tao lao," "san-hu
hua" [coral flower], "lo-te-ta," "chieh-
ku ts'ao" [bone-knitting herb], "lu-
ying," "ch'i-yeh ma," "ch'i-li ma."

Morphology: A perennial herb. Found
growing in wild areas, along outskirts
of villages and wasteland. Stem height
1-3 meters, spindle-shaped. Leaves opposite, odd-pinnate compound, leaflets
5-7, long elliptical-lanceolate, apexes
acute, base cuneate, margins dentate.
In summer, white flowers growing from
the top, inflorescence corymb. Berry
globular, black when ripe.

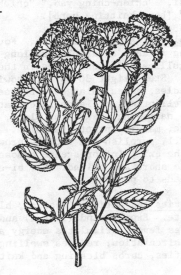

Properties and action: Slightly warm
in nature, slightly sweet and pleasant
to taste. Can reduce swelling and promote diuresis, stimulate circulation
and stop pain.

Conditions most used for: (1) Spasms
of the extremities, pain in the bones;
(2) traumatic injuries; (3) swelling of
lower extremities [beri-beri?]

Preparation: The whole plant is used,
1-2 liang each time, prepared in decoction. Or a suitable amount of the
fresh product may be crushed and used
as a poultice.

9. Chiu-t'ou Shih-tzu Ts'ao [Nine-headed lion grass]

Family: Acanthaceae

Scientific name: Dicliptera japonica
Makino.

Synonyms: "Chiu-chieh li," "ch'uan-pai
niu-hsi," "chien-ching yao," "chieh-ku
ts'ao" [bone-knitting herb].

Morphology: A perennial herb. Found
growing in damp shady places along mountain gullies and under trees in the
woods. Stem height 30-50 cm, showing
4 spindles, nodes enlarged. Leaves opposite, elliptical or lanceolate-ovate,
apexes narrowing, head tips blunt, bases
cuneate, margin intact, petioled. In
the fall, purplish-red flowers growing
from the axil, inflorescence cymose.
Capsule short and cylindrical, bi-cleft,
for seeds to pop out.

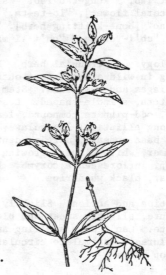

Properties and action: Cooling, bland
in taste. Expels wind (flatus) and
relieves fever, stimulates energy and
blood circulation, reduces swelling and
detoxifies, curbs bleeding and knits bones.

Conditions most used for: (1) Traumatic
injuries; (2) any type of swelling;
(3) snakebites.

Preparation: The whole plant is used,
5 ch'ien to 1 liang each time, prepared in decoction.

10. Chiu-li Kuang [Groundsel species]

Family: Compositae

Scientific name: Senecio scandens Buch-Ham.

Synonyms: "Chiu-li ming," "ch'ien-li chi," "huang-hua ts'ao" [yellow-flowered grass], "yeh chu-hua" [wild daisy], "t'ien ch'ing-hung," "wang-wei," "ch'eng-lin-hsien," "chou ya-kan," "pai-su kan," "chiu-fu kang," "hua wang-wei," "chiu-li kung," "tuan-tzu chiu-li-kuang," "o-yung shen-ken."

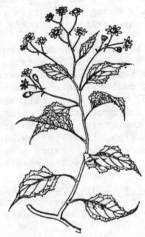

Morphology: A perennial herb. Found growing in shady and damp spots along roadsides. Stem curved and trailing, branching, scabrous. Leaves alternate, elliptical-lanceolate, apexes acuminate, margins irregularly dentate or slightly undulate. In the fall, yellow flowers growing from the end of stem. Achene roundish-cylindical.

Properties and action: Cooling, bitter-tasting, slightly toxic. Lowers fevers and detoxifies, promotes clear vision.

Conditions most used for: (1) Epidemic influenza, malaria; (2) boils and abscesses, acute conjunctivitis, dysentery, enteritis.

Preparation: The whole plant is used, 5 ch'ien to 1 liang each time, prepared in decoction. The fresh product can also be crushed for external use.

11. Shih-ta Kung-lao [Ten great merits]

Family: Berberidaceae

Scientific name: Mahonia japonica DC.

Synonyms: "Hua-nan shih-ta kung-lao,"
"mao-erh t'ou" [cat's head], "pu-kua
shan-shu," "t'u huang-pe" [native yellow
cedar], "tz'u-huang-lien" [prickly coptis].

Morphology: Evergreen shrub. Grows wild
in uplands. Stem height as much as 3 meters,
erect, coarse bark. Leaves clustered at
apex of stem, oddly-pinnate compound,
leaflets 9-15, ovate-elliptical, apexes,
acute, bases unsymmetrical, margins prickly
dentate. In the spring, flowers growing
from the stem tips, light yellow blossoms,
inflorescence racemose. Berry ovoid,
bluish-black, contains white powder.

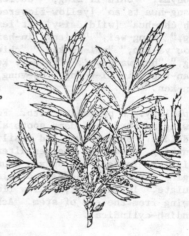

Properties and action: Cooling, bitter.
Lowers fever and detoxifies, reduces
phlegm. Also used as cough sedative.

Conditions most used for: (1) Bone-
breaking fevers, dizziness and tinnitus,
backache, weak lower extremities (knees);
(2) Dysentery, enteritis.

Preparation: Roots and stems are used,
5 ch'ien to 1 liang each time, prepared
in decoction.

12. Jen-Hsien [3-seeded mercury, copperleaf]

Family: Euphorbiaceae

Scientific name: Acalypha australis L.

Synonyms: "P'i-tao chen-chu, [skin-wrapped pearls], "hai-pang han-chu" [oyster-holding-a-pearl], "chen-chu ts'ao" [pearl brass/herb], "hai-tsang chu" [pearl-hidden-in-the-sea], "tieh hsien-ts'ai," "piao-li chen-chu," "tien-lei ts'ao" [snail grass], "hai-ti tsang chen-chu [pearl-hidden-in-bottom-of-sea].

Morphology: Annual herb. Found growing wild along roadsides, edges of fields, mountainsides. Stem height 30-50 cm, branching, longtidunally striped, scabrous. Leaves alternate, rhombic-ovate, ovate-lanceolate or elliptical, apexes acuminate, bases cuneate, margins denticulate at base, sometimes the whole margin. Blooms in summer, small axillary flowers appearing, inflorescence a short spikelet. Flower buds shell-like, deltoid semi-spherical capsule contained inside the bud, hence the name "oyster-holding-a-pearl."

Properties and action: Cooling, bitter and sharp tasting. Lowers fever and detoxifies, stops bleeding.

Conditions most used for: (1) Bacterial dysentery, enteritis and diarrhea; (2) Bleeding wounds.

Preparation: The whole plant is used, 5 ch'ien to 1 liang each time, prepared in decoction. The fresh product can also be crushed for external use as a poultice.

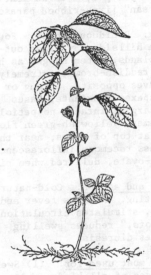

13. Liao-ko wang (Nan-ling Jao-hua)

Family: Thymelaeaceae

Scientific name: Wickstroemia indica A. C. Mey.

Synonyms: "Chiu-hsin ts'ao," "ti-mien ken," "shan yen-p'i," "ti-ku-ken," "t'ieh-ku san" [iron-ribbed parasol].

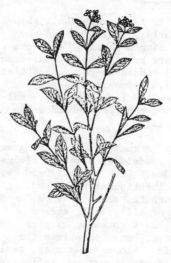

Morphology: Deciduous shrub. Found growing on hillsides, village outskirts, uplands. Stem height as high as 60 cm, reddish-brown, extremely fibrous. Leaves opposite, oblong or obovate, apexes acuminate, bases cuneate, margins intact, no petiole. In the summer, yellowish-green flowers appearing at top of stems, near the petiole-less racemose inflorescence. Fruit long-ovate, dull red when ripe.

Properties and action: Cold-natured, bitter tasting. Reduces fever and detoxifies, stimulates circulation and "de-clots," reduces swelling and promotes diuresis.

Conditions most used for: (1) Swellings and abscesses of all kinds, enlarged cervical nodes, mumps, and fungus infections of the scalp; (2) snake and insect bites; (3) traumatic injuries; (4) asthma.

Preparation: Roots are used, 3-4 ch'ien each time, prepared in decoction.

14. Ginseng (Panax quinquefolium)

Properties and action: Neutral, sweet and pleasant to taste. A tonic to supplement energy and calm the nerves, to produce more saliva and stimulate the appetite.

Conditions most used for: Deficiency of energy (wind) and blood, internal injuries caused by deficiency-activity [worry], convalescent weakness, no appetite, palpitation, insomnia and forgetfulness.

Preparation: Use 1-3 ch'ien each time. When necessary, 5 ch'ien of Tangshen (Campanumaea pilosula, Franch), a bluebell species, may be used as a substitute.

15. Ting-hsiang (Caryophyllus aromaticus, Linne)

Properties and action: Warm, sharp tasting. Warms the body center, alleviates pain, and curtails any bad effects on the body.

Conditions most used for: "Han" cold-type stomach vomiting, hiccups, pains in the heart and abdomen, hernia.

Preparation: Use 5 fen to 1.5 ch'ien each time.

16.   San-ch'i Ts'ao [Three-seven grass]

Family: Compositae

Scientific name: Gynura segetum (Lour.)
Merr.

Synonyms: "P'o-hsueh ts'ao" [blood
'breakdown' grass], "hsueh tang-ku'ei,"
"t'ien-ch'ing ti-hung" [sky-blue earth-
red], "tzu-jung san-ch'i," "san-hsueh
ts'ao" [blood-thinner grass], "ai-hsieh
san-ch'i," "chu-hsieh san-ch'i," "t'ieh
lo-han," "chen tse-lan," "wu-ch'i,"
"hsien-ts'ai t'eng," "t'u san-ch'i."

Morphology: Perennial herb. Found
growing in fertile and moist grassy
areas or in small shrub thickets along
ditch edges or along stream edges.
Stem erect, purplish-red when young,
with multiple branches, longitudinally
ridged. Basal leaves clustered, margins
dentate or pinnately compound, surface
dark green, underside purplish-red,
leaves along upper stem alternate,
pinnately compound, margins of lobes
shallowly parted or crenate, points
acute or acuminate. In the fall,
golden yellow flowers growing from
top of stem, inflorescence capitate.
Achene keeled.

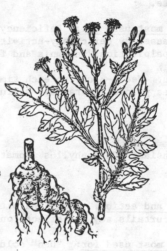

Properties and action: Neutral, sharp
tasting. As an anti-coagulant, resolves
clots. Stimulates circulation, and stops
bleeding. Clears fevers and detoxifies.

Conditions most used for: (1) Traumatic
injuries, amenorrhea; (2) hemoptysis,
hematemesis, epistaxis; (3) mastitis,
and other pus-forming diseases.

Preparation: The whole plant is used,
5 ch'ien to 1 liang each time, prepared
as decoction or crushed to be taken with
white wine. For external use, crush
and use a suitable amount as a poultice.

17. San-pai Ts'ao [Chinese Lizard's Tail]

Family: Saururaceae

Scientific name: Saururus chinensis
(Lour.) Baill.

Synonyms: "Pai-t'ou weng" [white-haired
old man], "hu-chi t'ui," "pai-chieh ou,"
"ch'ing-yu tan," "I-pai erh-pai," "shuang
tu she" [two single snakes].

Morphology: A perennial herb. Mostly
found growing in low damp places near
water. Rhizomes slender, adventitious
roots numerous. Stem erect, nodes
marked, surface striped. Leaves alternate, ovate or ovate-lanceolate, apexes
acute, bases cordate, margins intact;
when blooming 2-3 white leaves appear
at the apex of stem. In summer, light
yellow flowers growing from the stem
apex, inflorescence racemose, leaves
opposite. Capsule cracked open at
tip when ripe.

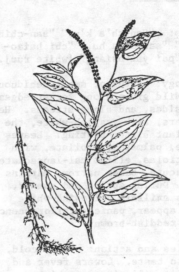

Properties and action: Cooling, slightly
sweet. Clears fever and detoxifies,
promotes diuresis and reduces inflammation.

Conditions most used for: (1) Edema,
nephritis-associated edema, nutritional
edema, inflammatory conditions and
calculus of the urinary system; (2)
rheumatoid arthritis; (3) boils and
abscesses, rashes and fungus infections
of the skin.

Preparation: The whole plant is used,
5 ch'ien to 1 liang each time, prepared in decoction. For external use,
the fresh grass may be crushed and
applied on affected areas.

18. San Ya-k'u [Rue species]

Family: Rutaceae

Scientific name: Evodia lepta (Spreng.) Merr.

Synonyms: "San-ch'a k'u," "san-chih ch'iang" "san-ch'a hu," "chi hsiao-feng," "pai yun-hsiang" [white rue].

Morphology: Shrub or small deciduous tree. Wild grown along forest edges, on hillsides, and along streams. Height 2-5 meters, bark grayish-white, the whole plant bitter-tasting. Leaves opposite, palmate trifoliate, with long petioles, elliptical-lanceolate, apexes acute, bases narrow, margins intact. During spring and summer, numerous axillary yellowish-white flowers appear, panicle inflorescence. Capsule reddish-brown.

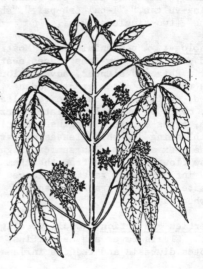

Properties and action: "Han" cold, bitter to taste. Lowers fever and detoxifies, alleviates itching.

Conditions most used for: (1) Epidemic influenza, meningitis, infectious hepatitis, sore throat; (2) rheumatoid arthritis pain, traumatic injuries; (3) chicken pox, hemorrhoids.

Preparation: Roots and leaves are used, 3-5 ch'ien each time, prepared in decoction.

19. San-k'e Chan [Chin's barberry]

Family: Berberidaceae

Scientific name: Berberis chengii Chen.

Synonyms: "Three needles," "huang lien" [coptis chinensis], "t'u huang-lien" [native coptis].

Morphology: Prickly evergreen shrub. Found growing on hilly slopes in shady and fertile spots. Roots thick and sturdy. Stem with numerous branches, older parts grayish-yellow, newer growth light yellow, deeply grooved. Leaves leathery, alternate or clustered, elliptical-obovate to obovate-elliptical, apexes acute or obtuse, barbed, bases gradually narrowing, leaf margins barbellate-dentate, basal leaves thick and prickly, forked. In the spring, small yellow flowers appear. Berry spheroid, purplish-red.

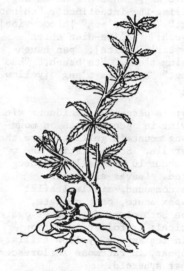

Properties and action: "Han" cold, bitter to taste. Antipyretic and detoxifying, anti-inflammatory and antibacterial.

Conditions most used for: (1) Acute gastroenteritis, gingivitis, laryngitis, conjunctivitis; (2) boils and abscesses, ulcers, burns; (3) traumatic injuries.

Preparation: Roots and stems are used, 2-4 ch'ien each time, prepared in decoction, or crushed and mixed with sesame oil or vaseline for use as ointment.

20. Ta Hsueh-t'eng [Big blood-vine]

Family: Sargentodoxaceae

Scientific name: Sargentodoxa cuneata (Oliv.) Rehder et Wils.

Synonyms: "Kuo hsueh-t'eng," "hung-t'eng," "hua hsueh-t'eng," "hsueh-kuan-ch'ang" [blood-filling-the-intestines[, "ch'uan-chien lung," "hsueh-t'eng" [blood-vine], "ta-huo-hsueh," "ch'ien-nien chien" [thousand-year's health], "pan hsueh-lien," "hsing t'eng," "ta hsueh," "huo hsueh-t'eng," "huang la-t'eng" [yellow wax-vine].

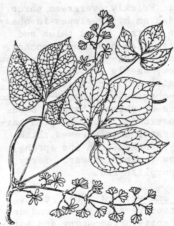

Morphology: A perennial deciduous vine. Found growing in open forests on mountains, along mountain gullies where the soil is fertile. Stem twisting and climbing, about 10 meters long, young branches red. Leaves alternate, trifoliate compound, middle leaflet obovate, apex acute, base cuneate, leaflets on both sides deltoid or ovate, nonsymmetrical; trifoliate venation marked. In the spring, yellow axillary flowers appear, in racemose inflorescence. Berry almost spheroid.

Properties and action: Neutral, slightly bitter. Blood stimulate and tonic.

Conditions most used for: (1) Amenorrhea in women, metrorrhagia, anemia, traumatic injuries; (2) rheumatoid arthritis; (3) hookworm disease, roundworm disease and filariasis.

Preparation: Stems are used, 5 ch'ien to 1 liang each time, in decoction or steeped in spirits.

21. Ta-ch'ing [verbena species]

Family: Verbenaceae

Scientific name: Clerodendron cyrtophyllum Turcz.

Synonyms: "Tan ch'in-chia," "tan p'o-p'o," "lu-tou ch'ing," "ch'ou-hsieh hsieh shu" [stink-leaf tree], "ch'ou ta-ch'ing," "ku-tsai hsieh," "tan p'o-niang," "ts'ai-sheng tzu," "ta pai-chieh."

Morphology: Deciduous shrub growing wild in shrub thickets on mountain slopes. Stem height reaching 3 meters. Single leaves opposite, long elliptical or ovate, apexes acuminate, bases almost rounded or mucronate, madrib on back raised, venation on both sides pubescent, unpleasant odor emitting when shaken. In summer, white flowers appear, inflorescence panicle or cymose. Drupe blue and globular.

Properties and action: "Han" cold, bitter to taste. Antipyretic and detoxifying, blood "cooling" and diuretic.

Conditions most used for: (1) Preventive for epidemic meningitis; (2) tonsillitis, acute pharyngitis, mumps; (3) snake and insect bites.

Preparation: Leaves and roots are used. Leaves 3-5 ch'ien, and roots 5 ch'ien to 1 liang used each time, prepared in decoction; or fresh leaves may be used crushed for painting on affected parts.

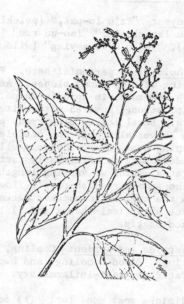

22. Ta-chi [Common or plumed thistle]

Family: Compositae

Scientific name: Cirsium japonicum Dc.

Synonyms: "Tz'u lo-pai," [prickly turnip], "shan lao-shu-le," "lao-hu tzu" [tiger's burs], "yeh p'u-kung-ying" [wild dandelion].

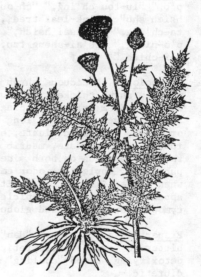

Morphology: A perennial herb. Found growing wild on sunny slopes. Adventitious roots numerous, in spindle shape. Stem erect, strong, covered with white woolly hairs. Basal leaves clustered, petioled; stem leaves alternate, no petioles, base clasping stem; leaves obovate elliptical-rounded, margins irregularly parted, lobes serrated, barbs of varying lengths at tips. In the summer reddish-purple flowers growing from the top, inflorescence racemose. Achene elliptical-shaped and flat, plumed at tip.

Properties and action: Cooling, and sharp-tasting. Blood "cooling" and hemostatic, diuretic and anti-inflammatory.

Conditions most used for: (1) Boils and carbuncles; (2) Acute appendicitis; (3) uterine bleeding, hematuria, nose bleed, hematemesis, traumatic bleeding.

Preparation: Dried roots are used, 1 liang each time in decoction.

23. Hsiao Mao-ken [Small crowfoot]

Family: Ranunculaceae

Scientific name: Ranunculus zuccarinii Mig.

Synonyms: "Mao-chao ts'ao" [cat's-claw grass], "huang-hua ts'ao" [yellow-flower grass].

Morphology: A perennial herb. Usually found growing along paddy field edges, village outskirts, grassy slopes. Height 5-15 cm. Subterranean web-like tuberous roots. Basal leaves tri-parted, long petioles, lobes again 2-3 parted or not parted at all, with a few teeth on margins, leaflets rounded or obovate, tips often dentate and shallowly parted, bases cuneate; stem leaves non-petioled, 3-parted deeply, lobes slender-linear. In the summer, yellow flowers appearing from top. Achene ovate, with short and slightly curved tip.

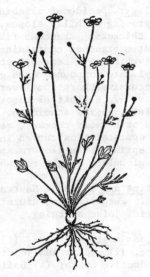

Properties and action: Neutral, biting, toxic. Dispels "congestion," alleviates pain, retards pterygium growth.

Conditions most used for: (1) Headache and toothache; (2) malaria; (3) enlarged glandular growths; (4) corneal pterygium.

Preparation: The whole plant is used, the fresh leaves crushed each time into a ball, and a horsebean-size amount is placed on the affected part or surrounding acupuncture points.

24. Hsiao-kuo Ch'iang-wei [Small-bloom rose]

Family: Rosaceae

Scientific name: Rosa cymosa Tratt.

Synonyms: "Ch'i chi-mei" [seven sisters], "ch'ing tz'u" [blue thorns].

Morphology: Deciduous climbing shrub.
Found growing on hilly slopes, roadsides
and in thickets. Branches fibrous and
fine, stem branches containing prickly
recursive thorns. Leaves leathery,
oddly-pinnate compound, axes grooved,
with recursive thorns on lowersurfaces;
leaflets 3-7, elliptical to ovate-
lanceolate, apexes acuminate, bases
rounded or broadly cuneate, margins
finely dentate, tips curved inward.
In the spring white flowers appear.
Achene globular, bright red when ripe.

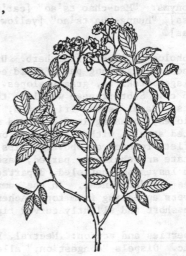

Properties and action: Neutral, sour
tasting. Purgative and diuretic, anti-
rheumatic, joint soothing.

Conditions most used for: (1) Blood
in urine; (2) rheumatism joint pain;
(3) productive cough; (4) boils.

Preparation: Roots, leaves and fruits
are used, 3 ch'ien to 1 liang each
time, prepared in decoction. A suitable amount may be used externally.

25. Hsiao-hui [Common fennel]

Family: Umbelliferae

Scientific name: Foeniculum vulgare Mill

Synonyms: "Hsiao-hui-hsiang" [fragrant
fennel], "Hui-hsiang hsieh" [fragrant
fennel leaves]

Morphology: Perennial herb. Wild
grown or cultivated in gardens. Whole
plant highly aromatic. Stem erect,
cylindrical. Basal leaves clustered,
stem leaves alternate, leaves 3 or 4
times pinnately compound, parted lobes
linear. In the fall, yellow flowers
appear in a compound umbellate inflorescence. Fruits suspended.

Properties and action: Neutral, sharp
and sweet tasting. A tonic that stimulates energy, promotes digestion, resolves
phlegm, and stimulates milk production.

Conditions most used for: (1) Gastroenteritis; (2) hernia; (3) indigestion
and abdominal pain.

Preparation: Fruits are used, 1-2 ch'ien
each time, prepared in decoction. Or
crushed and mixed with clear boiled
water for drinking.

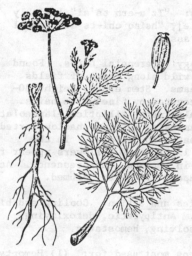

26. Hsiao-chi [Safflower species]

Family: Compositae

Scientific name: Cnicus segetum (Bunge)
Maxim.

Synonyms: "Tz'u-erh ts'ai" [prickly
vegetable], "hsiao chi-ts'ao" [small
onion-grass].

Morphology: Perennial herbs. Found
growing wild along edges of fields
and streams. Stem erect, height 30-
16 cm, covered by fine white hairs.
Leaves alternate, elliptical-lanceolate,
tips acuminate, margins shallow-parted
and crenate, no petioles. In the
summer, light purple flowers appear from
the tip in racemose inflorescence. Achene
oval-shaped, tip white, plumed.

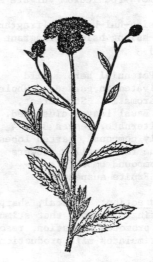

Properties and action: Cooling and bitter
tasting. Antipyretic, detoxifying,
clot-resolving, hemostatic.

Conditions most used for: (1) Hemoptysis,
hematemesis, metorrhagia; (2) boils and
carbuncles; (3) traumatic bleeding.

Preparation: The whole plant is used,
5 ch'ien to 1 liang each time, prepared in decoction.

27. Hsiao Huai-hua [Tick trefoil species]

Family: Leguminosae

Scientific name: Desmodium caudatum (Thunb) DC.

Synonyms: "Shan ma-huang" [mountain leech], "pa-jen ts'ao," "shui-chih ts'ao" [leech grass], "t'ou-tzu ts'ao," "o ma-huang" [hungry leech], "nien-I tz'u" [sticky thorns], "ts'ao hsieh-pan," "lu-pien chi" [roadside chicken], "lu-pein hsiao."

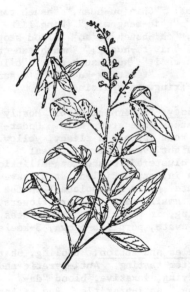

Morphology: Grassy shrub. Found growing in mountain wilds and grassy pastures. Stem erect, branching. Trifoliate compound leaves alternate, petioled, long elliptical or lanceolate, apexes acute, middle leaflet larger, midrib on back pubescent. In the summer white flowers appearing, in axillary or apical racemose inflorescences. Flat legumes glochidiate.

Properties and action: Neutral, bitter tasting. Antipyretic and detoxifying, analgesic for entrenched pain.

Conditions most used for: (1) Dysentery, gastroenteritis, mastitis, boils and carbuncles; (2) influenza fever, incomplete appearance of measles rash; (3) gastric and duodenal ulcers, and abdominal cramps in women.

Preparation: The whole plant is used, 3 ch'ien to 1 liang each time, prepared in decoction. Decoction can also be used for bathing skin in skin diseases.

28. T'u Ta-huang [Dock species]

Family: Polygonaceae

Scientific name: Rumex daiwoo Makino

Synonyms: "Chin pu-huan," "hsueh tang-k'uei," "chiu-meng wang" [king life-saver], "chi-hsueh ts'ao" [blood-stopping grass], "niu ta-huang," "hsueh san-ch'i," "lo-pai ch'i," "huo hsueh-tan," "t'ien san-ch'i," "t'u tang-kuei," "t'u san-ch'i," [ringworm medicine].

Morphology: Perennial herb. Mostly cultivated, some grown wild. Under-ground root large and fleshy, yellow. Stem height over 1 meter. Basal leaves clustered, ovate long-elliptical, margins intact, petioled; stem leaves alternate, ovate-lanceolate. In the summer, small green axillary flowers appearing, in panicle inflorescences. Achene ovate, purplish-brown, 3-keeled.

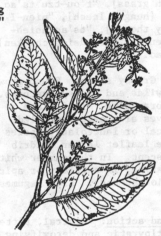

Properties and action: Cooling, sharp and bitter tasting. Anti-pyretic and detoxifying, laxative, blood "de-clotting," anti-pruritic. Bug killer.

Conditions most used for: (1) Constipation, abdominal cramps; (2) all kinds of boils and abscesses, fungus infections.

Preparation: Roots are used, 5 ch'ien each time, prepared in decoction. Suitable amount can also be used externally.

29. T'u ching-chieh [Chenapodium species]

Family: Chenpaodiaceae

Scientific name: Chenopodium ambrosioides
L.

Synonyms: "hu-ku hsiang" [fragrant tiger
bones], "t'u yen-ch'en," "shih-tzu ts'ao"
[lice-grass], "kao-tzu ts'ao," "shua-ch'ung
chieh" [insect-killing mustard], "kou-ch'ung
ts'ao" [hookworm herb].

Morphology: Annual herb. Found growing
along village outskirts and roadsides.
Stem erect, height attaining 1 meter,
spindled, emitting a fragrance when
crushed. Leave alternate, oblong-
rounded to oblong-rounded lanceolate,
margins crenate or undulate and sparsely
toothed, short-petioled. In summer and
fall, small greenish-white flowers growing from the axils and apexes of stems,
inflorescence spike. Fruit small
ascocarp.

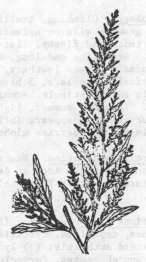

Properties and action: Neutral, biting
and bitter, fragrant. Anthelmintic,
stomachic, carminative, analgesic.

Conditions most used for: (1) Ancylostomiasis; (2) poisonous insect and spider
bites.

Preparation: The whole plant is used,
5 fen to 1 ch'ien each time, crushed
and mixed with boiling water for tea;
or stems and leaves may be boiled in
water for external use as compresses
or as soaks or baths.

30. T'u fu-ling (Greenbrier, catbrier) [China Root]

Family: Liliaceae

Scientific name: Smilax Glabra Roxb.

Synonyms: "kuang-yen pa-hsieh" [shiny
leaf smilax], "leng-fan tu'an" [ball-
of-leftover rice], "ti hu-ling," "shan
ku'ei-lai," "kou-lang-t'ou," "chiu-lao-
shu," "t'u pi-chieh."

Morphology: Climbing, trailing shrub.
Found growing wild on uplands. Root
tuber thick and fleshy, flat-round
nodes. Stem fine and long, smooth with
no thorns. Leaves leathery, alternate,
elliptical-lanceolate, 3 basal veins,
patiole short, stipule becoming 2 tendrils. In early summer, light yellow
axillary flowers appear, inflorescence
umbellate. Red berries globular.

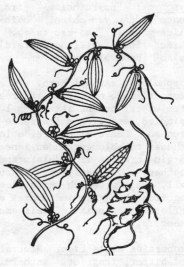

Properties and action: Neutral, bland
and cool tasting. Acts as detoxifier,
"moisture-promoter" (li-shih), stomach
tonic.

Conditions most used for: (1) Indigestion,
diarrhea, nephritis, cystitis; (2)
rheumatoid arthritis; (3) lymphadenopathy,
boils and abscesses, furuncles, syphilis.

Preparation: Stem tubers are used.
5 ch'ien to 1 liang each time, prepared
(boiled) in water for internal consumption.

31. T'u Tang-shen [Bluebell species]

Family: Campanulaceae

Scientific name: Campanumoea javanica Bl.

Synonyms: "Chin-ch'ien p'ao" [gold-coined
leopard], "man chieh-keng [trailing blue-
bell], "nai ch'an" [milky 'bluebell'].

Morphology: Perennial trailing herb.
Found growing wild along hillsides and
damp fertile areas along streams. Roots
fleshy, cylindrical. Stems fine and long,
entwining, a white milky juice seeping
out when broken. Leaves opposite, sometimes alternate, broadly ovate, apexes
obtuse, bases cordate, margins sparsely
toothed, petioles long. During summer
and fall, purplish-blue axillary flowers
appear. Globular berry purple when ripe.

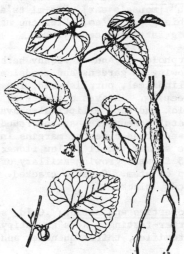

Properties and action: Slightly warm-
natured, taste bitter-sweet. A stomach
tonic that stops diarrhea, promotes
lactation.

Conditions most used for: (1) Spleen-
deficient diarrhea, general weakness;
(2) poor lactation (inadequate milk
supply).

Preparation: Roots are used, 1-2
liang each time, prepared in water
and taken as a decoction.

32. Ma-Ch'ih Hsien [Portulaca]

Family: Portulacaceae

Scientific name: Portulaca oleracea L.

Synonyms: "Kua-tzu ts'ai," "lao-shu erh" [mouse's ear], "Ta-mi ts'ai," "chiang-pan ts'ao," "fei-chu nan" [hog-fattening cedar].

Morphology: Annual fleshy herb. Found growing in gardens and roadsides. Stem cylindrical, purplish-red, lower section creeping. Leaves opposite or alternate, thick and fat, elliptical-obovate or spatulate-cuneate, apexes rounded-retuse, bases broad-cuneate, margins intact. In the summer, small yellow flowers appear, 3-5 flowers growing axillary or from the top of stem. Capsule cracked. Numerous seeds, black.

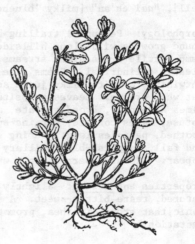

Properties and action: Cold, sour and bitter-tasting. Acts as antipyretic, detoxifier, thirst quencher and diuretic.

Conditions most used for: (1) Dysentery, enteritis; (2) urinary tract infections, leukorrhea; (3) hemorrhoids, erysipelas, boils and ulcers; (4) snake and insect bites.

Preparation: The whole plant is used, 1-2 liang each time, prepared and taken as decoction; or the fresh plant may be crushed for external application.

33. Ma-sang [Coriaria species]

Family: Coriariaceae

Scientific name: Coriaria sinica Maxim.

Synonyms: "Ha-mo shu" [frog-tree], "a-ssu-mu," "shang-t'ien t'i" [ladder-to-Heaven], "lien-hua hsien."

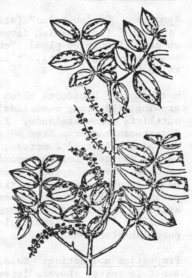

Morphology: Deciduous shrub. Found growing along hillsides, along gravelly rocks. Stem height 2-5 meters, tender branches squarish, red. Leaves opposite, elliptical or long-elliptical, apexes acuminate, bases rounded, margins intact, 3-ribbed venation fanning out from base, petioles short. Blooms in summer, axillary flowers, inflorescence race-mose. Achene bright red, black when ripe.

Properties and action: Cooling, sweet and bitter-tasting, toxic. Clears fevers and detoxifies, reduces swelling and stops pain. Also promotes healing, and acts as a vermifuge.

Conditions most used for: (1) Boils ulcers; (2) burn injuries; (3) ancylostomiasis.

Preparation: Leaves are used for medicine, 1-2 liang each time, prepared as a decoction or boiled in water for external use as a lotion or a soak. Or the fresh leaves may be crushed and used for a poultice.

34. Ma-ying tan [Prickly lantana, hedgeflower]

Family: Verbenaceae

Scientific name: Lantana camara L.

Synonyms: "ts'ou-ts'ao" [stink-grass],
"ju-I Hua" [as-you-wish flower], "wu-
se mei" [5-colored plum], "chu-shih
hua" [hog-dung flower], "t'ien-lan
ts'ao."

Morphology: Deciduous shrub. Found
growing wild along roadsides, village
outskirts and wastelands. Plant emits
disagreeable odor. Stem 4-keeled,
reaching height of 2 meters, with re-
curved thorns. Leaves opposite, ovate
or obtuse-ovate, apexes acuminate,
bases truncate, margins serrated,
petioled. Blooming in summer,
axillary flowers red, inflorescence
umbellate. Fruit fleshy, globoid,
purplish-black when ripe.

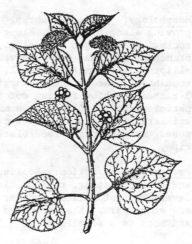

Properties and action: Cold, bitter-
sweet in taste. Lowers fever,
detoxifies, stops bleeding.

Conditions most used for: (1) Epidemic
parotiditis [mumps]; (2) neurodermatitis;
(3) traumatic injuries.

Preparation: Roots are used, 1-2 liang
each time, prepared in decoction; or
fresh leaves may be crushed for external
use.

35. Ma-pien Ts'ao [Vervain; verbena]

Family: Verbenaceae

Scientific name: Verbena officinalis L.

Synonyms: "Lung-ya ts'ao [dragon-teeth grass], "feng-t'ou tsao" [head-of-the-wind grass], "kou-ya ts'ao" [dog-teeth grass], "t'ui-hsueh ts'ao," "t'ieh ma-lien," "weng-mu hsi," "feng-ching ts'ao" "t'ieh ma-pien" [iron vervain], "t'ieh ma-hsien," "t'ieh ma-t'iao ken," "tzu-ting lung-ya" [purple-topped dragon sprout].

Morphology: Perennial herb. Found growing wild along wasted slopes, grass-lands, where soil is fertile. Stem rectangular, scabrous on keels and nodes. Single leaves opposite, 3-parted or irregularly pinnately-compound, mar-gins serrated, coarsely pubescent on both surfaces. Blooms in summer, flowers light purple or yellow, apical or axillary, inflorescence spiked. Capsule long ellipsoid.

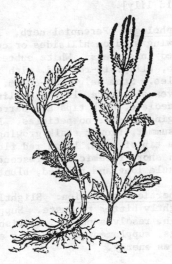

Properties and action: Cold, bitter to taste. Anti-coagulant, detoxifying, diuretic.

Conditions most used for: (1) Amenorrhea, traumatic injuries; (2) hepatitis, mastitis; (3) liver cirrhosis ascites, nephritic edema, urinary tract infections.

Preparation: The whole plant is used medicinally, 5 ch'ien to 1 liang each time, prepared in decoction. Fresh plant may be crushed for external use.

36. Shan-tan [Lily species]

Family: Liliaceae

Scientific name: Lilium concolor Salisb.

Synonyms: "Yao-pai-ho," "wo-tan,"
"hung-hua wo pai ho," "yeh pai-ho
[wild lily].

Morphology: Perennial herb. Found
growing wild on hillsides or cultivated in gardens. White subterranean
bulb, ellipsoid-rounded, with few
scales. Stem height 30-60 cm, erect.
Leaves alternate, linear or linear-
lanceolate, both tips are narrowed,
margins intact, no petioles. Blooms
in summer, flower stalk growing out
from tip of stem, large red flower,
with short racemic inflorescence.
Capsule long and rounded, bluntly angled.

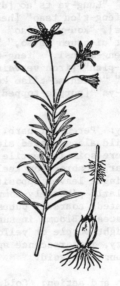

Properties and action: Slightly "cold,"
slightly bitter to taste. Suppresses
cough, resolves phlegm, nourishes the
lungs, supplements the vitals and restores energy.

Conditions most used for: (1) Lung
disease, hemoptysis; (2) fever due to
yin-deficiency; (3) anemia and shortness of breath.

Preparation: The subterranean bulb or
the whole plant may be used, 5 ch'ien
- 1 liang each time, prepared as decoction or further steamed with
sugar.

37. Shan Chi-chiao [Pondspice species]

Family: Lauraceae

Scientific name: Litsea cubeba (Lour) Pers.

Synonyms: "Pi-ch'eng-ch'ia," "ch'eng ch'ia-tzu," "shan ch'ia-tzu" [mountain eggplant], "shan ts'ang-tzu," "mu chiang tzu" [wood ginger], shan hu chiao [alpine pepper].

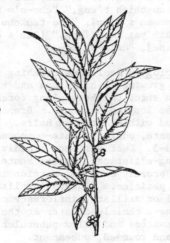

Morphology: Deciduous shrub or small tree. Found growing wild in mountain thickets. Plant emits a fragrant ginger odor. Bark grayish-brown, small branches turning black when dry. Leaves alternate, lanceolate, margins intact. Blooms in spring, flowers and leaves appearing simultaneously, light yellow, axillary inflorescence umbellate. Drupe spheroid.

Properties and action: Warm, peppery and sharp to taste. Loosens up phlegm, dispels "han" cold stimulates energy circulation and curtails swelling.

Conditions most used for: (1) Influenza headaches; (2) rheumatoid arthritis; (3) stomach-ache.

Preparation: The whole herb is used medicinally, 3-5 ch'ien each time, prepared in decoction.

38. Shan-chi Hsueh-t'eng [Wisteria species]

Family: Papiliona

Scientific name: Millettia dielsiana
Harms. et Diels.

Synonyms: "Hsiang-hua Yai tou-t'eng"
[fragrant cliff pea-vine], "lao-jen ken,"
"kuo-shan lung" [over-the-hill dragon],
"mao-tou-chieh t'eng," "chu-p'o t'eng,"
[hog-woman's vine], "hou-tzu chu p'i-ku,"
"ti-shih yai tou-t'eng," [Dee's cliff
pea vine], "hsia-pa tou."

Morphology: Deciduous climbing shrub.
Found growing on hillsides and highlands,
and in shrub thickets along forest edges.
Stem as long as 5 meters. Branches
covered with short brown hairs. Leaves
alternate, oddly pinnate-compound, leaflets 3-5. Leaf surfaces broadly lanceolate
to long-elliptical, apexes acute or obtuse,
bases broadly cuneate, margins intact, with
short petioles. Flowers purplish-red,
apical or axillary, inflorescence racemose,
forming a panicle cluster at the top,
flower stems and calyx puberulent. Legume
flat and rounded, pubescent.

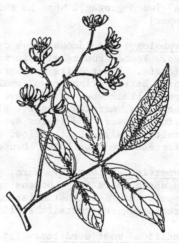

Properties and action: Warm, slightly
bitter and sweet. Stimulates blood and
energy, counteracts anemia, and strengthens
muscles and bone.

Conditions most used for: (1) Anemia,
blood deficiency and irregular menstrual
periods; (2) rheumatoid muscular aches
and pains, numbness of hands and feet
in blood deficiencies, infantile paralysis;
(3) "wet dreams."

Preparation: Roots and vine portions are
used medicinally, 4-6 ch'ien each time,
prepared in decoction; or prepared as a
wine potion.

39. Shan-yao [True yam species]

Family: Dioscoreaceae

Scientific name: Dioscorea batatas Deene.

Synonyms: "Huai-shan," "huai-shan yao,"
"tzu-t'i chi" [purple ladder], "shan-shu"
[mountain tuber], "yeh huai-shan," "t'u
yang-shen," "chiu huang-chiang," "yeh
pai-shu" [wild white potato].

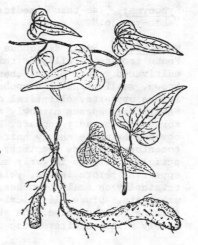

Morphology: Perennial growing herbaceous
vine. Cultivated or found growing wild
along hillslopes and in valleys. Stem
tuber thick and fleshy, cylindrical in
shape. Stem greenish-purple, slender and
entwining. Leaves opposite or trifoliate
whorled, ovate-lanceolate or deltoid-ovate,
apexes pointed, bases auricular-cordate,
axils frequently containing appendages,
petioles long and slender. Blooms in
summer, light purple axillary flowers
forming spike inflorescence. Capsule
3-angled and winged.

Properties and action: Neutral, sweet
tasting. Serves as stomach-spleen tonic
and anti-diarrheal agent, nourishes lungs
and complements the kidneys.

Conditions most used for: (1) Chronic
enteritis, dysentery, poor indigestion;
(2) asthma; (3) "wet dreams," excessive
perspiration, leukorrhea; (4) neurasthenia.

Preparation: Stem tubers are used medicinally. 3 ch'ien - 1 liang each time,
prepared in decoction.

40. Shan Chu-yu [Dogwood species]

<u>Family</u>: Cornaceae

<u>Scientific name</u>: Cornus officinalis S et Z.

<u>Synonyms</u>: "Yao-tsao" [medicinal date], "shan-you jo."

<u>Morphology</u>: Small deciduous shrub. Found growing in hillside thickets or cultivated. Bark of branches grayish-brown, small branches nonpubescent. Single leaves opposite, elliptical or long-elliptical, apexes narrowly acute, bases rounded or broadly cuneate, back surfaces covered by white shaggy hairs, rib-axils tomentose, margins complete, with short petioles. Blooms in early summer, flowers appearing before leaves, yellow, clustered terminally on small branches, inflorescences umbellate. Drupe elliptical-round, turning red when ripe, the skin reticulately wrinkled after being dried.

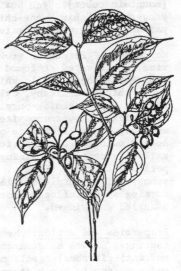

<u>Properties and action</u>: Slightly warm in nature, sour and biting to taste. Supplements the liver and kidneys, controls sperm ejaculation and excessive prespiration

<u>Conditions most used for</u>: (1) Backache and knee joint pains, dizziness and tinnitus, impotence and seminal emission, frequent micturition; (2) metrorrhagia; (3) excessive night sweats.

<u>Preparation</u>: Fruits are used medicinally, 3-5 ch'ien each time, prepared in decoction.

41. Shan P'i-hsieh [Yam species]

Family: Dioscoreaceae

Scientific name: Dioscorea tokoro Makino.

Synonyms: "Fen p'i-hsieh," "p'i-hsieh,"
"ch'ih-chieh," "pai-chih," "chu-mu,"
"pai pa-hsieh."

Morphology: A perennial vine-like herb.
Found growing wild on hillsides and shrub
thickets. Rhizome thick and fleshy, curved
or straight-cylindrical. Stems entwining,
slender and long. Leaves alternate, cordate,
apexes acute, bases cordate, 7-11 veined
longitudinally, with short petioles. Blooms
in summer, flower stalk axillary, holding
yellowish-green or purplish flowers, in
a spike inflorescence. Fruit a capsule.

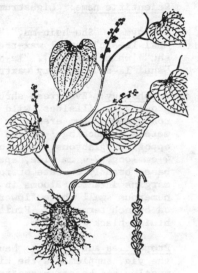

Properties and action: Neutral, bitter
to taste. Carminative and diuretic.

Conditions most used for: (1) Prostatitis,
and difficulty in urination; (2) rheumatoid
arthritis.

Preparation: Rhizomes are used medicinally,
3-5 ch'ien each time, prepared in
decoction.

42. Nu-chen [Waxy privet]

Family: Oleaceae

Scientific name: Ligustrum lucidum Ait.

Synonyms: "Shu-hsin-mu," "hsiao la-liu,"
"hsi la-shu" [small wax-tree], "pai la-
shu" [white waxtree], "la-shu"[waxtree],
"shui la-shu" [watery waxtree], "ju la-shu."

Morphology: Evergreen shrub. Found
growing on hillsides, wild places and
roadsides. Stem erect, as tall as 10
meters, branching. Leaves leathery,
opposite, glabrous, ovate or elliptical,
4 cm long, 2-4 cm wide, apexes acute,
bases broadly cuneate or rounded-obtuse,
margins intact. Blooms in summer,
numerous small white flowers appearing
on branch terminals. Fruit ellipsoid,
bluish-black when ripe.

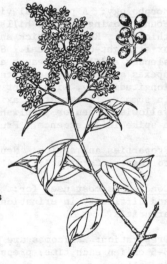

Properties and action: Neutral. Nourishes
the yin, supplements the kidneys, strengthens
muscles and bones, promotes clear vision
and hearing.

Conditions most used for: (1) Yin
deficiencies and internal heat, rheumatoid
pains and weakness of back and knee; (2)
deafness and blurred vision, palpitations
and insomnia; (3) constipation.

Preparation: Seeds are used medicinally,
2-5 ch'ien prepared in decoction.

43. Wan-nien Ch'ing [Evergreen]

Family: Liliaceae

Scientific name: Rohdea japonica Roth.

Synonyms: "Ch'ing-yu tan," "pao-ku ch'i," "chu-ken ch'i," "chin shih-tai," "k'ai-hou chien" [throat-opening arrow], "wu-sung ch'i," "hai-tai ch'ing," "o-pu-ch'ih," "niu ta-huang."

Morphology: Perennial evergreen herb. Found growing in wild lands, and damp and shady places along hillsides, or cultivated. Rhizome short and coarse, numerous fibrous roots emitting from the sides. Basal leaves clustered, thick, lanceolate, oblanceolate or ligulate, as long as 30 cm, apexes acute, bases gradually narrowing to become petioled, venation parallel, midrib obvious, leaf surfaces dark green, undersides light green, margins intact. Blooms in late spring, flower stalks emerging from leaf cluster, yellowish-white flowers terminal, forming short spike inflorescence. Fruit an orange-red berry.

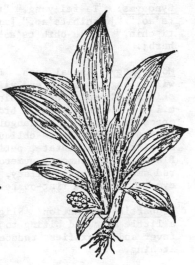

Properties and action: Cold, bitter yet slightly sweet to taste. Clears fever and detoxifies.

Conditions most used for: (1) Red and swollen sore throat, boils and abscesses; (2) early stages of epidemic encephalitis and diphtheria.

Preparation: Roots and leaves are used medicinally, 1-3 ch'ien each time, prepared in decoction. Roots can also be crushed with water and made into paste for external use.

44. Fei-yang Ts'ao [Spurge species]

Family: Euphorbiaceae

Scientific name: Euphorbia hirta L. var. typica L. C. Wheel.

Synonyms: "Ta fei-yang," "ta nai-chiang ts'ao," "ju-chih ts'ao," [milk herb], "ta-ti chin," "ta ju-chih ts'ao" [giant milk herb].

Morphology: Annual herb. Found growing wild along roadsides and village out-skirts. Creeping or climbing, secreting milky juice when stem is broken. Leaves opposite, ovate to rectangular-rounded, apexes rounded, bases obliquely inclined, margins finely dentate, petioles short. Blooms in the summer, numerous purplish-red small flowers axillary, inflorescence cymose. Capsule flat-ovate.

Properties and action: Slightly cooling, a little sour and biting to taste. Lowers fever and detoxifies, reduces flatus, stops itching.

Conditions most used for: (1) Enteritis, dysentery; (2) athlete's foot, other skin conditions.

Preparation: The whole plant is used medicinally, 5 ch'ien - 1 liang each time, prepared in decoction.

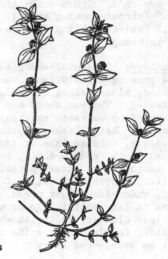

45. Ch'ien-chin T'eng [Priceless vine; Moonseed species]

Family: Menispermaceae

Scientific name: Stephania hernandifolia Walp.

Synonyms: "Shan wu-k'uei" [mountain black turtle], "pai yao" [white medicine], "chin-hsien tiao wu-k'uei" [black-turtle-hanging-on-a-gold-thread].

Morphology: A perennial deciduous vine. Found growing mostly on fertile spots of wild areas. Subterranean root tubers, dark brown externally, yellowish-white on the inside. Stem becoming woody when old, but green when young, 4-5 meters long. Single leaves alternate, peltate, ovate-rounded; margins intact, apexes obtuse, bases rounded or almost truncate, leaf surfaces dark green, backsides grayish-white. Blooms in the summer, flowers small and pale green. Drupe globular, red when ripe.

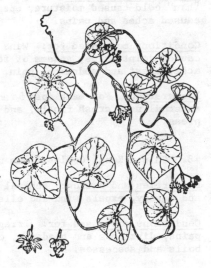

Properties and action: Cooling, bitter to taste, slightly toxic. Expels flatus, detoxifies, clears meridian passageways and stimulates muscles.

Conditions most used for: (1) Rheumatoid arthritis; (2) laryngitis, toothache, gingivitis; (3) deficient-activity abdominal pain.

Preparation: Root tubers are used medicinally, 2-5 ch'ien each time, prepared as decoction.

46. Ch'uan Pei [Szechuan fritillary]

Properties and action: Slightly cold, bitter and acrid to taste. Nourishes the lungs, resolves phlegm, lowers fever and dispels constipation.

Conditions most used for: (1) Chronic cough, "heated" [nonproductive?] cough and dry sputum, enlarged cervical nodes.

Preparation: For each preparation, 1-3 ch'ien, prepared as decoction.

47. Ch'uan Wu [Szechuan monkshood]

Properties and action: Slightly warm, biting to taste, very toxic. Eliminates "han" cold-caused moisture, opens up meridian passageways, alleviates cold caused aches and pains.

Conditions most used for: Wind and cold caused moisture -- numbness, wind caused joint pains, spasms of four extremities, hemiplegia, windblown headache, chest and abdominal pain.

Preparation: For each dose 5 fen - 1.5 ch'ien, prepared in decoction. For external use, crush finely, and mix with water or white wine for use as compress.

48. Ch'uan Kung [Conioselinum univattum]

Properties and action: Neutral and peppery to taste. Stimulates circulation and energy, expels wind and alleviates pain.

Conditions most used for: Irregular menstrual periods, post-partum contraction pains, dizziness and headache, cold numbness and muscular pain, inflammatory boils and abscesses.

Preparation: For each use, 1-3 ch'ien, prepared in decoction.

49. Ta-Feng-tzu [Common chaulmoogra]

Properties and action: Hot-natured, peppery to taste, highly toxic. "Dries" [excess] moisture, and kills and expels worms.

Conditions most used for: Leprosy, scabies, syphilitic ulcers.

Preparation: For internal use, 10-15 drops of chaulmoogra oil. A suitable amount may be used externally.

50. Ta-feng Ai

Properties and action: Cooling, bitter and peppery to taste, slightly toxic. Expels wind, clears meridians, and stimulates blood circulation.

Conditions most used for: Joint pains in influenza and rheumatism, post-partum gas pains, dysmenorrhea, traumatic injuries, pruritus.

Preparation: For internal use, 5 ch'ien - 1 liang each time, prepared as decoction. For external use, boiled in water and used for bathing the affected parts.

51. Ta Tou (Hei Tou) [Black soybean]

Properties and action: Neutral, pleasant to taste. Supplements the kidneys, and cultivates the heart (the nerves), expels gas and provides clear vision, stimulates blood circulation, promotes diuresis, lowers fever, and detoxifies.

Conditions most used for: Kidney-deficient enuresis, wind-caused dizziness, edema, food poisoning, overactive fetal activity in pregnant women.

Preparation: For internal use, 5 ch'ien - 1 liang each time, prepared in decoction.

52. Ta Hui (Pa-chiao Hui-hsiang) [Common fennel]

Properties and action: Slightly warming, peppery and fragrant. Warms the central organs, and dispels "han" cold, corrects energy and alleviates pain.

Conditions most used for: Hernia, gaseous belching, "han" cold-stomach and vomiting, "han" cold abdominal pain.

Preparation: For each dose, 5 fen - 1.5 ch'ien each time, prepared as decoction.

53. Ta-huang (Rheum officinale) [Rhubarb]

Properties and action: Cold, bitter to taste. Expels heat and corrects constipation, breaks down clots.

Conditions most used for: Constipation, moist-heat jaundice, heat-toxic boils and ulcers, worm-caused or indulgence-caused dysentery, blood clots [that need expulsion].

Preparation: For each preparation, 1.5 - 3 ch'ien made up as decoction. For external use, a suitable amount may be crushed and mixed with water for compress.

54. Ta Fu-p'i [Betelnut palm]

Properties and action: Slightly warm, biting to taste. Stimulates energy circulation and promotes diuresis, eliminates stagnation [constipation?]

Conditions most used for: Dyspepsia and constipation, edema and beri beri, diminished urinary output, and other stoppages.

Preparation: For each use, 1.5 ch'ien - 3 ch'ien, prepared as decoction.

55. Shan-tou Ken (Euchresta japonica)

Properties and action: "Han" cold, bitter to taste. Lowers fever and detoxifies.

Conditions most used for: Sore throat, toothache and tooth abscesses, hemorrhoids, boils and abscesses.

Preparation: For each use, 1.5 - 3 ch'ien prepared as decoction. For external purposes, a suitable amount may be used.

56. Shan Tz'u-ku (Tulipa edulis)

Properties and action: Cold-natured, sweet yet peppery to taste, slightly toxic. Lowers fever and detoxifies, resolves sputum and loosens (constipation).

Conditions most used for: Ulcers and abscesses, tubercular cervical nodes.

Preparation: For each use, 1 - 3 ch'ien prepared in decoction. For external purposes a suitable amount may be used.

57. T'u P'i-ch'ung (Land isopoda)

Properties and action: Slightly "han" cold, somewhat salty to taste, toxic. Alleviates amenorrhea, stops pain, stimulates lactation.

Conditions most used for: Traumatic injuries, "clotting" cramps in women, amenorrhea, and abdominal masses.

Preparation: For each use, 8 fen - 1.5 ch'ien, prepared as decoction. Or roast and crush into powder for consumption. Not to be used for pregnant women.

58. Ma-wei Sung (Pinus massoniana)

Properties and action: Warming, bitter to taste. Expels wind and "dries"
moisture.

Conditions most used for: Pains and aches associated with rheumatism.

Preparation: For each use, 3 - 5 ch'ien, prepared as decoction. For external
purposes, use a suitable amount.

59. Ma Po (Lycoperdon gemmatum)

Properties and action: Neutral, peppery to taste. Clears fever and detoxifies.

Conditions most used for: Sore throat, hoarseness and coughing, hemoptysis
and nosebleed, various ulcers and skin conditions.

Preparation: For each use, 1 - 1.5 ch'ien, prepared as decoction. For external purposes, use a suitable amount.

60. Fei Huang [Flying locust] (Tsa-meng)

Properties and action: Neutral, pleasant to taste. Supplements deficiencies
and complements the blood.

Conditions most used for: Lung-disease associated coughing and asthma,
post-partum anemia, and worms in children.

Preparation: For each use, 5 ch'ien - 1 liang. Burnt or sun-dried grasshoppers are crushed and fried with sauce, then taken with some boiled water.

61. Mu Kua [Papaya] (T'ieh-keng Hai-t'ang)

<u>Family</u>: Rosaceae

<u>Scientific name</u>: Chaenomeles lagenaria
Koidz.

<u>Synonyms</u>: "Tu mu-kua," "ch'un-an hsiao
mu-kua," "hsuan mu kua."

<u>Morphology</u>: A deciduous shrub. Mostly
cultivated, rarely found wild. Branches
spreading, thorned. Single leaves alternate,
almost non-petioled, ovate to long
elliptical, apexes sharply acute, bases
cuneate, margins finely serrated, surfaces smooth and glabrous, stipule
large. Blooms in the spring, axillary
flowers like those of the pear, appearing before or at the same time that the
leaves appear, several flowers clustered,
red. Fruit a yellowish-green ovoid or
globose "pear," smooth, fragrant.

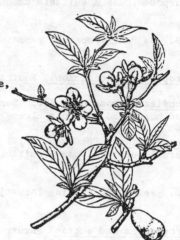

<u>Properties and action</u>: Warm, sour and
biting to taste. Fortifies the spleen
and resolves moisture, loosens up the
sinews and activates the muscles.

<u>Conditions most used for</u>: (1) Vomiting
and diarrhea, cholera-associated cramps;
(2) joint pains in the back and knee,
numbness in cases of beri beri.

<u>Preparation</u>: The fruits are used
medicinally, 2-4 ch'ien each time,
prepared in decoction.

62. Mu Fang-chi [Snailseed]

Family: Menispermaceae

Scientific name: Cocculus trilobus (Thunb) DC

Synonyms: "Kuang fang-chi," "hsiao ch'ing-t'eng" [small green vine], "ch'ing mu-hsiang," "Pai-shan fan-shu" [Pai-shan sweet potato], "T'ien fang-chi" [Yunnan cocculus], "t'eng ku-shen," "ch'ing t'eng," "t'u-shui hsing," "ch'ing t'eng-ken," "t'u fang-chi" [local cocculus], "she-tu hsiao" [snakebite neutralizer], "huang-shan t'eng" [yellow eel vine], "ching-feng t'eng," "fang-chi," "ch'uan-ku feng," "Kuang t'eng-tzu" [S. china vine], "chu'an-shan t'eng" [mountain pene-trating/boring vine], and "chu'an-shan chia" [crocodile].

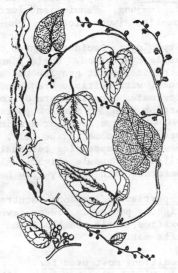

Morphology: Entwining deciduous vine. Found growing wild along hillsides and edges of gullies. Whole plant pubescent. Root an irregular round cylinder. Stem woody, up to 3 meters long, with fine longitudinal stripes. Single leaves alternate, ovate or ovate-rounded, apexes pointed, bases rounded, margins intact or undulate, few shallowly 3-parted, with petioles. In the summer, terminal or axillary yellowish-white flowers appear, forming a panicle inflorescence. Round drupe bluish-black, powdery white on surface.

Properties and action: Cooling, flavor bitter and peppery. Expels wind and eliminates moisture, opens meridian passageways and activates sinews, promotes diuresis and reduces inflammation, detoxifies.

Conditions most used for: (1) Rheumatoid arthritis; (2) nephritic edema, urinary tract infections; (3) snake and insect bites, other boils and ulcers of unknown origin.

63. Mu Fu-jung [Rose mallow species]

Family: Malvaceae

Scientific name: Hibiscus mutabilis L.

Synonyms: "Fu-jung hua," "ti'ieh ku-san," "ti fu-jung," "shui-lien" [water lotus], "mu-lien" [woody lotus], "chu-hsiang."

Morphology: Deciduous shrub or tree. Mostly cultivated. Whole plant covered with fine, short grayish hairs. Stems erect, with multiple branches. Leaves alternate, broadly ovate or rounded-ovate, margins with 3-5 shallow parts and obtuse toothed apexes acute or acuminate, bases cordate. Blooms in the fall, white or red flowers appearing terminally or axillary. Capsule slightly globose, tomentose with light yellow hairs.

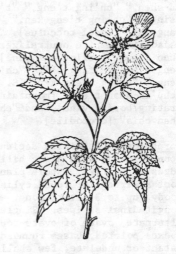

Properties and action: Neutral, flavor slightly peppery. Lowers fever and detoxifies, cools the blood and reduces inflammation.

Conditions most used for:
(1) Ulcers and abscesses; (2) burn injuries.

Preparation: Flowers and leaves are used medicinally, leaves crushed and mixed with strong tea for compresses; or flowers 1-2 ch'ien prepared in decoction.

64. Mu-t'ung [Trifoliate akebia]

Family: Lardizabalaceae

Scientific name: Akebia trifoliata (Thunb.) Koidz.

Synonyms: "Yang-k'ai-k'ou," "na-kua," "pa-yueh na," "huang-kou shen" [yellow dog's kidney], "pa-yueh tsa," "yang-tsa t'eng," "huang la-ku t'eng" [yellow wax-ribbed vine], "mu wang-kua," "tsa kua," "chu yao-tzu" [hog's kidneys], "pa-yueh kua" [August melon], "yu-chih-tzu."

Morphology: Deciduous vine. Found growing beneath forests or semi-shady and damp places in thickets. Stem entwining, reaching 6 meters or more, longitudinally striped and pock-marked. Leaves often clustered, trifoliate-compound, long petioles; small tri-foliate leaves leathery, ovate or long ovate-rounded, apexes elliptical and slightly dented, bases rounded or broadly cuneate, the whole margin per-haps slightly undulate. Purplish-red flowers appear in the spring, inflor-escence racemose. Berry purple, long cylindrical shape.

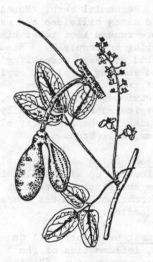

Properties and action: Slightly cold, bitter to taste. Settles heart fire [nerves], promotes moisture-heat, stimulates blood circulation.

Conditions most used for: (1) Moist-heat edema, micturition difficulties; (2) amenorrhea, inadequate lactation.

Preparation: Vine and fruit are used medicinally, 3-5 ch'ien each time, prepared in decoction.

65. Mu Tsei [Equisetum species]

Family: Equisitaceae

Scientific name: Equisetum hiemale L.

Synonyms: "Ts'ao-ts'ao," "che che ts'ao," "pi-t'ung ts'ao."

Morphology: Perennial herb. Found growing wild along hillsides and sandy areas. Subterranean root tuber blackish-brown, creeping horizontally. Stem multi-branched at base, resembling a cluster, and showing in midair obvious longitudinal grooves on surface, node separation obvious. In the summer, sporangium spike appears terminally, long elliptical in shape, erect, slightly acute at apex, dull brown.

Properties and action: Neutral, bitter to taste. Loosens up wind and clears fever, calms the liver and reduces pterygium formation, promotes diuresis and stops bleeding.

Conditions most used for: (1) Conjunctivitis, inflammation of the lacrimal ducts, pterygium; (2) influenza and colds, dysentery, edema; (3) hematuria, blood in stools, and metrorrhagia.

Preparation: The whole plant is used medicinally, 3-5 ch'ien each time, prepared as decoction.

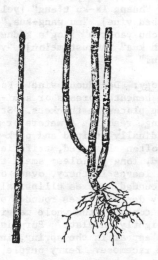

66. Mu Lan

Family: Leguminosae

Scientific name: Indigofera tinctoria
L.

Synonyms: "Ch'ing-tai," "yeh lan-chih-tzu" [wild blue twigs], "hsiao ch'ing," "ta ch'ing yeh," "ma-lan," "yeh huai-shu" [wild sophora], "Yin-tu lan" [Indian blue], "lan-ting" [blue dye], "huia-lan."

Morphology: Erect-standing shrub. Mostly found growing on hilly slopes, wild areas, and among weed patches along roadsides; also found cultivated. Stems erect, anoted, small branches covered by fine silvery white hairs. Leaves alternate, oddly pinnate compound, leaflets 7-15, opposite, long elliptical or obovate, apexes acute, bases cuneate, margins intact, back surfaces grayish-white, pubescent. Reddish-yellow flowers appearing in spring, forming racemic inflorescences. Legume slender and long, containing 5-12 seeds inside.

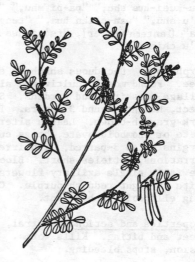

Properties and action: "Han" cold, salty to taste. Clears the liver to dispel depression, cools the blood and detoxifies, reduces inflammation and alleviates pain.

Conditions most used for: (1) Acute laryngitis, lymphoadenitis, mumps; (2) sudden high fevers; (3) swellings that are inflammed, scabies, heat rash.

Preparation: Roots and leaves are used medicinally, 5 ch'ien - liang of roots each time, prepared as decoction. Fresh leaves in suitable amount, crushed and used externally.

67. Mu Chin [Rose mallow species]

Family: Malvaceae

Scientific name: Hibiscus syriacus L.

Synonyms: "Mu Ching-hua," "chao-k'ai mu-lo" [morning-open-and-evening-close], "mu-kuei-hua shu," "pa-pi shu," "ts'a-ts'u shu," "wan-chien hua," "teng-chien hua" [lantern flower], "ts'ai-hua shu," "t'u chin p'i."

Morphology: Deciduous shrub or small tree. Found mostly cultivated along village outskirts and gardens. Stem erect, height around 3 meters. Tree bark grayish-brown. Leaves alternate, ovate or rhomboid-ovate, bases cuneate, margins often 3-parted, with irregular serrations, petioles short. Blooms in the fall, single axillary flowers in white or light reddish-purple. Capsule long ellipsoid, puberulent.

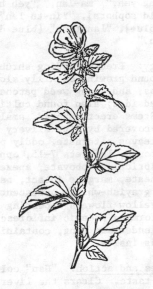

Properties and action: Neutral, flavor sweet and biting. Kills worms. Clears vision, stops bleeding.

Conditions most used for: (1) Dermaphytosis [root bark used]; (2) bloody stools accompanied by much gas, dizziness [flowers used].

Preparation: Root bark and blossoms are used medicinally, flowers 3-5 ch'ien each time, prepared as decoction. Root bark crushed and mixed with vinegar for external application.

68. Mu Pi

Family: Cucurbitaceae

Scientific name: Momordica cochinchinesis
(L) Spreng.

Synonyms: "T'u mu-pi," "mu-pieh-tzu,"
"mu-pieh t'eng," "mu-pieh kua."

Morphology: A perennial climbing vine-
like herb. Found growing under open
forests or among thickets. Subterranean
root and rhizome large and fleshy. Stem
slender, long and angled, with non-
branching spiral tendrils. Single
leaves alternate, ovate-rounded, 3-5
parted deeply, each lobe ovate,
apexes acute, bases on both sides
containing a protruding nectary, margins undulate. Blooms in the summer,
light-yellowish axillary flowers.
Fruit a long ellipsoid gourdish melon,
red, with numerous soft barbs on the
outside. Seeds black, flat, longitudinally striped.

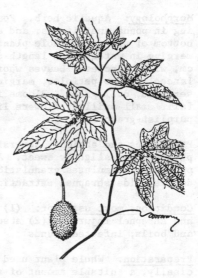

Properties and action: Warming, bitter
and slightly pleasant to taste, toxic.
Stimulates digestive function, detoxifies, promotes good appetite to put on
weight.

Conditions most used for: (1) Worms in
small children, as well as enteritis
and dysentery; (2) pus-forming ailments,
mastitis, hemorrhoids; (3) enlarged
lymph nodes, moles.

Preparation: Seeds are used medicinally
chiefly for external application. For
taking internally, care should be taken
(2-4 fen, prepared as decoction).

69. Shui Wang-sun

Family: Hydrocharitaceae

Scientific name: Hydrilla uerticillata
Casp. var roxburghii Casp.

Synonyms: "Hsia-kung ts'ao," "shui tsao"
[pondweed], "hei tsao" [black pondweed],
"hsia-mi ts'ao" [shrimp grass].

Morphology: Aquatic herb. Found growing in ponds and ditches, and along the
bottom of streams. Whole plant sub-
merging in water, stem length 60-70
cm, with branches. Leaves whorled,
lanceolate, no petioles, margins finely
serrated, dull green. Blooms in summer-
fall, small axillary flowers light
purplish-green.

Properties and action: Neutral, taste
pleasant and slightly sweet. Anti-
pyogenic, stimulates granulation, clears
debris, aids shrapnel extraction.

Conditions most used for: (1) Bullet
and shrapnel injuries; (2) abscesses
and boils, infected wounds.

Preparation: Whole plant used medicinally, a suitable amount of the fresh
product crushed for external application.

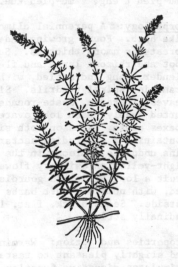

70. Shui Lung

Family: Onagraceae

Scientific name: Jussiaea repens L.

Synonyms: "Kuo-t'ang she" [pond-crossing snake], "shui-yang ts'ai," "ju-piao ts'ao" [fishbladder grass], "chia yung-ts'ai," "ch'an chien ts'ao" [cocoon grass].

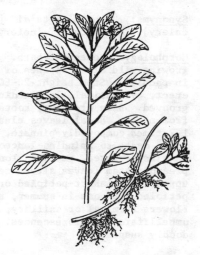

Morphology: Aquatic herb. Found growing mostly along water's edge, in ponds, and in ditches. Lower part of stem stoloniferous, the upper part floating on the water's surface, silk-like roots growing from nodes. Leaves alternate, obovate, apexes rounded or obtuse, bases narrowed, margins intact. Single axillary flowers, white. Capsule long and cylindrical.

Properties and action: Cooling, tastes pleasant and slightly sweet. Clears fever and detoxifies, cools the blood, promotes diuresis.

Conditions most used for: (1) Urinary tract infections; (2) boils and abscesses; (3) snakebites.

Preparation: The whole plant used medicinally, 5 ch'ien - 1 liang each time, prepared as decoction.

71. Shui Ch'in [Celery]

Family: Umbelliferae

Scientific name: Oenanthe stolonifera
DC

Synonyms: "Yeh ch'in-ts'ai" [wild
celery], "ch'in ts'ai" [celery].

Morphology: Perennial herb. Found
growing wild along ditches or cultivated
in paddies. Stem height 20-80 cm,
erect, cylindrical, longitudinally
grooved. Base creeping, roots growing
from nodes. Basal leaves clustered,
1-2 times compoundly pinnate, final
lobes ovate to spindled-lanceolate,
margins serrated, petioles long, ochrea
present; stem leaves alternate, smaller,
upper leaves short-petioled or non-
petioled. Blooms in summer, small white
flowers terminal or axillary, forming
umbelliferous inflorescences. Fruit
doubly suspended.

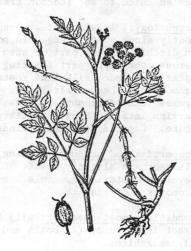

Properties and action: Neutral, pleasant to taste. Reduces fever and detoxifies, stops bleeding.

Conditions most used for: (1) Epidemic
influenza, fever and discomfort; (2)
jaundice; (3) hematuria; (4) metrorrhagia.

Preparation: The whole herb used medicinally, 5 ch'ien - 1 liang each time,
prepared as decoction.

72. Shu Ssu [Mint species]

Family: Labiatae

Scientific name: Stachys baicalensis
Fisch.

Synonyms: "Yeh tzu-ssu," "shan sheng-
ma," "wu lei-kung," "peng-t'ou ts'ao,"
"yen-hu ts'ao," shui chi-ssu," "yeh
yiu-ts'ai" [wild rape].

Morphology: Perennial herb. Found
growing along roadsides in wild places.
Stems erect, height 30-80 cm, elongate,
covered with white scabrous hairs.
Leaves opposite, non-petioled, long
elliptical-lanceolate, apexes obtuse,
bases cordate, margins serrated, surfaces wrinkled, blooms in the summer,
light purplish small flowers appearing
from the apex, forming spike-like
racemose inflorescence. Fruit a small
nut.

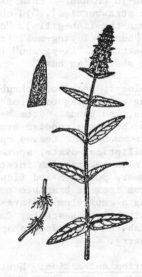

Properties and action: Cold-natured,
bitter and biting to taste. Can detoxify, stop bleeding, promote
diuresis.

Conditions most used for: (1) Metorrhagia;
(2) Hematuria; (3) jaundice; (4) bacterial dysentery.

Preparation: The whole plant is used
medicinally, 3-5 ch'ien each time,
prepared as decoction.

73. Shui Yang-mei [Madder species]

Family: Rubiaceae

Scientific name: Adina rubella Hance.

Synonyms: "Sha ching-tzu" [sand-thorn], "ch'uan-ju ch'uan," "chia yang-mei" [false strawberries], "ju ch'uan-sai [through-the-fish-gills], "chu'an-yu liu," "hung-p'i yang-mei" [red-skinned strawberries], "li-pa shu" [lattice-tree], shui-tu'an hua."

Morphology: Deciduous shrub. Found growing wild along edges of streams, ditches, and ponds. Stem height 1-2 meters, branches reddish-brown, smooth and non-pubescent. Leaves opposite, long elliptical-ovate, apexes acute, bases cuneate, margins intact. Blooms in summer, purplish-red flowers appearing from apex of branches and axils, forming a capitulum inflorescence, flower stem slightly pubescent. Capsule purplish-red when ripe, shaped like strawberry.

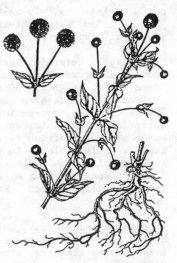

Properties and action: Neutral, bitter and biting to taste. Expels gas, stops diarrhea, stimulates circulation, and stops bleeding.

Conditions most used for: (1) Acute and chronic dysentery, enteritis; (2) mardsmus and other intestinal parasitical diseases; (3) ulcers; (4) traumatic bleeding.

Preparation: The whole inflorescence is used for medicinal purposes, 5 ch'ien - 1 liang each time, prepared as decoction; or inflorescences may be crushed and mixed with boiling water to be taken by mouth. A suitable amount may be used for external purposes.

74. Shui Ch'ang-p'u [Calamus species]

Family: Araceae

Scientific name: Acorus calamus L.

Synonyms: "Pai ch'ang-p'u" [white calamus], "ch'ang-p'u" [calamus], "ni ch'ang-p'u" [muddy calamus], "chien ch'ang-p'u" [sword calamus].

Morphology: Perennial aquatic herb. Usually found growing in paddy fields, and other damp areas along stream banks. Whole plant emitting characteristic fragrance. Rhizome thick and fleshy, subterranean stolon with numerous nodes, light red. Leaves clustered from rhizome, in parallel arrangement, lanceolate, midrib obvious, apexes acute, bases enclosing stem. Blooms in summer, yellowish-green flowers appearing from apex, forming a fleshy spandix inflorescence. Fruit an ovoid-round berry, red when ripe.

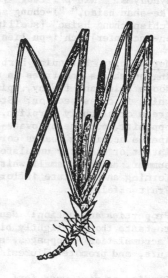

Properties and action: Neutral in nature, biting to taste. Expels gas, alleviates constipation, resolves phlegm, kills worms and detoxifies.

Conditions most used for: (1) Epilepsy and strokes; (2) rheumatoid arthritis; (3) stomach-ache, edema, toxic dysentery.

Preparation: Roots and stems are used medicinally, 1-2 ch'ien each time prepared in decoction. For external use, fresh roots and stems are crushed for application.

75. Nui-p'i Hsiao [Flycatcher species]

Family: Asclepiadaceae

Scientific name: Cynanchum caudatum Maxim.

Synonyms: "Niu-p'i tung" [cold oxhide], "ke-shan hsiao," "I-chung san-hsiao," "chien-chung hsiao" [swelling-reduction-on-encounter], ch'i-pu lien [7-step lotus].

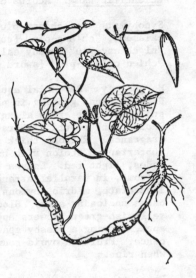

Morphology: Perennial herb. Found climbing on shrubs and trees in wild areas. Roots thick and fleshy, spindle-shaped, white in cross-section. Stem entwining, green or slightly purplish. Leaves opposite, cordate or ovate-cordate, apexes acuminate, bases cordate, margins intact or slightly undulate. Blooms in summer, axillary small white flowers forming an umbellate inflorescence. Fruit a follicle.

Properties and action: Neutral, soothing to taste though slightly bitter. Purges "accumulation" stoppages, eliminates moisture, and promotes diuresis.

Conditions most used for: (1) Liver cirrhosis ascitis, poor digestion, and "accumulation" stoppage caused abdominal pain; (2) gonorrhea and leukorrhea.

Preparation: Rhizomes are used medicinally, 5 ch'ien - 1 liang each time prepared in decoction.

76. Nui-nai Chiang [Spurge species]

Family: Euphorbiaceae

Scientific name: Euphorbia sieboldiana
Morr. et Decne.

Synonyms: "La-chiang ts'ao" [hot-sauce
herb].

Morphology: Perennial herb. Found
growing wild along embankments, and
edges of fields. Secretes white milky
juice when broken. Tap root cylindrical.
Stem erect, 20-40 cm in height, green
or slightly purplish. Leaves are
alternate, long oval or slightly obovate,
apexes slightly truncate or retuse,
bases cuneate, margins intact, no petioles.
In late spring, 5-9 flower stems appearing in clusters, each branch subdividing
further into two branches, showing 2
bracteal leaves at base of each branch,
opposite, deltoid ovate, forming a cymose
inflorescence, and 5 leaves whorled and
spreading at base of inflorescence. Capsule deltoid globular.

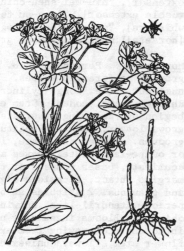

Properties and action: "Han" cold,
bitter to taste, toxic. Laxative
and diuretic.

Conditions most used for: (1) Schis-
tosomiasis-caused ascites, edema; (2)
constipation.

Preparation: Roots are used medicinally,
1 - 1.5 ch'ien each time, crushed and
swallowed with water.

77. Niu-wei Ts'ai [Oxtail greens]

Family: Liliaceae

Scientific name: Smilax nipponica Mig.

Synonyms: "Ta shen ching" [great muscle extensor], "niu-wei shen-ching" [oxtail muscle extensor], "lung-su ts'ao" [dragon's whiskers], "ma-wei shen-ching ts'ao" [horsetail muscle-extensor grass].

Morphology: Perennial herb. Found growing on forested slopes. Roots numerous, fine, long, cylindrical. Rhizome short, noded. Stem erect in beginning, becoming prostrate as it grows longer, showing longitudinal grooves. Leaves alternate, long ovate or ovate-lanceolate, apexes acute or acuminate, bases cuneate or rounded, margins intact, backsides light green and glaucous, 2 stipules at base of petiole, tendril-like, entwining other objects. Blooms in summer, umbellate inflorescence growing from axillary flower stem, flowers unisexed. Berry globular, black and powdery when ripe.

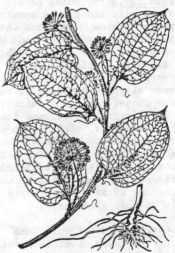

Properties and action: Neutral, pleasant taste. A muscle relaxant, it also stimulates circulation, expels gas and eliminates moisture.

Conditions most used for: (1) Arthritic pains, backache, (2) amenorrhea; (3) nightmares.

Preparation: Roots are used medicinally, 3-5 ch'ien each time, prepared in decoction.

78. Niu Pang [Great burdock]

Family: Compositae

Scientific name: Arctium lappa L.

Synonyms: "Niu-tzu," "ta-li-tzu," "sheng-ma," "niu-ting pao," "niu-pang-tzu."

Morphology: Biennial herb. Mostly cultivated. Roots fleshy. Stem multi-branching, height 1-2 meters. Basal leaves clustered, stem leaves opposite, large, broad-ovate or cordate, apexes rounded, bases cordate, leaf surfaces glossy, undersides pubescent with fine grayish-white hairs, margins irregularly dentate or slightly undulate. Blooms in summer, flowers light purple, in a capitulum inflorescence. Fruit achene, obovate, covered with stiff hairs.

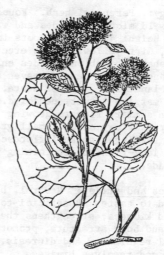

Properties and action: "Han" cold, bitter and slightly biting to taste. Clears fever, detoxifies, dispels wind.

Conditions most used for: (1) Influenza, tonsillitis; (2) boils and abscesses; (3) pertussis.

Preparation: Seeds, roots, and leaves are used medicinally, seeds 1-3 ch'ien each time, prepared in decoction; roots, leaves crushed for external application on affected parts.

79. Niu Hsi [Ox Knee]

Family: Amaranthaceae

Scientific name: Amaranthus bidentata Bl.

Synonyms: "Pai niu-hsi" [white ox-knee],
"t'u niu-hsi," "niu-ke-hsi."

Morphology: Perennial herb. Found
growing wild along roadsides and waste
places. Height 40-90 cm. Roots fine
and long, dirt yellow. Stems erect,
spindle-shaped or oblong, nodes enlarged,
young branches pubescent. Leaves opposite,
ovate or lanceolate, apexes acute, bases
cuneate, margins intact, petioled.
Blooms in summer, flowers growing from
apical or axillary stems, small green
flowers, forming a spike inflorescence.
Ascocarp long-rounded, containing 1
seed inside.

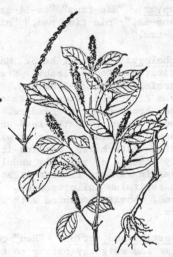

Properties and action: Neutral, bitter
and acrid to taste. Beneficial to the
liver and kidneys, strengthens the
muscles and bone structure, promotes
menstrual regularity and diuresis, pus
drainage and resolves bruises.

Conditions most used for: (1) as a
diphtheria preventive; (2) beri beri,
rheumatism pains; (3) impotency,
enuresis; (4) hematuria; (5) amenorrhea.

Preparation: Roots are used medicinally,
5 ch'ien each time, prepared in
decoction.

80. Wu Pao [Raspberry species]

Family: Rosaceae

Scientific name: Rubus tephordes Hance.

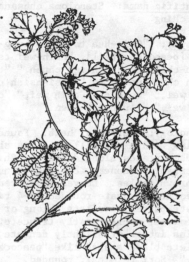

Synonyms: "Wu-lung pai-wei," "she wu-pao," "hei wu-pao" [blackberry], "tao shui-lien" [upside-down water-lotus), "wu-pao tz'u," "k'ou-szu p'u," "pa-yueh pao," "kuo-chiang lung" [crossing-the-river dragon], "ta wu-pao" [large black bubble].

Morphology: Climbing shrub. Found growing in sunny places in wild areas and roadsides. Stems, branches and petioles pubescent, covered with thorns and fine hairs. Leaves alternate, almost rounded, length and width almost equal, apexes acuminate, bases auricular, margins irregularly parted and serrated, leaves green on surface, white on backside, petioled. Blooms in summer, small white flowers growing from apex, forming a panicle inflorescence. Fruit a fleshy drupe, reddish-purple when ripe.

Properties and action: Neutral, sour and biting to taste. Stimulates circulation and stops bleeding, astringent.

Conditions most used for: (1) Traumatic injuries, pain in muscles and bones, numbness; (2) amenorrhea; (3) traumatic bleeding; (4) dysentery, diarrhea.

Preparation: Roots and leaves are used medicinally, 5 ch'ien - 2 liang each time, prepared in decoction. For external application, use a suitable amount.

81. Wu Chiu [Sphenomeris species]

Family: Pteridaceae

Scientific name: Stenoloma chusana
(L.) ching.

Synonyms: "Chin-hua ts'ao," "kung-chiao
wei" [peacock's tail], "chih-wei ts'ao,"
"chin-chih wei," "ch'ing chueh," "ta-
hsieh chin-hua ts'ao," "hsi-hsieh chin-
chih wei," "hsao chin-chih wei," "chi-
feng wei," "t'u huang-lien."

Morphology: Perennial herb. Found
growing wild along hillsides, in shady
and damp places along ditches. Rhizomes
subterranean runners, covered by numerous brown scales. Leaves clustered,
lanceolate to ovate-rounded, 3-4 times
pinnate-parted, leaflets oblong or
lanceolate, apexes mostly truncate,
margins intact or slightly dentate, 1
complete blade shaped like "peacock's
tail." Sori terminal, rounded.

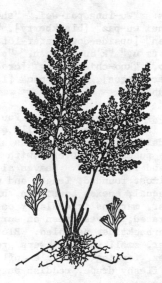

Properties and action: Cooling, bitter
to taste. Clears fevers and detoxifies,
reduces inflammation and stops bleeding.

Conditions most used for: (1) Colds
and influenza, bronchitis, pneumonia;
(2) enteritis, dysentery; (3) burns,
cuts, and skin sores.

Preparation: The whole plant is used
medicinally, 1-2 liang each time, prepared in decoction. For external
application, crush a suitable amount
of the fresh herb and apply to affected
part or dry the herb and pulverize to
obtain oil for external use.

82. Wu Yao [Allspice species]

Family: Lauraceae

Scientific name: Lindera strychnifolia
F. vill.

Synonyms: "Hsiang-hsieh shu" [fragrant-
leaf tree], "niu yen-ching" [cow's eyes],
"t'ai-wu," "hsiang-hsieh-tzu" [fragrant
leaves], "lei-kung shu" [thunder god
tree].

Morphology: Evergreen shrub or small
tree. Found growing in shrub thickets
along mountainsides. Roots fat and large,
small at both ends, forming a bead shape.
Young branches covered densely with rusty
colored fine hairs. Leaves alternate,
leathery or semi-leathery, broadly oval
or ovate, apexes acute or tail-like,
bases rounded or broadly cuneate, margins intact, 3-veined, petioled. Blooms
in summer, yellowish-green flowers growing from terminal and axillary stems,
forming umbellate inflorescences. Drupe
black and globular.

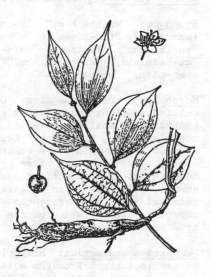

Properties and action: Warm-natured,
slightly biting to taste. Expels gas
and disperses cold, corrects energy
and relieves congestion, reduces inflammation and alleviates pain.

Conditions most used for: (1) Gastric
ulcers, gastritis, abdominal distension;
(2) apoplexy, headaches; (3) rheumatoid
back and leg pains; (4) hernia,
dysmenorrhea; (5) traumatic injuries.

Preparation: Roots are used medicinally,
1-3 ch'ien each time, prepared in decoction; for external use, crush leaves
for application on affected parts.

83. Wu Chiu [Tallow tree]

Family: Euphorbiaceae

Scientific name: Sapium sebiferum Roxb.

Synonyms: "Wu-shu kuo," "la-tzu shu"
[wax tree], "tao-hsueh mu," "wu-yu mu,"
"yu-tzu shu" [oil tree], "shiu-yu shu,"
"mu-hsin shu," "ku-ch'iu shu," "kan-
shan-pien," "mu-tzu shu."

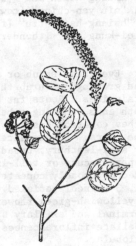

Morphology: Deciduous tree. Commonly
cultivated along roadsides or river
banks. Stem maximum height 15 meters,
containing sap, bark gray. Leaves
alternate, rhomboid-ovate or broadly
ovate, apexes awnlike, bases broadly
cuneate, margins intact. Blooms in
summer, yellowish-green flowers forming
terminal spike inflorescences. Fruit a
capsule. Seeds covered on the outside
by a white waxy layer.

Properties and action: Slightly warm,
bitter to taste. Promotes moisture
and relieves constipation, detoxifies and
stimulates pus drainage.

Conditions most used for: (1) Edema, constipation; (2) poisoning caused by 2 toxic
plants the smartweed Polygonum perfoliatum
and the spindle tree Tripterygium wilfordii
Hook; (3) snakebites; (4) skin diseases.

Preparation: Roots and leaves are used
medicinally, 1-2 liang each time prepared as decoction.

84. Wang-pu-liu-hsing [Cow soapwort]

Family: Carophyllaceae

Scientific name: Vaccaria pyramidate
Medic.

Synonyms: "Chin-kung hua" [Forbidden
Palace flower], "chien-chin hua," chin-
chien yen-t'ai [golden-lamp-on-silver
pedestal], "mai-lan-ts'ai."

Morphology: Annual or biennial herb.
Found growing wild on hillsides or
cultivated in gardens. Stem erect, height
attaining 60 cm, cylindrical, nodes enlarged.
Leaves opposite, ovate-lanceolate, apexes
acuminate, bases clasping stem, margins
intact. Blooms in late spring, light
red flowers forming a terminal cymose
inflorescence. Capsule ovate-round.
Seed globular and black.

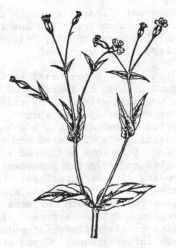

Properties and action: Neutral, pleasant
yet bitter to taste. Promotes menstrual
regularity and stimulates blood circulation, induces labor and promotes
lactation, reduces inflammation and
relieves pain.

Conditions most used for: (1) Abscesses
and ulcers; (2) sluggish labor in pregnant
women, menstrual irregularity, poor
lactation.

Preparation: Seeds are used medicinally,
3-5 ch'ien each time, prepared in
decoction.

85. Wang Kua [Cucumber]

Family: Cucurbitaceae

Scientific name: Trichosanthes cucumeroides
Maxim.

Synonyms: "Shan k'u-kua," "t'u-kua" [local
gourd], "shan ko," "k'u kua lien," "ya-len
kua" [duck-egg gourd], "tiao-kua" [hanging
melon], "chia kuo-lou."

Morphology: A perennial herbaceous vine.
Found growing in fertile and damp places
in mountain wilds. Root thick and fleshy,
long oval or spindle-shaped, longitudinally
striped, shaped like a k'u-kua [momordica],
several roots clustered around the rhizome
base. Stem long and slender, linear-
angled and slightly pubescent, tendrils
growing alongside petiole. Leaves alternate, palmate 3-5 parted, apexes acute,
bases cordate, both surfaces pubescent,
margine undulate-serrate. Blooms in summer,
white axillary flowers forming short racemose inflorescence. Gourd oval, turning
red when ripe.

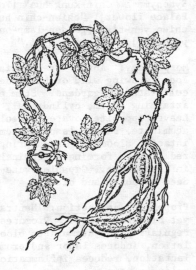

Properties and action: "Han" cold, bitter
to taste. Clears fevers and detoxifies,
reactivates blood and clears clots, reduces
inflammation and relieves pain.

Conditions most used for: (1) Poisonous
snakebites; (2) sore throat; (3) boils
and abscesses; (4) traumatic injuries.

Preparation: Roots are used medicinally,
3-5 ch'ien each time, prepared as decoction; or fresh fruits may be crushed
for external application to affected part.

86. T'ien-ming Ching

Family: Compositae

Scientific name: Carpesium abratanoides
L.

Synonyms: "Tu-niu chi," "ch'ou-hua niang-
tzu" [stink-flower lady], "ts'ou-mien
ts'ao" [wrinkled-face herb], "lai-ssu
ts'ao, "he-shih" [stork louse] "yeh-
yen" [wild tobacco].

Morphology: Perennial herb. Found
growing in virgin wilds, and in grassy
thickets along forest edges and roadsides.
Stem height 30-100 cm, erect, multi-
branching in upper section, covered by
fine hairs. Basal leaves broadly ovate,
wilting after flowers have bloomed; leaves
alternate, broadly oval or long oval,
apexes acute, bases cuneate, margins
intact or slightly irregular-serrate,
leaves in lower part having short petioles,
leaves in upper part non-petioled. Blooms
in the fall, axillary yellow flowers
forming capitulum inflorescence. Upper
part of achene secreting sticky fluid
that adheres easily to clothing.

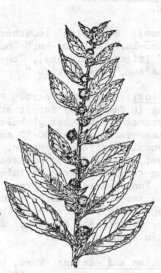

Properties and action: Warm-natured,
slightly bitter to taste. Loosens
up mucus, clears fever and detoxifies,
reduces inflammation and promotes
diuresis.

Conditions most used for: (1) Tonsillitis, bronchitis; (2) boils and ulcers,
snakebite.

Preparation: The whole plant is used
medicinally, 1-2 liang each time, prepared
as decoction. (Seeds are called "pei-he
shih," which can be used as a vermifuge
for expelling round worms, tapeworms,
pin worms. For each dose 1 ch'ien prepared in decoction.)

87. T'ien-nan Hsing [Dragon-arum species]

Family: Araseae

Scientific name: Arisaema consanguineum
Schott.

Synonyms: "Nan hsing" [southern star],
"she-pao-ku," "chu-pao-ku," "hu-chiang
ts'ao" [tiger-palm grass], "tu-hsieh-I-
chih ts'ang,""she yu-t'ou."

Morphology: Perennial herb. Found
growing in damp shady forest areas.
Subterranean stem tuber globular. Leaf
petioles erect, height 60-90 cm, fleshy,
dull purple stripes and spots, and 2 ochreae
at base; single-leafed, palmate compound,
growing terminally from petioles, leaflets
11-23, long-lanceolate, apexes pointed,
margins intact. Blooms in summer, flowers
forming spadix inflorescence, bracts light
purple, long-linear at apex. Berry bright
red when ripe, granular.

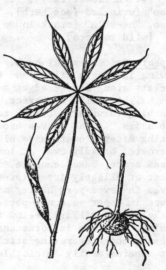

Properties and action: Warm, bitter and
biting to taste, toxic. Relieves spasms
and pain, loosens mucus, dispels clots and
reduces swelling.

Conditions most used for: (1) Epileptic
foaming at the mouth; (2) high fevers and
convulsions; (3) boils and abscesses;
(4) traumatic injuries.

Preparation: Stem tuber is used medicinally, 1-3 ch'ien of the processed stem
tuber each time, prepared in decoction.
The unprocessed stem tuber may be crushed
in suitable amounts for external use.

88. T'ien Kuei [Columbine species]

Family: Ranunculaceae

Scientific name: Semiaquilegia adoxoides
(DC) Makino.

Synonyms: "Ch'ien-nien lao-shu shih"
[Thousand-year rat droppings], "t'ien
ch'u-tzu," "t'u-kuei" [anemone], "tzu-
pei t'ien-kuei" [purple-backed columbine],
"lao-shu shih" [rat droppings], "han
t'ung-ch'ien tsao," "yeh wu-t'ou tzu,"
"chih t'ui" [chicken drumsticks], "hsia-
wu-tsung" [no-footprints-in-summer],
"t'ien kuei-tzu," "san-hsueh chu."

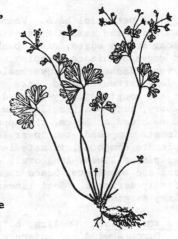

Morphology: Small perennial herb.
Found growing wild in damp and shady
waste places. Black subterranean stem
tuber spindle-shaped, resembling rat
droppings. Leaves clustered, with
slender and long petioles, 3-leaved
compound, leaflets flat, broadly cuneate,
deeply 3-parted, cuneate at base, surface
green, purplish on underside. Small white
terminal flowers appear in summer. Fruit
a follicle. Stem leaves wither by
summer's end, hence the term "shia-wu-
tsung" [no footprints in summer].

Properties and action: Cold-natured,
pleasant to taste. Clears fevers and
detoxifies, promotes diuresis.

Conditions most used for: (1) Abscesses;
(2) cystitis; (3) snakebite.

Preparation: Stem tuber is used medicinally, 5 ch'ien - 1 liang each time,
prepared as decoction.

89. Feng Ya Chueh [Coniogramme species]

Family: Pteridaceae

Scientific name: Coniogramme japonica (Thunb.) Diels.

Synonyms: "San-hsueh lien" [blood-'dispersing' lily], "huo-hsueh lien" [blood tonic lily].

Morphology: A perennial herb. Found growing on shady and damp places on hillsides, along stream edges, river banks, and field edges. Rhizome creeping, green, covered densely by brown scale. Petioles long, straw-colored, base pubescent and longitudinally-grooved. Leaves papery, long-oval, as long as 50 cm and as broad as 30 cm, the upper leaf 1-pinnate compound, the lower leaf often 2-pinnate compound, pinnate leaves 3-5 pairs; pinnae linear-long oval, apexes long and acuminate, bases cuneate, margins finely serrated. Sori linear, no covering, marginal.

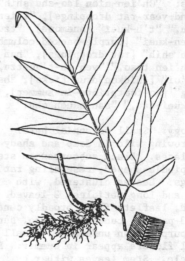

Properties and action: Cooling, bitter to taste. Dispels wind and moisture, cools the blood and disrupts clots [bruises].

Conditions most used for: (1) Aches and pains of muscles and bones, bloodshot eyes; (2) amenorrhea; (3) mastitis and other kinds of abscesses.

Preparation: Rhizomes or whole plant is used medicinally, 2-5 ch'ien each time, prepared in decoction, or decoction may be mixed with sweet wine for consumption.

90. Feng-wei Ts'ao [Bracken]

Family: Pteridaceae

Scientific name: Pteris multifida
Poir.

Synonyms: "Ching-k'ou-pien ts'ao" [well-side grass], "chin-chi wei," "hsien-chi wei," "san-pa ch'a," "yeh-chi wei" [wild chicken tail], "fei-ching ts'ao," "feng-wei lien," "hsi chi-chiao sha," "ta-hsien chi-wei."

Morphology: Perennial evergreen herb. Usually found growing along edges of wells, and in damp cracks in wild places. Underground taproot short and thick, covered densely by brown scales. Leaves clustered, petioles 10-30 cm long, leaves pinnately compound; leaves ovate-round, leaflets linear-lanceolate, leaves terminating in sori long ovate-rounded, sori cluster attached to margin on leaf underside, linear.

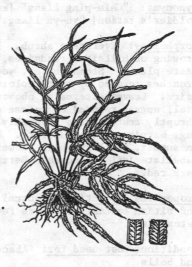

Properties and action: Cooling, acid and biting to taste. Clears fevers, detoxifies, stops bleeding, promotes tissue regeneration [or weight gain].

Conditions most used for: (1) Dysentery, hepatitis, urinary tract infections; (2) insecticide poisoning and poisoning by smartweed polygonum perfoliatum and the spindle tree tripterygium wilfordii; (3) traumatic bleeding.

Preparation: The whole plant is used medicinally, 1 liang each time, prepared as decoction.

91. Huo-pa Kuo [Pyracantha species]

<u>Family</u>: Rosaceae

<u>Scientific name</u>: Pyracantha fortuneana (Maxim) Li.

<u>Synonyms</u>: "Chiu-ping liang" [emergency soldier's ration] "yu-yu liang."

<u>Morphology</u>: Evergreen shrub. Found growing on hillside, roadsides, or waste places. Stems thorny, young branches covered by rusty colored soft hairs. Leaves alternate, obovate or oval, apexes rounded or retuse and abruptly acute, bases gradually narrowing, margins rounded-dentate. Blooms in summer, axillary white flowers forming umbellate inflorescences. Berry globular, dark red.

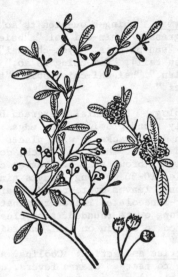

<u>Properties and action</u>: Neutral, sour and biting to taste. Clears fever and detoxifies.

<u>Conditions most used for</u>: Abscesses and boils.

<u>Preparation</u>: Fruit or leaves used medicinally, 2-5 ch'ien each time, prepared as decoction; or fresh leaves may be crushed in suitable amounts for external application.

92. Huo-t'an-wu [Chinese knotweed]

Family: Polygonaceae

Scientific name: Polygonum chinense L.

Synonyms: "ch'ih ti-li," "huo-t'an hsing"
[burning coal sparks], "wu-tu ts'ao" [five-
poison grass], "mao kan-che" [hairy sugar-
cane], "huo-t'an t'eng" [burning coal vine],
"lao-shu che."

Morphology: Perennial herb. Found growing wild along edges of ditches and
gullies. Stem rounded, height about 1.5
meters, trailing on ground, tender branches
reddish-purple. Leaves alternate, oval,
apexes obtuse, bases truncate or rounded,
margins intact or dentate, leaf surfaces
showing purple inverted "V"-shape lines.
Between summer and fall, small white or
light red terminal flowers forming panicle
or umbellate inflorescences. Small nut
triple-edged.

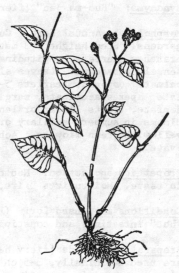

Properties and action: Cooling, slightly
acid to taste. Clears fevers, adds
moisture, aids indigestion, detoxifies.

Conditions most used for: (1) Enteritis,
dysentery; (2) sore and painful throats,
abscesses and weeping sores; (3) traumatic
injuries.

Preparation: The whole plant is used
medicinally, 1-2 liang each time, prepared as decoction; or fresh leaves may
be crushed for external use.

93. Huo Ma [Hemp -- Marihuana]

Family: Moraceae

Scientific name: Cannabis sativa L.

Synonyms: "Huo-ma jen" [fiery hemp seed]

Morphology: Annual herb. Cultivated in gardens. Stem height 1-3 meters, multiple branches, surface longitudinally grooved, densely pubescent. Leaves alternate, palmate compound, leaflets 5-11, lanceolate, apexes acuminate, margins coarsely dentate, bracts linear or lanceolate. Blooms in summer, axillary or terminal yellowish-green flowers. Achene flatovate.

Properties and action: Neutral, pleasant to taste. Moisturizes "fire," laxative.

Conditions most used for: (1) Overly "hot" intestines and constipation.

Preparation: Seeds [fiery hemp seeds] are used medicinally, 3-5 ch'ien each time, prepared in decoction.

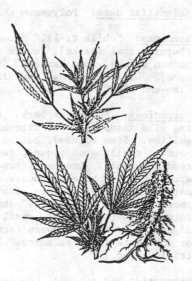

94. Mao-kuo hsuan-p'an-tzu [Hairy fruit abacus]

Family: Euphorbiaceae

Scientific name: Glochidion eriocarpum Champ.

Synonyms: "ch'i tai-pai," "ch'i ta-ku," [seven aunts], "ch'i ta-ku" [lacquer aunt], "ch'i-pao mu," "ch'i ta-kung."

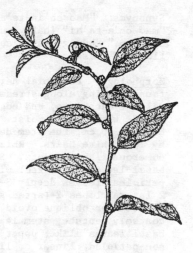

Morphology: Small deciduous shrub. Usually found growing on hillsides, waste places and roadsides. Stem erect, multi-branching, densely covered by light yellow, spreading coarse hairs. Leaves alternate, ovate or ovate-lanceolate, apexes acuminate, bases rounded, both sides coarsely pubescent. Axillary flowers appear in summer. Capsule ovate, 5-sided, covered by dense mat of long soft hairs, hence the term "mao-kuo hsuan-p'an-tzu" [hairy fruit abacus].

Properties and action: Neutral, bitter and biting to taste. Clears fevers, aids hydration, relaxes muscles and activates sinews, relieves itching, removes lacquer-poisons [allergic substance], stops diarrhea.

Conditions most used for: (1) Acute gastroenteritis, dysenteries; (2) hemoptysis; (3) rheumatoid arthritis pains, traumatic injuries; (4) allergic reactions to lacquer, burns, weeping dermatitis, styes.

Preparation: Roots and leaves are used medicinally, 5 ch'ien - 1 liang each time, prepared as decoction; a suitable amount of fresh leaves crushed for external use or cooked in water for soaks and baths.

95. Mao-ken [Japanese crowfoot]

Family: Ranunculaceae

Scientific name: Ranunculus japonicus
Thunb.

Synonyms: "Mao ch'in-ts'ai" [hairy celery],
"mao chia-ts'ai" [hairy mustard], "t'ien
chih-wu," "huang-hua ts'ao" [yellow-
flowered grass].

Morphology: Perennial herb. Usually
found growing along stream edges,
village outskirts, and edges of paddy
fields where it is moist. Height as
high as 80 cm, the stem densely covered
by long white hairs. Rhizome short,
numerous fibrous roots. Stem angled,
basal leaves clustered, with long
petioles; leaves deeply 3-parted, the
2 lateral lobes 2-Parted again, lobes
rhomboid or oblique ovoid, margins
coarsely dentate; stem leaves and
basal leaves alike; upper leaves
non-petioled, linear or linear-lanceolate. In spring-summer, small yellow
terminal flowers form cymose inflorescence. Obovate achene, slight oblique.

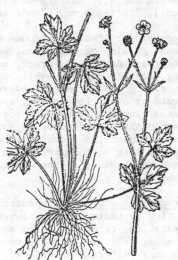

Properties and action: Warm, slightly
biting, toxic. Arrests malaria, dispels congestion, and kills worms.

Conditions most used for: (1) Malaria;
(2) tuberculosis of the cervical glands.

Preparation: The whole plant is used
medicinally. The fresh product crushed
into a mass each time the size of the
thumb and applied externally on affected
part or on acupuncture point location
(as a vermicide will kill maggots, mosquito
larvae, or the whole plant may be chopped
and thrown into outhouses or ditches).

96. Wa-wei

Family: Polypodiaceae

Scientific name: Lepisorus thunbergianus
(kaulf.) Ching.

Synonyms: "Ch'i-hsing chien" [seven-star
sword], "ku-p'ai ts'ao," "ku-p'ai shen-
chin."

Morphology: Perennial herb. Found
growing wild on rocky hillsides or trees.
Rhizome creeping, covered densely by
blackish-brown scales. Leaves parallel-
clustered, leathery and thick, linear
lanceolate, apexes acuminate, bases
gradually narrowing to form short petiole.
On the upper parts of both margins on
leaf under surface are yellow sori,
rounded like domino dots, arranged in 2
longitudinal columns.

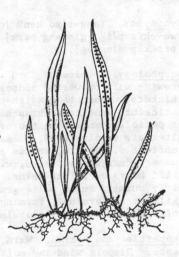

Properties and action: Slightly "han"
cold, and slightly bitter to taste.
Controls moisture, reduces inflammation,
and promotes diuresis.

Conditions most used for: (1) Urinary
tract infections; (2) bacterial dysentery;
(3) chronic bronchitis; (4) rheumatism.

Preparation: The whole plant is used
medicinally, 3-5 ch'ien each time,
prepared as decoction.

97. Wu Chia [Ginseng]

Family: Araliaceae

Scientific name: Acanthopanax gracilistylus,
W. W. Sm.

Synonyms: "Yang-t'ao ken" [carambola root],
"wu-chia p'i" [ginseng bark], "la wu-chia"
[prickly ginseng].

Morphology: Deciduous shrub. Found
growing wild on wasted slopes or shrub
thickets. Branches grayish-brown, with
noticeable lenticels, branches and bases
of petioles containing thorns. Leaves
alternate or clustered, palmate-compound,
leaflets 5, obovate, apexes acute, bases
cuneate, margins serrated, with sparse
stiff hairs over leaf veins. Blooms in
early summer, small white greenish flowers,
axillary or terminal, forming umbellate
inflorescence. Berry globular, purple.

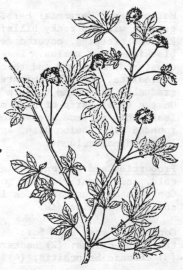

Properties and action: Warm, biting to
taste. Dispels wind and moisture,
strengthens sinews and bones, and back and
knees.

Conditions most used for: (1) Rheumatoid
arthritis, aches and pains in the back
and legs; (2) open sores on scrotum, beri
beri; (3) traumatic injuries.

Preparation: Roots and bark of stems
are used medicinally, 3-5 ch'ien each
time, prepared as decoction or steeped
in wine.

98. Yüan-pao Ts'ao [Hypericum species]

Family: Hypericaceae

Scientific name: Hypericum sampsonii Hance.

Synonyms: "Chiao-ku feng," "she k'ai-k'ou" [open-mouth snake], "shang-t'ien t'i [ladder-to heaven], "liu-chi-nu," "tui-yeh ts'ao," "ch'iao-tzu-feng," "ch'iao-tzu ts'ao," "tui-shih hsiao," "yeh han-yen" [wild drought tobacco], "chiao-chu ts'ao," I-tzu ts'ao," "hsiao lien-ch'iao [dwarf forsythia], "wang-pu-liu-hsing" [cow soapwort], "lan-ch'ang ts'ao [ulcerated-intestines grass], "chiao-tzu ts'ao."

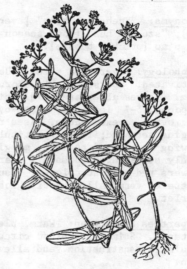

Morphology: A perennial herb. Found growing on wasted slopes and roadsides. Stem erect, cylindrical, multi-branching in upper section, non-pubescent, light reddish-brown. Leaves opposite, deltoid-lanceolate, apexes obtuse, bases joined, stem growing through (the leaf), two ends of leaf curled upward, like "yuan-pao" [paper cash burned for deceased], margins intact. Blooms in late summer, numerous terminal and axillary small yellow flowers, forming an umbellate inflorescence. Capsule ovate-rounded, dull brown.

Properties and action: Cold, bitter to taste. Cools the blood to stop bleeding, alleviates pain and knits bones, breaks down blood and injures the fetus, stimulates blood circulation and detoxifies, kills worms.

Conditions most used for: (1) Incomplete breakout of measles rash; (2) bacterial dysentery, diarrhea; (3) mastitis, poisonous snakebites, various infections and swellings; (4) hematemesis, epistaxis, burns, cuts; (5) menstrual irregularities, traumatic injuries, backache.

Preparation: The whole plant is used medicinally, 5 ch'ien - 1 liang each time, prepared as decoction; for external use, crushed fresh herbs for application on affected parts.

99. Yueh-chi Hua [Chinese rose]

<u>Family</u>: Rosaceae

<u>Scientific name</u>: Rosa chinensis Jacq.

<u>Synonyms</u>: "Yueh-yueh hung" [every-month red], "szu-chi hua" [four-season flower], "le p'ao [prickly bubble].

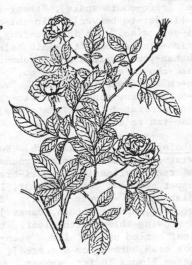

<u>Morphology</u>: Evergreen shrub. Usually cultivated. Sparse prickly thorns on stem. Leaves alternate, oddly pinnate compound, 5-7 leaflets, ovate-oval or long ovate, apexes acute, bases rounded, margins serrated; feathery stipule found growing at base of petiole, margins finely serrated. Blooms all year round, flowers red or rose colored. Usually clustered terminally. Berry globular, scarlet.

<u>Properties and action</u>: Warm, pleasant to taste. Stimulates blood circulation, regulates menstruation, and alleviates pain.

<u>Conditions most used for</u>: (1) Menstrual irregularity, dysmenorrhea, amenorrhea; (2) traumatic injuries, swellings and pains of back and legs.

<u>Preparation</u>: Flowers are usually used for medicinal purposes, roots and leaves less frequently, flowers 1-3 ch'ien, or roots and leaves 3-5 ch'ien, used each time, prepared in decoction.

100. Tan-shen [Sage species]

Family: Labiatae

Scientific name: Salvia miltiorrhiza L.

Synonyms: "Tzu tan-ken" [roots of purple sage], "hung ken" [red roots], "shu-wei ts'ao [rat-tail grass], "ch'ih shen" [scarlet sage], "pin-ma ts'ao [horse-racing grass].

Morphology: Perennial herb. Found growing on the sunny side of hillsides, and stream edges. Root cylindrical, scarlet red. Stem erect, 40-60 cm tall, multi-branching, rhomboid, greenish-purple, grooved, densely pubescent. Leaves opposite, oddly pinnate compound, leaflets ovate-round to oval-round, apexes acute, bases rounded, margins finely serrated. Blooms in the summer, bluish-purple terminal flowers forming a racemose inflorescence. Nut ovoid brown.

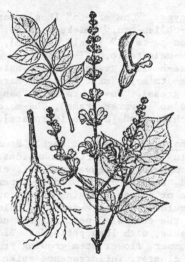

Properties and action: Slightly "han" cold, bitter to taste. Promotes menstrual regularity, invigorates blood, resolves bruises and aids granulation.

Conditions most used for: (1) Menstrual irregularity, uterine bleeding, abdominal pain; (2) neurasthenia, insomnia; (3) hepatitis, mastitis, hives.

Preparation: Roots are used medicinally, 3-5 ch'ien each time, prepared as decoction.

101. Ch'e-ch'ien [Plantago]

Family: Plantaginaceae

Scientific name: Plantago major Lim.

Synonyms: "Chu erh-to" [hog's ears],
"che-ch'ien-tzu," "ma-kuai ts'ao,"
"t'ien po-ts'ai" [field spinach],
"ch'a-hsin ts'ao," "I-ma ts'ao"
[horse-healing grass], "ha-mo-hsieh,"
"ha-mo ts'ao," "ma t'i ts'ao [horse-
hoof grass], "fu-tzu ts'ao," "pang-
ha ts'ao" [oyster grass], "ha-mo ching,"
"ya-chiao pan" [duck's footplate].

Morphology: Perennial herb. Found
growing in wild places, roadsides.
Rhizome short. Leaves radical, clustered, broadly ovate or oval, apexes
acute or obtuse, margins intact or
irregularly undulate-dentate, veins
5-7, the central 3 particularly noticeable, with long petioles. Blooms
in summer, flower stem growing from
leaf cluster, inflorescence spike,
flowers small and greenish-white.
Fruit a capsule. Seeds blackish-brown.

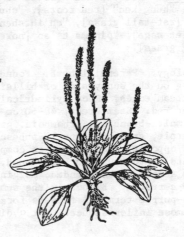

Properties and action: Cooling, pleasant
to taste. Clears fever and detoxifies,
promotes diuresis.

Conditions most used for: (1) Urinary
tract infections, prostatitis, acute
conjunctivitis; (2) nephrotic edema,
ureteral stones, difficult micturition.

Preparation: The whole plant is used
medicinally, 5 ch'ien - 1 liang each
time, or seeds alone 3-5 ch'ien, prepared as decoction.

102. Pa-tou [Croton]

Properties and action: Warm, biting to taste, highly toxic. Purgative.

Conditions most used for: "Han" cold constipation, ascites, chest congestion, epilepsy, mania, resistant cold-moist fungus infections.

Preparation: Crush and pulverize 1-3 li of croton bean, remove oil, swallow residue.

103. Pa-chi-t'ien [Bacopa monniera, Hyata]

Properties and action: Slightly warm, pleasant and somewhat biting to taste. Warms the kidneys and invigorates the yang energy.

Conditions most used for: Impotence, premature ejaculation, "wet dreams," backache, cold uterus [frigidity?], irregular menstruation, rheumatism.

Preparation: For each dose, 1-2 ch'ien, prepared as decoction.

104. Wu-tse ku [cuttlefish bones]

Properties and action: Slightly warm, salty to taste. Hemostatic.

Conditions most used for: "Wet dreams," metrorrhagia, leukorrhea, spotting, hyperacidity (stomach), traumatic bleeding, scrotal ulcers.

Preparation: Decoction of 1.5-3 ch'ien cuttlefish bones and water. Or pulverize and swallow with water.

105. Wu Mei [Black Prune] (Prunus mume Sieb et Zucc)

Properties and action: Neutral, sour to taste. Astringent and antipyretic, neutralizing [for stomach] and vermicidal.

Conditions most used for: Chronic diarrhea and dysentery, feverish thirst, achlorhydria, no appetite, residue coughing, chronic malaria, intestinal worms, abdominal pain.

Preparation: For each dose, 1-2 ch'ien, in decoction.

106. Shui Chi [Leeches]

Properties and action: Neutral, salty and bitter to taste. Loosens clots and invigorates the blood circulation.

Conditions most used for: Group of "disease-symptoms," fractures and bruises, amenorrhea.

Preparation: For each dose, 3-5 fen, prepared as decoction; or roasted leech, pulverized and swallowed with water.

107. Sheng-ma [Skunk bugbane] (Cimicifuga foetida)

Properties and action: Slightly "han" cold, pleasant yet bitter to taste. Purifies system and lifts the yang, clears fevers and detoxifies.

Conditions most used for: Rashes, measles, smallpox, erysipelas, sore throat, canker sores, eversion of anus following chronic diarrhea, metrorrhagia, uterine prolapse.

Preparation: For each dose, 5 fen - 2 ch'ien, prepared as decoction.

108. Wu-ling Chih [Bat Droppings]

Properties and action: Warm and pleasant to taste. Stimulates blood circulation, alleviates pain, and resolves bruises.

Conditions most used for: Pains associated with sluggish circulation of blood and energy, amenorrhea, dysmenorrhea metrorrhagia and abdominal cramps.

Preparation: For each dose, 1.5 - 3 ch'ien, prepared as decoction.

109. Pei Ho [Oyster shells]

Properties and action: "Han" cold, salty to taste. Clears pulmonary heat, resolves phlegm and stops coughing.

Conditions most used for: Coughing and wheezing, chest and haunch pains, pulmonary congestion, hemoptysis, neck tumors, nummular sputum, metrorrhagia.

Preparation: For each dose, 2-4 ch'ien, crushed into powder and prepared as decoction.

110. Wu-ming I [No-name difference]

Properties and action: Neutral, salty yet pleasant to taste. Invigorates blood and alleviates pain.

Conditions most used for: Traumatic injuries, boils and ulcers.

Preparation: For each dose, 8 fen to 1.5 ch'ien, pulverized and prepared as decoction. An appropriate amount used for external application.

111. Tan P'i [Bark of Root Peony]

Properties and action: Slightly chilling ["han" cold], biting and bitter to taste. Cools blood, dispels clots [by resolving bruises], clears fevers.

Conditions most used for: Menstrual irregularity, non-sweat recurrent fever, "heated" blood and disorderly circulation, hematemesis, epistaxis, bloody stools, boils and abscesses, bruises, typhus fever.

Preparation: For each dose, 1-3 ch'ien prepared as decoction.

112. Mang-hsiao, Hsuan-ming-fen [Glauber's Salt]

Properties and action: "Han" cold, salty. Purges heat, softens the "hard," hydrates the parch-dry [system], keeps bowels open.

Conditions most used for: Malnutrition and bloated abdomen, constipation, "solid" heat preventing loosening of sputum.

Preparation: For each dose, 1.5 - 3 ch'ien, to be taken with water.

113. Huo-hsiao Hsiao-shih [Saltpeter]

Properties and action: Warm, biting, bitter and salty to taste. Slightly toxic. Loosens the "knotted up."

Conditions most used for: Summer colds, "solid" abdominal masses, chest congestion, headache due to deficient kidneys and suppressed vitality.

Preparation: For each dose, 3-5 fen, pulverized. Swallow and take with water.

114. Mu-hsiang (Saussurea lappa Clarke)[Inula]

Properties and action: "Warm," biting and bitter to taste. Promotes energy circulation, alleviates pain.

Conditions most used for: Indigestion, distended abdomen, abdominal pains, stomach "growling," stomach-ache, vomiting, diarrhea, dysentery.

Preparation: For each dose, 8 fen to 1.5 ch'ien, in decoction. Or ground.

115. Mu Hu-tieh [Wood butterfly]

Properties and action: "Han" cold, bitter to taste.
Clears lung congestion, eases up speech, normalizes the liver.

Conditions most used for: Coughing and hoarseness, colic, "gassy" liver-stomach.

Preparation: For each dose, 3 fen to 1 ch'ien, in decoction.

116. T'ien-ma [Gastrodia elata]

Properties and action: Neutral, biting to taste. Dispels flatus, quiets spasm.

Conditions most used for: Lateral and frontal headaches, dizziness and fainting, "epileptic" spells, muddled speech, numbness, joint pains, infantile diarrhea, apprehension, convulsive spasms.

Preparation: For each dose, 2-4 ch'ien, in decoction.

117. T'ien-hsien-tzu [Scopolia japonica]

Properties and action: "Warm," pleasant to taste, but highly toxic. Relaxes spasms and alleviates pain.

Conditions most used for: Mania-depression, spasms, stomach-ache, chronic diarrhea and dysentery.

Preparation: Each dose 2-4 f'en, external application unlimited.

118. Pai-niu Tan [White Ox gallbladder]

Family: Compositae

Scientific name: Inula cappa DC

Synonyms: "Ta-ma hsiang," "mi-meng hua,"
"mao ch'ai-hu," "pai-mien feng" [white-
face wind], "kung pai-t'ou," "mao hsia-
ts'ai" [hairy scholar], "mao hsiang-kung,"
"yang erh-to" [sheep's ear], "pai tu-huo,"
"t'u meng-hua," "ke-shan hsiang [over-
the-hill fragrance], "t'u yen-ch'en,"
"mao lao-hu" [hairy tiger], "ch'ai-hu,"
"ta huang-hua" [giant yellow flowers].

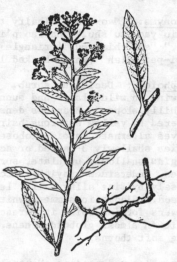

Morphology: A deciduous semi-shrub.
Mostly found growing on wasted places on
sunny hillsides and valleys. Stem erect,
height 1-2 meters, branches coarse and
strong, covered by fine white hairs.
Leaves alternate, long oval to almost
obovate, apexes acute, bases cuneate,
margins finely dentate, both sides
pubescent, hairs white, particularly
dense on underside. Blooms in the fall,
yellow terminal or axillary flowers
forming a capitulum inflorescence. Fruit
achene, covered with fine hairs.

Properties and action: Slightly warm
nature, biting to taste, fragrant. Resolves phlegm and relieves asthma, dispels clots and reduces inflammation,
dispels gas and alleviates pain, detoxifies
and promotes granulation.

Conditions most used for: (1) Headaches, post-partum colds and "wind
type" swelling; (2) leukorrhea, nephrotic edema; (3) rheumatoid pains
of back and legs, traumatic swelling and pain; (4) weeping sores of
skin, pruritus.

Preparation: Roots or whole plant used medicinally, 5 ch'ien - 1 liang of
dried roots, prepared as decoction; for external use, the whole plant
crushed or cooked in water for washing affected parts.

119. Pai-hsieh Yeh-t'ung [White-leafed wild t'ung-tree]

Family: Euphorbiaceae

Scientific name: Mallotus apelta (Lour.)
Muell-Arg.

Synonyms: "Mao-t'ung" [hairy t'ung-tree]
"chiu yao-tzu shu," "ha-lao p'i," "pa'pa
shu," "san-chiao mu" [triangle tree],
"pai-pei hsieh" [white-backed leaf].

Morphology: Deciduous shrub. Found
growing in wild places and sunny side
of hilly slopes. Branches densely
covered by yellow scabrous hairs.
Leaves alternate, ovoid-globose,
apexes shallowly 3-parted or acuminate,
margins shallowly undulate, surfaces
green, undersides grayish-white, covered
densely by fine silky hairs, leaf rib
raised. Blooms in summer, white terminal
flowers forming spike inflorescence.
Fruit an almost globoid achene, with
long soft thorns.

Properties and action: Neutral, slightly
bitter biting to taste. Can dispel
moisture, stabilizes "leaks" [vitality?
or impairment of certain body functions?],
detoxifies.

Conditions most used for: (1) Chronic hepatitis, hepatosplenomegaly,
leukorrhea, gonorrheal discharge; (2) uterine prolapse, prolapse of anus,
hernia; (3) boils and abscesses, tonsillitis, otitis media.

Preparation: Roots and leaves are used medicinally, 5 ch'ien - 1 liang each
time, prepared as decoction; for external use, fresh leaves and roots crushed
for application on affected parts.

120. Pai Chi [Bletilla species]

<u>Family</u>: Orchidaceae

<u>Scientific name</u>: Bletilla striata
(Thunb.) Reichb. f.

<u>Synonyms</u>: "Ti lei-ssu" [ground screw],
"yang-chiao ch'i," "chien-nien tsung"
[thousand-year palm], "chun-ch'iu-tzu,"
"I-tou-ts'ung," "pai chi-erh" [white
chicken], "p'i-yao tzu," "p'i-k'ou
yao," "li-chih-tzu."

<u>Morphology</u>: Perennial herb. Found
growing wild in sandy soil among grassy
patches on cool mountain slopes. Stem
tuber ovate or cylindrical, highly
sticky; psuedo-bulbs flat. Leaves
basally alternate, broadly lanceolate,
apexes long-acute, clasped by tubular
ochrea to stem in layers, margins intact, parallel venation. Blooms in
late spring, reddish-purple or yellowish-white flowers forming a capitulum
inflorescence. Fruit a tubular capsule, slightly pointed at both ends.

<u>Properties and action</u>: Neutral, bitter
to taste. Tonifies the lungs and stops
bleeding, reduces inflammation and promotes muscle regeneration [to stimulate
appetite and promote weight gain?].

<u>Conditions most used for</u>: (1) Hemoptysis
in tuberculosis, silicosis; (2) gastric
and duodenal ulcer bleeding; (3) traumatic
injuries, abscessed swellings, cracked
skin of hands and feet.

<u>Preparation</u>: Stem tuber is used medicinally,
1-3 ch'ien each time, prepared as decoction
or crushed into powder for taking internally.

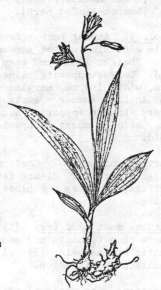

121. Pai-hua She-she Ts'ao [White-flowered snake-tongue grass]

Family: Rubiaceae

Scientific name: Olaenlandia diffusa
(Willd) Roxb.

Synonyms: "She-she ts'ao," "erh-hsieh
lu" [two-leaved humulus], "she-chen
ts'ao" [snake-needle grass], "chu-hsieh
ts'ai" [bamboo-leafed herb].

Morphology: Annual herb. Found growing
wild in weed clusters of gardens and
fields. Height 20-30 cm, stem prostrate,
angled. Leaves opposite, linear, length
1-3 cm, width 1-3 mm, margins intact.
Blooms in late summer - early fall, white
axillary flowers appearing singly or in
pairs, petioles short. Capsule a flat
globoid.

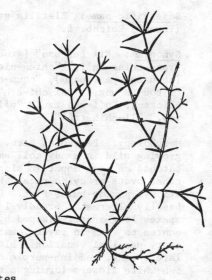

Properties and action: Cooling, pleasant
and light to taste. Clears fever and
detoxifies, tonifies the blood, and promotes
diuresis.

Conditions most used for: (1) Cancer;
(2) sore throat, boils and abscesses,
traumatic bruise pain; (3) poisonous
snakebites; (4) jaundice.

Preparation: The whole plant is used
medicinally, 1-2 liang each time, prepared as decoction.

122. Pai Fu-tzu

Family: Araceae

Scientific name: Typhonium giganteum
Engl.

Synonyms: "Tu-chiao lien" [one-corned
lotus], "tu-chiao lien" [single-foot
lotus].

Morphology: Perennial herb. Found
growing in moist and fertile spots in
the uplands. Subterranean stem tuber
ovate-globose or ovate-oval, varying
in size, covered externally by dull
brown scales, containing 6-8 nodes.
Leaves basal, 1-4; leaves folding
toward right in triangular form when
first emerging, hence the term "tu-chiao
lien"; petioles large and fleshy,
cylindrical, leaves deltoid-long ovate
or hastate-sagittate, apexes acuminate,
margins intact or slightly undulate.
Blooms in summer-fall, purplish flowers
forming a fleshy spadix inflorescence.
Fruit a berry.

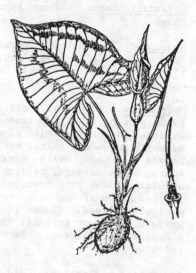

Properties and action: Highly warm, acrid
yet pleasant to taste, slightly toxic.
Dispels cold and moisture, brings up gas
and sputum, relieves spasms.

Conditions most used for: (1) Apoplexy
accompanied by frothing at the mouth,
contortions of mouth and eyes (cross-
eyed); (2) headaches, tetanus, numbness
and pain in rheumatism; (3) lymphadenopathy.

Preparation: Stem tuber is used medicinally,
8 fen - 1.5 ch'ien each time, prepared as
decoction. Can slso be prepared as poultice,
tincture, the liquid to be used externally.

123. Pai Ying [White nightshade]

Family: Solonaceae

Scientific name: Solanum lyratum Thunb

Synonyms: "Fu-kuei mu" [sorcerer's eyes], "pai ts'ao," "p'ai-feng t'eng," "pai-mao t'eng" [white-haired vine], "shu-yang-ch'uan," "wang-tung hung."

Morphology: Perennial trailing vine. Found growing on hill uplands, roadsides, gardens and woods. Whole plant covered by white pubescent hairs, stem climbing. Leaves alternate, ovate, apexes sharply acute, bases cordate, margins intact or undulate, lower part frequently contain-ing 1-2 pairs of obtuse parted leaves, auricular-shaped. Blooms in summer, white axillary or terminal flowers forming a cymose inflorescence. Berry globoid, red when ripe.

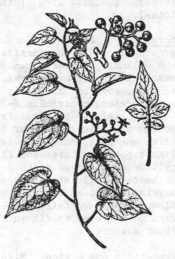

Properties and action: Cold, pleasant to taste. Clears fever, detoxifies.

Conditions most used for: (1) Leukorrhea; (2) abscesses, enlarged thyroid glands; (3) cancer of the esophagus and stomach.

Preparation: The whole plant is used medicinally, 5 ch'ien - 1 liang each time, prepared as decoction.

124. Pai-kuo (Yen-hsing) [Ginkgo]

<u>Family</u>: Ginkgoaceae

<u>Scientific name</u>: Ginkgo biloba L.

<u>Synonyms</u>: "Kung-sun shu," "Fei-o-hsieh"
[flying-moth leaf], "fu chi-chia [Buddha's
fingernails], "ya-chiao-pan" [duck-foot],
"ling-yen."

<u>Morphology</u>: Large deciduous tree. Found
growing on rich sandy soil, no resistance
to cold. Tree trunk erect, forming a
dense crown when old. Bark gray, deeply
cracked. Branches long and short. Leaves
on long branches single, on short branches
clustered. Leaves fan-shaped, bi-parted
at apex, bases cuneate, upper margins
undulate or irregularly shallow-parted,
both surfaces yellowish-green, containing numerous parallel veins. Blooms in
summer. Fruit seeds are drupes, obovate
or ellipsoid.

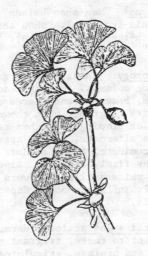

<u>Properties and action</u>: Neutral, pleasant
yet bitter and biting to taste. Exerts
an astringent affect on pulmonary energy,
stops coughing and asthma, stabilizes
spermatogenesis and stops leukorrhea.

<u>Conditions most used for</u>: (1) Pulmonary
tuberculosis; (2) seminal emissions,
leukorrhea, frequent micturition.

<u>Preparation</u>: Seeds, seedcoat or leaves
are used medicinally, 1-3 ch'ien each
time in decoction; or seeds may be pan
fried for eating.

125. Pai-chu Shu [White-bead tree]

Family: Ericaceae

Scientific name: Gaultheria cumingiana Vidal

Synonyms: "Man-shan hsiang" [whole-mountain-fragrant], "shou shan-hu" [search-the-mountain-lion], "lao ya-feng."

Morphology: Shrub. Found growing wild on uplands. Height reaching 3 meters, branches and leaves emitting a fruity fragrance when chewed. Stems erect or sloping, branches reddish. Leaves alternate, ovate, apexes long and acuminate, bases cordate or rounded, margins finely dentate. Blooms in the fall, white axillary flowers forming a panicle inflorescence. Capsule flat-globoid.

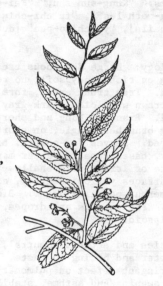

Properties and action: Warm, acrid and pleasant to taste, fragrant. Resolves clots and bruises, stimulates blood circulation, promotes bone-knitting and tissue repair.

Conditions most used for: (1) Liver cirrhosis and ascites; (2) traumatic injuries; (3) rheumatoid arthritis apins in joints and back.

Preparation: Rhizomes are used medicinally, 5 ch'ien - 1 liang each time, prepared as decoction.

126. Pai Lien [Ampelopsis species]

Family: Vitaceae

Scientific name: Ampelopsis japonica
(Thunb.) Makino

Synonyms: "Ch'i tzu-mei" [seven sisters],
"ssu-hsien tiao hu-lu" [gourd-hanging-
by-a-silk-thread], "yeh hung-shu" [wild
red yam], "chiu-tzu pu-li niang" [nine-
sons-inseparable-from-mother], "chi-p'o
pao-tan," "fei-chu ts'ai" [hog-fattening
vegetable].

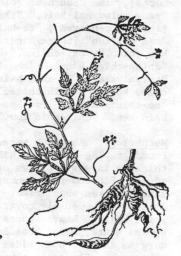

Morphology: Climbing vine. Found growing wild on mountainsides. Roots like
ovoid tubers, several clustered together.
Stem mostly branching. Leaves alternate,
palmate compound, 3-5 leaflets, some
leaflets pinnately-compound, pinnate
lobes ovate, apexes acuminate, margins
dentate. Blooms in summer, light yellow
flowers forming cymose inflorescence
growing opposite to leaves. Berry globoid,
white purplish-blue.

Properties and action: Neutral, bitter
to taste. Clears fever and detoxifies.
Alleviates pain and promotes muscle regeneration [putting on weight?].

Conditions most used for: (1) Tuberculous
cervical nodes; (2) bleeding from hemorrhoids;
(3) burn injuries.

Preparation: Roots are used medicinally,
3-5 ch'ien each time, prepared as decoction.
Suitable amount may be used externally.

127. Pai Wei [Milkweed species]

Family: Asclepiadaceae

Scientific name: Cynanchum stratum
Bunge

Synonyms: "Lao lung-chiao" [old dragon's
horns], "lao chun hsu" [old man's beard],
"yang chiao hsi-hsin," "shang-t'ien t'i,"
[ladder-to-heaven], "ta-hsiang sha,"
"san-pai ken" [three hundred roots], "chiu-
ken chiao," "pai-ch'ien," "tu-shen hsu,"
"chieh-chieh k'ung," "shu lao-chun hsu,"
"ta pai sha," "ke-shan hsiao," "shuang-
chiao kuo," "I-chih ch'ien" [one arrow],
"ho-chiang hsiao," "mu lao-chon," "hsi-
hsin ken," "chin-chin tou."

Morphology: An erect perennial herb.
Found growing mostly on hilly slopes,
thickets in waste places or along forest
edges. Fibrous roots numerous, fragrant,
easily broken when dried. Stems erect,
cylindrical, densely covered by fine
white hairs. Leaves opposite, broadly ovate,
apexes acute, bases broadly cuneate,
margins intact, both sides finely
pubescent. Blooms in summer, apical or
axillary purplish black flowers clustered.
Fruit a follicle.

Properties and action: "Han" cold, bitter
and salty to taste. Neutralizes blood
heat, stimulates salivation to supplement energy, stops coughing.

Conditions most used for: (1) Yin-deficiency
fevers, tuberculosis; (2) nephritis,
urinary tract infections, edema; (3) body
weakness, seminal emission, leukorrhea,
and other ailments seen during convalescence.

Preparation: Roots and stems are used
medicinally, 2-3 ch'ien each time, prepared as decoction.

- 672 -

128. Shih Wei [Pyrrosia species]

Family: Polypodiaceae

Scientific name: Pyrrosia lingua
(Thunb.) Farw.

Synonyms: "Shih-p'i"[rock bark], "shih-
lan," "fei-tao chien," [flying sword],
"shih-chien" [flint sword], "fei-hsin
ts'ao [lung heart grass], "hui-ch'uan
ts'ao," "hsiao mu-chi."

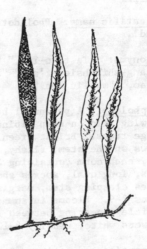

Morphology: Perennial herb. Found
growing in dark damp places on hilly
slopes, between rocky crevices, and
along cliffs. Rhizomes slender and
stoloniferous, covered densely by brown
scales. Leaves growing sparsely from
stem, coriaceous, narrow lanceolate,
apexes acuminate, bases narrow, margins
intact, leaf surfaces dark green, undersides
rusty colored, covered densely by
powdery and granular sori, petioles
noded at base, covered by stellate hairs.

Properties and action: Slightly "han"
cold, pleasant and bland in taste. Clears
fevers, promotes diuresis, and ease of
urination due to [gonorrhea?], stops
bleeding.

Conditions most used for: (1) Nephritic
edema, urinary tract infections, urinary
tract stones, hematuria; (2) "lung-fire"
caused hemoptysis.

Preparation: The whole plant is used
medicinally. For each dose, 3-5 ch'ien
of the dry herb or 1-2 ch'ien of the
fresh herb, prepared in decoction.

129. Shih Hsien-t'ao [Stony fairy's peach]

Family: Orchidaceae

Scientific name: Pholidota chinensis
Lindl.

Synonyms: "Ta tiao-lan," "fou-shih hu,"
"shang-shih hsien-t'ao," "ch'uan chia-
ts'ao," "ma-liu ken."

Morphology: A perennial herb. Found
growing wild on deep alpine cliffs or
large trees. Bright green psuedo-corm
grows on the stem, flashy, long-elliptical, each corm containing 2 small leaflets, long oval, apexes short and acute,
bases clasping stem, margins intact,
veins 7-9. Blooms in summer, flower
pedicle appearing between leaves,
flowers white, usually 8-12.

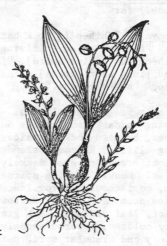

Properties and action: Cooling, pleasant
and bland to taste. Nourishes the yin
and moistens the lungs, cools the blood
and promotes salivation.

Conditions most used for: (1) Tuberculosis-associated hemoptysis; (2) gastroenteritis.

Preparation: The whole plant is used
medicinally, 1-2 liang each time, prepared in decoction.

130. Shih Ch'ang-p'u [Ginseng species]

Family: Araliaceae

Scientific name: Acorus gramineus
Soland.

Synonyms: "Shui chien-ts'ao" [aquatic
sword-grass], "tzu-erh" [purple ears],
"po ch'ang-p'u"

Morphology: A perennial evergreen
herb. Found growing wild on rocky
surfaces on mountain gullies. The
whole plant is fragrant. Underground
stem creeping, with whorled nodes.
Leaves clustered, linear, as long as 60
cm, margins intact. Blooms in summer,
flower pedicel appearing from leaf
cluster, small yellowish-green flowers
forming a spike inflorescence, containing leaflike spathe. Berry obovate.

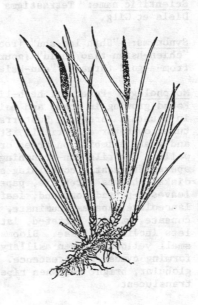

Properties and action: Warm, acrid-
tasting. Corrects energy, alleviates
pain, strengthens stomach function,
keep bowels open and resolves sputum.
Also acts as a vermicide.

Conditions most used for: (1) Pains
of the abdomen, back and sides, rheumatism
and numbness; (2) epilepsy, convulsive
comas; (3) purulent otitis media.

Preparation: Dried roots are used
medicinally, 3-5 ch'ien each time,
prepared in decoction; or fresh roots may
be crushed and the juice taken.

131. Shih Hou-tzu [Tetrastigma species]

Family: Vitaceae

Scientific name: Tetrastigma hemsleyanum Diels et Gilg.

Synonyms: "Shih lao-shu" [rock rat], "chien-hsien tiao hu-lu" [gourd-suspended-from-a-gold thread], "san-hsieh ch'ing."

Morphology: Perennial herb-like vine. Found growing in shady and moist places in mountain forests. Subterranean root tuber ovate or elliptical. Stem slender and weak, climbing on trees or cliff walls. Tendrils non-branching, red, apexes frequently containing suction disks. Leaves alternate, papery, petioled, leaves 3-parted compound, leaflets ovate lanceolate, apexes acuminate, bases cuneate, margins serrated, lateral leaf-lets inclined at base. Blooms in summer, small yellowish green axillary flowers forming cymose inflorescence. Berry globular, bright red when ripe, semi-translucent.

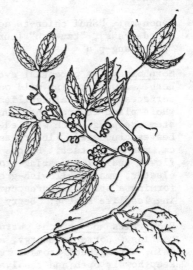

Properties and action: Cooling in nature, bitter yet pleasant to taste. Clears fevers and detoxifies, stimulates blood circulation and relaxes the muscles.

Conditions most used for: (1) Diphtheria; (2) boils and ulcers, traumatic bleeding, snakebites; (3) rheumatoid aches and pains in the back and legs.

Preparation: The root tuber is used medicinally, 2-5 ch'ien each time, prepared in decoction or steeped in wine. For external use a suitable amount is crushed and applied as poultice.

132. Shih Suan [Garlic]

Family: Amaryllidaceae

Synonyms: "Lao-ya suan" [crow's garlic], "wu-suan [black garlic], "yeh-suan" [wild onion], "tu ta-suan"

Morphology: A perennial herb. Found growing wild in the shade under trees on the
mountains. Subterranean globular corm
covered by thin purplish black film.
Leaves clustered 4-5, linear or fleshy,
margins intact. Blooms in summer, flower
pedicel extending from leaf cluster after
leaves have withered, supporting bright
red flowers forming an umbellate inflorescence. Capsule oval-shaped.

Properties and action: Warm, acrid, yet
pleasant to taste, toxic. Can detoxify,
reduce swelling, and kill worms.

Conditions most used for: (1) Sores,
boils and abscesses; (2) myofascitis,
(3) scabies and dermaphytoses.

Preparation: The corm is used medicinally,
5 fen each time, prepared as decoction.
For external use the fresh product is
crushed for application as a poultice.

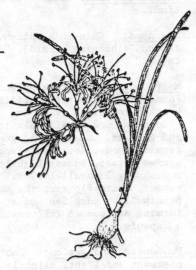

133. Shih Hu [Orchid species]

Family: Orchidaceae

Scientific name: Dendrobium nobile
Lindl.

Synonyms: "Chin-ch'a shih-hu," "tiao
lan-hua" [hanging orchid], "huang
ts'ao."

Morphology: Evergreen perennial herb.
Found growing on rocky cliffs or tree
trunks, to height of 30 cm. Stem erect,
clustered, noded, slightly inclined,
and grooved. Leaves 3-4, growing on
terminal node, long oval-lanceolate,
apexes obtuse, bases slightly narrow,
containing 5 parallel ribs. Blooms in
summer, white flowers, the sepals and
petals light purplish red at apexes,
forming a racemose inflorescence. Fruit
a capsule.

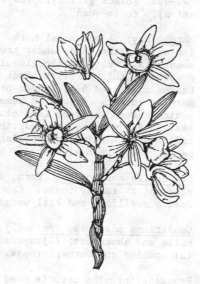

Properties and action: "Han" cold,
pleasant and light, slightly salty to
taste. As a stomachic, it nourishes
the yin, and promotes salivation.

Conditions most used for: (1) Restlessness and thirst, deficiency-fevers of
convalescence; (2) parchness of mouth
following fever.

Preparation: Stems are used medicinally,
3-5 ch'ien each time, prepared as
decoction.

134. Hsien Mao [Curculigo species]

Family: Curculigo family

Scientific name: Curculigo orchioides Gaertn.

Synonyms: "Tu-chiao hsien-mao," "tu-chiao huang-mao," "tu mao-ken," "tu-chiao ssu-mao," "tsung-se mao."

Morphology: Perennial herb. Found growing mostly on hilly slopes and wild places. Roots fleshy, cylindrical, with numerous side roots alongside the main tap root. Leaves basal, 3-6 lanceolate to linear-lanceolate, apexes acute, bases narrowing to form petioles, margins intact, containing parallel veins. Blooms in summer, axillary flower pedicel appearing to show terminal yellow flower. Capsule flashy.

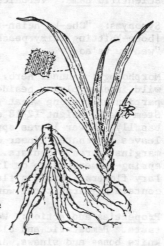

Properties and action: Warm, acrid to taste. Tonifies the kidneys and strengthens the yang, expels gas and eliminates moisture.

Conditions most used for: (1) Weak kidneys, impotency, enuresis; (2) joint pains.

Preparation: Roots are used medicinally, 3-5 ch'ien each time, prepared as decoction.

135. Hsien-t'ao Ts'ao [Fairy peach grass]

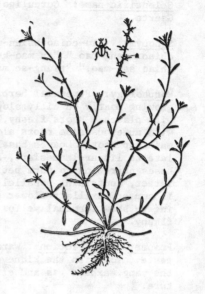

Family: Scrophulariaceae

Scientific name: Veronica peregrina L.

Synonyms: "Che-ku heisn-t'ao ts'ao"
[bone-knitting fairy peach grass],
"wen-mu ts'ao."

Morphology: Annual herb. Found growing
wild in damp places besides paddy fields,
particularly along wheat growing fields.
Stem erect, height 12-18 cm, branching
basally. Lower leaves opposite, upper
leaves alternate, linear lanceolate,
margins sparsely dentate. Blooms during
spring-summer, white or light red axillary flowers. Fruit a flat round capsule,
containing parasitical worms.

Properties and action: Warm, bitter to
taste. Hemostatic and blood-activating,
knits bones and sinews, and promotes menstrual regularity.

Conditions most used for: (1) Traumatic
injuries, fractures; (2) traumatic
[tubercular?] hemoptysis, dysmenorrhea.

Preparation: The whole plant is used
medicinally, 5 ch'ien - 1 liang each
time, prepared in decoction.

136. Hsien-he Ts'ao (Lung-ya Ts'ao) [Magic stork grass; dragon-tooth grass]

Family: Rosaceae

Scientific name: Agrimonia pilosa Ledeb.

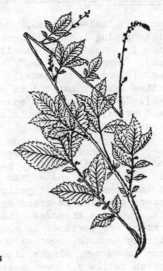

Synonyms: "Mao-chiao ying," "mao chiang-chun" [hairy general], "kua-huang ts'ao," "huang lung-wei" [yellow dragon's tail]; "she chih-tà," "she tao-t'ui," "lao-kuan tsui [heron's beak], "lu-pien huang," "tai- ying ch'i" [poky eagle's wing], "lu-pien chi" [roadside chicken], "mao-chi ken," "chiu-lo-ying," "wu-t'i feng" [5-hoofed wind], "fu-erh ts'ao" [tiger's eargrass], "k'u-ya ts'ao," "niu-t'ou ts'ao [ox-head grass], "lung-shu ts'ao," "chiao-erh nao" [birdbrain], "chi-chao sha," "t'ieh ma-pien" [iron horsewhip], "t'u-lu-feng," "hang-li ts'ao," "t'o-li ts'ao" [energy-weakening grass].

Morphology: Perennial herb. Found growing wild along hillsides and grassy thickets in waste places. Whole plant covered by fine white pubescent hairs. Stem striped or angled. Leaves alternate, oddly pinnate-compound, leaflets varying in size, alternate or opposite, ellipsoid lanceolate, coarsely dentate. Blooms in fall, terminal or axillary yellow flowers forming a cymose inflorescence. Achene and calyx both contain prickly thorns.

Properties and action: Slightly warm-natured, bitter and biting to taste. Hemostatic, antipyretic, and heat-reducing, also eliminates dampness [moisture].

Conditions most used for: (1) All bleeding ailments; (2) abdominal pain, sore throat, headache; (3) bloody and mucoid dysentery, bloody and white discharge; (4) heatstroke.

Preparation: The whole plant is used medicinally, 3 ch'ien - 1 liang each time, prepared in decoction.

137. Pan-pien Lien [One-half lotus]

Family: Campanulaceae

Scientific name: Lobelia radicans Thunb.

Synonyms: "Hsi-mi ts'ao," "chi-chieh so"
[quick-opening lock], "fei-ching ts'ao,"
"hsiao lien-hua ts'ao" [small lotus-flower
grass], "mien-feng ts'ao," "ch'iu-hsueh
ts'ao" [blood-blown grass], "fu-shui ts'ao"
[ascites herb], "kan-chi ts'ao" [marasmus
grass], "chao-tzu chin,""pai-la hua ts'ao"
[waxed grass], "chin-chu ts'ao," [golden
chrysanthemum grass].

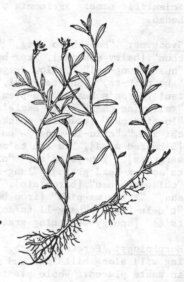

Morphology: Perennial vine-like herb.
Found growing wild in damp places along
paddy field edges and stream banks. Roots
fine and rounded, light yellow. Stem
slender, purplish in creeping section,
roots appearing at nodes. Leaves alternate,
linear or narrow-lanceolate, front ends
shallowly dentate, posterior ends intact.
Blooms in summer, single light red or
purplish axillary flower appearing, open
on one side, like 1/2 of lotus flower.
Fruit a capsule.

Properties and action: Neutral, slightly
acrid-tasting. Clears fever and detoxifies, resolves bruises, and promotes diuresis.

Conditions most used for: (1) Sores and
abscesses, poisonous snakebites, tooth
abscesses; (2) ascites, traumatic injuries.

Preparation: The whole plant is used medicinally, 1-2 liang each time, prepared as
decoction. Or fresh plant may be crushed
for use as poultice. Or boiled down to
concentrate for external application.

138. Pan-chih Lien (Ping-t'ou ts'ao) [Half-stick lotus]

Family: Labiatae

Scientific name: Scutellaria barbata Don.

Synonyms: "Wang-chiang ch'ing," "szu-fang ma-lan," "wa-erh ts'ao" [ear-scoop grass], "hsi-pien huang-ch'in" [stream-bank scutellaria], "hsia-hsieh han-hsin ts'ao."

Morphology: Annual herb. Mostly found growing on fertile and moist areas along paddy fields and streams. Stem height 20-50 cm, oblong, green or slightly purplish. Leaves opposite, ovoid or lanceolate, apexes obtuse, bases cuneate or straight, margins sparsely crenate or almost intact. Lower leaves on lower stems larger, with short petioles; upper leaves smaller, almost no petioles. Between spring and summer, axillary blue labiate flowers appearing to form a racemose inflorescence. Small knot is formed after blooming, shaped like an ear-scoop.

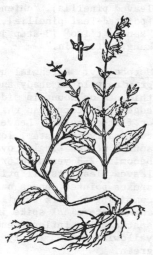

Properties and action: Slightly "han" cold, pleasant and bland to taste. Clears fever and cools blood, detoxifies, and promotes diuresis.

Conditions most used for: (1) Sore throat pain, boils; (2) schistosomiasis; (3) poisonous snakebites; (4) tumors.

Preparation: The whole plant is used medicinally, 1-2 liang each time, prepared in decoction; fresh product also crushed for external use.

139. Pan Hsia [Pinellia species]

Family: Araliaceae

Scientific name: Pinellia ternata (Thunb.) Breit.

Synonyms: "San-hsieh pan-hsia" [tri-leaved pinellia], "chien-hsieh pan-hsia [pointed-leaf pinellia], "ti tzu-ku," "san-pu t'iao" [3-step jump], "ti lei-kung," "fa-hsia."

Morphology: Perennial herb. Found growing wild in shady and damp grass thickets on mountain sides and stream edges. Subterranean rhizome globular or flat-globular. Leaves appearing terminally from stem, long petrioles, annual leaves single, ovate cordate, becoming 2-3 years later 3-leaflet compound leaves, leaflets elliptical-lanceolate, apexes pointed, bases narrow, 3 leaflets combining to form bulbils. Blooms in summer, terminal spike inflorescence, spathe below inflorescence, flowers yellowish green. Berry small ovate and green.

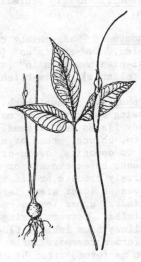

Properties and action: Warm, acrid-tasting, toxic. Strengthens the spleen and dries [neutralize] moisture, resolves phlegm and stops vomiting, stops bleeding and reduces inflammation.

Condition most used for: (1) Vomiting, poor digestion; (2) bronchitis; (3) traumatic bleeding, poisonous snakebites, swollen abscesses; (4) rheumatism and arthralgia.

Preparation: Tuberous stems are used medicinally, 1-3 ch'ien each time, prepared in decoction; for external use, the fresh herb crushed and applied as a poultice.

140. Szu-hsieh Lu [Four-leaved humulus]

Family: Rubiaceae

Scientific name: Galium gracile Bunge

Synonyms: "Hsiao chu tzu ts'ao" [little saw-grass], "szu-ling hsiang-ts'ao" [four-angled fragrant grass].

Morphology: A perennial herb. Found growing wild along village outskirts, and grassy thickets along ditches. Stem slender and fine, upper section erect, base frequently prostrate. Leaves elliptical and small, 4-whorled to each node. Blooms in summer, axillary flower pedicel appearing with fine and small light yellow flowers, the corolla 4-parted. Fruit small grains.

Properties and action: Neutral, pleasant to taste. Clears fever, detoxifies, reduces swelling and alleviates pain, promotes diuresis.

Conditions most used for: (1) Boils and abscesses; (2) bloody and mucoid dysentery, gonorrhea, "red" and "white" discharge [bloody and mucus discharge]; (3) cancerous tumors; (4) infantile marismus.

Preparation: The whole plant is used medicinally, 5 ch'ien - 1 liang each time, prepared as decoction.

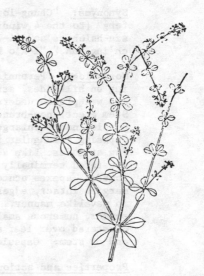

141. Szu-k'uai Wa [Four pieces of tile]

Family: Primulaceae

Scientific name: Lysimachia paridiformis
Franch.

Synonyms: "Chung-lou p'ai-ts'ao," "szu-san
feng" [to the 4 winds], "szu-p'ien wa,"
szu-hsieh ts'ao" [4-leaved grass], "szu
ch'ing-hua," "I-k'o hsing."

Morphology: Perennial herb. Found growing on hillsides, stream edges, and damp
and wet places underneath forest trees.
Stem erect, non-branching, base reddish-
purple, nodes enlarged and widely spaced,
opposing triangular regressed leaves growing at nodes, like scales. Leaves 4,
clustered terminally on stem, obovate-
rounded, apexes acute, bases cuneate,
margins intact, edges frequently curled
in wavelike manner. Blooms in early
summer, numerous small yellow flowers
clustered over leaf axils on terminal
end of stem. Capsule globular.

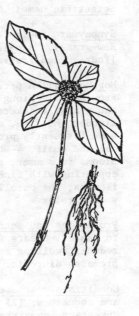

Properties and action: Warm, sour and
biting to taste. Expels gas and disperses cold, activates blood and alleviates
pain, stills coughing and brings up
sputum.

Conditions most used for: (1) Pulmonary
tuberculosis, "wind-cold" coughing; (2)
rheumatoid arthritis, traumatic injuries;
(3) stomach ache, enteritis; (4) snake
bites, abscess swellings.

Preparation: The whole plant is used
medicinally, 5 ch'ien - 1 liang each
time, in decoction; for external application, the fresh herb crushed and prepared
as poultice.

142. Lung-tan Ts'ao [Gentian]

Family: Gentianaceae

Scientific name: Gentiana scabra Bunge.

Synonyms: "Lung-tan" [dragon's gall-bladder], "tan ts'ao," "szu-hsieh ts'ao" [4-leaved grass].

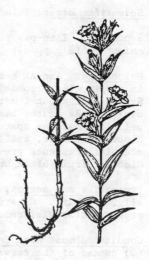

Morphology: A perennial herb. Found growing on wasted slopes, and grassland shrub thickets. Subterranean perennial roots numerous, fleshy, slender and fine. Stem branching, slightly 4-angled, green. Leaves opposite, nonpetioled, shape ovate-lanceolate, apexes acute, bases clasping stem, margins intact. Blooms in fall-winter, blue flowers, singly or clustered, to form terminal cymose inflorescence. Capsule long and rounded.

Properties and action: "Han" cold, bitter and biting to taste. Purges liver fire, clears damp heat.

Conditions most used for: (1) Acute hepatitis, acute conjunctivitis, acute tonsillitis; (2) high fever convulsions; (3) vaginal pruritis and discharge, open sores of the scrotum, abscesses and boils.

Preparation: The whole plant is used medicinally, 1-3 ch'ien each time, prepared in decoction.

143. Lung Kuei [Black nightshade]

Family: Solanaceae

Scientific name: Solanum nigrum L.

Synonyms: "Tien-pao ts'ao," "yeh la-chiao" [wild pepper], "t'ien ch'ieh-tzu."

Morphology: Annual herb. Found growing in virgin wilds, roadsides, and gardens. Stem height about 1 meter. Leaves alternate, oval, apexes acute, bases extending to petioles, margins sparsely undulate-crenate. Blooms in summer, axillary umbellate-racemose inflorescence presenting white flowers. Globular fruit black when ripe.

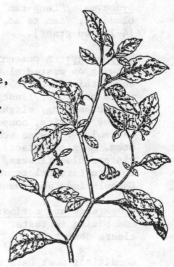

Properties and action: Slightly "han" cold, slightly toxic. Clears fever, detoxifies, promotes diuresis, reduces swelling.

Conditions most used for: (1) Leukorrhea; (2) cancer of the cervix; (3) abscesses and open sores.

Preparation: The whole plant is used medicinally, 3-5 ch'ien each time, prepared in decoction. For external bathing, the herb is boiled in water, solution used.

144. Ai [Mugwort]

Family: Compositae

Scientific name: Artemesia vulgaris L.

Synonyms: "Sheng-ai," "hsi-ai" [fine
mugwort], "ai-kao," "wu-yueh ai" [May
mugwort], "shan ai" [mountain mugwort],
"huang-hua ai" [yellow-flowered mugwort].

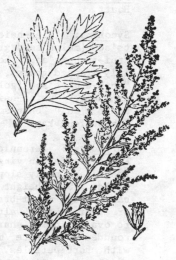

Morphology: Perennial herb. Cultivated
in gardens and along roadsides. The
whole plant emits fragrance. Stem erect,
attaining height of 1 meter, covered
slightly by fine grayish hairs. Leaves
alternate, ovate-rounded, pinnately compound,
lobes elliptical-rounded, lanceolate or
linear, apexes acute, margins intact or
dentate, both surfaces covered by fine
gray hairs. Blooms in the fall, light
yellow small flowers appearing terminally,
forming capitulum inflorescence, that
group to form a panicle inflorescence.
Fruit an achene.

Properties and action: Slightly warm
in nature, bitter to taste, but fragrant.
Can quiet the fetus, stops bleeding,
dispels gas and "cold."

Conditions most used for: (1) Excessive
fetal activity, and post-partum abdominal
cramps; (2) hematemesis, continuous
spotting, irregular menstruation; (3)
"cold" pain in the epigastric area;
(4) skin conditions.

Preparation: Leaves are used medicinally,
3-5 ch'ien each time, prepared as decoction; or a suitable amount may be
cooked for bathing external parts.

145. Kua-tzu Chin [Japanese milkwort]

Family: Polygalaceae

Scientific name: Polygala japonica
Houtt.

Synonyms: "Tieh-hsien feng," "kua-tzu
ts'ao" [melon seed grass], "kua-tzu lien,"
"tui-yueh ts'ao," "ho-pao ts'ao" [water
lily-wrapped grass], "shiu-kua-tzu lien,"
"chin-chu ts'ao" [golden bead-grass], "nu-
erh hung," "ch'en-hsiang ts'ao," "chien-
hsien k'ou," "chin so-yao" [golden key],
"ch'ou-feng kan."

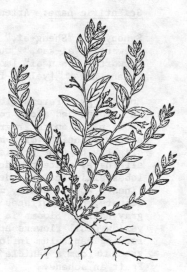

Morphology: Perennial evergreen herb.
Found growing in virgin wilds, along
roadsides, hilly slopes and edges of
fields. Stem height reaching 25 cm,
base woody, multi-branching, inclined
or erect. Leaves alternate, ellipsoid
to ovate, apexes sharply acute, bases
rounded or cuneate, margins intact,
with short petioles. Blooms in summer,
axillary purplish-white flowers forming
a racemose inflorescence. Capsule broadly
ovate-rounded and flat, margins winged.

Properties and action: "Han" cold,
pleasant and bitter to taste. Carminative in action, brings up phlegm and stops
coughing, reduces inflammation and detoxifies.

Conditions most used for: (1) Upper
respiratory tract infections, inadequate
measles eruption; (2) palpitation and insomnia; (3) traumatic injuries, snakebites.

Preparation: The whole plant is used
medicinally, 5 ch'ien - 1 liang each time,
prepared as decoction.

146. Hsieh-hsia Chu [Pearl-under-the-leaf]

Family: Euphorbiaceae

Scientific name: Phyllanthus urinaria L.

Synonyms: "Chen-chu ts'ao" [pearl grass], "chu-tzu hsieh," "jih-k'ao yeh-pi" (open-by-day and closed-by-night], "hsieh-hou chu" [pearl behind the leaf], "shih-tzu chen-chu ts'ao."

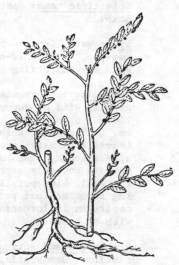

Morphology: Annual herb. Found growing wild along village outskirts, between fields and damp grasslands. Stem multi-branching, height about 30 cm, longitudinally angled. Leaved alternate, pinnate arrangement, leaves oblong or oval, apexes obtuse acute, bases rounded, margins intact. Blooms in summer, axillary reddish-brown or white flowers. Small globular capsules found growing below leaves, hence the term "pearl-under-the-leaf."

Properties and action: Cooling, slightly biting to taste. Purifies the liver and promotes clear vision, purges worms, and promotes diuresis.

Conditions most used for: (1) Hepatitis, jaundice, (2) conjunctivitis; (3) enteritis and diarrhea, infantile marasmus; (4) urinary tract infections, nephritic edema.

Preparation: The whole plant is used medicinally, 5 ch'ien - 1 liang each time, prepared in decoction.

147. T'ien-pien Chu [Field aster]

Family: Compositae

Scientific name: Aster trinervius
Roxb.

Synonyms: "Lan chu-hua" [blue aster],
"ma-lan," "ju ch'iu-ch'uan," "huang-
shan ch'uan [string-of-yellow-eels].

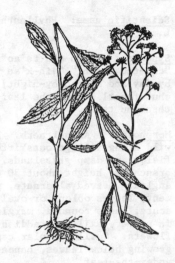

Morphology: Perennial herb. Found
growing wild on sunny roadside locations. Stem erect, height about 80
cm, cylindrical, shiny and smooth.
Leaves alternate, oval to lanceolate,
apexes acute, bases narrowly cuneate,
margins coarsely serrated. Blooms in
the fall, blue purplish flowers growing from terminal pedicle, to form a
capitulum inflorescence. Achene flat
with no hairs.

Properties and action: Neutral, acrid-
tasting. Hemostatic, anti-inflammatory,
and detoxifying.

Conditions most used for: (1) Hematemesis,
epistaxis, traumatic bleeding; (2) boils,
erysipelas, poisonous snakebites; (3)
infectious hepatitis.

Preparation: The whole plant is used medicinally, 1 liang each time, prepared in
decoction. Fresh herbs may also be
crushed for external applications.

148. Yu Chu [Solomon's seal]

Family: Liliaceae

Scientific name: Polygonatum officinale All.

Synonyms: "Wei-jui," "wei shen"

Morphology: Perennial herb. Found growing on hilly slopes, in shady and damp grass thickets. Underground stem fleshy, cylindrical, creeping, with many nodes from which adventitious roots grow. Stem angled. Leaves alternate, parallel-veined, narrow-oval or long-oval, apexes acute, bases cuneate, margins inact, leaf surface green, leaf underside pale white. In summer, white or light green flowers emerge from leaf axils. Berry globular, becoming dull purple after ripening.

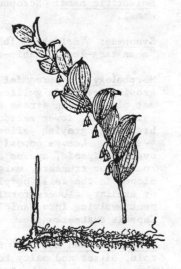

Properties and action: Neutral, pleasant to taste. Builds-nourishes the yin, and resolves fever, moistens the lungs and quells coughing.

Conditions most used for: (1) Body weakness and hidrosis, debilitating chronic cough; (2) parched mouth and aversion to heat.

Preparation: Rhizomes are used medicinally, 5 ch'ien - 1 liang each time, prepared in decoction.

149. Hsuan Shen [Figwort species]

Family: Scrophulariaceae

Scientific name: Scrophularia ningpoensis Hemsl.

Synonyms: "Hei-shen" [black figwort], "shan tang-kuei," "shih-t'ao ts'ao."

Morphology: A perennial herb. Found growing mostly in gullies, thickets or wet places along stream edges. Roots cylindrical, lower sections frequently branching, grayish yellow. Stem erect, 4-angled. Leaves opposite, ovate or ovate-ellipsoid, apexes acuminate, bases rounded or truncate, margins crenate. Blooms in the fall, purplish-red terminal or axillary flowers forming cymose arrangement evolving into panicle inflorescence. Capsule ovate-rounded.

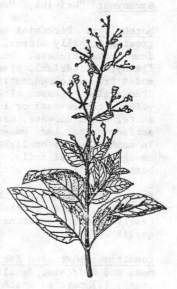

Properties and action: Slightly "han" cold, bitter and salty to taste. Nourishes the yin and lowers heat, moisturizes heat-dryness and promotes salivation.

Conditions most used for: (1) Sore and painful throat, thirstiness; (2) cervical nodes, constipation, and burning urination.

Preparation: Roots are used medicinally, 3 ch'ien - 1 liang each time, prepared in decoction.

150. Ta-p'o-wan Hua-hua (yeh mien-hua) [Broken-bowl flower; wild cotton]

Family: Ranunculaceae

Scientific name: Anemone vitifolia Buch-Ham.

Synonyms: "Tieh-kao" [iron wormwood], "ch'ing-shui tan," "hsiao yeh-mien-hua" [small wild cotton].

Morphology: Perennial herb. Found growing on hillsides, roadsides, and stream edges. Roots deep brown. Stem erect, with forklike branches. Compound leaves appearing in triple; leaflets ovate-rounded or oblique-ovate, apexes acute, bases cordate or auricular, margins rounded-dentate, leaf surface green, slightly pubescent, leaf underside grayish white, hairs more dense, petioles long. Blooms in the fall, white or pink flowers growing singly from the branching joint. Achene covered densely by long silky hairs.

Properties and action: "Warm-natured" bitter to taste, highly toxic. Can kill worms and bugs, suppresses malaria, and treats/cures pterygium.

Conditions most used for: (1) Malaria; (2) red eyes, beginning pterygium; (3) toothache.

Preparation: The whole plant or fresh root and leaves are used medicinally. Crush and assemble into small balls the size of the little finger. To treat malaria place ball over the "ta-chiu" point (big vertebra point); for eye ailments apply over the "nei-kuan" point (for the right eye apply poultice over point to the left, and for treating the left eye apply poultice over point to the right), then bandage in place with gauze bandage. When the skin feels burning sensation and becomes red, take these poultice balls down, the blisters produced indicating therapeutic action having been produced. For toothache, take a section of fresh root and place over the affected painful tooth. For use as a vermicide or maggot-killing agent, the whole plant may be chopped up and thrown into maggot-surviving areas.

- 695 -

151. Tung Kuei [Winter mallow]

Family: Malvaceae

Scientific name: Malva verticillata L.

Synonyms: "Tung hsien-ts'ai"

Morphology: Biennial herb. Mostly
cultivated. Stem erect, with coarse
hairs. Leaves alternate, with long
petioles, pubescent on both sides,
palmate 5-7, shallowly lobed, each
lobe obtuse-rounded at apex, margins
crenate, with 5-7 main ribs. Blooms
in late spring, small light red flowers
clustered at axilla. Fruit a capsule,
found growing inside the calyx.

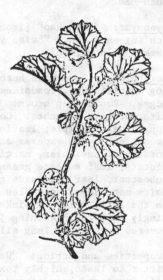

Properties and action: Slightly "han"
cold, pleasant and bland to taste.
Mild laxative, it also stimulates
milk production [in nursing mothers].

Conditions most used for: (1) Edema,
difficult urination, constipation;
(2) inadequate milk supply.

Preparation: The whole plant or seeds
are used medicinally, 3-5 ch'ien of
the whole herb each time, prepared as
decoction; or seeds 3-5 ch'ien, also
prepared as decoction.

152. Tung-kua P'i [Peel of Chinese waxgourd (winter melon)], Benincasa
hispida Cogn.

Properties and action: Slightly "han" cold, pleasant to taste. Clears
lungs and resolves phlegm, facilitates pus drainage and moisturizes.

Conditions most used for: In lung abscess to promote expectoration of
purulent and blood-stained sputum; in ulcerations of the intestines to
relieve abdominal pain, constipation and retention of purulent mucus,
and difficulties in bowel movement and urination.

Preparation: For each dose, 3-5 ch'ien prepared as decoction.

153. Ya Tsao [Teeth crushed into powder?]

Properties and action: Warm, acrid and salty to taste, slightly toxic.
Relieves constipation, loosens up mucus, and kills insects.

Conditions most used for: Lockjaw in convulsions, epilepsy, laryngeal spasms,
coughing and asthma. Used externally for scabies, ringworm, skin sores and
ulcers.

Preparation: For each dose, 3-5 fen prepared as decoction. For external
application, use an appropriate amount.

154. Kan Ts'ao [Licorice, Glycyrrhiza species]

Properties and action: Neutral, pleasant to taste. Revitalizes the center
and supplements energy, detoxifies and loosens phlegm.

Conditions most used for: Splenic and gastric imbalance, abdominal pain,
vomiting and diarrhea, productive cough, parched and sore throat, and swollen
abscesses.

Preparation: For each dose, 5 fen to 3 ch'ien, prepared as decoction.

155. Lung Ch'ih ["Dragon's teeth"]

Properties and action: Cooling, acrid to taste. Used as a tranquilizer to
calm nerves.

Conditions most used for: Convulsions, spasms, epilepsy, extreme nervousness,
insomnia and frequent dreams at night.

Preparation: For each dose, 3-5 ch'ien, prepared as decoction.

156. Lung Ku ["Dragon bones"]

Properties and action: Slightly "han" cold, acrid and pleasant to taste. Quells "yang" dominance, controls convulsions, stabilizes "acridity," and stops perspiration.

Conditions most used for: Restlessness and apprehension, spasms and insomnia, premature seminal emission and metrorrhagia, chronic diarrhea and rectal prolapse, and excessive perspiration.

Preparation: For each dose, 3 ch'ien - 1 liang, prepared as decoction.

157. Lung-yen Ju [Nephelium longana Camb.]

Properties and action: Neutral and pleasant to taste. Tonifies the spleen, cultivates the heart, and supplements the intellect.

Conditions most used for: Anemia, hyperactive mental activity, forgetfulness.

Preparation: For each dose, 1.5 - 3 ch'ien, in decoction.

158. Ku-shan-lung

Properties and action: "Han" cold and bitter, slightly toxic. Clears fevers, promotes normal hydration, purges [excess] fire, neutralizes poisons, and alleviates pain. Also acts as a vermicide.

Conditions most used for: Headache, stomach-ache, diarrhea and dysentery, malaria, boils and abscesses, and open skin sores.

Preparation: For each dose, 3 ch'ien - 1 liang, in decoction. A proper amount may be used externally.

159. Shih-chueh-ming [Abalone shell]

Properties and action: Neutral and salty to taste. Neutralizes the liver and lowers fevers, clears ptygerium and restores vision.

Conditions most used for: Dizziness, convulsions and spasms, blurred vision, glaucoma and cataracts.

Preparation: For each dose, 5 ch'ien - 1 liang, in decoction.

160. Shih-ka [Gypsum]

Properties and action: Very "han" cold, biting yet pleasant to taste.
Clears fevers.

Conditions most used for: High fever, headache and restlessness, great
thirst, delirium, lung-heated wheezing and coughing, bloodshot and sore
throat.

Preparation: For each dose, 3 ch'ien - 1 liang, prepared in decoction.

161. Pai Ch'ih [Angelica anomala, Pall.]

Properties and action: Warm-natured, acrid to taste. Clears the inner
organs and dispels gas, warms [excessive] hydration and promotes pus drainage.

Conditions most used for: Colds and headache, head "stuffiness" and coryza,
"spotting" and luekorrhea, boils and abscesses.

Preparation: For each dose, 1-3 ch'ien, prepared in decoction.

162. Pai Ch'ien [Cynanchum japonicum variation]

Properties and action: Slightly "han" cold, bitter and acried to taste.
Clears chest congestion, brings up phlegm and stops coughing.

Conditions most used for: Productive coughing, lung congestion, fullness
of chest and sides, shortness of breath, and rasping throat.

Preparation: For each dose, 1.5 - 3 ch'ien, prepared as decoction.

163. Pai-hsien P'i [Leucobrya species]

Properties and action: "Han" cold, bitter to taste. Clears fever and
detoxifies, suppresses gas and neutralizes "moisture" (excessive hydration).

Conditions most used for: Seasonal fevers and "poisons" [allergies?], fungus
infections and parasitical infestations, "wet" fever related jaundice,
painful swelling of the genitals.

Preparation: For each dose, 1.5 - 3 ch'ien, prepared in decoction. For
external use, any amount crushed for preparation into poultice.

- 699 -

164. Pai-t'ou Weng [White Anemone]

Properties and action: Slightly "han" cold, bitter to taste. Cools the
blood and neutralizes poisons.

Conditions most used for: Feverish toxins-caused dysentery, bloody dysentery
and abdominal cramps.

Preparation: For each dose, 1-3 ch'ien, prepared as decoction.

165. Pai Shao [White peony] Paeoma albiflora Pallas var. tricocarpa Bunga

Properties and action: Slightly "han" cold, bitter and biting to taste.
Purifies the "yin," and restores liver balance, neutralizes the blood and
alleviates pain.

Conditions most used for: Anemia and liver dominance, dizziness, pains in
sides and abdomen, bloody and mucoid dysentery, menstrual irregularity.

Preparation: For each dose, 3 ch'ien prepared as decoction.

166. Pai-shu [Atractylis ovata]

Properties and action: Warm-natured, bitter yet pleasant to taste. Supplements
spleen, benefits energy, converts [excessive] moisture, and promotes diuresis.

Conditions most used for: Spleen-deficient diarrheas, indigestion, edema,
chest tightness and abdominal distension, vomiting.

Preparation: For each dose, 1.5 - 3 ch'ien prepared as decoction.

167. Hsien-hu-so [Corydalis ternata, Makino]

Properties and action: Has warming properties, acrid and bitter to taste.
Stimulates energy and blood circulation, alleviates pain.

Conditions most used for: Stomach-ache and abdominal pain, hernia-caused
pain, poor circulation of blood and energy, body aches, dysmenorrhea, post-
partum pain due to clots, and traumatic-injury pain.

Preparation: For each dose, 1.5 - 3 ch'ien, prepared as decoction.

168. Ti-erh Ts'ao [St. Johnswort species]

<u>Family</u>: Guttiferae

<u>Scientific name</u>: Hypericum japonicum.
Thunb.

<u>Synonyms</u>: "Sha-tzu ts'ao," "kuang-ming
ts'ao," "t'ien-chi hsien" [paddy-field
amaranth], "chiao-she ts'ao [bird-tongue
grass], "ts'ui-sha ts'ao" [gravel grass],
"chin so-shih" [golden key], "yang-ho
ts'ao," "hsiao wang-pu-liu-hsing,"
"hsi-hsieh huang," "kuan-yin lien"
[goddess-of-mercy lotus].

<u>Morphology</u>: Annual herb. Found growing
along roadsides, and wet places along
ditches. Stem erect, height 20-40 cm,
slightly 4-angled. Single leaves alternate and opposite, non-petioled, apexes
obtuse, bases clasping stem slightly,
margins intact, leaf surfaces containing
transparent little dots. In summer, small
yellow flowers appear terminally to
form cymose inflorescence. Capsule long-
ellipsoid.

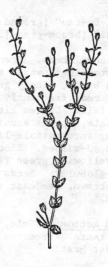

<u>Properties and action</u>: "Cooling," slightly
pleasant to taste. Clears fever and detoxifies, reduces swelling and resolves
bruises.

<u>Conditions most used for</u>: (1) Acute
hepatitis, pain in the liver region,
appendicitis; (2) boils and abscesses,
mastitis, snakebites.

<u>Preparation</u>: The whole plant is used
medicinally, 5 ch'ien - 1 liang each
time, prepared in decoction; for external
application, a suitable amount may be
crushed for the purpose.

169. Ti Fu [Summer cypress]

Family: Chenopodiaceae

Scientific name: Kochia scoparia Schrad.

Synonyms: "Ti-fu-tzu" [ground cover],
"sao-chou ts'ai" [broom-grass].

Morphology: Annual herb. Stem height
1.5 meters, extending upwards and branching off like a broom, finely grooved,
green or light red, frequently changing
to red in the fall. Leaves alternate,
linear lanceolate, apexes acuminate,
bases narrowing into petiole-like shape,
margins intact, 3-ribbed. Blooms in
July-August, yellowish green flowers.
Ascocarp flat-globular. Seeds obovate,
flat and palm-brown, seedcoat thin,
easily crushed.

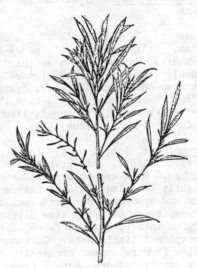

Properties and action: "Cold," pleasant
yet bitter to taste. Promotes diuresis,
eliminates moist heat.

Conditions most used for: (1) Gonorrhea,
baldness; (2) scabies and sores.

Preparation: Usually a suitable amount
is boiled in water and the preparation
is used for bathing the skin, or 1-3
ch'ien may be prepared as decoction.

170. Ti Tan-t'ou [Elephant's foot]

<u>Family</u>: Compositae

<u>Scientific name</u>: Elephantopus scaber L.

<u>Synonyms</u>: "Ti-tan ts'ao," "mo-ti-tan,"
"t'ien chieh-ts'ai" [heavenly mustard],
"ts'ao hsieh-ti" [straw sandals],"tieh
teng-ch'u" [iron lamp post], "chia p'u-
kung-ying" [false dandelion].

<u>Morphology</u>: Perennial herb. Usually
found growing on hillsides, grass
meadows, riverbanks and roadsides.
Stem height 30-60 cm, branching into
2. Basal leaves covering the ground,
spatulate or long ellipsoid-lanceolate,
apexes obtuse, bases gradually narrowing, margins crenate; stem leaves few,
extremely small. Blooms in summer,
light purple flowers appearing in
terminal style to form a capitulum
inflorescence. Achene angled, covered
by stiff hairs.

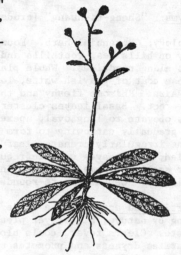

<u>Properties and action</u>: "Han" cold,
acrid and bitter to taste. Clears
fever and detoxifies, reduces swelling
and promotes pus drainage.

<u>Conditions most used for</u>: (1) Colds
and influenza, pharyngitis; (2) dysentery,
gastroenteritis; (3) edema, acute gonorrhea;
(4) swollen abscesses, snakebites.

<u>Preparation</u>: The whole plant is used
medicinally, 5 ch'ien - 1 liang each
time, prepared in decoction.

171. Ti-huang [Figwort species]

Family: Scrophulariaceae

Scientific name: Rehmannia glutinosa
(Gaertn.) Libosch.

Synonyms: "Sheng-ti-huang" [crude figwort].

Morphology: Perennial herb. Found growing
mostly on hillsides, foothills and waste
places along roadsides. Whole plant covered
by dense coat of grayish white, long and
soft hairs. Rhizome fleshy and thick.
Stems erect. Basal leaves clustered,
leaves obovate to long oval, apexes obtuse,
bases gradually narrowing to form long petiole,
margins irregularly crenate, leaf surfaces
wrinkled, stem leaves seen infrequently,
rather small. Blooms in the spring, purplish
red flowers. Capsule ovate-rounded.

Properties and action: The crude figwort
cooling by nature, bitter yet pleasant
to taste. Clears fever, cools blood,
moisturizes dryness and promotes salivation.
The processed figwort warm by nature, pleasant to taste. Nourishes the yin and supplements the blood.

Conditions most used for: (1) High fever
and restlessness, parchness of mouth; (2)
diphtheria, tonsillitis; (3) various types
of bleeding due to too much heat in the
blood; (4) constipation or difficult urination (Use the crude product for above
conditions). (5) Anemia, dizziness, seminal
emission; (6) menstrual irregularity,
post-partum hemorrhage; (7) deficient-yin
caused wheezing and coughing. (The processed
product is used for the above conditions).

Preparation: For each dose, 3 ch'ien - 1
liang, prepared in decoction.

172. Ti-yu [Burnet, bloodwort]

Family: Rosaceae

Scientific name: Sanguisorba officinalis
L.

Synonyms: "Yeh sheng-ma," [wild bugbane],
"hung ti-yu" [red bloodwort], "yen ti-chi,"
"hsueh chien-ts'ao," [bloody arrow-grass].

Morphology: Perennial herb. Found growing on uplands and plains. Perennial roots
thick. Stem erect, height 20-150 cm, finely
angled and shallowly grooved. Leaves alternate, oddly pinnate compound, leaflets
long oval, apexes obtuse, bases truncate,
margins serrated; basal leaves larger,
with long petioles, stem leaves smaller,
petioles almost absent, bases clasping
stem, stipules on both sides encircling.
Blooms in fall, dark purplish red terminal
flowers obovate or rounded, forming a spike
inflorescence. Achene ovate and 4-angled.

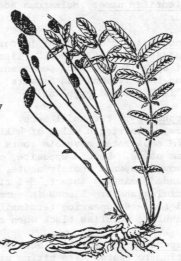

Properties and action: Slightly "han"
cold, bitter tasting. Clears fever and
detoxifies, cools the blood and stops
bleeding.

Conditions most used for: (1) Acute
bacillary dysentery, burn injuries;
(2) gastrointestinal bleeding, bleeding
hemorrhoids, uterine bleeding.

Preparation: Roots are used medicinally,
5 ch'ien - 1 liang each time, prepared
as decoction; or dried roots may be
crushed and taken by mouth; or sesame
oil may be mixed with the powdered root
for applying on external cuts and
injuries.

173. Ti-shen [Melastoma species]

Family: Melastomataceae

Scientific name: Melastoma dodecandrum
Lour.

Synonyms: "P'u ti-chin" [groundcover
brocade], "shan ti-shen," "lien ti-shen,"
"ti shih-liu" [ground pomegranate], "ti
hung-hua" [ground red flowers], "ti-
ch'ieh" [ground eggplant].

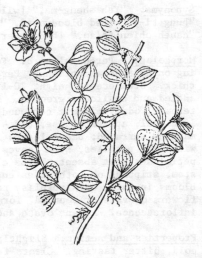

Morphology: Perennial herb. Found
growing on virgin wilds of hillsides.
Stem prostrate, moveable roots growing
from nodes. Leaves opposite, obovate
or oval, apexes sharply acute, bases
rounded, margins intact, 3-5 ribs,
petioles short. Blooms in summer, purplish
red flowers appearing terminally. Fruit
globular, purplish black when ripe.

Properties and action: Neutral, sour and
biting to taste. Its biting properties
stop dysentery, relax sinews and stimulate circulation, supplement the blood
and quiet the fetus.

Conditions most used for: (1) Enteritis,
dysentery; (2) apins in back and legs,
rheumatism; (3) excessive menstruation;
(4) an overly active fetus.

Preparation: The whole plant is used
medicinally, 5 ch'ien - 1 liang each
time, prepared in decoction.

174. Ti Chin [Euphorbia species]

Family: Euphorbiaceae

Scientific name: Euphorbia humifusa Willd.

Synonyms: "P'u ti-hung" [red carpet],
"ch'ien-hsieh ts'ao" [thousand-leaf grass],
"hsien-t'ao ts'ao" [peach-of-the-god's
grass], "nai-chiang ts'ao" [milky grass],
"p'u ti-chin" [ground cover brocade].

Morphology: Annual herb. Found growing
along stream edges, roadsides, and hillsides. Stem fine and slender, creeping,
multiple-branched. Leaves opposite,
interspaced or alternate, long oval,
apex rounded-obtuse, margins doubly
serrated. Stem leaves oozing white
milky fluid when broken. Blooms in late
summer, small axillary flowers, yellowish brown. Small capsule globular.

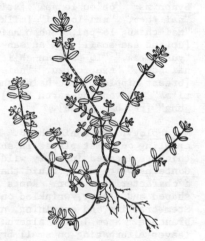

Properties and action: Neutral, bitter
tasting. Eliminates moisture and detoxifies, promotes diuresis, stops
bleeding.

Conditions most used for: (1) Jaundice,
dysentery, enteritis; (2) poisonous snake
bits; (3) traumatic bleeding.

Preparation: The whole plant is used
medicinally, 1-3 liang each time, prepared in decoction.

175. Yang Ju [Goat's milk]

Family: Campanulaceae

Scientific name: Codonopsis lanceolata
Benth. et Hook.

Synonyms: "ch'ou lo'pai" [stinky turnip],
"nai shen," "nai-lo-pai" [milky turnip],
"nai-chiang lo-pai," "shan hai-lei"
[upland sea-snail], "p'an san-ch'i,"
"yu fu tzu," "lo-pai san-ch'i," "niu-
nai shen," "niu fu-tzu," "nai chien-t'ou"
[breast nipple], "ssu-hsieh shen," "t'ien-
ti ma" [heaven-and-earth hemp], "hung mao-
jung" [red hat plume].

Morphology: Perennial herb. Found
crawling on moist places in shrub
thickets located in hilly wilds.
Contains white milky fluid that emits
a characteristic odor. Roots spindle-
shaped and fleshy, wrinkled on outside.
Stem crawling and entwining, numerous
branches. Stem leaves alternate, single
leaves alternating on small branches,
4 or more leaves clustered or whorled, long
or obovate, margins almost intact or
slightly undulate-dentate. Blooms in
summer-fall, yellowish white on upper
side, purple on back side. Capsule
green, cone-shaped.

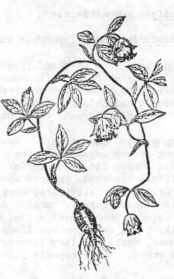

Properties and action: Neutral, pleasant
to taste. Clears the lungs, detoxifies,
regulates menstruation, and stimulates
milk production.

Conditions most used for: (1) Lung
abscess; (2) milk-flow obstruction,
amenorrhea; (3) acute and inflamed boils
and abscesses, lymphadenopathy.

Preparation: The root tuber is used
medicinally, 5 ch'ien - 1 liang each
time, prepared in decoction.

176. Yang-t'i Ts'ao [Goatsfoot grass]

Family: Compositae

Scientific name: Emilia sonchifolia
(L.) DC

Synonyms: "I-tien hung" [a-drop-of-red],
"hsieh-hsia hung" [leaf-underside-red],
"yeh chieh-lan" [wild broccoli], "la-pa
hung-ts'ao" [red trumpet-grass], "hsiao
p'u-kung-ying" [dwarf dandelion].

Morphology: Annual herb. Found growing
wild in village outskirts, gardens, and
along roadsides. Whole plant containing
white milky juice. Height 20-40 cm.
Basal leaves irregularly pinnate-parted,
stem leaves ovate lanceolate, apexes
obtuse, base clasping stem, margins
irregularly serrated, leaf reddish
purple on underside. Blooms in summer,
reddish purple flowers appearing terminally
to form a capitulum inflorescence. Achene
narrow and cylindrical in shape, covered
by white hairs.

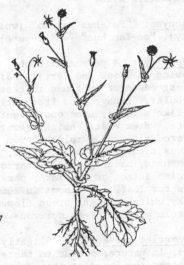

Properties and action: Cooling bitter
to taste. Clears fever, detoxifies,
promotes diuresis.

Conditions most used for: (1) Colds
and influenza, pharyngitis, laryngitis,
boils and abscesses; (2) enteritis,
dysentery; (3) traumatic injuries; (4)
poisonous snakebites.

Preparation: The whole plant is used
medicinally, 1 - 2 liang each time,
prepared as decoction.

177. Pai-ho [Lily species]

Family: Liliaceae

Scientific name: Lilium brownii var. Colchesteri Wils.

Synonyms: "Pai-hua pai-ho" [white-flower lily], "pa-fan hua" [white-petaled flower].

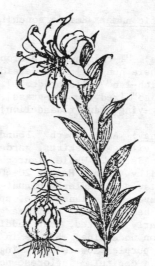

Morphology: A perennial herb. Found growing in loose and fertile soil along forest edges or in grass thickets. Corm globular, fleshy, apex frequently opening up like a lotus, numerous adventitious roots. Stem erect, height about 1 cm, covered often by purplish brown spots. Leaves alternate, oblanceolate, apexes acuminate, bases gradually narrowing, margins intact or undulate, parallel ribs for leaf, 5. Blooms in summer, milky white or light brown flowers. Capsule green. Seeds numerous.

Properties and action: Slightly "han" cold, in nature, bitter to taste. Moistens the lungs to stop coughing, clears fever and calms nerves, promotes diuresis.

Conditions most used for: (1) Coughing and hematemesis due to deficiency-condition; (2) anxiety, apprehension; (3) edema difficult urination.

Preparation: For each dose, 2-4 ch'ien, prepared as decoction, or steamed for juice to be taken by mouth.

178. Pai-pu [Stemona species]

Family: Stemonaceae

Scientific name: Stemona tuberosa Lour.

Synonyms: "Tui-hsieh pai-pu," "ta-chun ken-yao" [spring drug-root], "niu pai-pu" [oxen stemona], "chiu-ch'ung ken" [nine-layered roots], "pai-t'iao ken" [hundred roots].

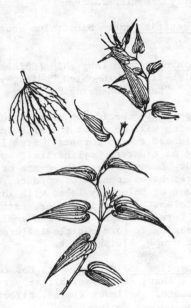

Morphology: Perennial climbing herb. Found growing mostly in thickets on sunny slopes. Fleshy root tuber growing horizontally, spindle-shaped or cylindrical. Upper stem section entwining, finely-grooved longitudinally. Leaves opposite or whorled, broad ovate, apexes acuminate, bases shallowly chordate, margins intact or slightly undulate. Blooms in the spring. Single axillary light purple flowers appearing on wiry peduncles, base and petiole connected. Capsule obovate and flat.

Properties and action: Slightly warming, pleasant and bitter to taste. Warms the lungs, expel gas, quiets coughing, kills bugs.

Conditions most used for: (1) Pulmonary tuberculosis, bronchitis, pertussis; (2) epidemic diseases; (3) head lice and ringworm; (4) intestinal parasites.

Preparation: Root tubers are used medicinally, 3-5 ch'ien each time, prepared in decoction. For external use, cook an appropriate amount or steep in alcohol for use as an externally applied agent.

179 Fang-chi [Levant berry]

Family: Menispermaceae

Scientific name: Sinomenium acutum
Rhed. et Wils.

Synonyms: "Han fang chi" [Chinese cocculus],
"chieh-li," "shih-chieh," "fang-yuan," "fang
tzu," "tsai-chun-hsing."

Morphology: Deciduous vine. Found
growing wild in shrub thickets in
hills and sparse forests. Stem length as
long as 6 meters, cylindrical, woody and
hard. Leaves alternate, ovate or broad-
ovate, bases rounded or cordate, margins
intact or palmately lobed with long
petioles. Blooms in summer, axillary
and terminal light green and small flowers
appearing to form panicle inflorescences.
Flat drupe, bluish black.

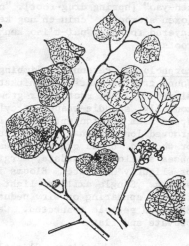

Properties and action: (1) Has cold-
chill [han] qualities, bitter yet acrid
to taste. Relieves flatus, alleviates
pain, purges "moist heat."

Conditions most used for: (1) Edema;
(2) moisture related beri beri; (3)
rheumatoid arthritis.

Preparation: Roots are used medicinally,
3-5 ch'ien each time, in decoction.

180. Chu-hsieh Chiao [Bamboo-leafed pepper]

Family: Rutaceae

Scientific name: Zanthoxylum planispinum
Sieb. et Zucc.

Synonyms: "Ch'ou hua-chia" [stinky pepper],
"kou hua-chiao," "ch'ou hu-chiao," "szu-
liang ma" [four ounces hemp], "yeh hua-chiao"
[wild pepper], "san-hsieh hua chiao" [3-
leafed pepper], "shan hu-chiao" [mountain
pepper], "t'u hua-chiao," "ju chiao-tzu,"
"hua-chiao," "yu chiao," "chuan hua-chiao"
[Szechuan pepper].

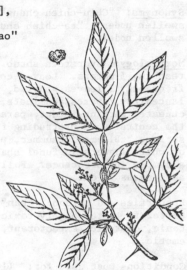

Morphology: Evergreen shrub. Found
growing on hillside slopes, and shrub
thickets along roadsides. Whole plant
emits an aromatic fragrance. Tree bark
greyish-white, branches, twigs, undersides of leaves and petiole ribs all
covered by long and straight flat thorns.
Leaves alternate, oddly pinnate-compound,
extending from base of leaves to form a
narrow wing, leaflets 3-7 oval or long
lanceolate, apexes acuminate, bases
cuneate, margins intact. Blooms in
early summer, light yellow flowers forming
a panicle inflorescence. Fruit globular,
red when ripe. Seed black, lustrous.

Properties and action: Warm-natured,
acrid to taste. Dispels cold and
eliminates moisture and strengthens
the stomach. Also a vermifuge.

Conditions most used for: (1) Stomach-ache,
gastrointestinal disturbances, ascariasis;
(2) rheumatoid arthritis, traumatic bruises
and aches; (3) Swellings and abscesses of
unknown origin, poisonous snakebites.

Preparation: Seeds or roots are used
medicinally, 1-3 ch'ien of roots, or 7-
14 seeds, prepared in decoction. Suitable
amount may be used for external purposes.

181. Chia-chu-t'ao [Dogbane, oleander]

Family: Apocynaceae

Scientific name: Nerium indicum Mill.

Synonyms: "Chiu-chieh chung" [nine
swollen nodes], "ta-chieh chung [large
swollen node].

Morphology: Evergreen shrub. Height
reaching 5 meters. Leaves coriaceous,
frequently 3 leaves whorled, linear
lanceolate, apexes acuminate, bases
cuneate, margins intact, parallel veins,
the central vein protruding from back
surface. Blooms in summer, peach red
or white flowers in funel shape forming
a cymose inflorescence. Follicle 2,
as long as 18 cm.

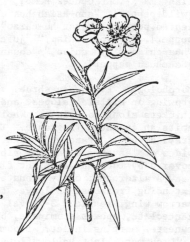

Properties and action: "Han" cold,
bitter to taste, highly toxic. Cardio-
tonic, diuretic, expectorant, perspirant,
emetic.

Conditions most used for: (1) heart
disease, heart failure; (2) traumatic
bruises and swellings; (3) ringworm,
resistant fungus infections; (4) insecticide for killing flies and maggots.

Preparation: Leaves are used medicinally,
dried under low temperature, after which
the dry leaves are crushed for taking
by mouth: 1-1.2 fen the first day, 0.8-1.2
fen the second and third day, divided into
2-3 doses in each instance. Dosage reduced to 3 li (0.3 fen) divided in 2 doses,
after the patient's condition improves.
The medication is stopped when symptoms
have all disappeared. A suitable amount
may be used externally.

182. Hung-hua [Safflower, bastard saffron]

Family: Compositae

Scientific name: Carthamus tinctorius L.

Synonyms: "Hung lan-hua" [red orchid], 'huang lan" [yellow orchid].

Morphology: Annual or biennial herb. Height as much as 90 cm, the whole plant quite cleancut. Stem erect, greenish white, with fine and shallow grooves. Leaves alternate, ovate or broad ovate-lanceolate, apexes acute, bases gradually narrowing, clasping stem, margins irregularly shallow-parted, apexes of parted lobes like a pointed thorn. Large capitulum inflorescence terminal, flowers red and tubular. Achene white, black, four-angled.

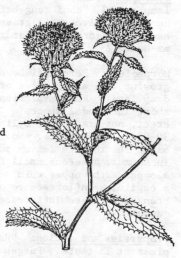

Properties and action: Warm, acrid to taste. Resolves bruises and stimulates tissue regeneration. Activates and clears meridian channels.

Conditions most used for: (1) amenorrhea, unexpelled dead fetus, and prolonged post-partum discharge; (2) traumatic injuries, and painful bruises.

Preparation: Flowers are used medicinally, 5 - 2 - ch'ien each time, prepared as decoction.

183. Teng-hsin Ts'ao [Rush, lamp-wick rush]

Family: Juncaceae

Scientific name: Juncus effusus L.

Synonyms: "Shui teng-ts'ao," [water
lamp grass], "shui teng-hsin," "wu-
ku ts'ao" [five-grain grass], "lung-
hsu ts'ao" [dragon's beardgrass], "t'u
ma-huang."

Morphology: Perennial herb. Found
growing wild along edges of swamps and
damp lands. Rhizomes creeping, with
short internodal spaces. Culms clustered,
erect, non-branching, cylindrical, height
30-90 cm, pith white. No leaves on culms,
basal sheath-like leaves purplish brown.
In summer, numerous small flowers appear
alongside the upper culm section, forming
a capitulum inflorescence or a non-
branching cymose inflorescence. Fruit a
capsule.

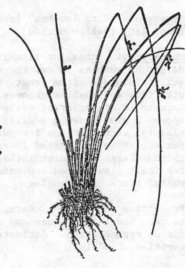

Properties and action: "Han" cold,
pleasant to taste. Purges "heart fire,"
calms nerves, promotes diuresis.

Conditions most used for: (1) Acute
convulsions and fright in small children;
(2) jaundice; (3) difficult urination;
(4) restlessness and insomnia.

Preparation: The whole plant is used
medicinally, 5 ch'ien-1 liang each time,
prepared in decoction.

184. Hsi-ho Liu (Ch'eng-liu) [Chinese tamarisk]

Family: Tamaricacea

Scientific name: Tamarix chinensis
Lour.

Synonyms: "Kuan-yin liu" [Goddess-of-
mercy tamarisk], "kuang-hsieh liu"
[shiny-leaf tamarisk].

Morphology: Small deciduous shrub.
Mostly found cultivated along roadsides and stream edges. Stems erect,
multiple branches, small branches
slender and drooping. Leaves small,
alternate, scaly lanceolate, bases
clasping stem. Blooms in summer,
pink flowers forming a panicle inflorescence. Fruit a capsule.

Properties and action: Neutral, pleasant
yet salty to taste. Clears fevers, aids
measles rash surfacing, detoxifies and
promotes diuresis.

Conditions most used for: (1) Influenza;
(2) measles, chickenpox; (3) alcoholic
intoxication; (4) rheumatoid arthritis.

Preparation: Branches and leaves are
used medicinally, 3-5 ch'ien each time,
prepared in decoction.

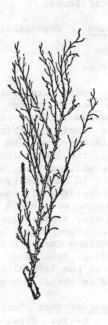

185. Kuan-yi꞉   ꞉ien [Lotus like the Kuan-Yin's cushion]

Family: Marattiaceae

Scientific name: Angiopteris fokiensis Hieron

Synonyms: None

Morphology: Large perennial evergreen herb. Found mostly growing in dark and shady places in the forest and along stream edges. Rhizomes thick, fleshy and tuberous, clustered to form a column. Leaves basal, the large-sized ones double pinnate-compound, petioles sturdy and strong, about 50 cm primary pinnae 5-7 pairs, oblanceolate, alternate; the secondary pinnae or pinnule 35-40 pairs, oval lanceolate, apexes acute, bases oval, margins presenting a new pattern of shallow triangular serrations, leaf veins spreading, branching. Sori brown, distributed on the lateral margins of the pinnules on their undersides.

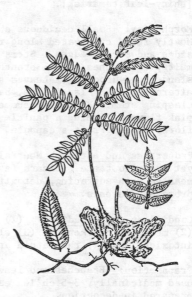

Properties and action: Cooling, pleasant yet bitter to taste. Expels gas and flatus, detoxifies, stops coughing.

Conditions most used for: (1) Consumption, apprehension and restlessness; (2) boils and ulcers, snakebites; (3) dry (hot) cough.

Preparation: Rhizomes containing petioles are used medicinally, 3-5 ch'ien each time, in decoction; or a suitable amount of the fresh herb may be crushed and used externally.

186. Kuo-lu Huang [Primrose species]

Family: Primulaceae

Scientific name: Lysimachia christinae Hance.

Synonyms: "Szechwan ta-chin-ch'ien ts'ao" [Szechwan golden-coin grass], "lu-pien huang" [yellow by the roadside], "ti huang-hua," "chin-hua ts'ai" [golden-blossom herb], "hsien-jen tui-tso ts'ao" [fairies-sitting-opposite-each-other-grass], "jan-chin t'eng," [soft-sinew vine], ch'ien-li ma" [1000-kilometer horse], "wu-sung ts'ao [centipede grass], "t'eng-huang po-lo" [yellow-vined pineapple], "p'ien-ti huang" [ground-all-covered yellow], "shuang t'ung ch'ien" [double copper cash], "t'ung-ch'ien ts'ao [copper-cash grass], "mao-hsieh hsien," "no-mi ts'ao" [glutinous rice herb], "pu-liao ts'ao" [unpredictable grass], "p'an yu ts'ao."

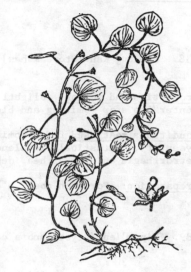

Morphology: Perennial herb. Found growing in grassy thickets along roadsides. The whole plant sparsely pubescent. Stems soft and weak, prostrate. Leaves, calyx, and corolla covered by black dots and stripes. Leaves opposite, ovate or cordate, apexes obtuse, bases rounded or cordate, margins intact, length of petiole and leaves approximately the same. Blooms in summer, single axillary yellow flower. Capsule globular.

Properties and action: Cooling, bitter and sour. Detoxifies and reduces inflammation, promotes diuresis.

Conditions most used for: (1) Mushroom poisoning, drug poisoning; (2) pus-forming inflammations, burn injuries, abscesses, poisonous snakebites; (3) stones of the urinary tract, gallbladder stones.

187. Fang-feng,(Siler divaricatum, Benth et Hook)

Properties and action: "Warm," acrid yet pleasant to taste. Promotes perspiration, suppresses gas and flatus, overcomes moisture.

Conditions most used for: Influenza, headache, chills, rheumatoid numbness, joint pains, tetanus.

Preparation: For each dose, 1-3 ch'ien, prepared in decoction.

188. Fu-lung Kan [Stove ashes]

Properties and action: Slightly warm, pleasant to taste. Warms the "body center" to stop vomiting and bleeding.

Conditions most used for: Vomiting and regurgitation stomach-ache and "cold dysentery," intestinal flatulence and bleeding, hematemesis and hematuria, metrorrhagia and leukorrhea, debilitating diarrheas.

Preparation: For each dose, 5 ch'ien to 1 liang, prepared in decoction.

189. Pin p'ien (Dryobalanops camphora Coleb) [Camphor]

Properties and action: Slightly "han" cold, acrid and bitter to taste. Clears body passageways and dispels fire [heat], eliminates pterygiums and restores vision, reduces edema and alleviates pain.

Conditions most used for: Laryngeal numbness and pharyngeal edema, canker sores and ulcers. Conjunctivitis and pterygiums, heatstroke, coma, convulsions, vomiting and diarrhea in cholera.

Preparation: Product not used in decoction, though prepared mostly in pill or powder form, the amount determined by the original prescription.

190. Tang-kuei (Angelica polymorpha Maxim var. sinensis)

Properties and action: Warm natured, acrid and bitter though pleasant to taste. Supplements blood and stimulates circulation. Mildly laxative, it also moistens "dryness" in the system.

Conditions most used for: Menstrual irregularity, metrorrhagia, meridian and passageway obstructions, rheumatism, boils and ulcers, traumatic injuries, anemia, dryness [dehydration] and constipation.

Preparation: For each dose, 2-4 ch'ien, prepared in decoction.

191. Ch'ueh-ming tzu (Cassia tora L.)

Properties and action: Slightly "han" cold, bitter yet pleasant to taste. Purifies the liver and supports the kidneys. Expels gas and clarifies vision.

Conditions most used for: Headache, swollen and red eyes, dizziness, pterygiums.

Preparation: For each dose, 1.5-3 ch'ien, prepared in decoction.

192. Ju-ku'ei [Cinnamon]

Properties and action: Very "hot." Pleasant, yet acrid to taste. Warms the kidneys, and supplements the body fire. Dispels cold and alleviates pain.

Conditions most used for: Cold visceral organs and chronic diarrhea, cold and pain in heart and abdomen, inadequate yang element in kidneys, chilled lungs and coughing and wheezing, lumbago, and vaginal cancer [?].

Preparation: For each dose, 0.3 to 1 ch'ien, prepared in decoction.

193. Hsueh-chih [Resin from Calamus draco, Willd]

Properties and action: Neutral, pleasant yet salty to taste. Resolves bruises, promotes tissue granulation. Also stimulates blood circulation and alleviates pain. External use stops bleeding and aids healing.

Conditions most used for: Menstrual irregularities, chest pains, post-partum abdominal cramps, traumatic injuries.

Preparation: For each dose, 3-6 fen, prepared in decoction. For external use, a suitable amount.

194. Ch'uan-hsieh [Whole scorpion]

Properties and action: Neutral, pleasant yet acrid to taste. Toxic. Dispels flatus and relieves spasms.

Conditions most used for: Stroke and hemiplegia, nystagmus, infantile convulsions, spasms, tetanus, leprosy.

Preparation: For each dose, 3-5 fen of whole scorpion, or 3-8 scorpion tails, prepared in decoction.

195. Pai-ts'ao Hsiang [Stove soot]

Properties and action: "Warm-natured," but acrid-tasting. Stops bleeding, resolves [cures?] marasmus.

Conditions most used for: Hematemesis, epistaxis, metrorrhagia, leukorrhea, indigestion, diarrhea, canker sores in the throat and mouth.

Preparation: For each dose, 0.5-1.5 ch'ien, prepared in decoction.

196. Liu Chi-nu (Senecio palmatus Pall)

Properties and action: "Warm-natured," bitter-tasting. Stimulates circulation and alleviates pain.

Conditions most used for: Amenorrhea, abdominal distention and cramps, traumatic injuries, bruises and swellings.

Preparation: For each dose, 1.5-3 ch'ien, prepared in decoction.

197. Chi-shih T'eng [Paederia species]

Family: Rubiaceae

Scientific name: Paederia scandens
(Lour.) Merrill.

Synonyms: "Ch'ou teng" [stink vine],
"kuang chu-tzu" [shiny beads],"ch'ing
t'eng," "ya-pa teng."

Morphology: Perennial herb-like vine.
Found growing in wild places, hillsides,
or shrub thickets. Base of stem woody,
climbing. Rubbing stem leaves or fruit
precipitates a disagreeable odor that
smells like chicken droppings. Leaves
opposite, oval, apexes acuminate, bases
cuneate or rounded-obtuse, margins intact. In the fall, terminal or
axillary white purplish flowers appearing to form panicle inflorescence. Nut
globular, yellow when ripe, glabrous.

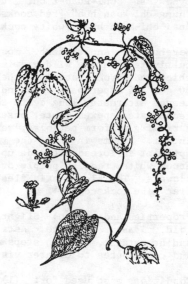

Properties and action: Neutral, sour
but slightly biting to taste. Expels
gas and flatus, eliminates moisture,
detoxifies, relieves overeating, kills
worms.

Conditions most used for: (1) rheumatoid
arthritis; (2) abdominal pain, overeating; (3) boils, abscesses and poisonous snake bites.

Preparation: The whole plant is used
medicinally, 1-2 liang each time, prepared in decoction.

198. Chi-kuan Hua [Cockscomb]

Family: Amaranthaceae

Scientific name: Celosia cristate L.

Synonyms: "Chi-kuan-t'ou," "chi-t'ou,"
"hung chi-kuan hua" [red cockscomb],
"pai chi-kuan hua" [white cockscomb].

Morphology: Annual herb. Mostly found
cultivated, rarely wild-growing. Stem
thick and strong, attaining height of
80 cm, its upper part flat and level.
Leaves alternate, long ovate to ovate-
lanceolate, apexes acute, bases gradually
narrowing to form petioles, margins
intact. Blooms in fall, the terminal
spikelet inflorescence made up of numerous white, reddish purple or yellow
flowers. The floral axis fleshy, and
flat like cockscomb.

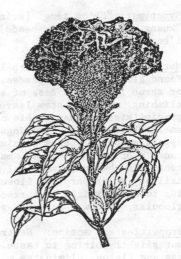

Properties and action: Slightly "han"
cold, pleasant to taste. Astringent
and hemostatic, it also stops diarrhea
and contributes to clearer vision.

Conditions most used for: (1) Dysentery;
(2) bleeding hemorrhoids, metrarrhagia,
leukorrea; (3) red eyes and other pains
and aches.

Preparation: The flowers are used
medicinally, 3-5 ch'ien each time,
prepared in decoction.

199. Mai Tung

Family: Liliaceae

Scientific name: Ophiopogon japonicus
ker-gaw.

Synonyms: "Chiu'tzu ts'ao" [onion grass],
"hsiao yang-hu-tzu ts'ao" [small goatee
grass], "yang-shih ts'ao" [goat's dung
grass], "yen-men-tung," "wei-tai ts'ao."

Morphology: Perennial herb. Found growing in mountain wilds or in damp and shady
places in the forest. Rhizomes short, containing slender and fine roots, the central
or lower part of the fibrous roots expanding to form spindle-shaped rhizome.
Basal leaves clustered, coriaceous, slender
and long-linear, apexes acute or acuminate,
base sections gradually narrowing into
petioles, margins like leaf sheaths.
Blooms in summer, terminal flowering stem
presenting with light purple flowers on
top to form a racemose inflorescence.
Fruit globular.

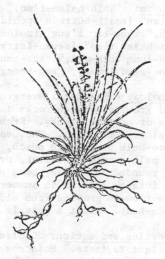

Properties and action: Has slightly
"han" cold properties; pleasant yet
slightly bitter to taste. Tonifies the
lungs and nourishes the stomach, stops
coughing and resolves phlegm, nourishes
the yin and promotes salivation.

Conditions most used for: (1) Chronic
bronchitis, hemoptysis in pulmonary
tuberculosis; (2) restlessness and
thirst, laryngitis, pertussis.

Preparation: Root tubers are used
medicinally, 1.5 - 3 ch'ien each time,
prepared in decoction.

200. Mai-Hu

Family: Orchidaceae

Scientific name: Bulbophyllum inconspicuum
Maxim.

Synonyms: "Shih hsien-t'ao," "hsiao k'ou-tzu lan" [small-buttons orchid], "tzu-shang hsieh," "kua-tzu t'eng" [melon-seed vine], "ch'i-hsien t'ao" [seven-fairy peach], "shih-lung shih-wei," "kua-tzu lien" [melon-seed lotus], "ken-shang tzu."

Morphology: Perennial evergreen herb. Found growing between rocks in mountainous areas or on tree trunks. Stem slender and creeping, horizontal. The ovate-rounded pseudo-bulb similar to peach, fleshy. Each bulb growing one leaf, ovate-rounded, apex rounded or retuse, base narrow, margins intact. Blooms in summer, small white flowers growing from side of pesudo-bulb. Fruit a capsule.

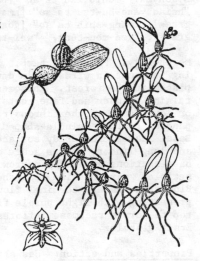

Properties and action: Cooling, pleasant and light to taste. Moistens the lungs and resolves phlegm, nourishes the yin and the stomach.

Conditions most used for: (1) Hemoptysis in pulmonary tuberculosis; (2) cancer of the stomach.

Preparation: The whole plant is used medicinally, 1 liang each time, prepared in decoction.

201. Tu-chung T'eng

Family: Apocynaceae

Scientific name: Parabarium micranthus (Wall.) Pierre.

Synonyms: "Pai-p'i chiao-t'eng" [white-bark rubber vine], "chiu-niu t'eng [nine-oxen vine], "t'u tu-chung."

Morphology: Evergreen woody vine. Found growing in valleys, stream edges, or shrub thickets. Bark smooth, a milky white fluid under bark. Numerous branches, young branches covered by short hairs that shed as branch becomes more mature. Single leaves opposite, oval-oblong, apexes acuminate, base rounded, margins intact. Blooms in summer, white flowers forming a racemose inflorescence. Follicle cracks open when ripe, exposing many white hairs and brown seeds.

Properties and action: Neutral, bitter to taste, slightly toxic. Quells gas and flatus, stimulates blood circulation, strengthens sinews and bones, and strengthens the back and knees.

Conditions most used for: (1) Rheumatoid numbness and pain, lumbago due to deficient kidney function, strained back muscles; (2) fractures, torsion injuries, and hemorrhage due to wound injuries.

Preparation: Roots and the mature vine are used medicinally, 3-5 ch'ien each time, prepared in decoction.

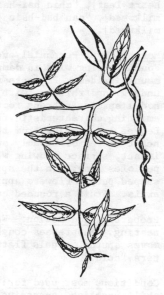

202. Tu-heng [Asarum species]

Family: Aristolochiaceae

Scientific name: Asarum blumei Duch.

Synonyms: "Ma-t'i hsi-hsin" [horse-hoof heart leaf], "chia hsi-hsin" [pseudo-milkweed], "nan hsi-hsin [southern milkweed].

Morphology: Perennial evergreen herb. Found growing wild in damp shady spots on mountainsides. Presents a horizontal underground rhizome, with short inter-nodal spaces, fibrous roots numerous, emitting characteristic fragrance. Leaves 1-3 growing from the rhizome, heart-shaped or broadly oval, margins intact, surface showing white spots, petioles long. In the spring, bell-shaped purple flowers appearing from axils. Fruit a rounded capsule.

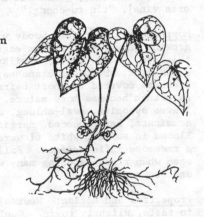

Properties and action: Warm, acrid tasting. Suppresses cough and re-moves sputum, expels flatus and scat-ters "cold."

Conditions most used for: (1) Wind-chill coughing, excessive salivation; (2) enlarged lymphatic nodes of the neck; (3) edema; (4) rheumatism, traumatic injuries.

Preparation: Roots are used medi-cinally 2-3 ch'ien for each dose, prepared in decoction.

203. Lien-ch'ien Ts'ao [Ground-ivy]

Family: Labiatae

Scientific name: Glechoma hederaceae L.

Synonyms: "T'ou-ku hsiao," "szu-fang hsiao," "ju tsa-tzu ts'ao" "chin-ch'ien ts'ao" [golden-coin grass], "hu po-ho" [hairy mint], "ch'uan-ch'ang ts'ao" [wall-penetrating grass], "chieh-chieh sheng," "hsing-tzu ts'ao" [star-grass], "man-shan-hsiang [the whole-mountain-is-fragrant], "ma-chiao ts'ao" [horse-hoof grass], "man-t'ien hsing" [stars all over the sky], "hsi-ch'uan ts'ao," "ch'iang-tao ts'ao" [robber grass], "ch'uan-hua t'ung-ch'ien ts'ao," "p'ien-ti-hsiang."

Morphology: Perennial creeping herb. Stem oblong and slender, creeping on surface of ground mostly, fibrous roots growing from node wherever it touches the ground. Leaves opposite, reniform or rounded, apexes rounded and obtuse, bases cordate, margins broken by coarse blunt teeth, with long petioles. In spring and summer, light purplish-red flowers appear as axillary flowers. Nut small, almost globoid.

Properties and action: Slightly warm, acrid-tasting, clears fever and promotes diuresis, stimulates blood circulation and dissolves bruises, reduces inflammation and alleviates pain, and detoxifies.

Conditions most used for: (1) Influenza; (2) infantile marasmus; (3) stones in the urinary tract; (4) traumatic injuries, fractures, rheumatoid arthritis; (5) swollen abscesses, sores.

Preparation: The whole plant is used medicinally, 5 ch'ien - 1 liang each time, but 1-2 liang if used fresh, prepared in decoction. A suitable amount may be used for external application.

- 729 -

204. Lien-ch'iao [Weeping forsythia]

Family: Oleaceae

Scientific name: Forsythia suspensa Vahl.

Synonyms: "Lien-chiao tzu," "erh-ts'ao" [ear-grass]

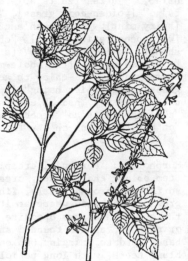

Morphology: Deciduous shrub, attaining height of 3 meters. Stem erect, branches spreading or drooping, smaller branches spindle-shaped, internodal spaces empty of pith, which is only present in the nodal parts. Leaves opposite, single-leafed or trifoliate, ovate-rounded to long ellipti-cal-ovate, apexes acute, margins serrated, bases broadly cuneate or rounded, with petioles. Flowers appearing from axils, gloden yellow. Capsule narrow-ovate, slightly flat.

Properties and action: Slightly "han" cold, bitter to taste. Clears fever and detoxifies, reduces swelling, promotes drainage and diuresis.

Conditions most used for: (1) Influenza, colds, measles, chicken-pox; (2) in-fantile paralysis; (3) lymphadenitis, erysipelas, boils and ulcers. It is also an important drug used for the control of stroke.

Preparation: The fruits are used medi-cinally, 1.5-3 ch'ien for each dose, prepared in decoction.

205. Yuan-hua

Family: Thymelaceae

Scientific name: Daphne genkwa S{. et Z.

Synonyms: "Ch'un chiang-tzu," "chiu-lung hua" [nine-dragon flower], "fou-chang ts'ao," "huang ta-chi" [yellow spurge], "su sang" [Szechuan mulberry], "ti mien-hua" [groundcover cotton], "ju tu" [fish poison], lao-c'hu hua" [mouse-flower], "ch'u-shui t'ou-t'ung hua," "wen-t'ou hua," "erh ts'ao," "pi-hua," "ching-kuang shu" [all-clean tree], "fan-t'eng shu" [turnover vine-tree], "ni-ch'iu shu," "pan-pao shu," "yang hua-wei," "chen t'ien-tai," "ta-pu-szu" [cannot beat to death], "ta-chiu-chia" [great life saver], "chin yao tai" [golden belt], "tzu ching-hua," "shou-shan hu."

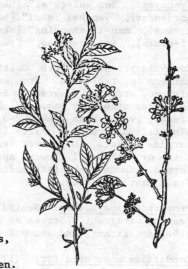

Morphology: Deciduous shrub. Found growing wild along field edges, hillsides, and valleys. Stem erect, multi-branching, bark quite fibrous, not easily broken. Leaves opposite, a few alternate, oval to long oval-rounded, apexes acuminate, bases cuneate, margins intact. Blooms in spring, flowers appearing before leaves, light purple. Fruit a drupe, white when ripe.

Properties and action: Warm, acrid-tasting, toxic. As a purgative and diuretic, it also helps resolve bruises and clots.

Conditions most used for: (1) Ascites, edema; (2) traumatic injuries.

Preparation: Flowers and roots are used medicinally, 0.5-1 ch'ien each time, prepared in decoction. Should be avoided by the pregnant woman.

206. Yuan-sui (Hu-sui) [Coriander]

Family: Umbelliferae

Scientific name: Coriandrum sativum L.

Synonyms: "Yen sui-ts'ai" [banquet coriander], "yen-hsi ts'ai" [banquet greens], "man-t'ien hsing" [sky-full-of-stars], "yen ko-ts'ao," "yuan-hsin."

Morphology: Annual herb. Cultivated in gardens for table use. Stem erect, striped, strongly fragrant. Basal leaves 1-2 times pinnately compound, lobes broadly ovate; stem leaves 2-3 times pinnately compound, leaflets linear, margins intact. In summer, terminal white or pink small flowers appear to form a compound umbellate inflorescence. Fruit nearly globose.

Properties and action: Neutral, acrid-tasting, fragrant. Serves as a carmina-tive, detoxicant, and stomach tonic.

Conditions most used for: (1) Measles; (2) stomach-ache, nausea; (3) painful hernia.

Preparation: The whole plant is used medicinally, 5 ch'ien-1 liang each time, in decoction; or the decoction may be used externally to bathe affected parts.

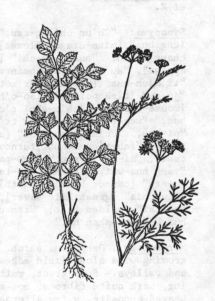

207. Lu [Reed]

Family: Graminea

Scientific name: Phragmites communis
Trin.

Synonyms: "Lu-ken," "wei-ken" [roots
of bulrushes], "lu-chu ken," "lu mao-
ken" [hairy roots of reed].

Morphology: Large perennial herb. Found
growing along river banks, stream banks,
lake beaches and other wet areas. Subterranean stem creeping horizontally, thick,
hollow between nodes. Stem erect, cylindrical, smooth and hollow inside. Leaves alternate, in two rows, ochrea clasping stem;
leaves linear-lanceolate, length 30-50 cm.
Blooms in the fall, terminal brownish-
purple or dull purple flowers appearing
to form a panicle inflorescence. Fruit
a capsule.

Properties and action: Cold-natured, but
pleasant to taste. Clears fevers and detoxifies, promotes salivation to stop
thirst, found to promote diuresis.

Conditions most used for: (1) Thirst in
fevers, nausea and vomiting; (2) hematuria
and burning urination.

Preparation: Roots are used medicinally,
1-2 liang each time, prepared in decoction.

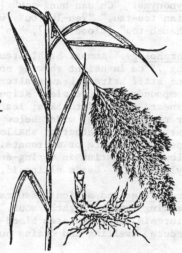

208. Ch'ih Hsiao-tou [Kidney bean species]

Family: Leguminosae

Scientific name: Phaseolus angularis Wight.

Synonyms: "Ch'uan hung-tou" [scarlet bean],
"fan tou-tzu," "yeh-lu-tou" [wild mung bean],
"hsueh-tou" [blood bean], "ts'ai-tou."

Morphology: Annual herb, stem erect, attaining 75 cm in height showing noticeable long
and stiff hairs. Leaves alternate, trifoliate
compound; long petioles, stipules slightly
linear, attached to base; leaflets ovate
or rhombic-ovate, wider below the central
part, margins intact or shallowly 3-lobed,
apexes acuminate or mucronate. Yellow
flowers appearing in spring-summer. Legume
cylindrical. Seeds ellipsoid, scarlet.

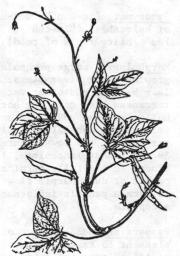

Properties and action: Neutral, pleasant
tasting though slightly sour. Promotes
diuresis and stimulates blood circulation,
reduces swelling and drains pus.

Conditions most used for: (1) Edematous
beri-beri; (2) dysentery; (3) sores and
abscesses.

Preparation: Seeds are used medicinally,
3-5 ch'ien each time, prepared in decoction.

209. Hsin-I

Family: Magnoliaceae

Scientific name: Magnolia liliflora
Desr.

Synonyms: "Mu-lan" [magnolia], "tzu
yu-lan," "mu-pi" [wood brush], "mu lien-
hua" [woody lotus], "ying-ch'un hua"
[spring-welcoming flower], "pai-hua-
shu hua."

Morphology: Large-sized deciduous shrub.
Height 1-3 meters. Trunk bark grayish-
white, bark of small branches frequently
a dark dull purple, lenticels noticeable.
Leaves alternate, broadly obovate, apexes
acute, bases cuneate, margins intact, leaf
margins and veins covered by fine pubescent
down, petioles short. Purple flowers appearing in summer, bell-shaped. Fruit a
follicle, broad-oblong-rounded, light
brown.

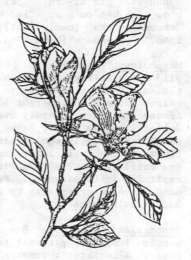

Properties and action: Warm-natured,
acrid tasting. Dispels wind-heat [fever],
alleviates pain by controlling or [dampen-
ing] the wind.

Conditions most used for: (1) Headache,
running nose.

Preparation: The buds are used medicinally,
8 fen - 1.5 ch'ien, prepared in decoction
each time. For external use, a suitable
amount may be crushed for use as plugs for
nose.

210. Ts'ang-erh [Burweed]

Family: Compositae

Scientific name: Xanthium strumarium L.

Synonyms: "Ts'ai-erh," "pai-chih-t'ou p'o," "chih-t'ou p'o," "lao ts'ang-tzu," "chuan-mao tzu" [curly fuzz], shih ma-t'ou," "pai-hua shih-mu-t'ou."

Morphology: Annual herb. Found growing wild along village outskirts and waste places. Whole plant covered by short white hairs. Stem erect, height 30–90 cm. Leaves alternate, broadly ovate or ovate-deltate, apexes acute, bases cordate, margins showing irregular serrations. Blooms in the fall, light green terminal and axillary flowers appearing to form capitulum inflorescences. Fruit ellipsoid, covered externally by small stiff and prickly hairs.

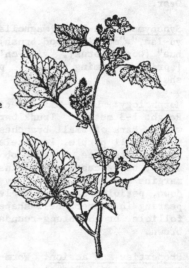

Properties and action: Has a slightly warming property, pleasant to taste, toxic. Alleviates rheumatism, stops pain, and relieves constipation.

Conditions most used for: (1) Colds, sinusitis; (2) leprosy; (3) rheumatism; (4) [skin] pruritus.

Preparation: Fruits or the whole plant is used medicinally, 5 ch'ien-1 liang of the plant, or 2–3 ch'ien of the seeds, prepared in decoction. For external use a suitable amount may be steeped, and the solution used for bathing the affected parts.

211. Yuan-chih [Polygala species]

Family: Polygalaceae

Scientific name: Polygala tenuifolia
Willd.

Synonyms: "Hsi-hsieh yan-chih" [small-
leaf polygala].

Morphology: Perennial herb. Found growing wild along hillsides, roadsides, and
meadows. Root thick and fleshy, cylindrical. Culms clustered, height about 20-40
cm, base slightly woody. Leaves alternate,
linear or linear-lanceolate, apexes acuminate, bases cuneate, margins intact.
Blooms in the summer, purple axillary or
terminal flowers appearing to form race-
most inflorescences. Capsule flat, margins
winged.

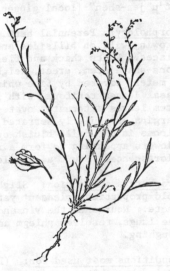

Properties and action: Has warming
properties, acrid yet pleasant to taste.
Calms nerves, resolves phlegm and reduces swelling [of abscesses].

Conditions most used for: (1) Apprehension and forgetfulness, insomnia and
tendency for dreaming; (2) "cold" sputum
cough, moisture-related abscesses and
sores.

Preparation: Roots are used medicinally,
2-3 ch'ien each time, prepared in decoction.

212. Sha-Shen (Hsing-hsieh sha-shen) [Adenophora species]

Family: Campanulaceae

Scientific name: Adenophora stricta Miq.

Synonyms: "Yu ya-shen," "pao ya-shen,"
"t'u jen-shen" [local ginseng].

Morphology: Perennial herb. Found
growing wild on hillsides and hilly
places. Roots thick and fleshy, a long
cone-shape stem, erect, height attaining
1 meter, covered by fine white hairs.
Basal leaves reniform, with long petioles;
stem leaves alternate, ovate-rounded,
margins irregularly serrated, no petioles.
Blooms in the fall, bluish-purple axillary
flowers appearing to form a racemose inflorescence. Fruit a capsule.

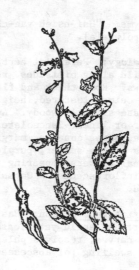

Properties and action: Slightly "han"
cold properties, pleasant yet bitter to
taste. Nourishes the yin and purifies
the lungs, resolves phlegm and stops
coughing.

Conditions most used for: (1) Tuberculosis, bronchitis, whooping cough; (2)
vomiting and coughing up of blood.

Preparation: Roots are used medicinally,
3-5 ch'ien each time, prepared in decoction.

213. Chien [Euryale species]

Family: Nymphaeaceae

Scientific name: Euryale ferox Salisb.

Synonyms: "Chien-shih," "chi-t'ou lien"
[chicken-head water-lily], "La ho-hsieh"
[prickly water-lily leaf], "t'ien-ch'ing
ti-hung" [sky-blue earth-red], "shui-
liang hsieh."

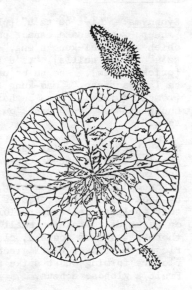

Morphology: Annual aquatic herb, covered
completely by thorns. Subterranean stem
short and thick, with many white fibrous
roots. Leaves rounded or peltate-cordate,
floating on the water's surface; margins
folded upwards to form a disc, leaf surface
green, underside purple. Blooms in summer-
fall, purplish-red flowers opening at noon,
and fading by dusk. Fruit a sponge-like
berry, shaped like the head of a chicken.
Seeds the size of a lima bean.

Properties and action: Neutral, pleasant
yet acrid to taste. Fortifies the spleen
and strengthens the kidneys, stops diarrhea
and seminal emission.

Conditions most used for: (1) Diarrhea,
incontinence of urine; (2) seminal emission,
leukorrhea; (3) joint pains in lower extremities and backache; (4) thirst, chronic
fever (use stems); (5) hernia (use roots);
(6) non-expulsion of placenta (use leaves).

Preparation: Seeds 2-4 ch'ien are mostly
used in decoction; roots and stems 3-6
ch'ien, or leaves 5 ch'ien - 1 liang, are
also used in decoction.

214. Kung-pan-kuei (Kuan-hsieh liao) [Tearthumb]

Family: Polygonaceae

Scientific name: Polygonum perfoliatum L.

Synonyms: "Li-t'ou tz'u" [plow thorn],
"she-pu-kuo" [snake cannot pass], "chi-
chieh-so," "lei-kung t'eng," "lao-hu
tz'u" [tiger quills], "tz'u li-t'ou"
[prickly plow], "she pu ch'uan," "pai
ta lao-ya hsuan," "mao-kung tz'u"
[tomcat quills], "niao pu hsi," "pu-
chung ts'ao," "yueh pan-k'ou," mao-tzu
ts'u."

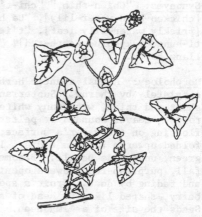

Morphology: Perennial herb. Found
growing wild in out-of-the-way places
and in shrub thickets. Stem climbing
or creeping, multi-branching, covered
by hook-like thorns. Leaves alternate,
soft, peltate-deltate, petioles and ribs
on backside containing small hook-like
thorns, stipules rounded, clasping stem.
Blooms in summer, small greenish-white
flowers forming short spike inflorescences.
Fruit a globose achene.

Properties and action: Neutral, sour and
slightly acrid to taste. Clears fever
and detoxifies, promotes diuresis and
stimulates blood circulation.

Conditions most used for: (1) Dysenteries,
enteritis; (2) boils and abscesses, poisonous snakebites; (3) hematuria, cloudy
urine; (4) traumatic injuries.

Preparation: The whole plant is used
medicinally, 5 ch'ien - 1 liang each
time, prepared in decoction.

- 740 -

215. Mu-ching [Vitex species]

Family: Verbenaceae

Scientific name: Vitex cannabifolia Sieb. et Zucc.

Synonyms: "Huang-ching" [yellow vitex], "hsiao-ching," "nai-chu" [milk ulcer], "ch'ang-shan," "yeh niu-hsi" [wild ox-knee] "t'u ch'ang-shan" [local clerodendron species], "ch'i-hsieh huang-ching."

Morphology: Deciduous shrub. Found growing on hilly slopes or roadsides. Stem oblong, multi-branching. Leaves opposite, palmate-compound, usually 5 leaflets, leaflets oval, apexes long-acute, bases cuneate, margins serrated. Blooms in summer, terminal light purplish flowers appearing to form panicle inflorescences. Drupe globose, brown.

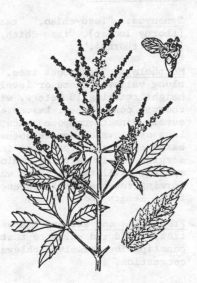

Properties and action: Has warming properties, slightly bitter and acrid to taste. Promotes perspiration, clears fever, eliminates moisture, and resolves phlegm.

Conditions most used for: (1) Dysenteries, enteritis; (2) malaria, heat stroke; (3) arthralgia.

Preparation: Roots, leaves and fruits are used medicinally, 5 ch'ien-1 liang each time in decoction.

216. Tsao-hsia [Chinese locust]

Family: Leguminosae

Scientific name: Gleditsia sinensis Lam.

Synonyms: "Tsao-chiao," "tsao-chiao tz'u"
[thorny locust], "tsao-chieh," "tsao-tz'u"
[soapy thorns].'

Morphology: Deciduous tree. Found growing
along valley streams or level land. Stem
height reaching 15 meters, with thick
thorns, cone-shaped. Leaves alternate,
evenly pinnate compound once, leaflets
long oval-ovate, apexes obtuse or sharp,
bases cuneate, often-times inclined,
margins finely serrated. Blooms in
spring, axillary yellowish white flowers
forming racemose inflorescences. Legumes
flat, length about 30 cm.

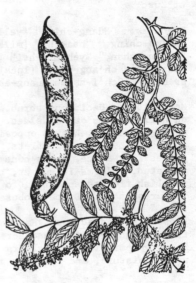

Properties and action: Has warming properties, acrid and salty to taste. Relieves
constipation, resolves phlegm, and loosens
congestion.

Conditions most used for: (1) Stroke and
lockjaw; (2) acute numbness of the throat;
(3) epilepsy.

Preparation: Legumes or thorns from stem
are used medicinally, 1-3 ch'ien each time,
in decoction; or a suitable amount may be
crushed and used for blowing into the
nostrils.

217. Ho-shou-wu [Polygonum species]

Family: Polygonaceae

Scientific name: Polygonum multiflorum
Thunb.

Synonyms: "Wai hung-t'eng" [outside-
scarlet-vine], "hsieh tou-tou," "Ho hsiang-
kung [Minister Ho], "ma-kan shih," "chi-shih
t'eng" [chicken-droppings vine], "ch'en-t'o
hsiao," "shen-t'ou ts'ao," "tieh ch'en-t'o"
[iron scale-weight], "li-erhts'ai," "t'u
tou-chi."

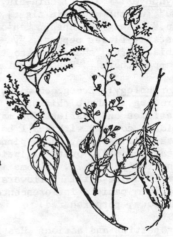

Morphology: A perennial deciduous vine.
Found growing along stream banks and in
valley shrub thickets. Has fibrous roots
and large fat root tubers that sometimes
connect together in one lump, surface purplish
black, yellowish white on the inside. Stem
climbing, suspended in mid-air. Single
leaves alternate, with long petioles,
leaves narrow ovate or cordate, margins intact. Blooms in the fall, axillary or
terminal small white flowers appearing to
form panicle inflorescences. Achene
ellipsoid.

Properties and action: Has warming properties, bitter and acrid yet pleasant to taste.
Roots and leaves tonify the liver and kidneys,
fortify the blood, strengthen muscles and
bone and keep the hair black; stems [night-
crossover vine] calm nerves, and keep "lo"
passageways open.

Conditions most used for: (1) Rickets, anemia and premature graying [of hair],
backache and pains and aches of the knee joint; (2) neurasthenia; (3) lymphadenitis, traumatic bruises.

Preparation: Root tubers, stems, and leaves are used medicinally, 3-5 ch'ien
each time, in decoction. A suitable amount may be used externally.

218. Liang-mien Chen [Two-sided needle]

Family: Rutaceae

Scientific name: Zanthoxylum nitidum (Lam) DC.

Synonyms: "Jih-ti chin-niu," "shang-shan hu" [up-the-mountain tiger], "hsia-shan-hu," "liang-pei chen," "ch'ou-hua chiao" [stinky-flower pepper], "yu-chiao," "hua-chiao tz'u" "shan-hu-chiao tz'u" [mountain pepper-thorn], "Yeh hua-chiao."

Morphology: Evergreen woody vine. Found growing in shrub thickets. Young branches, petioles and leaflets (on main rib, both sides) covered with small hook-like thorns. Leaves alternate, oddly pinnate compound, leaflets 5-11, ovate-elliptical, margins shallowly toothed. Blooms in summer, small white axillary flowers appearing to form panicle inflorescences. Capsule globose, purplish red.

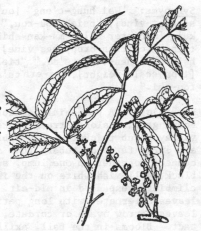

Properties and action: Has slightly warm-ing properties, acrid and bitter to taste, slightly toxic. Eliminates flatus and de-toxifies, reduces inflammation and alleviates pain.

Conditions most used for: (1) Stomach-ache; (2) rheumatoid arthralgia, back-strain, and bruises; (3) tetanus, burns, poisonous snakebites.

Preparation: Roots are used medicinally, 2-3 ch'ien each time, in decoction (avoid taking the same time that acid food stuffs are eaten).

219. Wu Chu-yu [Evodia species]

<u>Family</u>: Rutaceae

<u>Scientific name</u>: Evodia rutaecarpa.

<u>Synonyms</u>: "Wu-yu," "ch'ou la-tzu shu"
[stinky pepperweed], "ch'a-la," "ch-ang
chu-yu," "ch'u yao-tzu" [crooked herb],
"ch'i la-tzu," "ch'ou pao-tzu."

<u>Morphology</u>: Small deciduous tree.
Found growing wild or cultivated on uplands. Height as much as 8 meters, young
branches purplish brown. Leaves opposite,
oddly pinnate compound, leaflets 5-9,
oval-ovate, apexes acute, bases cuneate,
margins intact. Blooms in summer, small
yellowish white terminal flowers appearing to form cymose inflorescences. Capsule
flat and globose, purplish red when ripe.
Seeds black.

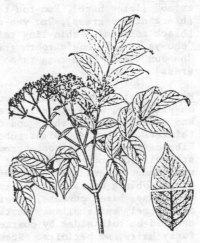

<u>Properties and action</u>: Has warming proper-
ties, acrid and bitter to taste. Warms
the central organs and dispels chilling
influences, corrects energy and loosens
any congestion.

<u>Conditions most used for</u>: (1) Gastroenteritis,
abdominal pain; (2) post-partum hot pains;
(3) beri beri edema.

<u>Preparation</u>: Fruits are used medicinally,
1-2 ch'ien each time, in decoction.

220. Han-lien Ts'ao [Eclipta species]

Family: Compositae

Scientific name: Eclipta prostrata L.

Synonyms: "Shui han-lien," "lien-tzu ts'ao" [lotus herb], "mo-tou ts'ao" [black dipper grass], "mo yen-ts'ao" [black tobacco], "chin-ling ts'ao," "chu-ya ts'ao" [hog's tooth grass], "hu-sun t'ou," "pin-tung ts'ao" [ice grass].

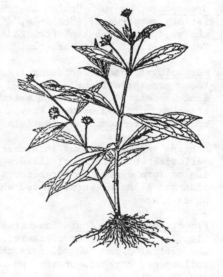

Morphology: Annual herb. Found growing on hillsides, wild places, stream edges, and roadsides among shady and damp grass thickets. The whole plant pubescent. Fibrous adventitious roots growing from stoloniferous nodes, stem soft and fine, with numerous branches. Leaves opposite, linear-oblong or lanceolate, apexes acute or obtuse, bases cuneate, margins intact or sparsely and shallowly dentate, leaves covered on both sides by coarse white fuzzy hairs, no petioles. Stem leaves when broken ooze white milky fluid that turns black. Blooms in summer, small white axillary or terminal flowers appearing to form capitulum inflorescences. Achene ellipsoid and flat.

Properties and action: Neutral, sour yet pleasant to taste. Tonifies the lungs, strengthens the kidneys, clears fever and detoxifies, cools the blood and stops bleeding.

Conditions most used for: (1) Pulmonary tuberculosis; (2) hepatitis, gastroenteritis, conjunctivitis, cystitis, urinary tract inflammation, boils and abscesses, poisonous snakebites; (3) hemoptysis, hematemesis, bloody stools, hematuria, expistaxis and traumatic bleeding.

Preparation: The whole plant is used medicinally, 5 ch'ien-2 liang each time in decoction; fresh plant can also be crushed for external application.

221. Chu-ma [False Nettle]

Family: Urticaceae

Scientific name: Boehmeria nivea (L.)
Gaud.

Synonyms: "Ch'ing-ma" [blue nettle],
"pai-ma" [white nettle], "yeh-ma" [wild
nettle].

Morphology: Perennial herb. Mostly
cultivated. Single stem, cylindrical.
Leaves alternate, broadly ovate or
ovate-rounded, margins coarsely serrated,
leaf surfaces coarse, underside densely
covered by white hairs. Blooms in the
fall, axillary yellowish white flowers
appearing to form panicle inflorescences.
Achene ellipsoid.

Properties and action: Has chilling
properties, bitter yet pleasant to
taste. Clears fevers, stops bleeding,
promotes pus drainage, and quiets a
restless fetus.

Conditions most used for: (1) Hematuria,
emaciation; (2) bleeding from wound injuries; (3) abdominal pain due to abnormal
fetal activity, leukorrhea.

Preparation: Roots, stems and leaves are
used medicinally, roots 1 liang, or stem
and leaves 5 ch'ien, each time prepared
as decoction. For external application
a suitable amount may be crushed.

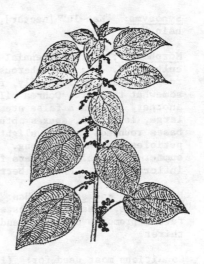

222. Pa-chiao [Banana]

Family: Musaceae

Scientific name: Musa basjoo Sieb. et Zucc.

Synonyms: "Kan-lu" [nectar], "pa-chiao hsin."

Morphology: Large perennial herb. Mostly cultivated. Rhizome tuberous, fat, side roots running horizontally, fibrous roots somewhat thicker. Ochrea pile up on one another, to form a false stem. Leaves large, long oval, apexes obtusely pointed, bases rounded, margins slightly undulate, petioles coarse and strong. Blooms in summer-fall, yellow flowers forming spike inflorescences. Fruit a berry, 3-angled.

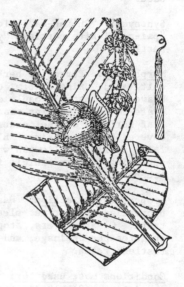

Properties and action: Has "han" cold properties, pleasant to taste. Resolves fever, promotes diuresis, and alleviates thirst.

Conditions most used for: (1) Beri beri, constipation; (2) jaundice, restlessness [due to heat]; (3) leukorrhea; (4) croton bean poisoning.

Preparation: Roots are used medicinally, 1-2 liang each time, in decoction.

223. Hua Chiao [Prickly ash species]

Family: Rutaceae

Scientific name: Zanthoxylum bungeanum Max.

Synonyms: "Chin-chiao."

Morphology: Large shrub or small tree. Height 3-7 meters. Stem-trunk usually showing enlarged thorns, base of thorns slightly flat. Leaves alternate, oddly pinnate compound, the main petiole and undersides of leaflets frequently sites of small upward-growing thorns; leaflets ovate or ovate elongated, margins coarsely serrated, with large transparent points found between serrations, the terminal leaflet being larger. Blooms in summer, yellowish green flowers forming corymb or panicle inflorescences. Capsule globose, red to purplish red. Seeds black and lustrous.

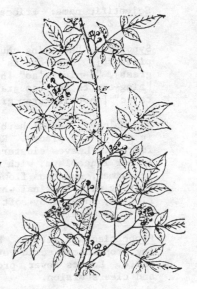

Properties and action: Has warming properties, acrid tasting and toxic. Warms the central organs and dispels chill-cold, counteracts moisture and acts as a vermicide against parasites.

Conditions most used for: (1) Chills and pains in the abdomen, vomiting, cold-damp diarrhea and dysentery; (2) ascariasis caused abdominal pain; (3) moist sores on the skin.

Preparation: The capsule peels or seeds are used medicinally, 0.8-1.5 ch'ien each time, pulverized, then mixed with water before taking by mouth.

224. Ku-ching Ts'ao [Pipewort species]

Family: Eriocaulaceae

Scientific name: Eriocaulon sieboldianum
S. et Z.

Synonyms: "Ku-ching chu" [pearl-of-pipewort], "chen-chu ts'ao [pearly
grass], "I-niu ts'ao" [button-grass],
"ting-tzu ts'ao [top grass], "liu-hsing
ts'ao" [shooting-star grass].

Morphology: Annual herb. Found growing
in damp shady places. Roots white and
fibrous. Leaves clustered, numerous
linear lanceolate, with many basal veins.
In summer, numerous flower pedicels appearing with terminal white globoid ovate
flowers, covered by soft white hairs.
Fruit a capsule.

Properties and action: Has slightly warming properties, acrid yet pleasant to
taste. Lowers fever, promotes diuresis,
and clears vision.

Preparation: Whole plant is used medicinally, 1-2 liang each time, in decoction.

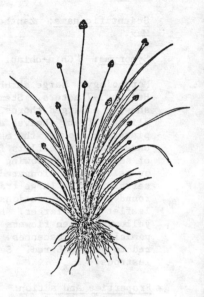

225. Shan [Fir]

Properties and action: Has warming properties, acrid to taste. Analgesic
and hemostatic.

Conditions most used for: Hernia pain, toothache, bleeding sores, burns,
and cholera-associated cramps.

Preparation: Roots are used medicinally, 1-2 liang each time prepared
as decoction.

226. Ho-tzu [Terminalia chebula Retz.]

Properties and action: Has warming properties, bitter, sour and peppery
to taste. Roughens [stimulates] intestines, strengthens lungs, and lowers
[excessive] energy [output].

Conditions most used for: Chronic cough and hoarseness [loss of voice],
chronic diarrhea and dysentery, prolapse of rectum, intestinal flatus and
bloody stools, metrorrhagia and leukorrhea, seminal emission and excessive
prespiration.

Preparation: For each dose 0.8-1.5 ch'ien, prepared as decoction.

227. Ch'ih-shao [water chestnut] (Heleocharis plantaginea R. Br.)

Properties and action: Has slightly cooling properties, sour and bitter to
taste. Purges liver fire, and resolves bruises and clots.

Conditions most used for: Pain in abdomen and haunches, malnutrition [due
to worms?], anemia, hernia and gassy stomach, inflamed swellings, pink [red]
eye, amenorrhea.

Preparation: For each dose, 1.5-3 ch'ien, prepared in decoction.

228. Su-mu [Logwood]

Properties and action: Neutral, pleasant yet salty to taste. Stimulates blood circulation and resolves clots, alleviates pain and relieves swelling.

Conditions most used for: Postpartum clots, amenorrhea and abdominal pain, painful swelling and traumatic injuries.

Preparation: For each dose, 1.5-3 ch'ien, prepared in decoction. For external use, crush and apply.

229. Hsing-jen [Almond]

Properties and action: Has warming properties, acrid yet pleasant to taste. Resolves phlegm and quiets cough, lowers [excessive] energy, and lubricates the intestines.

Conditions most used for: Colds and coughing, unproductive coughing, dyspnea and asthma, constipation.

Preparation: For each dose, 1.5-3 ch'ien, prepared in decoction.

230. Chi-nei-chin [Gold-in-Chicken]

Properties and action: Neutral, pleasant to taste. Stomach tonic to aid digestion.

Conditions most used for: Overeating, vomiting, diarrhea, marasmus in children

Preparation: For each dose, 1-3 ch'ien, prepared in decoction.

231. Ch'en P'i [Dried tangerine/orange peel]

Properties and action: Has warming properties, bitter and acrid to taste. Corrects energy circulation, strengthens the spleen, counteracts moisture [excessive, in body], and resolves phlegm.

Conditions most used for: Fullness in chest and abdomen, regurgitation and vomiting, chest and abdominal pains, poor appetite, productive coughing, indigestion, and diarrhea.

Preparation: For each dose, 1-3 ch'ien, prepared in decoction.

232. Ts'ang-shu [Atractylis ovata]

Properties and action: Has warming properties, pleasant yet acrid to taste. Tonifies the spleen, counteracts [excessive] moisture, removes gas and discharge.

Conditions most used for: Chills, rheumatism, diarrhea, edema, fullness in chest and abdomen, weakness of legs.

Preparation: For each dose, 1.5 - 3 ch'ien, prepared in decoction.

233. Tu-chung [Eucommia ulmoides, Oliv.]

Properties and action: Has warming properties, pleasant to taste. Tonifies liver and kidneys and strengthens muscles and bones.

Conditions most used for: Lumbago, knee-joint pain, weakness of muscles and lower extremities, back strain [due to added strain of pregnancy], and abortion resulting from overactive fetus.

Preparation: For each dose, 3-5 ch'ien prepared in decoction.

234. Ku-ya [Rice-grain sprouts]

Properties and action: Has warming properties, pleasant to taste. Nourishes the stomach, strengthens the spleen, balances the central organs and aids digestion.

Conditions most used for: Weak stomach and spleen, poor appetite, indigestion, and fullness in chest and abdomen.

Preparation: For each dose, 3-5 ch'ien, prepared in decoction.

235. Mai-ya [Malt]

Properties and action: Has slightly cooling properties, salty and pleasant to taste. Aids digestion, balances the central organs and controls lactation.

Conditions most used for: Indigestion, fullness in chest and abdomen. Poor appetites and fullness of lactating breasts.

Preparation: For each dose, 3-5 ch'ien, prepared in decoction.

236. Kuei-pan [Tortoise shell]

Properties and action: Neutral, pleasant to taste. Nourishes the yin and moderates the yang.

Conditions most used for: Inadequate kidney yin function, fatigue, chronic cough, seminal emission, metrorrhagia, leukorrhea, pains and aches of back and legs, yin deficiency and flatus, chronic dysentery, malaria, hemorrhoids, and non-closure of fontanels in infants.

Preparation: For each dose, 3-5 ch'ien, prepared in decoction.

237. Ch'eng-hsiang [Aquilaria agallocha, Roxb.]

Properties and action: Has slightly warming properties, acrid tasting. Lowers energy [activity], reinforces the kidneys, regulates central organs, and alleviates pain.

Conditions most used for: Abdominal pain, tightness of chest, vomiting and regurgitation, diarrhea, asthma.

Preparation: For each dose, 0.3-1 ch'ien, prepared in decoction.

238. Ju-hsiang [Pistachio]

Properties and action: Has warming properties, bitter and acrid to taste. Stimulates circulation of blood, resolves bruises and clots, relieves pain.

Conditions most used for: Amenorrhea and dysmenorrhea, traumatic injuries and pain, sores, ulcers and abscesses, chest and abdominal pain, and rheumatism.

Preparation: For each dose, 0.8-2 ch'ien, prepared in decoction.

239. Mo-yao [Myrrh]

Properties and action: Neutral, bitter to taste. Reduces swelling and localizes pain.

Conditions most used for: Traumatic injuries and pain, carbuncles, abscesses and sores, pains in the chest and abdomen region, rheumatism, amenorrhea and dysmenorrhea.

Preparation: For each dose, 0.8-2 ch'ien, in decoction.

240. Chiang-t'i [Ginger sprouts]

Properties and action: Neutral, acrid to taste, unpleasant odor. Vermicidical, it also eliminates marasmus [as the result].

Conditions most used for: Marasmus and helminthiasis and related diarrhea/dysentery.

Preparation: For each dose, 1-2 ch'ien, in decoction.

241. Pu-ku-chih [Psorales corylifolia L.]

Properties and action: Has warming properties, acrid tasting. Tonifies the kidneys and promotes the yang.

Conditions most used for: Kidney deficiency and impotence, seminal emission and premature ejaculation, lumbago and pains in the knee joint, polyuria.

Preparation: For each dose, 1-3 ch'ien, in decoction.

242. Mu-li (Ostrea cucullata, Born.) [Oyster shell]

Properties and action: Has slightly chilling properties, salty and acrid to taste. Moderates the yang, and stabilizes [body chemistry?], clears fever and breaks up congestion.

Conditions most used for: Hypertension and dizziness, seminal emission, tuberculous cervical nodes, and hidrosis.

Preparation: For each dose, 0.3-1 liang, pulverized and prepared in decoction.

243. Tou-ch'ih [Salted black bean]

Properties and action: Has chilling properties, bitter to taste. Relaxes muscles, promotes perspiration, clears fever and eliminates apprehension.

Conditions most used for: Fever, headache, and restlessness connected with colds, chest discomfort, macula and measles.

Preparation: For each dose, 3-4 ch'ien, in decoction.

244. A-chiao [Special glue prepared from donkey hide cooked in spring water from Tung-a Hsien, Shantung Province]

Properties and action: Neutral, pleasant to taste. Blood tonic that is hemostatic, nourishes the yin and moisturizes the lungs.

Conditions most used for: Metrorrhagia, hemoptysis, yin-deficient anemia, fever-caused yin damage.

Preparation: For each dose, 1.5-3 ch'ien, dissolved in water and taken by mouth.

245. Hua-jui Shih [pulverized stone similar to sulfur]

Properties and action: Neutral, sour and biting to taste. Hemostatic.

Conditions most used for: Hematemesis, hemoptysis, metrorrhagia and subsequent anemia in women, bleeding from cuts.

Preparation: For each dose, 3-5 ch'ien, prepared in decoction. Use an appropriate amount for external purposes.

246. Tou-k'ou [Amomum costatum, Roxb.]

Properties and action: Has heating properties, acrid to taste. Stimulates energy circulation, warms the stomach, aids digestion, and neutralizes ill effects of alcohol.

Conditions most used for: Chills-associated abdominal pain, vomiting and regurgitation, abdominal distension, hiccups, indigestion, drunken stupor.

Preparation: For each dose, 0.5-2 ch'ien, in decoction.

247. Chin-ssu Ts'ao [Golden-thread grass]

Family: Graminea

Scientific name: Pogonatherum crinitum (Thunb.) Kunth.

Synonyms: "Huang-mao ts'ao" [yellow hairy grass], "mao-wei ts'ao" [cat's tail grass], "mao-mao ts'ao" [cat's-hair grass], "chu-kao ts'ao," "chin-ssu mao" [golden-thread feathergrass].

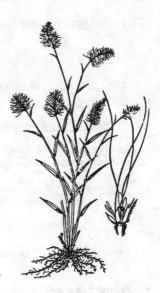

Morphology: Perennial herb. Found growing in rock crevices on slopes of foothills. Culms clustered, erect, height reaching 20 cm, nodes covered by white hairs. Leaves alternate, linear-lanceolate, margins of ochrea slightly pubescent. Blooms in the summer-fall flowers forming terminal spike inflorescences, spikes covered by dense tuft of yellowish brown awns, shaped like "cat's tail." Caryopsis small, long-ellipsoid.

Properties and action: Has cooling properties, light and pleasant to taste. Clears fevers, detoxifies, and promotes diuresis.

Conditions most used for: (1) Urinary tract infections; (2) influenza-caused fever; (3) jaundice, edema.

Preparation: The whole plant is used medicinally, 1-2 liang each time in decoction.

248. Chin-kuo Lan (Yuan-hsieh chin-kuo lan) [Tinospora species]

Family: Menispermaceae

Scientific name: Tinospora capillipes
Giagnep.

Synonyms: "Shan tzu-ku," "ti-tan" [earth
egg], "p'o shih-chu" [broken rock pearl],
"ch'ing niu-tan" [blue ox-gall], "p'o yen-
chu," "chiu niu-tan," "ti-tan."

Morphology: A perennial evergreen vine.
Found growing wild in shady and damp
places between rock crevices on hillsides.
Subterranean root tubers, ovate-rounded,
frequently joined, several together. Stem
climbing, encircling other objects. Leaves
alternate, long ovate, apexes acute, bases
cordate, margins intact. Blooms in spring-
summer, axillary small white flowers forming panicle inflorescences. Berry globose,
red.

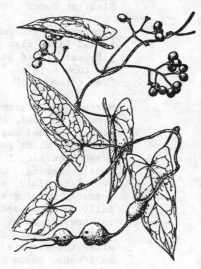

Properties action: Has cold-chill [han]
properties, bitter to taste. Clears fevers
and detoxifies, reduces inflammation and
alleviates pain.

Conditions most used for: (1) Laryngitis;
(2) boils and abscesses, dysentery; (3)
poisonous snakebites.

Preparation: Tuberous roots are used
medicinally, 2-3 ch'ien each time, in
decoction. A suitable amount may be used
for external purposes.

249. Chin Wa-erh [Golden ear scoop]

Family: Compositae

Scientific name: Carpesium divaricatum
Sieb. et Zucc.

Synonyms: "Yeh yen," "tieh chua-tzu
ts'ao" [iron claw-grass], "yeh hsiang-
jih-kuei" [wild sunflowers], "huang ku-
niu ta-cha ts'ao," "tieh-ku-hsiao,"
"fan t'ien yin," "mu yeh-yen ts'ao."

Morphology: Perennial herb. Found
growing in cool, shady and damp waste
places, roadsides, wilds, and hillsides.
The whole plant pubescent. Stem erect,
height reaching 1 meter, upper part
multibranching. Leaves alternate,
oval-lanceolate, apexes acute, bases
cuneate, margins intact. Blooms in the
fall, terminal and axillary capitulum
inflorescences of yellow flowers, the floral
receptacle assuming an ear-scoop shape
after the flowers have withered. Fruit
an achene, seeds sticky.

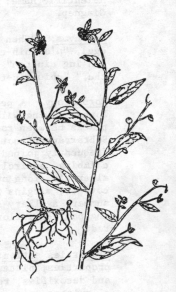

Properties and action: Has chilling
properties, bitter to taste. Clears
fevers and detoxifies, eliminates flatus
and also acts as a vermicide.

Conditions most used for: (1) Acute
enteritis, abdominal pains; (2) abscesses;
(3) poisonous snakebites; (4) arthralgia.

Preparation: Roots or the whole plant
may be used medicinally, 3-5 ch'ien each
time in decoction.

250. Chin-ts'ang Hsiao-ts'ao [Bugleweed species]

Family: Labiatae

Scientific name: Ajuga decumbens Thunb.

Synonyms: "Fu-ti chin-ku ts'ao" [creeping
sinew grass], "hsueh-li-k'ai-hua" [flowers-
blooming-in-the-snow], "ch'ing shih-t'eng
[blue rock vine], "peng hua," "I-chien teng"
[a lamp], "yeh-lu yu-hua," "t'ien-ch'ing
ti-hung," "hsieh-hsia hung" [red-under-the-
leaf], "pa-pa ts'ao" [creeping grass],
"ch'ing ju-tan" [blue fish bladder].

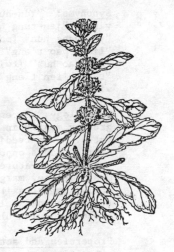

Morphology: Perennial herb. Found growing
in primitive wilds, hillsides, and roadsides. Whole plant pubescent. Basal
branches creeping. Leaves opposite,
obovate or long oval, apexes rounded-
obtuse or obtuse, bases narrowing
gradually, margins undulate-crenate,
tender leaves frequently purplish red on
underside. Blooms in spring-summer,
axillary white or light purple flowers,
in verticulate arrangement. Nut ovate,
black, small.

Properties and action: Has cooling
properties, pleasant to taste. Clears
fevers and detoxifies, promotes tissue
regeneration and stops bleeding.

Conditions most used for: (1) Boils and
abscesses, burn injuries, poisonous
snakebites; (2) traumatic bleeding,
epistaxis.

Preparation: The whole plant is used
medicinally. Usually a suitable amount
of the fresh plant is crushed for external application, or the juice is used
for rubbing onto affected parts. For internal consumption, 5 ch'ien - 1 liang
can also be used in decoction.

251. Chin-yen Hua (Jen-tung) [Honeysuckle]

Family: Caprifoliaceae

Scientific name: Lonicera japonica
Thunb.

Synonyms: "Yen-hua t'eng" [silver-flower
vine], "jen-tung hua," "jen-tung t'eng,"
"yen-yang hua" [mandarin duck flower],
"liang-pao t'eng" [double-precious vine],
"erh-pao hua" [twice-precious flower],
"tso-ch'ien t'eng" [left encircling
vine].

Morphology: Perennial woody vine. Found
growing mostly in wild places or cultivated. Stem reddish brown, softly pubescent. Leaves opposite, papery, ovate,
apexes short-acute, bases rounded or almost cordate, margins intact. Blooms in
early summer, axillary white flowers later
turning golden yellow, fragrant. Berry
globose, bluish black.

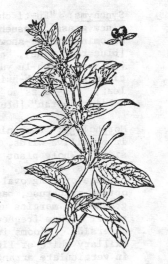

Properties and action: Has cooling
properties, pleasant yet bitter to taste.
Clears fevers and detoxifies.

Conditions most used for: (1) Colds,
laryngitis; (2) bacterial dysentery,
enteritis; (3) infected boils, skin
sores, and lymphadenitis; (4) rheumatism.

Preparation: Flowers and vine are used
medicinally, flowers 3-5 ch'ien each
time, or vines 1-2 liang each time,
prepared in decoction.

252. Chin-ch'ien Ts'ao [Golden coin tickclover]

Family: Leguminosae

Scientific name: Desmodium styracifolium
(Osbeck.) Merr.

Synonyms: "Chia hua-sheng" [false peanut],
"t'ung-ch'ien ts'ao" [copper-coin grass],
"lo-ti chin-ch'ien."

Morphology: Perennial herb. Found growing wild on hillsides and low-growing
thickets in waste places. The whole plant
covered by downy hairs. Stem branching
or decumbent. Leaves alternate, 3-compound,
the center leaf larger, rounded like a
golden coin, apex slightly retuse, base
cordate, margins intact. Blooms in
summer-fall, small purplish terminal and
axillary flowers, fragrant, forming racemose inflorescences. Legumes 4-5 noded,
covered by fine downy hairs.

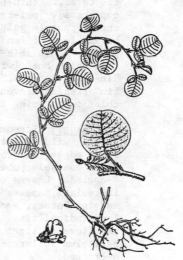

Properties and action: Has cooling
properties, pleasant and light to taste.
Clears fevers, promotes diuresis, relieves
gonorrhea.

Conditions most used for: (1) Stones in
the urinary system, gall-bladder stones;
(2) acute and chronic hepatitis.

Preparation: The whole plant is used
medicinally, 1-2 liang each time in
decoction.

253. Chin Chin-hsiang

Family: Melastomataceae

Scientific name: Osbeckia chinensis L.

Synonyms: "Chang-t'ien kuan," "hua-t'an ts'ao" [sputum-resolving grass], "kuan-tzu ts'ao," "chin-pei ts'ao" [golden-cup grass], "pei-tzu ts'ao," "tzu chin-chung" [purple golden-bell], "t'ien-hsiang lu," "t'ien hu-lu" [heaven's gourd], "chin shih-liu" [golden pomegranate], "liu-hsieh hua" [willow-leaf flower], "lu-liu-hsieh hua," "hsiang-t'ien shih-liu" [facing-heaven pomegranate], "chiu-chien teng" [nine lights].

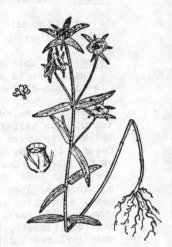

Morphology: Perennial herb. Found growing wild on hilly places, paddy field edges, and roadsides. The whole plant coarsely pubescent. Stem erect, 4-angled. Leaves opposite, linear lanceolate, apexes acuminate, bases obtuse, margins intact, each leaf containing 3 longitudinal ribs. Blooms in summer, terminal flowers, light purple or white, forming capitulum inflorescences. Fruit a capsule, 4-cracked.

Properties and action: Neutral, light in taste. Clears fevers and promotes adequate hydration, relieves coughing and resolves phlegm.

Conditions most used for: (1) Watery diarrhea and dysentery; (2) excessive sputum production in coughing.

Preparation: The whole plant is used medicinally, 1-2 liang each time, in decoction.

254. Chin Ying-tzu [Rosa species]

Family: Rosaceae

Scientific name: Rosa laevigata Michx.

Synonyms: "Chi-liang tz'u." [chicken-
feed thorns], "tz'u li-tzu" [prickly
pear], "shan shih-liu" [mountain
pomegranate], "pai yu-tai," "teng-lung
kuo" [lantern fruit], "chi-pa t'ui,"
"chi-t'o ya," "tz'u t'eng-la" [prickly
vine], "tz'u lang-tzu shu," "t'ang
tz'u-kuo" [sweet prickly fruit], "tz'u
kuo-kuo" [prickly fruit], "t'ang-lang-
tzu shu," "t'ang kuan-tzu," "ting-lang."

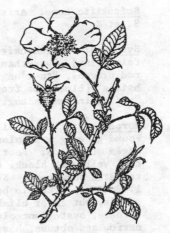

Morphology: Climbing shrub. Found
growing mostly in shrub thickets in wild
places. Stem and branches reddish brown,
very thorny. Leaves 3-pinnate compound,
alternate, central leaflet larger than
2 lateral leaflets, ovate-oval, apexes
acuminate, bases broadly cuneate, margins
finely serrate, central ribs on back of
leaves thorny. Blooms in summer, single
white flowers appearing terminally from
new growth, large and fragrant. Fruit shaped
like flower vase, with prickly hairs,
sweet and edible.

Properties and action: Neutral, slightly
pleasant yet acrid to taste. Detoxifies,
stabilizes the kidneys, and aids menstrual
regularity.

Conditions most used for: (1) Chronic
dysentery, urinary tract infections; (2)
wet dreams, prolapse of uterus; (3) menstrual irregularities, traumatic injuries.

Preparation: Roots, fruits, and leaves are
used medicinally, roots or fruits 5 ch'ien
- 1 liang each time in decoction. Fresh
leaves may be crushed for external use.

255. Ch'ing Mu-hsiang (Ma-tou-ling) [Birthwort species]

Family: Aristolochiaceae

Scientific name: Aristolochia debilis
S. et Z.

Synonyms: "T'ien-hsien t'eng" [heavenly
fairy vine], "wan-chang lung" [thousand-
rod dragon], "tu-t'ung p'a," "ch'ing-t'eng
hsiang" [blue vine fragrance], "sha yao,"
"pai ch'ing-mu-hsiang."

Morphology: Perennial vine-like herb.
Found growing wild along roadsides and
edges of fields. Root irregularly cylindrical, yellowish black, emitting a characteristic fragrance. Stem length reaching
1.5 meters, erect in beginning, a dull
purple, but later climbing. Leaves alternate, ovate-lanceolate or ovate, apexes
narrow and obtuse, bases cordate, both
sides forming drooping-ear shapes, margins
intact, with long petioles. Blooms in
summer, single axillary flowers a purplish
green, resembling trumpets. Capsule globose
or oval.

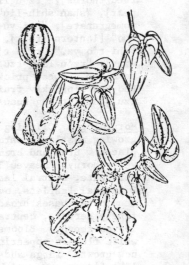

Properties and action: Has warming properties, acrid and bitter to taste. Dispels
flatus, stimulates energy circulation, tonifies the stomach, and relieves coughing.

Conditions most used for: (1) Vomiting,
abdominal pains; (2) coughing, wheezing;
(3) sore throat; (4) poisonous snakebites.

Preparation: Roots, stems, and fruit are
used medicinally, 3-5 ch'ien each time in
decoction.

256. Ch'ing Chu [Pepper Species]

Family: Piperaceae

Scientific name: Piper betle L.

Synonyms: "Chu hsieh," "chu-ch'ing," "wei-hsieh" [withering leaf], "pin-lang chu."

Morphology: Evergreen climbing vine. Mostly cultivated. Stem containing noticeably large nodes which send out roots. Leaves alternate, ovate, apexes acute, bases cordate, margins intact, each leaf containing 7 basal veins, emitting fragrance when crushed, petioled. Flowers unisexual, spike inflorescence axillary. Fruit ovate.

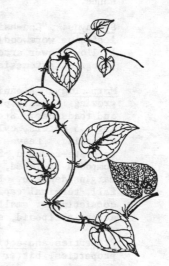

Properties and action: Has warming properties, acrid and slightly pleasant to taste. Dispels flatus, stops coughing, reduces inflammation and alleviates itching.

Conditions most used for: (1) Coughing; (2) rheumatic pains; (3) edema in pregnancy and moist sores.

Preparation: Leaves and stems are used medicinally, 5 ch'ien-1 liang each time in decoction; or a suitable amount of fresh leaves may be crushed for external application.

257. Ch'ing Kao [Blue Wormwood]

Family: Compositae

Scientific name: Artemesia apiaceae
Hance.

Synonyms: "Chu-hsieh ch'ing kao" [daisy-
leaf blue wormwood], "huang-kua kao"
[yellow-flower artemesia], "hsiang kao"
[fragrant artemesia].

Morphology: Biennial herb. Found
growing in waste places, field edges
and roadsides. Stem erect, height reaching 1.5 meters, cylindrical, multi-
branching. Leaves alternate, ovate
to ovate-rounded, 3 times pinnately
compound or lobed, small lobes linear,
margins dentate. Blooms in summer-
fall, terminal capitulum inflorescence
consisting of small light yellow flowers.
Achene ellipsoid, smooth.

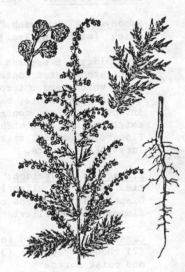

Properties and action: Has "han" cold
properties, bitter to taste, fragrant.
Clears fevers, detoxifies, exerts
vermicidal action, prevents malaria,
tonifies the stomach.

Conditions most used for: (1) Thirst,
hidrosis in chronic fevers, frequent
bloody urination; (2) vomiting and
diarrhea, abdominal pain, abdominal
distention; (3) jaundice; (4) acute
and chronic convulsive attacks; (5)
skin diseases.

Preparation: The whole plant is used
medicinally, 5 ch'ien - 1 liang each
time, in decoction.

258. Hu-erh Ts'ao (Saxifrage species) [Tiger-ear grass]

<u>Family</u>: Saxifragaceae

<u>Scientific name</u>: Saxifraga sarmentosa L.

<u>Synonyms</u>: "Fu-erh ts'ao" [Buddha's-ear
grass], "t'ien ho-hsieh [heavenly water-
lily leaf], "shih ho-hsieh [stony water-
lily leaf], "szu-szu ts'ao" [thready
grass], "chin-hsien tiao fu-jung" [hibiscus
hanging-on-a-golden-thread], "hsieh-ho
ts'ao" [crab-shell grass], "ch'a-erh
ts'ao," "mao erh-to" [cat's ear].

<u>Morphology</u>: Perennial evergreen herb.
Found growing wild along rock edges,
and shady damp places along ditches.
Leaves clustered, rounded or reniform,
fleshy and thick, pubescent, apexes
rounded, bases cordate or truncate,
margins undulated, blooms in summer,
axillary racemose inflorescence consisting of terminal white flowers at
end of flower style. Capsule ovate-
rounded.

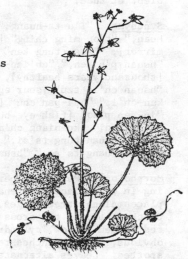

<u>Properties and action</u>: Has cold-chill
properties, slightly bitter and acrid to
taste. Clears fevers and detoxifies, promotes pus drainage.

<u>Conditions most used for</u>: (1) Boils
and abscesses, poisonous snakebites;
(2) otitis media, acute attacks of convul-
sion; (3) hematemesis.

<u>Preparation</u>: The whole plant is used
medicinally. For external use the
fresh plant may be crushed or extracted
for juice.

259. Hu Chang [Knotweed species]

Family: Polygonaceae

Scientific name: Polygonum cuspidatum
Sieb. et Zucc.

Synonyms: "T'u ta-huang," "chin-pu-
huan," "t'ou-ming ching" [transparent
mirror], "hsuan tung ken" [acid pipe root],
"hsuan p'u ken," "ch'ien-nien chien"
[thousand-years healthy], "t'u sheng-ma"
"hsuan ch'ia tzu" [sour eggplant], "chu-
ken-ch'i," "hua-pan chu" [spotted bamboo],
"ju-yen p'ao" [fish-eye bubble], "ma-
hsuan kan," "ku-niang ch'a" [young maid's
tea], "hsuan-tung ts'ai," "ch'u-tung ts'ao,"
"hsuan-kuang ts'ao," "hsuan-pa ken."

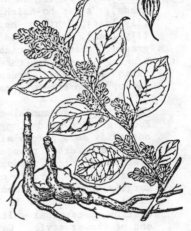

Morphology: Perennial herb. Found growing in wild places and shady and damp
places along stream edges. Root bark
blackish brown, the cross section a dull
red. Stem hollow, cylindrical, nodes
obvious, young branches red or purple-
spotted. Leaves alternate, oval or ovate-
oval, apexes obtuse or short-acute, bases
cuneate, margins intact. Blooms in the
fall, small white axillary flowers appearing
to form racemose inflorescences. Achene
3-angled, dull brown.

Properties and action: Has cooling
properties, acid and bitter to taste,
slightly toxic. Clears fevers and detoxifies, eliminates bruises [stagnant
blood] and promotes tissue regeneration.

Conditions most used for: (1) Burn injuries, boils and abscesses, poisonous
snakebites; (2) acute hepatitis, appendicitis; (3) traumatic injuries, and
menstrual irregularities.

Preparation: Roots and leaves are used medicinally, roots 3-5 ch'ien in
decoction; fresh leaves may be crushed for external application; or dried
root may be pulverized for sprinkling on affected parts.

260. Mao Ken [Cogongrass]

Family: Graminea

Scientific name: Imperata cylindrica
var. major (Nees) C. E. Hubb.

Synonyms: "Pai mao-ken" [white cogongrass],
"pa-ken tsao" [base-of-dike grass], "ssu
mao-ken" [silky cogongrass], "ch'uan-shan-
chia," "ch'uan-shan-hu," "yeh-lu-hua"
[wild reed-flower], "huang mao ts'ao
[yellow hair grass], "t'u ma-ken," "chuan-
ti-lung" [tunnelling dragon], "kan-shan
pien," "kuo-shan lung," "ch'uan-shan lung,"
"ta-ma-ken."

Morphology: Perennial herb. Found growing in wild places, roadsides, and field
edges. Rhizomes horizontal, covered externally by scales. Leaves clustered,
linear or linear-lanceolate, margins
coarse. Blooms in summer, flower style
appearing from leaf cluster to form
panicle inflorescence, densely covered
by silky white hairs.

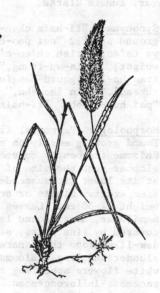

Properties and action: Has chilling
[han] properties, pleasant and light
to taste. Clears fevers, stops bleeding, promotes diuresis, allays thirst.

Conditions most used for: (1) Hemoptysis,
hematemesis, epistaxis, hematuria; (2)
nephritic edema, urinary tract infections;
(3) high fevers and thirst.

Preparation: Roots and flowers are used
medicinally, roots 5 ch'ien - 1 liang, or
flowers 1-3 ch'ien, each time in decoction.

261. Mao-kao Ts'ai [Sundew species]

Family: Droseraceae

Scientific name: Drosera peltata Sm.
var. lunata Clarke.

Synonyms: "Ti-hsia chen-chu" [under-
ground pearl], "nei pao-chu," "shih lung-
ya ts'ao," "tieh ch'en-t'o" [iron scale
weight], "hsia-wu-tsung," "chin-hsien
tiao hu-lu" [gourd-hanging-on-gold-
thread], "chin lao-shu," "lao-hu-tzu,"
"pai hua-hsieh," "ti-hsia ming-chu."

Morphology: Perennial fragile herb.
Found growing mostly on sunny hillsides.
Rhizome frequently curved, with small
globose root the size of a lima bean
at its lower tip suspended like a pearl.
Stem erect. Single or branching above,
height 12-30 cm. Leaves alternate,
semilunar, margins and leaf surfaces densely
covered by fine hairs, secretions forming
dew-like drops that snare insects; petioles
slender and long. Blooms in summer, small
white flowers appearing terminally to form
racemose inflorescences. Capsule cracked
on the backside.

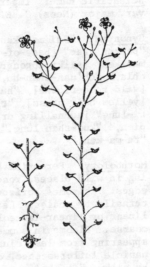

Properties and action: Has warming properties, pleasant but slightly bitter
to taste, slightly toxic. Eliminates flatus and [excessive] moisture, stimulates blood circulation and alleviates pain.

Conditions most used for: (1) Rheumatoid pains of back and leg, temporal
headaches, traumatic injuries; (2) dysentery; (3) cervical nodes enlargement.

Preparation: Roots or the whole plant is used medicinally. Used mostly for
external purposes (roots or the whole plant is crushed, mixed with water to
make pills about the size of horsebeans, that are placed in the middle of
plasters or adhesive to be applied on painful parts, to be kept there until
local sensation of heat is felt before removal. If the skin blisters after
the plaster has been removed, protect area with gauze.) For internal consumption, take 1-4 granules.

262. K'u Shen [Sophora species]

Family: Leguminosae

Scientific name: Sophora flavescens Ait.

Synonyms: "Ti huai," "shui huai" [aquatic sophora], "k'u-ku" [bitter bones], "niu shen."

Morphology: Deciduous shrub. Mostly found growing on hillsides and sunny slopes. Root thick and long, yellow. Stem cylindrical, with irregular longitudinal furrows, small branches pubescent. Leaves alternate, oddly pinnate compound, leaf axis pubescent, leaflets opposite or almost opposite, long oval or broadly lanceolate, apexes obtuse, bases cuneate or obtuse, margins intact, leaf undersides pubescent, petioled. Blooms in early summer, light yellow or yellow disc-like flowers, axillary or terminal, forming racemose inflorescences. Legumes, seeds black and globose.

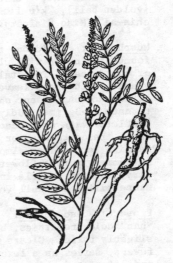

Properties and action: Has chill-cold properties, bitter to taste. Clears fevers and detoxifies, removes flatus and counteracts moisture.

Conditions most used for: (1) Enteritis, bacterial dysentery; (2) bleeding hemorrhoids, bloody vaginal discharge and luekorrhea; (3) hives, scabies, carbuncles, weeping rash.

Preparation: Roots are used medicinally, 2-5 ch'ien each time in decoction. For external purposes the decoction may be used for bathing the affected parts.

263. K'u Lien [China-tree (mahogany?)]

Family: Meliaceae

Scientific name: Melia azedarach L.

Synonyms: "Tz'u-hua shu" [purple-flower tree], "shen-shu," "chin ling-tzu [golden bell], "k'u lien-ya," "t'u-erh chia-ai" (Miao dialect).

Morphology: Deciduous tree. Mostly found growing in wild places, roadsides or cultivated. Tree tall, bark dull brown, young branches and leaves both emitting bitter and unpleasant odor. Leaves alternate, 2-3 times oddly pinnate compound, leaflets ovate or lanceolate, apexes sharp, bases rounded or obtuse-rounded, margins serrated or almost intact. Blooms in summer, purple flowers, terminal or axillary, forming panicle inflorescences. Drupe ellipsoid, dull yellow.

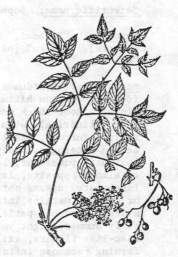

Properties and action: Has slightly "han" cold properties, bitter to taste, slightly toxic. Clears moisture-related fevers, serves as a laxative and vermicide, and alleviates abdominal pain.

Conditions most used for: (1) Abdominal pain due to parasitical worm infestation; (2) hernia; (3) ringworm and weeping lesions.

Preparation: Fruit and bark of root are used medicinally, fruit 2-4 ch'ien, or root bark 5 ch'ien - 1 liang, each time in decoction; or crushed and mixed with boiling water for internal consumption; or decoction used for bathing affected parts.

264. K'u Chi [Ground-cherry]

<u>Family</u>: Solanaceae

<u>Scientific name</u>: Physalis pubescens Linn.

<u>Synonyms</u>: "Hsiang-ling ts'ao" [tinkling bell grass], "t-ien-pao-tzu," "wang-mu chu," "wu-ts'ang-pa shu," "teng-lung ts'ao" [lantern grass], "hsiang-pao-tzu," "pai-t'ien pao-tzu," "hsiao t'ien-pao-tzu."

<u>Morphology</u>: Annual herb. Found grow-ing in wild places, roadsides and gardens. Height 30-60 cm, the whole plant pubescent. Stem inclined or erect, mostly branching. Leaves alternate, broadly ovate, apexes acute, bases obtuse-rounded, margins intact or slightly undulate, petioled. Blooms in summer, small light yellow axillary flowers appearing singly, the calyx increasing in size during fruit formation, pouch-like, angled, enveloping the fruit. Berry globose.

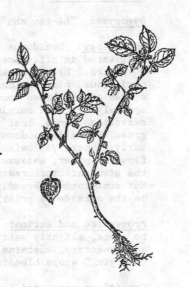

<u>Properties and action</u>: Has "chill" properties, bitter to taste. As a vermicide, cough sedative, diuretic, and antipyretic, also detoxifies.

<u>Conditions most used for</u>: (1) Abscesses and carbuncles; (2) sore throat; (3) pemphigus.

<u>Preparation</u>: The whole plant is used medicinally, 5 ch'ien - 1 liang each time, in decoction.

265. Pan-li (Li) [Chestnut]

Family: Fagaceae

Scientific name: Castanea mollisima Bl.

Synonyms: "Li-tzu shu" [chestnut tree]

Morphology: Deciduous tree. Mostly
cultivated in hilly areas. Height to
20 meters. Leaves alternate, thinly
coriaceous, oval or long oval-lanceolate,
apexes acute, bases rounded or cuneate,
sparsely serrated margins, points of
serrations awned, leaf surfaces dark
green, backsides a downy white. In
early summer, yellowish brown axillary
flowers appear, unisexual on same branch,
the staminate inflorescence spike-shaped.
Nut semi-rounded broadly ovate, covered
on the outside by prickly burrs.

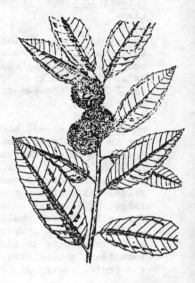

Properties and action: Neutral, pleasant
to taste, slightly salty. Stops diarrhea
and dysentery, sustains the stomach and
the "yin," stops bleeding.

Conditions most used for: (1) Diarrhea,
uncontrollable epistaxis, dysentery; (2)
regurgitation, profound thirst.

Preparation: The furry globe (burr)
is used medicinally, 5 ch'ien - 1 liang,
or root bark 1-2 liang, in decoction
each time.

266. Pan-lan Ken (Ma Lan) [Strobilanthes species]

Family: Acanthaceae

Scientific name: Strobilanthes flaccidifolius
Nees.

Synonyms: "Lan-ting" [indigo blue].

Morphology: Perennial shrub-like herb.
Found growing wild in hilly areas. Stem
erect, bluntly angled; height attaining 1
meter. Leaves opposite, ovate long-oval,
apexes, acute, bases narrowed, margins
serrated. Blooms in summer, light purple
terminal and axillary flowers appearing
to form sparse spike inflorescences.
Fruit a capsule.

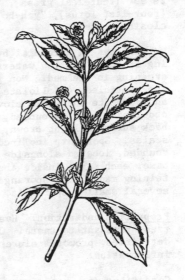

Properties and action: Has "chill"
properties, bitter to taste. Clears
fevers and detoxifies.

Conditions most used for: (1) Epidemic
mumps, sore throat; (2) erysipelas, fever
caused rashes.

Preparation: Roots and leaves are used
medicinally, 5 ch'ien - 1 liang each
time, in decoction.

267. P'ing [Pepperwort]

Family: Marsileaceae

Scientific name: Marsilea quadrifolia L.

Synonyms: "T'ien tzu ts'ao," "szu-heish ts'ao" [four-leaf grass], "szu-hsieh lien" [four-leaf lotus], "yeh-ho ts'ao [night-closing grass].

Morphology: A perennial herb. Found growing in quiet shallow waters, rhizomes creeping in the mud. Non productive leaves long petioled, 4-foliolate, leaflets paired and opposite in 4-leaf clover arrangement, obdeltoid, apexes rounded, margins intact, back surfaces light brown, with gland-like scales. Sporocarp inclined-ovate or rounded, located alongside petiole near the base, each sorus inside the sporocarp containing many large sporangia surrounded by several smaller sporangia.

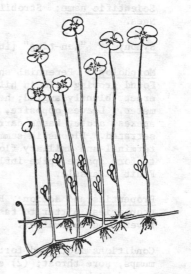

Properties and action: Has cooling properties, pleasant to taste. Clears fevers and detoxifies, promotes diuresis and reduces inflammation.

Conditions most used for: (1) Boils and abscesses; (2) poisonous snakebites; (3) trauma-caused back pain.

Preparation: The whole plant is used medicinally. A suitable amount can be crushed and used for external application. Or 3-5 ch'ien may be used in decoction.

268. Pao-shih Lien [Stone-clasping lotus]

Family: Polypodiaceae

Scientific name: Lepidogrammitis drymoglossoides (Bak.) Ching.

Synonyms: "Ju-pi chin-hsing," "kua-tzu
chin" [melon-seed gold], "jo shih-hu,"
"yen kua-tzu ts'ao" [rock melon grass],
"ch'a-pu-lan," "kua-tzu lien" [melon
seed lotus], "shih kua-tzu lien" [stony
melon seed lotus].

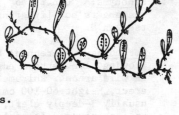

Morphology: Perennial herb. Found
growing wild on shady and damp rock cliffs.
Rhizome horizontal, sparsely covered by
light brown scales. Leaves seen in 2
forms: nutrient leaves ovate-rounded;
spore leaves lingulate or spatulate.
Sori rounded, distributed along both
sides of central rib.

Properties and action: Has "han" cold
properties, light and pleasant to taste.
Clears fevers and detoxifies, moisturizes
the lungs and stops coughing.

Conditions most used for: (1) Coughing
and hemoptysis; (2) jaundice; (3) traumatic injuries.

Preparation: The whole plant is used
medicinally, 3-5 ch'ien each dose, in
decoction.

269. P'ei Lan [Thoroughwort]

Family: Compositae

Scientific name: Eupatorium fortunei Turcz.

Synonyms: "Lan ts'ao" [orchid grass], "hsiang ts'ao" [fragrant grass], "hsiang tse-lan."

Morphology: Perennial herb. Found growing along stream edges or wet spots in wild areas. Rhizome horizontal, stem erect, height 60-100 cm. Leaves opposite, usually 3-deeply cleft, clefts long-rounded or long rounded-lanceolate, with short petioles, apexes gradually pointed, margins serrated, sparsely pubescent along ribs, emitting a fragrance when shaken. Blooms in the fall, purplish-red flowers appearing to form capitulum inflorescences arranged to resemble cymose inflorescences. Achene cylindrical, blackish-brown when ripe.

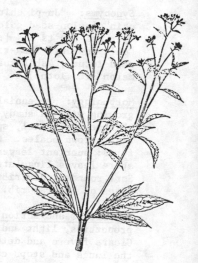

Properties and action: Neutral, slightly acrid to taste. Relieves [excess] moisture and resolves impurities, moderates central organs and stimulates the appetite.

Conditions most used for: (1) Heat exhaustion headache, fever without perspiration, tightness of chest and abdominal distention; (2) regurgitation, halitosis, and a greasy feeling in mouth.

Preparation: Stem and leaves are used medicinally, 2-4 ch'ien each time, in decoction.

270. Tse Lan (Ti-kua-erh miao) [Water-horehound; bugleweed]

Family: Labiatae

Scientific name: Lycopus lucidus Turcz.
var. hirtus Regel.

Synonyms: "Ti sun" [ground sprouts], "kan-
lu tzu" [nectar].

Morphology: Perennial herb. Found growing
along stream edges or in damp places in the
wilds. Subterranean stem creeping, large
and spindle-shaped. Stem erect, 4-angled,
hollow, surface pruplish red, with short
fine hairs over angles and nodes. Leaves
opposite, broadly lanceolate, apexes acute
or acuminate, bases cuneate, margins sharply
serrate or finely serrate, both sides
pubescent. In the fall, white axillary
flowers appearing to form verticillate
inflorescences. Fruit an achene, flat.

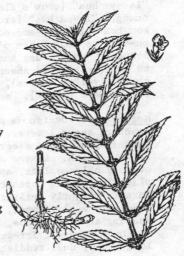

Properties and action: Has slightly warming
properties, bitter to taste. Stimulates
blood circulation and breaks up stagnant
blood clots, soothes the liver and reduces
edema.

Conditions most used for: (1) Menstrual
irregularities, metrorrhagia, dysmenorrhea;
(2) abscesses, congestive edema, abdominal
distention.

Preparation: The whole plant is used
medicinally, 1.5-3 ch'ien each time, in
decoction.

271. Nao-yang Hua (Yang tsun-chu) [Azalea]

Family: Ericaceae

Scientific name: Rhododendron molle G. Don.

Synonyms: "San-ch'ien-san," "pa-li ma,"
"shou-shan hu" [mountain searching tiger],
"ch'u-shan piao," "lao-hu hua" [tiger flower],
"tso-shan hu," "shui lan-hua" [aquatic orchid],
"lao-ya hua" [crow's flower], "ying shan-
huang," "la-pa hua" [trumpet flower], "p'ao-
kou hua" [leopard-and-dog flower], "yang-
pu-shih ts'ao," "shan p'i-p'a" [upland
loquat], "nao-ch'ung hua," "ching-yang
ts'ao" [frightened-sheep grass], "huang tu-
chuan" [yellow azalea], "kou-t'ou hua,"
[dog's-head flower], "men-t'ou hua."

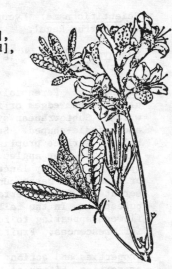

Morphology: Deciduous shrub. Height
reaching about 1 meter. Small branches
densely pubescent, older branches grayish
brown, smooth. Leaves alternate, long
oval or oblanceolate, apexes obtuse and
slightly convex, bases cuneate, margins
intact, slightly ciliate, short-petioled.
Blooms in early summer, yellow flowers appearing at branch tips, 5-merous, in bell
or funnel shapes, irregular. Capsule
long-ovoid, dull reddish brown when ripe.

Properties and action: Has warming
properties, acrid to taste, greatly
toxic. Purges flatus and dispels cold
[han], neutralizes moisture and kills
insects, stops itching and reduces
swelling.

Conditions most used for: (1) Rheumatoid
arthritis, traumatic injuries, malaria;
(2) caries; (3) insecticide for killing
maggots, mosquito larvae, and
oncomelania snails.

Preparation: Flowers and roots are used
medicinally, flowers usually for external
use; roots 5 fen - 1 ch'ien in decoction.

272. Tz'u Hsien-ts'ai [Thorny amaranth]

Family: Amaranthaceae

Scientific name: Amaranthus spinosus L.

Synonyms: "Le hsien-ts'ai," "yeh hsien-ts'ai" [wild amaranth], "ma-shih hsien," "yeh le-hsien."

Morphology: Annual herb. Found growing extensively in primative and wild places. Stem erect, height attaining 70 cm, purplish red, branching. Leaves alternate, ovate or long-ovate, apexes obtuse, bases cuneate, margins intact, petioled, with 1 pair of thorns at base of petiole. In summer-fall, terminal or axillary spike inflorescence of small green flowers appear. Sporocarp globose.

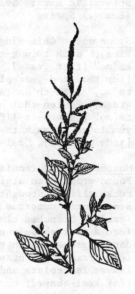

Properties and action: Has slightly chilling properties, light and pleasant to taste. Clears fevers and neutralizes [excess] moisture, acts as an astringent and stops diarrhea.

Conditions most used for: (1) Dysentery, enteritis; (2) poisonous snakebites.

Preparation: The whole plant is used medicinally, 1-2 liang each time, in decoction.

273. Chuan Pai [Spike moss species]

Family: Selaginellaceae

Scientific name: Selaginella tamariscina (Beauv.) Spring.

Synonyms: "Chiu-ming wang" [life-saver king], "shih hsiung-ti," "ch'uan-t'ou ts'ao" [fist grass], "wan-nien sung" [ten thousand-year pine], "fan-yang ts'ao," "szu ch'un ts'ao" [four-spring grass], "chien-shui huo," "hui-yang ts'ao" [return-to-life grass], "huan-yun ts'ao," "shih ta-pu-szu," "yu-pai" [jade cypress], "pai-jih huan-yang."

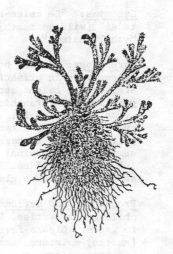

Morphology: Perennial evergreen herb. Found growing on alpine rocks or between rocky cliffs, drought resistant. Main stem short, numerous fibrous roots. Terminal branches clustered, curling into a fist shape when dried. Leaves dense, gathering in tile overlap pattern arranged on branches; lateral leaves lanceolate and drill-like, back of leaf keel-shaped; central leaves in 2 rows, long ovate-lanceolate, both sides inequally inclined. Sporangia at terminal tips like spikes.

Properties and action: Neutral, acrid tasting. Astringent and hemostatic.

Conditions most used for: (1) Traumatic bleeding, hemoptysis in pulmonary disease, gastrointestinal bleeding, metrorrhagia, hematuria, persistence of post-partum lochial discharge; (2) rectal prolapse, leukorrhea.

Preparation: The whole plant is used medicinally, 3-5 ch'ien each time, in decoction.

274. Yu T'ung

Family: Euphorbiaceae

Scientific name: Aleurites fordii Hemsl.

Synonyms: "T'ung-yu shu" [t'ung-oil
tree], "t'ung-tzu shu," "ying-tzu t'ung."

Morphology: A deciduous shrub. Mostly
cultivated in valleys and level places.
Height 3-10 meters. Bark smooth, gray,
upper part usually branched into 2-3
forks. Leaves alternate, coriaceous,
ovate-cordate, sometimes shallowly 3-cleft,
apexes acuminate, bases cordate or truncate,
with 2 glands located where the leaf
joins with the petiole. Flowers white,
blooming before leaves appear, base of
petals orange-red spotted and striped,
panicle inflorescences compounding into
cymose inflorescences. Drupe globose,
tip acute. Seeds broad ovate-rounded.

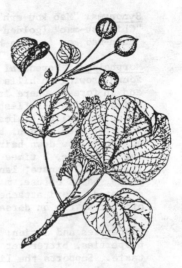

Properties and action: Has cooling
properties, pleasant to taste but
slightly acrid, slightly toxic. Produces emesis and reduces swelling,
vermicidal against scabies mite.

Conditions most used for: (1) Overeating and abdominal fullness, moisture-
based edema; (2) traumatic bleeding; (3)
scabies; (4) burns; (5) masturbation
and seminal emission [?] in boys.

Preparation: Flowers, fruit and leaves
are used medicinally. A suitable amount
of t'ung oil may be mixed for external
application.

275. Kou-chi [Dog's Spine]

Family: Dicksoniaceae

Scientific name: Cibotium barometz (L.) J. Sm.

Synonyms: "Mao kou-erh" [hairy puppy], "Chin-ssu-mao" [golden-silky hair], "chin-mao kou [golden-haired dog].

Morphology: Perennial evergreen herb. Found growing on hillsides, gullies, and in forests where it is shady and damp. Rhizome thick and fleshy, densely covered by golden-yellow scales. Leaves clustered, long-petioled, brown, bases covered by golden-yellow down hair, leaves broad ovate-deltate, 3 times pinnately compound, leaflets alternate, lanceolate, apexes acute, bases obtuse, margins finely serrated. Sori attached to both sides of central rib on dorsal side of leaf.

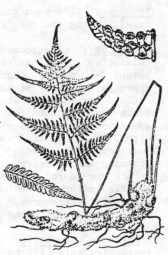

Properties and action: Has warning properties, bitter yet pleasant to taste. Supports the liver and kidneys, strengthens the back and knees, and eliminates rheumatism.

Conditions most used for: (1) Rheumatoid arthritis, backache and pains in the leg, numbness of hands and feet; (2) traumatic bleeding.

Preparation: Roots, stems or downy hairs used medicinally, roots and stems 3-5 ch'ien each time in concoction. Downy hairs are used for application on wounds to stop bleeding.

276. Ju-hsing Ts'ao (Ch'i ts'ai) [Fishy-odor grass]

Family: Saururaceae

Scientific name: Houttuynia cordata Thunb.

Synonyms: "Ch'ou mu-tan" [stinky peony], "ch'ou ling-tan," "la-tzu ts'ao" [pepper grass], "nai-t'ou ts'ao" [nipple grass], "chi-ken," "chi-erh ken," "ch'ou ts'ao" [stink-grass], "chi-erh ken" [chicken root].

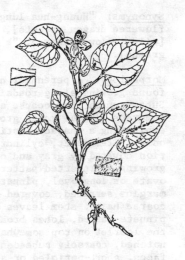

Morphology: A perennial herb. Found growing on shady and damp hillsides, stream edges, and roadsides. Whole plant smells fishy. Rhizome creeping subterraneanly, noded, numerous fibrous roots. Stem erect, cylindrical, purple. Leaves alternate, ovate-rounded, apexes acuminate, bases broadly cordate, margins intact. Blooms in summer, white flowers appearing terminally at end of branches, forming spike inflorescences. Fruit a capsule, cracked at tip.

Properties and action: Has cooling properties, acrid to taste, slightly toxic. Clears fevers and detoxifies, promotes diuresis and reduces swelling.

Conditions most used for: (1) Upper respiratory tract infections, lung abscess; (2) inflammatory conditions and other infections of the urinary tract; (3) poisonous snakebites.

Preparation: The whole plant is used medicinally; for the whole plant, 5 ch'ien - 1 liang each time; fresh herb, 2-4 liang in decoction; also crushed fresh for external application.

277. Pai-chiang (Huang-hua pai-chiang)

Family: Valerianaceae

Scientific name: Patrinia scabiosaefolia
Fisch.

Synonyms: "Huang-hua lung-ya" [yellow-
flowered dragon sprouts], "yeh huang-hua"
[wild yellow flowers], "k'u ts'ai" [bitter
greens].

Morphology: A perennial herb. Mostly
found growing along roadsides or wild places.
Subterranean stem coarse and thick, with
numerous fibrous roots growing from side,
exhibiting a characteristically unpleasant
odor. Stem erect, cylindrical, lower section covered by gray and coarse downy hairs
growing in inverted pattern. Basal leaves
ovate or long oval, pinnately compound,
margins serrated, covered sparsely by
coarse hairs; stem leaves smaller, opposite,
pinnate-parted, lobes broadly lanceolate,
the leaflet on top somewhat larger, apexes
notched, coarsely pubescent on both surfaces, short-petioled or almost non-petioled;
upper leaf petioles clasping stem at bases.
In late summer, small yellow flowers appearing terminally at stem, forming umbellate
inflorescence. Achene an ellipsoid.

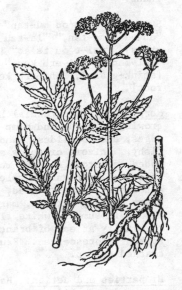

Properties and action: Neutral, bitter to
taste. Clears fevers and detoxifies, breaks
up clots and stimulates circulation, eliminates swelling.

Conditions most used for: (1) Appendicitis,
conjunctivitis, enteritis, and dysentery;
(2) boils and abscesses of unknown origin;
(3) post-partum abdominal cramps.

Preparation: Roots or whole plants are used medicinally, 5 ch'ien - 1 liang
each time, in decoction. Fresh tender leaves crushed may be used for external
application over affected parts.

278. Ch'ing-tai [Indigo flower]

Properties and action: Has "chilling" [han] properties, salty to taste. Clears fevers, cools blood, and detoxifies.

Conditions most used for: Fevers, rashes, hematemesis, hemoptysis, infantile convulsions, abscesses, erysipelas.

Preparation: For each dose, 5 fen to 1 ch'ien, in decoction. Suitable amount may be used for external purposes.

279. Ch'ing p'i [Dried tangerine peel]

Properties and action: Has warming properties, bitter and acrid to taste. Loosens up stagnant energy and breaks up body congestion, clears the liver and alleviates pain.

Conditions most used for: Epigastric pain, hepatic congestion, pain in chest and sides, distension, hernia, breast congestion, chronic malaria.

Preparation: For each dose, 1-3 ch'ien, in decoction.

280. Ch'ing-kuo [Olive, Canarium album]

Properties and action: Neutral, pleasant yet acrid to taste. Purifies the lungs, eliminates apprehension, stimulates appetite and promotes salivation.

Conditions most used for: Sore throat, thirst and restlessness, globefish poisoning, and alcohol intoxication.

Preparation: For each dose, 1.5-3 ch'ien, in decoction. Or, one plum may be kept in mouth for sucking.

281. Ts'ao [Date]

Properties and action: Neutral, pleasant to taste. Strengthens the spleen and stomach, moisturizes the heart and lungs, and regulates various medications [taken].

Conditions most used for: Weak stomach and spleen, anemia, inadequate energy [fatigue] and salivation.

Preparation: For each dose, 2-5 ch'ien, in decoction.

282. K'un-pu [Laminaria]

Properties and action: Has "cold-chill" [han] properties, salty to taste. Softens the "hard," and promotes moisturization.

Conditions most used for: Enlarged lymph nodes, tumors, edema, congestion, and painful testicles.

Preparation: For each dose, 1.5-3 ch'ien, in decoction.

283. Chih-mu [Anemarrhena asphodeloides Bunge]

Properties and action: Has "han" cold properties, bitter to taste. Nourishes the yin, lowers fever, counteracts excess "fire-parchness" by moisturizing, and lubricates the intestines [by being mildly laxative].

Conditions most used for: Heat and thirst [dehydration?], yin-deficiency and an overheated system, constipation and difficult elimination of urine.

Preparation: For each dose, 1.5-3 ch'ien, in decoction.

284. Lu Kan-shih [A precious mineral]

Properties and action: Neutral, pleasant to taste. Eliminates dampness and rot, cures pterygiums and stops bleeding.

Conditions most used for: "Pink-eye" and pterygiums, conjunctivitis, incurable ulcers, weeping dermatitis.

Preparation: For external application only.

285. Yu-chin [Curcuma longa, L. ?]

Properties and action: Has "han" cold properties, acrid to taste. Stimulates energy circulation and relieves congestion, cools the blood and resolves bruises and clots.

Conditions most used for: Stagnation in blood and energy circulation, pain in chest, abdomen and muscles, hematemesis, epistaxis, hematuria, menstrual irregularities, coma due to mania and fever.

Preparation: For each dose, 1-3 ch'ien, in decoction.

286. Yu-li Jen [Seed of Prunus japonica, Thunb.]

Properties and action: Neutral, acrid and bitter, yet pleasant to taste. Expels flatus, supports energy, and counteracts excessive moisture when used externally.

Conditions most used for: Sluggish colon, constipation, edema, and inadequate elimination of urine.

Preparation: For each dose, 1-3 ch'ien, in decoction.

287. Sung-hua Fen [Pine cone pollen]

Properties and action: Neutral, pleasant to taste. Expels gas and benefits energy [circulation]. Used externally to counteract [excess] moisture.

Conditions most used for: Dizziness, puffiness of face. Used externally, for various boils and draining sores.

Preparation: For each dose, 1-2 ch'ien, in decoction. For external use, an appropriate amount.

288. Shih-chun-tzu [Quisqualis indica L.]

Properties and action: Neutral, pleasant to taste. Eliminates malnutrition and kills intestinal parasites.

Conditions most used for: Marasmus in children, abdominal distention and pain, poor food digestion, and intestinal parasite infestations.

Preparation: For each dose, 1.5-3 ch'ien, in decoction.

289. Hsi Hsin [Asarum sieboldi, Mig.]

Properties and action: Neutral, acrid to taste. Dispels gas-chill [feng-han] symptoms, promotes moisturization of the body system.

Conditions most used for: Stuffy nose, toothache, headache, rheumatic pains and aches, productive coughing and wheezing.

Preparation: For each dose, 0.3-1 ch'ien, in decoction.

290. Tse-hsieh [Plantain species, Alisma plantago L. var. par. viglomum Torr.]

Properties and action: Has "han" chilling properties, pleasant to taste. Neutralizes moisture-heat [in system] and promotes diuresis.

Conditions most used for: Moisture-based fever, difficult urination, edema and ascites, vomiting, diarrhea, excessive sputum production, beri beri, and "wu-lin" [five disease conditions involving the urinary tract -- kidney stones, polyuria, hematuria, bladder distension and chyluria ?]

Preparation: For each dose, 2-4 ch'ien, in decoction.

291. Yeh-ming sha [Bat droppings]

Properties and action: Has "han" chilling properties, acrid to taste. Stimulates blood circulation and improves vision.

Conditions most used for: Poor vision, cataracts, marasmus in children.

Preparation: For each dose, 1-3 ch'ien, in decoction.

292. Ming-fan [Alum]

Properties and action: Has "han" chilling properties, sour to taste. Resolves phlegm, neutralizes [excess] moisture, expels flatus, lowers fever, detoxifies and kills parasites, stops bleeding and alleviates pain.

Conditions most used for: Numbness of throat, epilepsy, hypersalivation, excessive phlegm, leukorrhea, jaundice, epistaxis. For external use, on scabies, open sores, stomatitis and canker sores.

Preparation: For each dose, 2-5 fen, in decoction. For external application, use a suitable amount.

293. Chiang-huo [Angelica sylvestris L.]

Properties and action: Has warming properties, acrid and bitter to taste. Promotes perspiration, dispels gas and overcomes [excess] moisture.

Conditions most used for: Influenza chills, headache, anhidrosis, rheumatism, boils and abscesses.

Preparation: For each dose, 1-3 ch'ien, in decoction.

294. Tse-pai (Including: Pai-tzu jen) [Thuja orientalis L.]

Properties and action: Has "han" chilling properties, bitter and acrid,
yet pleasant to taste. Cools the blood and stops bleeding.

Conditions most used for: Hematemesis, epistaxis, blood in stools, hematuria,
and metrorrhagia.

Preparation: For each dose, 2-4 ch'ien, in decoction.

Note: Pai-tzu jen [Seeds of Thuja orientalis]

     Neutral, pleasant to taste. Calms nerves, and counteracts [excess]
heating in system. Used mostly to treat apprehension, insomnia, seminal
emission, hidrosis, and constipation. For each dose, use 1-3 ch'ien, in
decoction.

295. Hu-t'ao [Walnut]

Family: Juglandaceae

Scientific name: Juglans regia L.

Synonyms: "Ho-t'ao."

Morphology: Deciduous tree. Likes
warm and moist fertile soil, mostly
cultivated in level places. Height
20-meters. Branches long, spreading
to form a broad-ovate tree crown. Bark
silvery gray, lenticels projecting
noticeably. Leaves alternate, oddly
pinnate compound, leaflets usually
5-9, long rounded-ovate or elliptical
obovate, apexes obtuse or sharply
acute, bases rounded or inclined,
margins intact or sparsely serrated,
petioles hairy. Blooms in summer,
forming a drooping spike. Drupe
globose, its outer skin hard.

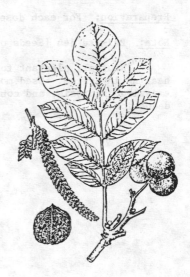

Properties and action: Has warming
properties, pleasant to taste. Supplements the kidneys and stimulates the
semen, moisturizes the lungs and stops
coughing, reduces inflammation and
alleviates pain.

Conditions most used for: (1) Deficient
and chill-based wheezing and coughing;
(2) constipation and hard feces; (3)
seminal emission, impotency; (4)
swelling and aches in back and legs.

Preparation: Seeds and seedcoats are
used medicinally, in proper amounts to
be taken internally.

296. Hu-t'o-tzu [Oleaster species]

Family: Elaeagnaceae

Scientific name: Elaeagnus pungens Thunb.

Synonyms: "Ch'iang-mi shu," "pan ch'un-tzu," "pan chu'an-tzu," "t'ien pang-ch'ui" [sweet hammer].

Morphology: Evergreen shrub. Found growing in wild places or hillsides. Height attaining 3 meters, branches spreading. Leaves alternate, long elliptical, apexes obtuse, bases rounded, margins undulate, under-surfaces silvery white, mixed with brown spots. In the fall, axillary white flowers appearing in clusters, forming cymose inflorescences. Drupe ellipsoid, covered by gray or brown scaly spots.

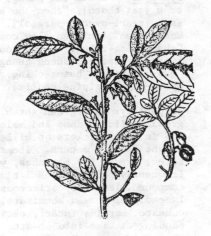

Properties and action: Neutral, acid and biting to taste. Stops coughing, relieves asthma, controls diarrhea.

Conditions most used for: (1) Coughing, asthma; (2) indigestion, diarrhea; (3) hemorrhoids.

Preparation: Stem and leaves are used medicinally, 1 liang each time, in decoction.

297. Nan-t'ien-chu

Family: Berberidaceae

Scientific name: Nandina domestica Thunb.

Synonyms: "T'ien-chu-huang," "lao-shu
tz'u [rat thorn], "chen-chu kai liang-
san" [pearl-over-a-parasol], "chi-chao
Huang-lien" [chicken-claw coptis],
"shan huang-ching," "hung kou-tzu"
[scarlet puppy], "sheng huang-ching,"
"nan-chu ken," "huang-ching," "shan
huang-lien" [alpine coptis].

Morphology: Evergreen shrub. Found
growing wild in damp and moist ravines,
and in weed thickets on hillside.
Height about 2 meters. Stems clustered, erect, few branches, young branches
frequently red. Leaves 3 times pinnate-
compound, leaflets coriaceous, elliptical
lanceolate, apexes acuminate, bases
cuneate, margins intact, petioles expanding at base into sheaths clasping
stem. In summer, small terminal white
flowers appearing at end of branches,
forming panicle inflorescences. Berry
globose, scarlet when ripe.

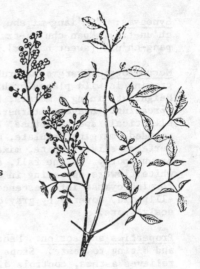

Properties and action: Neutral, bitter
to taste, berry toxic. Clears fevers,
quiets coughing, strengthens the stomach
and stops diarrhea, opens up meridian and
"lo" passageways, and strengthens bone
and muscle.

Conditions most used for: (1) Fever in
influenza, acute bronchitis, whooping
cough; (2) indigestion, acute gastroenteritis; (3) tooth abscess; (4) pain
in bones and muscles, traumatic injuries.

Preparation: Roots and stems are used
medicinally, 3-5 ch'ien each time, in
decoction.

298. Nan Wu-wei-tzu

Family: Magnoliaceae

Scientific name: Kadsura peltigera Rehd.
et wils.

Synonyms: "P'an-ch'u nan-wu-wei-tzu,"
"feng-sha t'eng" [wind-and-sand vine],
"huang niu-t'eng" [yellow ox-vine],
"hung t'eng-tzu" [red vine], "hsiao-hsieh
nan-wu-wei," "hsiao chu'an" [little drill],
"chien-ku-feng."

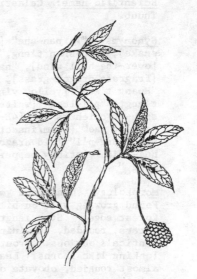

Morphology: Evergreen entwining vine.
Found growing wild along stream edges
or damp and shady thickets. Length may
be as much as 4 meters long. Stem exuding
a sticky secretion, smooth and nonpubescent.
Single leaves alternate, oval or long
oval-lanceolate, apexes acuminate, bases
cuneate, margins sparsely serrated. In
summer, light yellow flowers appear singly
from leaf axils. Fruit dull red, berry,
merged in globose shape.

Properties and action: Has warming properties, bitter and acrid, yet pleasant to
taste. Nourishes and supplements, quiets
coughing, expels flatus, breaks up congestion, and alleviates pain.

Conditions most used for: (1) Chronic
gastroenteritis, gastric and duodenal
ulcers; (2) rheumatoid arthritis, traumatic
injuries, dysmenorrhea; (3) coughing due
to "deficient" lungs, neurasthenia.

Preparation: Fruits or roots, stems and
leaves are used medicinally, fruits 5
fen - 1.5 fen, or roots, stems, leaves
3 - 3 ch'ien, in decoction.

299. Nan she t'eng [Spindle-tree species]

Family: Celastraceae

Scientific name: Celastrus articulatus Thunb.

Synonyms: "Ta nan-she" [great southern snake], "kuo-shan t'eng," "kuo-shan feng" [over-the-hill wind], "hsiang lung-ts'ao" [fragrant dragon-grass], "Nan-she feng," "Huang t'eng" [yellow vine], "ta-lun t'eng," "pai-lung" [white dragon], "szu-shih-pa chieh ts'ao" [48-section grass], "ch'ung yao" [worm/insect medicine], "lao lung-p'i" [old dragon-hide], "ch'ou hua-chiao" [stinky pepper], "chuan-shan lung."

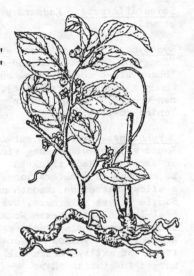

Morphology: Deciduous woody vine. Found growing wild on hillsides and forest edges. Stem length reaching 5 meters, rounded, entwining upwards, lenticels obvious, sprouting scales looking like thorns. Leaves alternate, almost rounded, obovate or long elliptical-obovate, apexes obtuse or acute, bases cuneate or rounded, margins finely serrated, with short petioles. In summer, light yellow flowers appearing from leaf axils to form cymose inflorescences. Fruit a capsule, turning brownish-yellow when ripe.

Properties and action: Has warming properties, neutral to taste. Relieves inflammation and detoxifies, stimulates blood circulation to open up meridian passageways, expels flatus-associated moisture, and strengthens sinews and bones.

Conditions most used for: (1) Paralysis, numbness of four extremities; (2) headache, toothache; (3) spontaneous abscess formation, and snakebites.

Preparation: Roots, stems, and leaves are used medicinally, roots and stems 1-2 liang each time in concoction; or fresh leaves crushed in appropriate amounts for external application.

300. Hsiang-fu (Sha-ts'ao) [Sedge species]

Family: Cyperaceae

Scientific name: Cyperus rotundus, L.

Synonyms: "Hsiang fu-tzu," "hui-t'ou ch'ing," "tiao ma tsung," "huai-mao ts'ao," "t'ien-t'ou ts'ao" [field sedge].

Morphology: A perennial herb. Found growing wild on hillsides and roadsides. Rhizome creeping, apex a fat and thick spindle-shaped tuber. Culm erect, 3-angled, height 30-60 cm. Leaves linear, fine, with parallel venation, apexes acute, margins intact. In summer, terminal brown flowers forming compound spike inflorescences. Achene 3-angled.

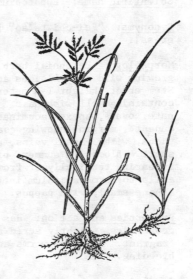

Properties and action: Neutral, acrid and slightly bitter to taste, fragrant. Corrects energy circulation and relieves congestion, restores menstrual regularity and alleviates pain, strengthens the stomach and relieves distension.

Conditions most used for: (1) Chest pain, side pains, abdominal pains, stomach pains and nausea and vomiting; (2) menstrual irregularity, dysmenorrhea; (3) traumatic injuries.

Preparation: Rhizomes are used medicinally, 3-5 ch'ien each time in decoction. For external use, an appropriate amount of the fresh material may be crushed for applying on affected parts.

301. Hsiang Tse-lan

Family: Compositae

Scientific name: Eupatorium odoratum L.

Synonyms: "Fei-chi ts'ao" [airplane grass].

Morphology: Perennial herb. Found growing wild on hillsides and roadsides. Stem erect, height 1-3 meters, few branches containing yellowish hair. Leaves alternate, ovate, apexes acuminate, bases cuneate, margins showing coarse serrations, with 3-basal veins, petioles short. Blooms in summer, pink flowers appearing terminally or from leaf axils to form capitulum inflorescences. Achene small, with pappus.

Properties and action: Has warming properties, slightly acrid to taste, fragrant. Destroys worms and stops bleeding.

Conditions most used for: (1) As control leptospirosis; (2) bleeding caused by leech bites.

Preparation: The whole plant is used medicinally, 5 ch'ien - 1 liang each time in decoction; or fresh leaves may be crushed for external application to wound.

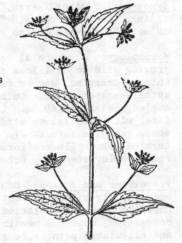

302. Hsiang P'u [Sweet flag]

Family: Typhaceae

Scientific name: Typha latifolia L.

Synonyms: "Kan-p'u," "huan-hsieh
hsiang-p'u" [broad-leaf fragrant
typha], "mao la-chu" [hairy candle],
"shui la-chu" [water candle].

Morphology: Perennial acquatic herb.
Found growing in swamps. Rhizome subterranean, white. Stem single, erect,
cylindrical, hard and smooth. Leaves
clustered, long broad-linear, margins
intact, lower section sheath-like,
clasping stem. In summer, fleshy spike
inflorescences appear terminally, with
2-3 leaf-like bracts. Yellow staminate
spike appearing terminally at end of
branches; lower section presenting
cylindrical pistillate spikes, like candles,
sienna brown. Fruit small.

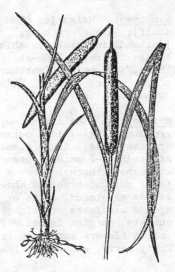

Properties and action: Has cooling
properties, pleasant to taste. Stops
bleeding, promotes diuresis, reduces
swelling and promotes pus drainage.

Conditions most used for: (1) Hemoptysis,
hematemesis, epistaxis, bloody stools,
hematuria, vaginal bleeding, bleeding
hemorrhoids; (2) cystitis, urethratitis;
(3) menstrual irregularities, metrorrhagia
and leukorrhea.

Preparation: Pollen (p'u-huang) is used
medicinally, 8 fen - 3 ch'ien each time,
in decoction.

303. Chou-ch'i

<u>Family</u>: Solanaceae

<u>Scientific name</u>: Lycium chinense Mill.

<u>Synonyms</u>: "Hsien-jen chang" [fairy's
staff], "niang-erh hung," "shua-ya lan"
[duck-killing orchid], shih shou-shu [rocky
longevity tree], "kou-chu ts'ai," "t'ien-
ching," "ti hsien" [earthly fairy], "ti-ku-
p'i," "yeh chou-ch'i," "t'u chou-ch'i,"
"hsueh ch'i-tzu."

<u>Morphology</u>: Small deciduous shrub. Found
growing along village outskirts, roadsides
or cultivated. Stems clustered, height
attaining 1-2 meters, branches slender,
with short thorns. Leaves alternate,
lower part of branches showing several
leaves clustered, ovate or ovate-lanceolate,
apexes acuminate or slightly obtuse, bases
cuneate, margins intact. In summer, light
purple flowers appearing from leaf axils.
Fruit berry, ellipsoid, fresh bright red.

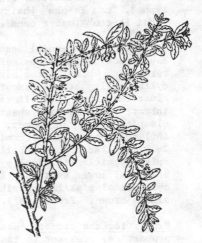

<u>Properties and action</u>: Fruit has neutral
properties, pleasant to taste. Strengthens
the kidneys and restores semen, nourishes
the liver and clears vision. Root bark
has "han" chill properties, bitter to
taste. Cools the blood and purges fire,
clears pulmonary "heat."

<u>Conditions most used for</u>: (1) Pulmonary
tuberculosis, pneumonia in small children;
(root bark often used) (2) nutritional-
deficiency eye diseases, diabetes; (3)
inadequate liver and kidney function,
seminal emission (fruits mostly used).

<u>Preparation</u>: Fruits and root bark are
used medicinally, 3-5 ch'ien each time,
in decoction.

304. Chou-ku [Holly species]

Family: Aquifoliaceae

Scientific name: Ilex cornuta Lindl.

Synonyms: "Mao-kung la" [tom-cat thorn],
"kou-kung la" [male dog thorn], "lao-shu
la" [rat thorn], "yang-chiao la" [prickly
goat horn], "niao-pu-su" [no-sleep bird],
"mao-erh la" [kitten thorn], "shih-ta
kung-loa" [ten great achievements], "lao-
hu la" [tiger's thorn].

Morphology: Evergreen shrub or small
deciduous tree. Growing in wild places,
and alongside mountain paths in full
sunshine. Height frequently 1-3 meters,
stem multi-branching. Leaves whorled,
coriaceous, long elliptic, apexes 2-3
sharp thorned, margins along bases also
fringed with similar thorns 1-2, leaf
surfaces deep green, lustrous. In
summer, small axillary yellow-white
flowers appearing to form cymose inflorescences. Globular drupe bright
red.

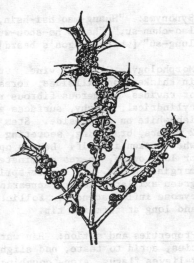

Properties and action: Has cooling
properties, slightly bitter to taste.
Brings down "deficient" fevers, strengthens
back and knee.

Conditions most used for: (1) Recurring
fever in pulmonary tuberculosis,
tubercular lymph nodes; (2) joint
pains, lumbago.

Preparation: The whole plant is used
medicinally; for roots, leaves, and
stems, 4 ch'ien - 1 liang, or fruit
3 ch'ien, in decoction.

305. Wa-erh T'eng [Species of milkweed; toad vine]

Family: Asclepiadaceae

Scientific name: Tylophora ovata (Lindl.)
Hook.

Synonyms: "Huang-mao hsi-hsin," "t'eng
lao-chun-su," "hsiao ho-shou-wu," "pai
lung-su" [white dragon's beard].

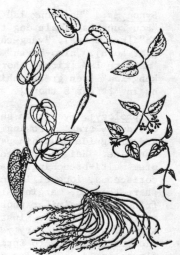

Morphology: Climbing vine. Growing
in thickets on hillsides, forest edges
or ravines. Numerous fibrous roots,
cylindrical, fleshy, surfaces gray, yellowish-white on the inside. Stem length about
2 meters, branching, secreting a milky fluid
when broken in half. Leaves opposite, ovate
or long ovate, apexes acuminate, bases cordate,
margins intact. In summer-spring yellowish-
green axillary flowers appearing to form
cymose inflorescences. Follicles, 2, pointed
and long at terminal tip.

Properties and action: Has warming properties, acrid to taste, and slightly toxic.
Relieves flatus, stops coughing, resolves
phlegm, promotes vomiting, and breaks down
clots.

Conditions most used for: (1) Asthma and
coughing; (2) traumatic injuries, rheumatoid
backaches; (3) pain in the stomach and
abdomen; (4) poisonous snakebites.

Preparation: Roots are used medicinally,
3-5 ch'ien each time, in decoction.

306. Chih-tzu [Gardenia]

<u>Family</u>: Rubiaceae

<u>Scientific name</u>: Gardenia jasminoides
Ellis.

<u>Synonyms</u>: "Huang chih-tzu" [yellow
gardenia], "shan chih" [mountain
gardenia], "pai ch'an" [white toad], "mu-
tan shan-chih," "shan chih-tzu."

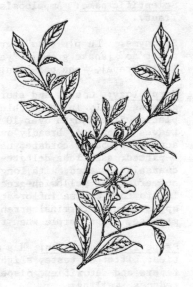

<u>Morphology</u>: Evergreen shrub. Found
growing in damp semi-shade on hillsides
and beneath forests. Trunk height
reaching 2 meters. Leaves opposite,
oblong-rounded or ovate-lanceolate,
apexes short and acute, bases cuneate,
margins intact, short-petioled, leaf
surfaces dark green and lustrous, dorsal
surfaces light green with ribs very noticeable. In summer, axillary or terminal
white flowers appearing like butterflies
on pedestal when in bloom. Berry ovate
or long ovate, with 6-8 winged grooves,
orange-red when ripe.

<u>Properties and action</u>: Has cooling proper-
ties, bitter to taste. Clears fevers and
purges fire, cools the blood and detoxifies.

<u>Conditions most used for</u>: (1) Hepatitis
with jaundice, high fevers associated
with influenza; (2) styes, canker sores,
toothache, mastitis; (3) epistaxis,
hematemesis, hematuria; (4) bacterial
dysentery; (5) snakebites.

<u>Preparation</u>: Roots and fruits are used
medicinally. Roots 1-2 liang, or fruit
1-4 ch'ien, in decoction.

307. Pa-shan Hu (shan p'u-t'ao) [Over-the-hill tiger (mountain grape)]

Family: Vitaceae

Scientific name: Ampelopsis brevipedunculata
Trautv.

Synonyms: "Lu p'u-t'ao" [green grape], "she
p'u-t'ao" [snake grape], "yeh p'u-t'ao"
[wild grape], "she pai-lien."

Morphology: Coarse and sturdy vine. Found
growing mostly in shrub thickets of wild
places. Stem length over 10 meters, noded.
Leaves alternate, broadly ovate, apexes
acuminate, bases cordate, usually shallowly
3-parted, each lobe deltate-ovate, margins
coarsely serrated, with long petioles. In
summer, small yellowish-green flowers appearing to form cymose inflorescences in axillary
opposition or terminal arrangement. Berry
globose, light purple when ripe.

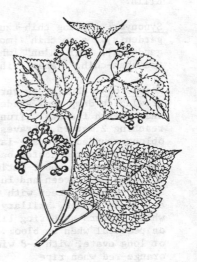

Properties and action: Has cooling properties, bitter to taste, slightly toxic. Clears
fevers and detoxifies, dispels clots and
reduces swelling.

Conditions most used for: (1) Abscesses,
boils and ulcers; (2) traumatic bruises
and aches.

Preparation: Fresh fruit or roots and leaves
are used mostly externally, a suitable amount
crushed or prepared in decoction for bathing affected parts; roots (woody centers)
may be prepared in decoction for taking by
mouth, 5 ch'ien - 1 liang each dose.

308. Ts'ao-wu [Monkshood species]

Family: Ranunculaceae

Scientific name: Aconitum chinense Pext.

Synonyms: "Kuang-wu" [shiny aconite], "wu-t'ou" [aconite], "hua wu-t'ou" [Chinese aconite].

Morphology: Perennial herb. Found growing mostly along edges of hillside thickets or in wasted upland meadows. Root tuber spindle-shaped or obovate, usually joined in two's, black-brown exteriors, side roots fibrous. Stem erect, angled. Leaves alternate, ovate-rounded, deeply 3-cleft, the central lobe spindle-shaped cuneate, apex again shallowly 3-parted, and 2 lateral lobes again 2-parted, the margins of all parted lobes coarsely dentate. In summer, terminal or axillary bluish purple flowers appearing to form panicle inflorescences. Fruit a follicle, long-rounded.

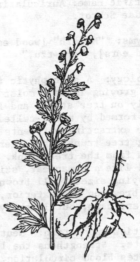

Properties and action: Has heating properties, acrid yet pleasant to taste, greatly toxic. Relieves flatus and dispels moisture, disperses "han" cold, alleviates pain, promotes hidrosis and diuresis.

Conditions most used for: (1) Wind-chill numbness, spasms of the hands and feet, paraplegia; (2) hernia pain, abdominal pain due to excess vin-cold; (3) uterine cancer, arthiritis, sciatica.

Preparation: Roots are used medicinally. The crude drug cannot be taken internally, but must be soaked a week in clear water, after which it is mixed with 4 percent fresh ginger and 2 percent licorice, crushed and soaked-bleached for 1-2 days (the water must cover the ingredients being soaked). Then the contents are steamed, sliced, and dried before being used in prescriptions. For each dose 1 - 1.5 ch'ien in decoction.

309. Hei Mu-erh [Black 'wood-ear']

Family: Auricularineae [subfamily]

Scientific name: Auricularia auricula
-- Judae Schrot.

Synonyms: "Mu erh" [wood ears], "yun-erh"
[cloud ears], "erh-tzu."

Morphology: A saprophytic fungus.
Found growing in damp moist forests,
usually on tree stumps and logged timber.
Plant formed by multi-celled hyphae, the
hyphae extracting nutrients from the de-
caying tree trunk, and later extending
spores from the tree trunk. The spores
shaped like a human ear, sticky, smooth,
of varying sizes, dull brown internally,
light brown on the exterior, sticky when
moist and damp, but leathery when dried.

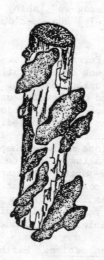

Properties and action: Neutral, pleasant
to taste. Strengthens the lungs and
activates blood circulation.

Conditions most used for: (1) Metrorrhagia, urinary tract diseases, dysentery
with blood; (2) traumatic injuries; (3)
gas in the gastrointestinal tract and
bleeding hemorrhoids.

Preparation: Spores are used medicinally, 2 ch'ien - 1 liang each time,
steamed and consumed.

310. Lo Shih [Climbing dogbane species]

Family: Apocynaceae

Scientific name: Trachelosperum jasminoides Lem.

Synonyms: "Kuo-ch'iang feng" [over-the-wall wind], "yuan-pi t'eng" [wall climbing vine], "shih-nan t'eng," "tieh-hsien ts'ao" [wiregrass], "feng t'eng" [wind vine], "che-ku ts'ao" [bone fracture grass], "chiao-chiao feng" "lo-shih t'eng" [rock connecting vine].

Morphology: Evergreen climbing woody vine. Found growing as a weed in gardens, on walls or trees. Stem cylindrical, as long as 10 meters, aerial roots present, entwining other objects. Leaves opposite, oval-rounded, apexes acute or obtuse-rounded, bases cuneate, margins intact, with short petioles. In summer, axillary while flowers appearing to form cymose inflorescences. Fruit a follicle, slender.

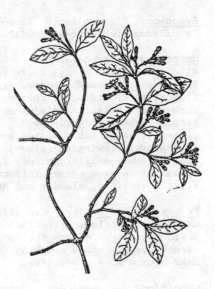

Properties and action: Neutral, bitter to taste. Keeps meridians and related passageways clear, beneficial to joints, clears fevers and detoxifies.

Conditions most used for: (1) Rheumatoid arthritis; (2) sore throats, and various boils and abscesses.

Preparation: Vines and stems are used medicinally, 5 ch'ien - 1 liang each time, in decoction.

311. Liu-hsieh Pai-ch'ien [Willow-leafed cynachum]

Family: Asclepiadaceae

Scientific name: Cynanchum stauntoni
(Decne.) Hand.-Mazz.

Synonyms: "Pai-ch'ien," "Yang-huo ken,"
"shui yang-liu" [Acquatic willow].

Morphology: Perennial herb. Growing
wild along water's edge where shady
and damp. Rhizomes slender, creeping,
fine roots clustered at rhizome node.
Stem erect, height attaining 60 cm, few
branches, base slightly woody. Leaves
opposite, lanceolate, apexes acute, bases
gradually narrowing, margins intact. In
summer, small axillary purple flowers
appearing to form cymose inflorescences.
Fruit a follicle, slender and angled.

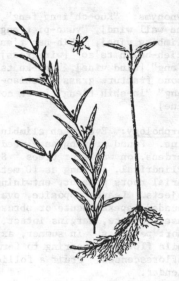

Properties and action: Has slightly
warming properties, bitter and slightly
acrid to taste. Clears the lungs, lowers
excess energy, stops coughing, and helps
make sputum more productive.

Conditions most used for: Coughing, asthma,
dyspnea.

Preparation: Roots and rhizomes are used
medicinally, 3-5 ch'ien each dose, in
decoction.

312. Kuan-tsung [Holly fern species]

Family: Aspidiaceae

Scientific name: Cyrtomium fortunei J. Sm.

Synonyms: "Hei kou-chi" [black dog's back], "Feng-wei ts'ao [tailwind grass], "kuan-chung," "Fu-shih kuan-tsung."

Morphology: Perennial fern. Found growing mostly along the sides of ditches and roadways, and rocky crevices where damp and shady. Rhizomes short and thick, densely covered by reddish-brown scales, ovate, lustrous. Leaves clustered, petioles densely covered by scales. Leaves oddly pinnate-compound, leaflets alternate, scythe-shaped, apexes acuminate, bases rounded or the superior border auricular, margins finely dentate. Brown sori scattered on dorsal surface of leaves.

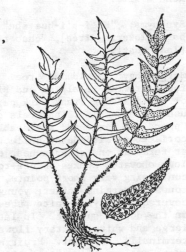

Properties and action: Has slightly "han"-cooling properties, bitter to taste. Clears fevers, disperses clots, detoxifies, and kills helminths.

Conditions most used for: (1) As a preventive for influenza and measles; (2) hookworm disease, tapeworm disease, ascariasis, and filariasis; (3) acute infectious hepatitis, and various bleeding ailments.

Preparation: Rhizomes are used medicinally, 3-5 ch'ien each time, in decoction.

313. Hou-p'o [Magnolia species]

Family: Magnoliaceae

Scientific name: Magnolia officinalis
Rehd & Wils.

Synonyms: "Kuei-p'i-hua shu" [cinnamon-
bark flowering tree], "chao teng-kan"
[lamp post].

Morphology: Deciduous tree. Usually
found growing in alpine and hilly areas,
or cultivated. Trunk bark purplish-brown,
usually branching, lenticels obvious.
Upper leaf large and noticeable. Leaves
coriaceous, alternate, collecting densely
at terminal end of branches, obovate or
long obovate, apexes obtuse-rounded or
containing very short points, bases
cuneate, margins intact; young leaves
covered by grayish-white pubescent hairs
on the dorsal surface. In late spring,
large and white solitary flowers appearing
terminally, fragrant. Fruit a follicle,
ovate-oval or long ovate-elliptic.

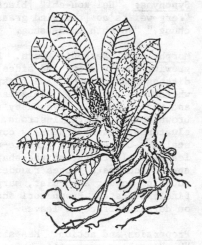

Properties and action: Has warming
properties, bitter and acrid to taste.
Neutralizes excess moisture, dispels
fullness, corrects energy and lubricates
the intestines.

Conditions most used for: (1) Abdominal
distension, constipation; (2) gastroenteritis, dysentery; (3) excessive sputum
production, asthma, and coughing (use the
dried bark); (4) gas pains in the
stomach and liver (use flowers).

Preparation: Dried bark and flowers are
used medicinally, 1-3 ch'ien for dried
bark, and 8 fen - 1.5 ch'ien blossoms,
in decoction.

314. Ch'u-ch'ung Chu [Pyrethrum]

Family: Compositae

Scientific name: Chrysanthemum
cinerariaefolium Vis.

Synonyms: "Pai-hua ch'u-ch'ung chu"
[white-flowered pyrethrum].

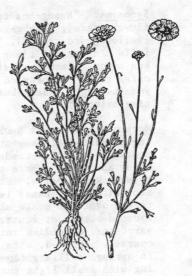

Morphology: Perennial herb. Likes growing in rich soil with highly decayed
matter. Whole plant grayish-green,
covered by grayish hairs. Tap root
cone shaped, side roots numerous.
Basal leaves clustered, stem leaves alternate, 2-3 times pinnately compound, completely cleft, pinnae cleft to central
rib, linear, apexes mostly notched,
bases narrowing gradually into petioles,
dorsal sides of leaf densely covered
by fine white downy hairs. In summer,
white flowers appearing as solitary
capitulum inflorescences, terminal.
Fruit cone-shaped achene, angled.

Properties and action: Has warming
properties, toxic. Vermicidal.

Preparation: (1) Killing maggots:
dry flowers and pulverize, throw into
excreta. (2) For use against mosquitos:
after the whole plant has been dried,
crush and prepare into a fumigant.

315. P'u-fu Ching [Creeping violet]

<u>Family</u>: Violaceae

<u>Scientific name</u>: Viola diffusa Ging.

<u>Synonyms</u>: "Huang-hua ts'ao" [yellow-flower grass], "huang-kua ts'ai" [yellow gourd greens], "yeh po-ho" [wild mint], "hsi t'ung ts'ao," "ya-kua t'eng," "mao-mao hsiang," "t'ien-ching ts'ao" [courtyard grass], "lu-yueh hsiang," "huang-kua hsiang," "ti ting-hsiang."

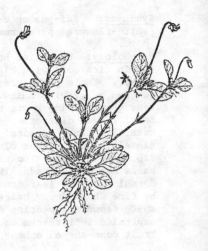

<u>Morphology</u>: Annual herb. Found growing on wasted slopes, stream edges, sparse forests and roadsides where shady and damp. Whole plant covered by soft white hairs. Stems creeping, stoloniferous. Basal leaves clustered, ovate or ovate-elliptic, apexes rounded-obtuse or acute, bases gradually narrowing, extending into wings, margins coarsely serrated, with long petioles. In spring, axillary flower style appearing with small light purplish or white flowers. Capsule long-elliptic.

<u>Properties and action</u>: Has cooling properties, bitter and acid to taste. Detoxifies, nourishes the blood and aids tissue regeneraton.

<u>Conditions most used for</u>: (1) Aplastic anemia, leukemia; (2) mastitis, mumps, ginseng [Pinellia ternata] poisoning, poisonous snakebites; (3) traumatic injuries, boils and abscesses.

<u>Preparation</u>: The whole plant is used medicinally, 1-2 liang each time in decoction; or the fresh product may be crushed for external application.

316. Yin-ch'en [Wormwood species]

Family: Compositae

Scientific name: Artemesia capillaris Thunb.

Synonyms: "Mien yin-ch'en" [fluffy wormword], "hsiang kao" [fragrant wormwood], "yeh-lan kao," "ch'ing kao-tzu," "hsiao ch'ing-kao" [small wormwood], "kou-mao ch'ing-kao," "hsi yin-ch'en," "niu-wei yin-ch'en" [ox-tail wormwood], "shua-ch'ung yao" [bug-killing drug].

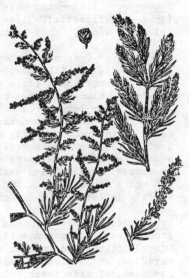

Morphology: Perennial herb. Found growing wild along roadsides, grassy thickets along stream edges. Stem erect, multi-branched, smaller branches finely pubescent. Leaves alternate, 2-3 times pinnately compound, pinnae finely linear, densely covered by white hairs; petioles short, bases expanding to clasp stem. In late summer, small greenish-yellow capitulate flowers appearing to form panicle inflorescences. Achene long-rounded.

Properties and action. Has slightly cold properties, bitter to taste. Clears moisture-fevers, promotes diuresis.

Conditions most used for: (1) Jaundice, difficult urination; (2) pruritus.

Preparation: The whole plant is used medicinally, 3-5 ch'ien each time, in decoction.

317. Wei-ling-hsien [Chinese clematis]

Family: Ranunculaceae

Scientific name: Clematis chinensis Osb.

Synonyms: "Tieh-chiao wei-ling-hsien" [iron-foot clematis], "ling-hsien t'eng" [clematis vine], "ch'i-ts'un feng."

Morphology: Perennial woody herb. Found growing wild on hillsides, along stream edges. Subterranean roots slender and long, clustered, blackish brown on the exterior. Stem length reaching 5 meters, black when dried, with noticeable stripes. Leaves opposite, pinnately compound, leaflets 3-5, ovate-lanceolate, apexes acute, bases cuneate, margins intact. In summer, terminal and axillary greenish white flowers appearing to form panicle inflorescences. Achene flat.

Properties and action: Has warming properties, bitter and acrid to taste. Dispels flatus and removes moisture, clears meridians and activates related passageways, alleviates pain.

Conditions most used for: (1) Rheumatoid arthritis; (2) cold-type stomach-ache; (3) fishbone stuck in throat; (4) tetanus.

Preparation: Roots are used medicinally, 3-5 ch'ien each time, in decoction.

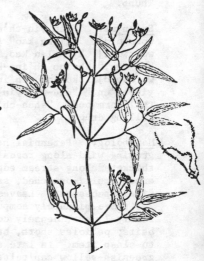

318. K'an-mai Niang [Foxtail]

Family: Graminea

Scientific name: Alopecurus aequalis
Sobol.

Synonyms: "Shan kao-liang," "Niu-t'ou
meng" [ox-head strength].

Morphology: Biennial herb. Found
growing mostly in paddy fields and wet
places alongside ditches. Fibrous roots
fine. Culms clustered, cylindrical,
hollow interiors, fragile, frequently
bending nodes, with fine longitudinal
grooves. Leaves linear, flat, length
3-10 cm, width 0.2-0.6 cm, sheath
somewhat enlarged. In early spring,
small terminal grayish-green flowers
appearing to form panicle-spike inflorescences. Caryopsis length 0.1
cm.

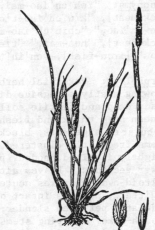

Properties and action: Neutral, light
and pleasant to taste. Promotes
diuresis, reduces swelling, and detoxifies.

Conditions most used for: (1) Chickenpox,
edema; (2) snakebites.

Preparation: The whole plant is used
medicinally, 3-5 ch'ien each time, in
decoction.

319. Ch'iao-mai San-ch'i [Buckwheat species]

Family: Polygonaceae

Scientific name: Fagopyrum cymosum
Meisn.

Synonyms: "Yeh ch'iao-mai," [wild
buckwheat], "k'u ch'iao-t'ou," "yeh
nan-ch'iao," "chin ch'iao-mai" [golden
buckwheat], "hua-mai," "tieh chu'an-
t'ou" [iron-fist], "ch'ih ti'li."

Morphology: Perennial herb. Found
growing mostly alongside ditches on
shady damp and fertile soil. Subterranean stem thick and fleshy, with
globular enlargements, blackish-brown.
Stems frequently clustered, erect or
slightly inclined, noded, purple in
lower sections. Leaves alternate,
deltoid-ovate, apexes acute, bases
sagittate, margins intact or slightly
undulate, petioles slender; stipules
sheath-like, clasping stems. In the
fall, terminal and axillary white
flowers appearing to form panicle
inflorescences. Achene 3-angled,
blackish brown.

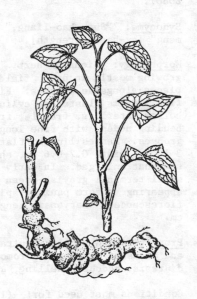

Properties and action: Neutral, acid
and slightly bitter to taste. Stimulates
energy and blood circulation, reduces
swelling and alleviates pain.

Conditions most used for: (1) Traumatic
injuries, lumbago; (2) menstrual irregularities, dysmenorrhea; (3) purulent inflammation; (4) snake and insect bites.

Preparation: Roots or the whole plant
are used medicinally, 1-2 liang each
time, in decoction.

320. K'un-ming Chi-hsueh T'eng [Kunming chicken-blood vine]

Family: Leguminosae

Scientific name: Millettia reticulata Benth.

Synonyms: "Hsueh-fang t'eng," "hsueh kuan-p'i" [blood-soaked bark], "lao-shu tou," "ch'ing-p'i huo-hsueh," "lan t'eng," "huang-t'eng" [yellow vine], "yen tou-chia" [rock peas], "kuo-shan lung," "shan tou-chiao," "yen tou chiao," "lei-kung kua-shih p'ien" [thunder god's dung scraper], "ch-hsueh-t'eng" [chicken blood vine].

Morphology: Evergreen woody vine. Found growing mostly in wild places, and hidden valleys in shady and damp places. Rhizome, when cut open, secreting a bloody red liquid, circular. Leaves alternate, oddly pinnate-compound, leaflets 7-9, ovate-elliptic, apexes obtuse, slightly retuse, margins intact, bases rounded. In summer, purplish red flowers appearing to form panicle inflorescences. Legume slender and long.

Properties and action: Has warming properties, bitter to taste. Stimulates energy circulation and supplements the blood, clears meridians and activates associated passageways, warms the back and knees, and strengthens bone and muscle.

Conditions most used for: (1) Shortness of breath and blood, anemia in women, menstrual irregularities, vaginal discharge [bloody discharge and leukorrhea]; (2) numbness and paralysis, backache and pain in the knees; (3) seminal emission, gonorrhea; (4) stomachache.

Preparation: Roots and vines are used medicinally, 5 ch'ien - 1 liang each time in decoction.

- 819 -

321. P'i-p'a Hsieh [Loquat leaves]

Family: Rosaceae

Scientific name: Eriobotrya japonica
Linal.

Synonyms: "P'i-p'a shu-hsieh" [loquat
tree leaf].

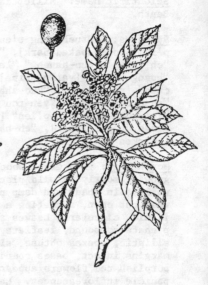

Morphology: Small evergreen shrub. Growing in uplands or cultivated. Trunk
greyish-brown, branches dense, short
strong branches densely covered by rusty
fine hairs. Leaves alternate, coriaceous,
obovate to long elliptic, apexes acute
or acuminate, bases cuneate, margins
sparsely dentate; leaf surfaces dark
green, lustrous, densely pubescent
dorsally with rust-colored hairs, ribs
marked, projecting on dorsal surfaces.
In winter, dense clusters of terminal
white flowers appearing to form panicle
inflorescences, densely pubescent.
Fruit pear-shaped or rounded, yellow or
orange-colored when ripe.

Properties and action: Neutral, bitter
to taste. Neutralizes stomach, lowers
[excess] energy, quiets coughs and resolves phlegm.

Conditions most used for: (1) Cough with
productive sputum; (2) hemoptysis; (3)
pertussis.

Preparation: Leaves are used medicinally,
2-4 ch'ien, in decoction.

322. Hsi Ts'ao [Madder]

Family: Rubiaceae

Scientific name: Rubia cordifolia L.

Synonyms: "Huo-hsueh ts'ao" [blood pick-up grass], "Hung hsi-ts'ao" [red madder], "feng-che ts'ao" [windmill grass], "szu-lun ts'ao" [four-wheeled grass], "chu-tzu ts'ao" [saw grass], "hsiao-huo-hsueh."

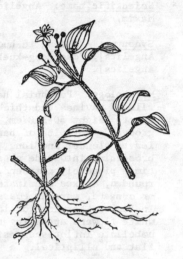

Morphology: Perennial climbing herb. growing wild under cover of damp wet upland forests. Stem creeping, 4-angled, with recursive thorns. Leaflets whorled, ovate-deltoid, apexes acute, bases rounded or cordate, margins intact. Blooms in summer, light yellow terminal and axillary flowers forming cymose inflorescence. Berry globose, bluish black when ripe.

Properties and action: Cooling, bitter to taste. Stops bleeding, alleviates pain, promotes diuresis and reduces inflammation.

Conditions most used for: (1) Traumatic injuries, rheumatoid arthritis; (2) dysmenorrhea and abdominal pain; (3) jaundice, edema.

Preparation: Roots are used medicinally, 3-5 ch'ien each dose, in decoction.

323. Tu-huo [Angelica species]

Family: Umbelliferae

Scientific name: Angelica pubescens
Maxim.

Synonyms: "Hsiang tu-huo" [fragrant
Angelica], "mao tang-kuei" [hairy
angelica].

Morphology: Perennial herb. Growing
wild in ravines and thickets. Stem
erect, height 50-150 cm, longitudinally
grooved. Petioles of basal and lower
leaves slender and long, bases of petioles
broadening into wide sheaths; leaves 2-3
times pinnately compound, leaflets ovate-
rounded, apexes acuminate, bases rounded
or cuneate, margins coarsely serrated.
In summer, terminal or laterally growing
white flowers appearing to form compound
umbellate inflorescences. Fruit winged,
flat and elliptical.

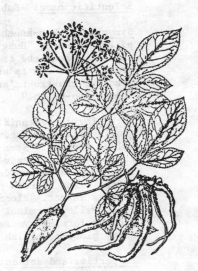

Properties and action: Has warming properties, acrid to taste. Relieves flatus and
dispels "han" chill, opens up "lo" passageways and alleviates pain.

Conditions most used for: (1) Rheumatoid
arthritis, rheumatism; (2) headache, toothache; (3) abscesses.

Preparation: Roots and rhizomes are used
medicinally, 1.5-3 ch'ien each time, in
decoction.

324. Ch'ien-hu [Hogfennel species]

Family: Umbelliferae

Scientific name: Peucedanum pracruptorum Dunn.

Synonyms: "Yen ch'uan-kung," "chi-chiao Ch'ien-hu" [chicken claw hogfennel].

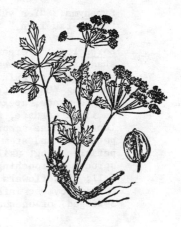

Morphology: Perennial herb. Growing wild in the sun among damp thickets on hill-sides and waste places. Roots thick and sturdy, with remnant fibers of decayed sheaths at base. Upper stem branching. Basal leaves rounded to broadly rounded, 2-times pinnately compound, with long petioles, base of petioles enlarging to form sheaths clasping the stem; stem leaves smaller, petioles short. In fall, terminal or axillary white flowers ap-pearing to form unbellate inflorescences. Fruit ovate-rounded, 3-angled, marginal lobe developing into wings.

Properties and action: Slightly cold [han], bitter to taste. Loosens up flatus, clears fevers, lowers excess energy and resolves phlegm.

Conditions most used for: (1) Colds, heache; (2) Coughing and asthma, tightness in chest [dyspnea].

Preparation: Roots are used medicinally, 2-3 ch'ien, in decoction.

325. Ch'iu Hai-t'ang [Begonia species]

Family: Begoniaceae

Scientific name: Begonia evanstana
Andr.

Synonyms: "Yen yuan-tzu" [rock pill],
"chiao-tzu lien," "yin-yang tzu."

Morphology: Perennial herb. Growing on
shady slopes or wet places. Subterranean
stem tuber globular. Stem erect, height
reaching 60 cm. Leaves alternate, inclined-ovate, apexes sharply acute, bases
inclined cordate, margins finely serrate,
leaf surfaces scabrous, the leaf undersides,
petioles, and stem nodes all purplish red,
petioles long; axillary buds growing new
sprouts on touching the ground. In the
fall, pink flowers at terminal stem
forming cymose inflorescences. Fruit
3-winged, of unequal size.

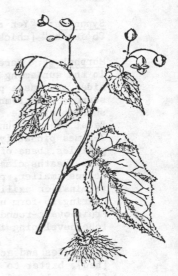

Properties and action: Has cooling
properties, acid and acrid to taste.
Stimulates energy and blood circulation,
reduces swelling, alleviates rain, and
relieves spasms.

Conditions most used for: (1) Traumatic
pain, hematemesis; (2) gonorrhea, and
post-partum vaginal discharge; (3)
amenorrhea; (4) snakebites.

Preparation: Tuberous roots and fruits
are used medicinally, 1-3 ch'ien each
time, in decoction.

326. Chen-chu Feng [Beauty-berry]

Family: Verbenaceae

Scientific name: Callicarpa pedunculata
R. Br.

Synonyms: "Tzu-chu ts'ao" [purple-bead
grass], "Tzu-chu shu" [purple-bead tree].

Morphology: Deciduous shrub. Growing wild
in alpine forests. Stem height reaching
3 meters, smaller branches covered by yellowish brown hairs. Leaves opposite, ovate-
elliptic or elliptic, apexes acuminate,
bases obtuse, rounded or broadly cuneate,
margins serrated, dorsal surface covered
densely by downy hairs and glandular dots,
petioles short. In the fall, small purple
axillary flowers appearing to form cymose
inflorescences. Berry purplish red.

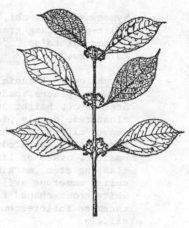

Properties and action: Neutral, acrid
and bitter to taste. Hemostatic and
analgesic. Also resolves clots and
bruises, and reduces swelling.

Conditions most used for: (1) Hemptysis,
hematemesis, epistaxis, hematuria, traumatic
bleeding; (2) traumatic injuries and rheumatoid arthritis.

Preparation: The whole plant is used
medicinally, 5 ch'ien- 1 liang in decoction.
Or, the whole plant may be crushed for
application over wound.

327. Chi Ts'ai [shepherd's purse; shovelweed]

Family: Cruciferae

Scientific name: Capsella bursa pastoris
Medic.

Synonyms: "Sha-chi," "hu-sheng ts'ao"
[life-protecting grass], "san-yueh-san,"
"shang-chi ts'ao," "chi-ju ts'ai," "ti-
ts'ai-tzu."

Morphology: Biennial herb. Growing wild
in waste places, paddy edges, and roadsides.
Stem erect, height 30-40 cm. Basal leaves
clustered, deeply pinnate-cleft; stem
leaves alternate, shallowly parted, margins
irregularly serrated; upper stem leaves
smaller, ovate or linear-lanceolate, bases
clasping stem, margins serrated. In
spring numerous axillary or terminal small
white cross-shaped flowers appearing to form
racemose inflorescence. Fruit an obdeltate
silicle.

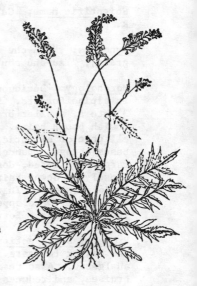

Properties and action: Neutral, rather
pleasant to taste. Hemostatic and diuretic.

Conditions most used for: (1) Hemoptysis,
hematemesis, hematuria, post-partum uterine
bleeding and metrorrhagia; (2) Nephritic
edema, difficult urination, chyluria.

Preparation: The whole plant is used medicinally, 2-4 liang each time, in decoction.

328. Fei Ts'ai [Sedum species]

<u>Family</u>: Crassulaceae

<u>Scientific name</u>: Sedum kamtschaticum
Fisch.

<u>Synonyms</u>: "San-ch'i," "ma san-ch'i,"
"t'ien-ch'i," "hu-chiao ch'i," "t'ung-
ta-pu-szu" [brass-cannot kill], "shai-
pu-kan" [sun-cannot dry].

<u>Morphology</u>: Perennial fleshy herb.
Cultivated mostly in gardens, also
growing wild on rocky areas. Stems
clustered, green, fleshy, height as
much as 25 cm. Leaves alterate, oval-
rounded, obovate to spatulate, apexes
obtuse, bases narrow-cuneate, margins
serrated, non-petioled. In summer,
yellow terminal flowers appearing to
form corymb inflorescences. Follicle
red or brown.

<u>Properties and action</u>: Has cooling
properties, acidic. Cools blood and
stimulates circulation, reduces inflammatdon
and alleviates pain.

<u>Conditions most used for</u>: (1) Traumatic
injuries, bleeding cuts; (2) burns;
(3) poisonous snakebites.

<u>Preparation</u>: Whole plant is used
medicinally, 1-2 liang each time, in
decoction. Or, fresh plant may be
crushed for external application.

329. Chi-chu [Horenia species]

Family: Rhamnaceae

Scientific name: Horenia dulcies Thunb.

Synonyms: "Chi-kua-tzu," "chi-chao li"
[chicken-claw pear], "kuai ts'ao-tzu"
[hanging date], "chi-chao" [chicken claw],
"chi-chao t'ang-shu."

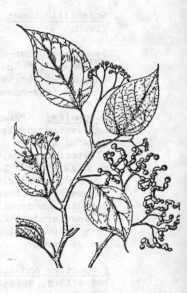

Morphology: Deciduous tree. Growing wild
in forests. Bark greyish brown, pores
marked. Leaves alternate, ovate-elliptic,
apexes long acute, bases rounded or cordate
finely mucronate-dentate, main rib 3-parted
from base. In summer, small terminal
or axillary yellowish green flowers appearing
to form short cymose inflorescences. Drupe
greyish-brown, globose; stem of fruit
twisted, purplish red, sweet and palatable.

Properties and action: Neutral, rather
pleasant to taste. Clears fevers, produces
mild laxative action, relieves spasms.

Conditions most used for: (1) Restlessness
and constipation; (2) infantile convulsions.

Preparation: Fruit and peel are used medicinally, fruits 5 ch'ien - 1 liang, or dried
peel 1-2 liang, in decoction.

330. Kou T'eng [Uncaria species]

Family: Rubiaceae

Scientific name: Uncaria rhynchophylla
(Mig.) Jacks.

Synonyms: "Ying-chao-feng" [eagle-claw
wind], "nei-hsiao," "shuang-k'ou" [double
hook], "shuang-k'ou t'eng" [double-hook
vine], "lao-ying chao" [old eagle's claw],
"tao-kua chin-k'ou," "tao-kua tz'u,"
"tiao k'ou t'eng" [hanging hook-vine],
"k'ou-erh."

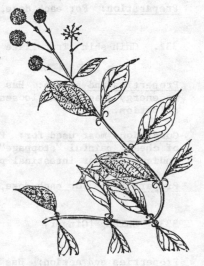

Morphology: Climbing shrub. Growing
wild in valleys and on slopes. Stem
smooth, non-pubescent, small branches
rounded-oblong. Leaves opposite, ovate
or oval, apexes acute, bases cuneate,
margins intact or slightly undulate, with
singly curved or doubly-curved thorns
growing from axils. In late summer, small
terminal or axillary yellowish green
flowers appearing to form capitulum inflorescences. Capsule spindle-shaped,
winged.

Properties and action: Has "han" cold
properties, pleasant yet slightly bitter
to taste. Clears fevers, soothes the liver,
stops gas [flatus] formation, and relieves
convulsions.

Conditions most used for: (1) Infantile
convulsions, headache; (2) dizziness,
hypertension, apoplexy.

Preparation: Curved thorns on stem are
used medicinally, 3-5 ch'ien for each
dose, in decoction (do not overcook).

331. Chi-ho [Trifoliate orange (Poncircus trifoliata) dried peels]

Properties and action: Has slightly "han" properties, bitter and acid to taste. Breaks up energy stagnation, loosens sputum, and aids digestion.

Conditions most used for: Pulmonary congestion, energy stagnation around heart-abdomen region, lumbago, indigestion.

Preparation: For each dose, 1-3 ch'ien, in decoction.

332. Chih-shih [Trifoliate orange (Poncircus trifoliata) unripe fruit]

Properties and action: Has "han" cold properties, bitter to taste. Breaks up energy stagnation, loosens up sputum, aids digestion and relieves con-stipation.

Conditions most used for: Pulmonary congestion [with much phlegm], tightness of chest, painful "stoppage" in gastrointestinal tract [intestinal obstruction?] indigestion [or intestinal parasites?], constipation.

Preparation: For each dose, 1-3 ch'ien, in decoction.

333. Chiang [Ginger]

Properties and action: Has warming properties, acrid to taste. Warms the central region and dispels "han" cold.

Conditions most used for: Yang deficiences, slow pulse, cold extremities, deficient-cold stomach-spleen, diarrhea, moderate cold-caused abdominal pain, moist coughs.

Preparation: For each dose, 0.5-1.5 ch'ien, in decoction. (Fresh ginger tends to dispel "han"-cold, roasted ginger tends to warm and stop bleeding, but action of toasted ginger somewhat weaker than roasted ginger. Ginger peelings tend to moderate the spleen and promote diuresis; ginger juice tends to resolve phlegm and relieve constipation.)

334. Pan-ta-hai

Properties and action: Has "han" cold properties, pleasant and light to taste. Clears fevers, detoxifies, and keeps bowels open.

Conditions most used for: Dry coughs and hoarseness, aches and pains in bones, nosebleeds, "pink" [red] eye, wind-fire dominant toothache, hemorrhoids, and "fiery" triple-warmer.

Preparation: For each dose, 2-3 pan-ta-hai taken with boiled water, or prepared as decoction.

335. Sha-jen [Amomum xanthioides Wallich (fruit of)]

Properties and action: Has warming properties, acrid to taste. Stimulates energy circulation, regulates the center [central organs?], and alleviates pain.

Conditions most used for: Indigestion and gas collection in somach-spleen, cramps, abdominal distension [intestinal parasites?] hiccups, and vomiting, "han"-cold dominant diarrhea and dysentery.

Preparation: For each dose, 0.5-2 ch'ien, in decoction.

336. Nan-kua Tz'u [Seeds of Cucurbita moschata Duch. var. toonas Makino]

Properties and action: Warm, pleasant to taste. Vermicidal.

Conditions most used for: Abdominal cramps and distension due to intestinal worms.

Preparation: For each dose, 1-2 liang, eaten fresh or roasted.

337. Shen-ch'u

Properties and action: Warm, pleasant yet acrid to taste. Aids digestion, purges worms [?].

Conditions most used for: Tightness and distension of chest and abdomen, indigestion, diarrhea.

Preparation: For each dose, 1.5-3 ch'ien, in decoction.

338. Hu-lu-pa [Trigonella foenumgraecum L. (seeds of)]

Properties and action: Has warming properties, bitter to taste. Warms the yang element inherent in the kidneys, and dispels cold moisture.

Conditions most used for: Hernia pain, kidney deficiency and seminal emission, "cold" uterus, various abdominal pains, "cold" type diarrheas.

Preparation: For each dose, 1.5-3 ch'ien, in decoction.

339. Ching-chieh [Nepeta japonica Maxim.]

Properties and action: Has warming properties, acrid to taste. Diaphoretic, carminative, and blood regulator. Also hemostatic when roasted black.

Conditions most used for: Colds and fever, severe chills and headaches, sore throat, syphilitic sores, scabies, post-partum anemia, apoplexy and lockjaw, hematemesis, nosebleeds, bloody stools, metrorrhagia.

Preparation: ; For each dose, 1.5-3 ch'ien, in decoction.

340. Pien-tou [Dolichos lablab L.]

Properties and action: Slightly warming, pleasant to taste. Moderates the central organs, dispels moisture, cools [clears summer heat], and detoxifies.

Conditions most used for: Summer moisture and cholera, vomiting, diarrhea and thirst, leukorrhea, gonorrhea, alcoholic intoxication and globefish poisoning.

Preparation: For each dose, 1.5-4 ch'ien, in decoction.

341. Fu-ling [Poria cocos Wolf.]

Properties and action: Neutral, pleasant and light to taste. Breaks
down moisture and promotes diuresis, benefits the stomach/spleen, settles
nerves.

Conditions most used for: Moisture dominance in kidney deficiency, edema,
pulmonary congestion, vomiting and diarrhea, difficult urination, apprehension
and insomnia (outer covering tends to promote diuresis and reduce edema;
scarlet fu-ling tends to circulate moisture and to reduce moisture [based]
heat, "fu-shen" [the part of fungus around roots of pine tree] tends to
relieve apprehension and settle the nerves.

[No preparation]

342. Chung Ju-Shih

Properties and action: Has warming properties, pleasant to taste. Warms
the lungs, stimulates the yang, promotes lactation.

Conditions most used for: Tuberculosis cough, excessive sputum, dyspnea,
non-lactation, impotency and seminal emission, cold and numbness in back
and legs.

Preparation: For each dose, 3-5 ch'ien, in decoction.

343. Lai-fu-tsu [Raphanus sativus L. var. macropodus Makino]

Properties and action: Neutral, acrid yet pleasant to taste. Resolves
phlegm, cures intestinal parasites.

Conditions most used for: Indigestion [intestinal parasites?], abdominal
distension, hiccups, excessive sputum, asthma, abdominal pain, diarrhea.

Preparation: For each dose, 1.5-3 ch'ien, in decoction.

344. Hu-chiao [Pepper]

Properties and action: Has warm properties, acrid to taste. Warms the
central organs and dispels cold, eliminates abdominal distension and
alleviates pain.

Conditions most used for: "Han"-cold stomach caused vomiting and diarrhea,
"cold" sputum and abdominal fullness [due to marasmus or intestinal worms?],
"cold energy dominance, "cold" diarrhea and dysentery, "yin-cold" abdominal
pain, food, (fish, meat, crab, mushroom) poisoning.

Preparation: For each dose, 0.5 - 1 ch'ien, in decoction.

345. Ch'ou Mu-tan [Clerodendron species]

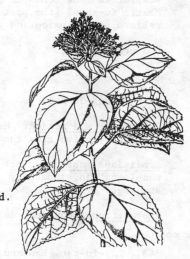

Family: Verbenaceae

Scientific name: Clerodendron bungei Steud.

Synonyms: "Ta hung-p'ao" [great scarlet cloak], "ch'ou feng-ken," "ta-hung-hua" [big red flower], "ch'ou wu-t'ung," "feng-hsien ts'ao" [meeting-the-fairy herb], "lao-ch'ung-hsiao," "ta-feng ts'ao" [big-wind herb].

Morphology: Deciduous shrub. Found growing in waste places, hillsides, and damp and shady roadsides. Height 1-2 meters. Root yellowish-white. Leaves opposite, broadly ovate, apexes acute, bases cordate, margins serrated but slightly undulate, leaf surfaces coarse, undersides smooth and shiny, emitting an unpleasant odor when crushed. In the fall, terminal red flowers appearing to form cymose inflorescence. Berry almost globose.

Properties and action: Has slightly warming properties, pleasant to taste. Expels flatus, reduces swelling, kills intestinal parasites, alleviates pain.

Conditions most used for: (1) Rheumatoid arthritis, hives; (2) traumatic injuries, hypertension, pus-forming infections; (3) filariasis, ancylostomiasis; (4) headache, toothache, pain in the abdomen.

Preparation: Roots, leaves and stems are used medicinally, 5 ch'ien - 2 liang each time in decoction; or crushed fresh leaves for external application or decocted and used for bathing affected areas.

346. Ch'ou Wu-t'ung (Hai-chou ch'ang-shan) [Clerodendron species]

Family: Verbenaceae

Scientific name: Clerodendron trichotomum Thunb.

Synonyms: "Ai t'ung-tzu," [dwarf t'ung], "yen t'ung-tzu," "pao-hua t'ung" [bubbly-flower t'ung], "pa-chiao wu-t'ung."

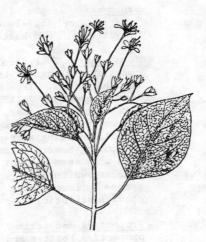

Morphology: Deciduous shrub or small tree. Found growing wild on uplands. Stem erect, height reaching about 5 meters, surface grayish-white, young branches angular. Leaves opposite, broadly ovate to elliptic, apexes acuminate, bases cuneate to truncate, margins intact or undulate-dentate. Blooms in the fall, terminal or axillary cymose inflorescences, white or pink flowers. Berry blue, flat drupe.

Properties and action: Neutral, bitter-tasting. Relieves rheumatism, lowers blood pressure.

Conditions most used for: (1) Rhematoid arthritis; (2) hypertension.

Preparation: Roots and leaves are used medicinally, 1-2 liang each time, in decoction.

347. An Eucalyptus

Family: Myrtaceae

Scientific name: Eucalyptus robusta Sm.

Synonyms: "An-shu" [eucalyptus tree], "ta-hsieh an" [big-leaf eucalyptus], "yu-chia-la," "ta-hsieh chia-li shu."

Morphology: Evergreen tree. Mostly cultivated alongside highways or out in open spaces. Tree bark thick and coarse, grooved, dull brown. Leaves alternate, coriaceous, ovate-lanceolate, apexes acuminate, bases cuneate, margins intact, emitting a fragrance when pinched, presenting numerous transparent glandular dots when seen against the sun. In summer, axillary white flowers appearing to form cymose inflorescences. Fruit a capsule, obovate-elliptic.

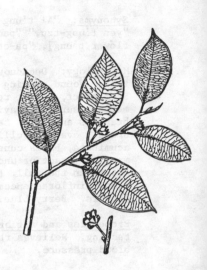

Properties and action: Has cooling properties, bitter and acrid to taste, fragrant. Clears fevers and detoxifies, resolves sputum and stops coughing, kills worms.

Conditions most used for: (1) Preventive for epidemic influenza and epidemic encephalitis, treatment for colds; (2) enteritis, dysentery; (3) cellulitis, abscesses, mastitis, erysipelas, boils, chronic ulcerations and gas gangrene.

Preparation: Leaves are used medicinally, 5 ch'ien - 1 liang each time in decoction. Fresh leaf decoction or crushed fresh leaves may be used externally.

348. She-kan [Blackberry-lily]

Family: Iridaceae

Scientific name: Belamcanda chinensis
(L.) DC.

Synonyms: "Lǎo-chun shan" [the lord's
fan], "yeh-kuei shan" [wild devil's fan],
"k'ai-hou chien" [throat-splitting sword],
"pien chu," I-shan feng," "shang-shan hu,"
"kao shou-shan," "hsien-jen chiang" [fairy's
palm], "feng-huang ts'ao," "yeh chiang"
[wild ginger], "liang-mien-tzu" [double-face].

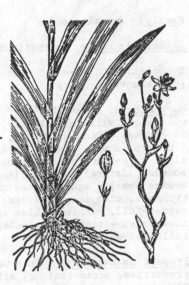

Morphology: A perennial herb. Found
growing in damp rich soil of mountain
wilds. Rhizome creeping, yellow,
numerous fibrous roots. Leaves alternate, in 2 rows, flat, in stack-of-sword
arrangement, apexes acuminate, bases
sheath-like, margins intact. In summer,
terminal racemose inflorescence appearing
with orange colored flowers, with red
spots. Fruit a capsule, obovate, 3-
angled.

Properties and action: Has "han" cold
properties, bitter-tasting, slightly
toxic. Clears fevers and detoxifies,
clears the lungs and stops coughing,
relieves blood congestion and inflammation.

Conditions most used for: (1) Sore
throat, tonsillitis, early breast
abscess; (2) coughing and wheezing,
excessive mucus production; (3) mad
dog bites, poisonous snake bites.

Preparation: Roots are used medicinally,
3-5 ch'ien each time, in decoction.

349. Hsien-niu [Morning glory]

Family: Convolvulaceae

Scientific name: Pharbitis nil Choisy.

Synonyms: "Ch'ou-niu," "hei hsien-niu" [black morning-glory].

Morphology: Annual herb. Found growing wild along village outskirts, cultivated in gardens. Stem entwining, as long as 5 meters, downy. Leaves alternate, 3-cleft to center, central lobe ovate-rounded, lateral lobes inclined-ovate, apexes sharply acute, bases cordate or truncate, with long petioles. Between summer-fall, purple or blue axillary flowers appearing, funnel-shaped. Seeds yellowish-white or black.

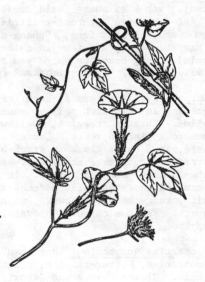

Properties and action: Has warming [hot] properties, acrid-tasting, slightly toxic. Diuretic, expectorant, and vermicidal.

Conditions most used for: (1) Ascites-caused dyspnea; (2) raspy throat and beri beri; (3) constipation and intestinal worms.

Preparation: Seeds are used medicinally, 1-3 ch'ien each time, in decoction.

350. Hsu Ch'ang-hsing [Species of milkweed family]

Family: Asclepiadaceae

Scientific name: Pycnostelma paniculatum
(Bunge.) K. Schum.

Synonyms: "Yao-chu hsiao," "tiao-ju kan"
[fishing pole], "tzu-tung ts'ao" [self-
moving grass], "lao-chun su" [the lord's
beard], "chu-hsieh hsi-hsin," "yao-pien
chu," "yao-chiao ch'ing," "lao-ching shu,"
"san-pai ken" [three hundred roots],
"shang-t'ien t'i" [ladder-to-yeaven],
"lien-ch'iao" [weeping forsythia], "I-
chih chien" [an arrow], "hsiang yao-
pien," "liao-chi chu," "hsiao-yao chu."

Morphology: Perennial herb. Found growing wild in reed thickets. Height reaching 80 cm. Subterranean rhizome short,
numerous fibrous roots. Stem slender,
erect, a few branches. Leaves opposite,
lanceolate to linear, apexes acute, bases
narrowing gradually, margins intact. In
summer, terminal or axillary small flowers,
yellow, appearing to form cymose inflorescences. Fruit a follicle, long-
angled.

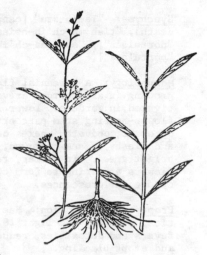

Properties and action: Has warming properties, acrid tasting, fragrant. Expels
flatus and removes moisture, stimulates
energy and blood circulation, alleviates
pain.

Conditions most used for: (1) Rhematoid
arthritis, lumbago; (2) abdominal pain
and vomiting, acute gastroenteritis,
hepatitis, liver cirrhosis ascites; (3)
snake bites; (4) traumatic injuries.

Preparation: Roots or whole plants are
used medicinally, 3-5 ch'ien each time,
in decoction.

351. Yuan-hsieh Fu-chia Ts'ao [Round-leafed Buddha's nails]

<u>Family</u>: Crassulaceae

<u>Scientific name</u>: Sedum makinoi Maxim.

<u>Synonyms</u>: "Ta-pu-szu" [cannot-beat-to-death], "tieh ma-ch'ih-hsien" [iron "portulaca"], "shih ma-ch'ih-hsien" [stony "portulaca"].

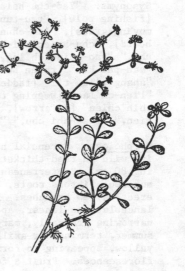

<u>Morphology</u>: A perennial fleshy herb. Found growing in alpine rock crevices, also cultivated in gardens. Lower stem creeping, flower-bearing stem part erect. Leaves opposite, obovate, apexes obtuse, thick and fleshy, bases narrowed, margins intact, bright green. In summer, terminal yellow flowers appearing to form corymb-like cymose inflorescences.

<u>Properties and action</u>: Has cooling properties, pleasant and light to taste. Clears fevers and detoxifies, reduces swelling and stops bleeding.

<u>Conditions most used for</u>: (1) Traumatic injuries, gunshot wounds, traumatic bleeding; (2) pain and swelling from boils and abscesses.

<u>Preparation</u>: The whole plant is used medicinally, usually the fresh product crushed and applied externally.

352. I-mu Ts'ao (Ch'ung-wei) [Motherwort]

Family: Labiatae

Scientific name: Leonurus heterophyllus Sweet.

Synonyms: "Hsueh-hua I-mu-ts'ao" [bloody-flower motherwort], "yu-pa ts'ai," I-mu kao," "yeh yu-ma."

Morphology: Annual or biennial herb. Found growing wild in waste places, hillsides, roadsides, and gardens. Height about 1 meter, stem erect, oblong, multi-branching. Single leaves opposite, bases rounded, lower stem leaves oval, upper stem leaves linear-lanceolate, with shallow clefts, pinnate parted or palmate parted, margins sparsely serrated. In summer, axillary flowers appearing in pink or purplish-red. Small nut 3-angled.

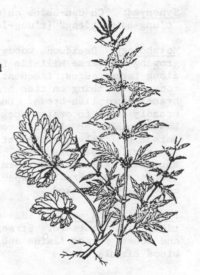

Properties and action: Has slightly warming properties, acrid and bitter to taste. Stimulates blood circulation and regulates menstrual periods. Seed helps improve vision.

Conditions most used for: (1) Menstrual irregularities, non-clearance of post-partum lochia, uterine functional bleeding; (2) atherosclerosis, hypertension; (3) conjunctivitis; (4) night blindness.

Preparation: The whole plant and fruits are used medicinally, whole plant 5 ch'ien - 1 liang, or fruit 3-5 ch'ien, each time in decoction. The whole plant can also be prepared into an extract for taking internally.

353. Ch'uan-ti Feng [Cleft-wall climbing hydrangea]

Family: Saxifragaceae

Scientific name: Schizophragma integrifolia
Oliv.

Synonyms: "Ch'uan-hsieh ch'uan-ti-feng,"
"t'ung-hsieh t'eng" [t'ung-leaf vine].

Morphology: Deciduous woody vine. Found
growing in sparse hillside forests or
along forest edges, frequently crawling on
rocks or climbing on tree branches. Small
branches purplish-brown. Leaves opposite,
broadly ovate to ovate, apexes acuminate,
bases rounded or slightly cordate, margins
intact or finely serrated at random above
mid-section, petioles long. Flowers white,
appearing terminally to form corymb inflorescences. Fruit a capsule, inverted
cone-shaped, cracked.

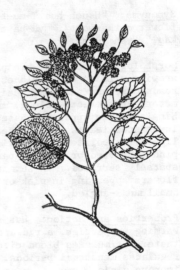

Properties and action: Has cooling properties, light to taste. Strengthens muscle
and bones, purges flatus and activates
blood circulation.

Conditions most used for: (1) Aches and
pains of extremity joints, rheumatism
associated pains and aches in bones and
muscle; (2) filariasis.

Preparation: Roots and vine are used
medicinally, 5 ch'ien - 1 liang each
time, in decoction.

354. Tieh Sao-chou [Bush-clover species]

Family: Leguminosae

Scientific name: Lespedeza cuneata (Dum. Cours) G. Don.

Synonyms: "Feng chiao wei" [wind-crossing tail], "kan-ch'ung pien" [worm-driving whip], "yeh-kuan-men" [lock-door-at-night], "hua-shih ts'ao," "hsiao yeh-kuan men."

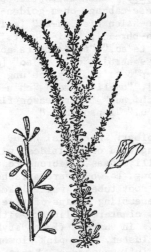

Morphology: Semi-shrub. Found growing wild in waste places, hillsides, and roadsides where sunny. Stem height reaching 1 meter, upper part with numerous branches. Leaves alternate, 3-lobed compound, leaflets linear-cuneate, apexes retuse, with small sharp points in middle, main rib on dorsal surface marked. In late summer, yellow axillary flowers appearing to form racemose inflorescences. Fruit a capsule, inclined ovate.

Properties and action: Has cooling properties, pleasant yet biting to taste. Strengthens the kidneys, kills intestinal worms, and detoxifies.

Conditions most used for: (1) Tuberculosis of testicles, hernia, enuresis; (2) dental caries toothache, infantile marasmus/ascariasis; (3) snake and dog bites, skin ulcerations; (4) dysentery, enteritis.

Preparation: The whole plant is used medicinally, 5 ch'ien - 2 liang each time, in decoction.

355. Fen-t'iao-erh Ts'ao [Colic-root, stargrass]

Family: Liliaceae

Scientific name: Aletris spicata (Thunb.)
Franch.

Synonyms: "Chin-hsien tiao pai ts'ai"
[Chinese-cabbage-on-a-golden-thread],
"chien-hsien tiao yu-mi" [maize-on-a-
golden-thread], "fei-feng ts'ao," "fei-
ching ts'ao," "fei-yung ts'ao" [lung
abscess herb], "ch'u ts'ao" [maggot grass],
"ch'u-p'o ts'ao," "ya-ch'ung ts'ao" [borer
grass], "ma-li ts'ao," "ch'u-che ts'ao,"
"szu-chi hua" [four-season flowers], "I-
wo ch'u," "I-pao ch'u."

Morphology: Perennial herb. Found
growing wild on hillsides, wild places
and hilly areas. Fibrous roots slender
and long, to which are attached numerous
small root tubers, white like maggots
and resembling grains of rice. Basal
leaves clustered, linear, with parallel
veins. In summer, flower style from
leaf cluster, with pink flowers forming
spike inflorescences. Fruit a capsule,
ellipsoid.

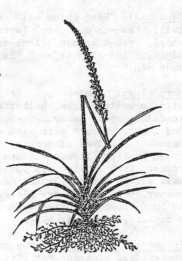

Properties and action: Neutral, pleasant tasting. Moistens the lungs and
stops coughing, kills intestinal worms.

Conditions most used for: (1) Coughing
and wheezing, or spitting up of blood
and pus associated with pulmonary diseases;
(2) ascariasis, marasmus in children.

Preparation: Roots are used medicinally,
5 ch'ien - 1 liang each time, in decoction. Several chin of the whole plant
may be chopped up and thrown into excreta
crock for killing maggots.

356. Yen-fu Mu [Sumac species]

Family: Anacardiaceae

Scientific name: Rhus semilata Murr.

Synonyms: "Wu-p'ei tzu" [sumac], "shan yen-ch'ing," "fei-t'ien wu-sung" [flying centipede], "p'o liang-san" [broken parasol], "wu-hsieh shu," "k'u-yin-chi," "ou-chieh shu," "ch'i-p'ei tzu," "pao-mu shu," "p'i-la mu-hsieh" [waxy tree-leaf], "yen-suan pai," "yen-hsiang pai."

Morphology: Small shurb. Mostly found growing along edges of hillsides forests. Height reaching 8 meters. Tree bark greyish-brown, with reddish brown spots, young branches pubescent. Leaves in spiral-like alternate arrangement, oddly pinnate-compound, leaf axis frequently winged, the site often of bug infestation. Leaflets 7-13, long ovate to oval, apexes acute, the part close to the stem rounded or cuneate, slightly inclined, margins serrated, undersurfaces densely covered by greyish-brown fine hairs, almost non-petioled. In the fall, terminal white flowers appearing to form panicle inflorescences. Drupe flat, red when ripe.

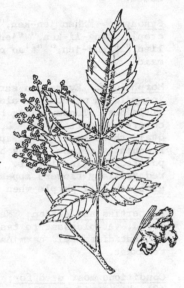

Properties and action: Has cooling properties, salty to taste. Reduces inflammation and detoxifies, stimulates blood circulation and removes stagnation and blood clots.

Conditions most used for: (1) Laryngitis, purulent inflammations, poisonous snake-bites; (2) hemoptysis; (3) stomach-ache; (4) traumatic fratures.

Preparation: Roots and leaves are used medicinally, For roots, 1-2 liang in decoction. For external purposes, a suitable amount may be used.

357. T'ao-chin Niang [Myrtle species]

Family: Myrtaceae

Scientific name: Rhodomyrtus tomentosa
Hassk.

Synonyms: "Shan jen-ken," "tou-jen" [bean
crop], "tang-li-ken," "jen-tzu," "shiu tao
lien," "kang-jen," "t'ao niang" [peach
maid].

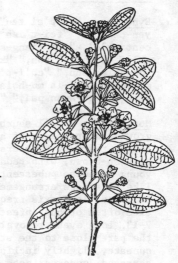

Morphology: Evergreen shrub. Found growing wild on mountains, along roadsides and
hillsides. Tender young branches densely
covered by soft hairs. Leaves opposite,
oval, three basal ribs, apexes obtuse,
frequently retuse, bases broadly cuneate-
pointed, margins intact. In summer, purplish-
red axillary flowers appearing. Berry
globose, dull purple when ripe.

Properties and action: Neutral, slightly
acrid, yet pleasant to taste. Astringent
and antidiarrheal, carminative and muscle
relaxant.

Conditions most used for: (1) Watery stools;
(2) rheumatoid arthritis.

Preparation: Roots and leaves are used
medicinally, 5 ch'ien - 1 liang, in
decoction.

358. Hai-chin-sha [Species of climbing fern]

Family: Schizaeaceae

Scientific name: Lygodium japonicum
(Thunb.) Sw.

Synonyms: "Pan-k'ou ch'ao" [pigeon's
nest], "men-t'ien-yun [sky-full-of-
clouds], "hai-yen-sha," "ha-mo t'eng"
[toad vine], "yin-chin t'eng" [sinew-
hardening vine], "mang-ku t'eng," "hsi-
niu t'eng," "wang-t'eng ts'ao," "tieh-
ssu mang" [wire netting], "tieh-hsien
ts'ao" [wiregrass], "shan-pu-ken,"
"tieh-hsien t'eng" [wire vine].

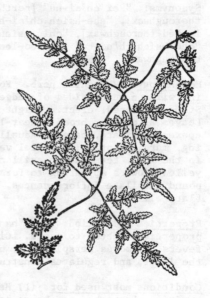

Morphology: Perennial climbing herb.
Found growing wild in shrub thickets on
hillsides and along roadsides. Stem
slender and long, frequently entwining
other objects. Leaves coriaceous,
alternate, 2-3 times pinnately compound,
leaflets alternate, in deltoid arrangement. In late summer, sori appearing on
underside of leaflet apexes, in spike
arrangement, sori ovate, sporangium
golden yellow, the "hai-chih-sha"
[golden sand describing the sporangium].

Properties and action: Has "han" cold
properties, pleasant to taste. Clears
fevers and detoxifies, promotes diuresis,
eases urination.

Conditions most used for: (1) Colds, high
fevers in infants; (2) urinary tract
infections, stone formation, and nephritic
edema.

Preparation: The whole plant or sporangium
is used medicinally. The whole plant, 5
ch'ien - 1 liang, or sporangium, 1 - 3
ch'ien, in decoction.

359. Ch'ai-hu [Thoroughwax species]

Family: Umbelliferae

Scientific name: Bupleurum chinense DC.

Synonyms: "Pei ch'ai-hu" [northern
thoroughwax], "she-hsieh ch'ai-hu" [snake-
leafed thoroughwax], "chiu-hsieh ch'ai-hu,"
"chu-hsieh ch'ai-hu" [bamboo-leaf
thoroughwax].

Morphology: Perennial herb. Found growing wild on sunny sides of sedge thickets.
Stems clustered, erect. Height 40-70 cm.
Leaves alternate, broad linear-lanceolate,
apexes acuminate, bases gradually narrowing, margins intact, parallel veins 7-9.
In the fall, terminal or axillary small
yellow flowers appearing to form compound unbellate inflorescences. Fruit
flat, ellipsoid.

Properties and action: Has "han" cold
properties, bitter to taste. Clears
fevers, promotes perspiration, neutralizes
the liver, and regulates menstruation.

Conditions most used for: (1) Headache,
vomiting, backache, parchness and bitter
taste in mouth as the result of colds;
(2) malaria; (3) stagnation of liver
energy; irregular menstruation.

Preparation: The whole plant or leaves
are used medicinally, 3-5 ch'ien each time,
in decoction.

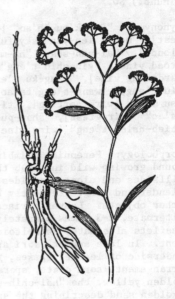

360. Hsia-k'u Ts'ao [Common selfheal]

Family: Labiatae

Scientific name: Brunella vulgaris L.

Synonyms: "Niu-k'u ts'ao" [oxen grass],
"lo-ch'ui ts'ao" [hammer grass], "tung-
feng" [east wind], "ti-k'u-niu," "teng-
lung ts'ao [lantern grass], "kuang-ku
ts'ao."

Morphology: Perennial herb. Found
growing wild along roadsides and hilly
slopes. Height reaching 40 cm. Stem
erect, oblong, multibranching, covered
by fine white hairs. Leaves opposite,
ovate or ovate-lanceolate, apexes acute,
bases cuneate, margins slightly undulate-
dentate or almost intact, both surfaces
pubescent: lower stem leaves petioled,
upper leaves non-etioled. In summer,
small terminal white or purple labiate
flowers appearing to form spike inflorescences.
Nut obovate, brown.

Properties and action: Has cooling properties, bitter to taste. Clears the liver
and relieves congestion, promotes diuresis
and reduces edema.

Conditions most used for: (1) Lymphadenopathy, goiter; (2) hypertension, conjunctivitis; (3) edema, difficult urination,
abscesses and swellings.

Preparation: Spikes are used medicinally,
2-5 ch'ien each time, in decoction.

361. T'ung Ts'ao (T'ung-t'o Mu) [Species of ginseng]

Family: Araliaceae

Scientific name: Tetrapanax papyrifera (Hook) koch.

Synonyms: "T'ung ts'ao" [pithy grass], "hua-ts'ao," "ta-t'ung."

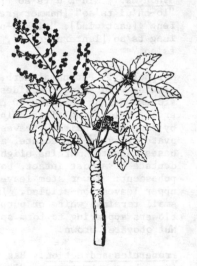

Morphology: Deciduous shrub. Found growing wild on hillsides or in woods or shrub thickets. Stem thick and sturdy, height reaching 6 meters, few branches, brittle, the pith white and spongy. Leaves rather large, alternate, clustering stem terminal, palmate 5-7 cleft, bases cordate, margins serrated; stipules 2, membranous, bases clasping the stem. In winter, axillary greenish white flowers in umbellate arrangement appearing to form large panicle inflorescences. Berry globose.

Properties and action: Has "han" cold properties, pleasant and light to taste. Clears fever, promotes diuresis, and stimulates lactation.

Conditions most used for: (1) Cystitis, difficult urination; (2) nonlactation.

Preparation: The spongy pith is used medicinally, 1-3 ch'ien, in decoction.

362. Ling-ling Ts'ao (Tsao-chui) [Species of chickweed]

<u>Family</u>: Carophyllaceae

<u>Scientific name</u>: Arenaria serpyllifolia L.

<u>Synonyms</u>: "Hsiao wu-hsin ts'ai" [small hollow greens], "ta-hsieh mi-hsi ts'ao," "o-pu-shih ts'ao" [gooseweed].

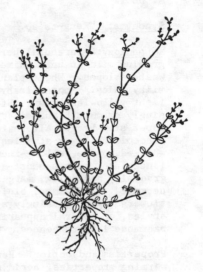

<u>Morphology</u>: Annual herb. Found growing on roadsides, along ditches, and in wild places. Whole plant pubescent. Stem branching from base, lower branch sections prostrate, upper sections erect or inclined, height 5-25 cm, all branches papillose. Leaves opposite, rounded-ovate, apexes acute, bases rounded-obtuse, margins intact. In summer, terminal white flowers appearing to form cymose inflorescences. Capsule rounded-globoid.

<u>Properties and action</u>: Has cooling properties, bitter and neutral to taste. Clears fevers and detoxifies, alleviates coughing and promotes diuresis.

<u>Conditions most used for</u>: (1) Pulmonary tuberculosis and associated coughing; (2) pterygium of the eyes.

<u>Preparation</u>: The whole plant is used medicinally, 5 ch'ien - 1 liang, in decoction. For external purposes, add leek (chiu ts'ai) and crush; insert crushed mixture into nostrils.

363. Chieh-keng [Balloon flower]

Family: Campanulaceae

Scientific name: Platycodon grandiflorum
A. DC.

Synonyms: "Keng-ts'ao."

Morphology: Perennial herb. Found
growing wild in unreclaimed places and
wasted slopes. Whole plant contains a
milky juice. Roots fleshy, cylindrical,
light yellowish-brown. Stem erect,
singly or multibranched, cylindrical.
Upper stem leaves alternate, narrowly
lanceolate; lower stem leaves 3-4
whorled, ovate, oblong-rounded to ovate-
lanceolate, apexes short-acute, bases
gradually narrowing, margins sharply
serrated. In summer, bluish-purple
flowers appearing singly at terminal
styles, or several appearing to form
racemose inflorescences. Capsule obovate.

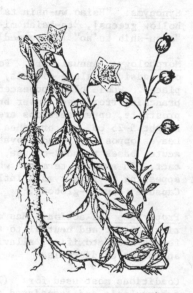

Properties and action: Has slightly
warming properties, acrid to taste.
Clears the lungs and throat, resolves
phlegm and stops coughing, reduces
swelling and promotes pus drainage.

Conditions most used for: (1) Coughing
due to acute bronchitis, pneumonia, or
colds; (2) acute laryngitis, lung abscess.

Preparation: Roots are used medicinally,
1-3 ch'ien each time, in decoction.

364.   Chi-hsueh Ts'ao [Centella species]

Family: Umbelliferae

Scientific name: Centella asiatica (L.) Urb.

Synonyms: "Kang-kuo lung," "p'o-t'ung-ch'ien" [Broken copper coin], "k'ou-tzu ts'ao" [button grass], "hsi-hsieh ma-t'i ts'ao" [small-leafed horsehoof grass], "ta-hsing-tzu ts'ao," "ma-t'i ts'ao" [horsehoof grass], "pan-pien ch'ien" [half-a-coin], "ma-chiao ts'ao," "mi-ch'ien ts'ao," "teng-chien ch'ing" [lantern grass], "yeh tung hsien-ts'ai," "ti fou-p'ing" [ground duckweed], "chin-ch'ien ts'ao" [golden coin grass], "p'an-lung ts'ao," "chieh-chieh lien," "she-p'i ts'ao" [snakeskin grass], "peng-ta-wan," "ta-hsieh ma-t'i ts'ao" [big-leaf horsehoof grass].

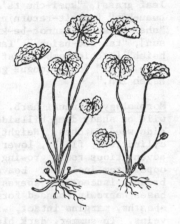

Morphology: Perennial herb. Found growing wild along roadsides, on shady and damp hillsides, or in grass thickets. Stem slender and delicate, creeping. Leaves 3-4 growing from nodes. Ovate-rounded or reniform, apexes rounded-obtuse, bases cordate, margins undulate-crenate. In summer, small purple axillary flowers appearing to form umbellate inflorescences. Fruit flat-rounded, purplish red.

Properties and action: Has cooling properties, pleasant to taste. Clears fevers and detoxifies.

Conditions most used for: (1) Upper respiratory tract infections, pleuritis; (2) acute infections and purulent inflammations.

Preparation: Whole plant is used medicinally, 5 ch'ien - 2 liang each time, in decoction; or fresh product crushed in suitable amounts for external use.

365. Ya-chih Ts'ao [Common spiderwort]

Family: Commelinaceae

Scientific name: Commelina communis L.

Synonyms: "Chu-hsieh ts'ao" [bamboo-
leaf grass], "kuei-chu ts'ao," "yeh-
huan-hun" [spirit-returning-at-night],
"shai-pu-ssu" [cannot-be-killed-by
sun], "tan chu-hsieh," "lan-hua chu-
hsieh" [orchid-bamboo-leaf], "ya-hsieh-
t'ou ts'ai" [duck-tongue grass], "chu-
hsieh lan."

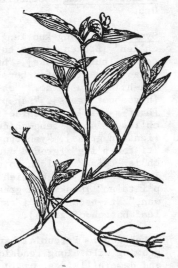

Morphology: Annual herb. Found growing
wild on shady damp hillsides or in roadside weed patches. Height 30 cm. Stem
cylindrical, fleshy, lower part creeping,
adventitious roots growing from nodes,
upper stem inclined. Leaves alternate,
broadly lanceolate, apexes short-acute,
bases narrowly rounded forming membranous
sheaths, margins intact, with parallel
veins. In summer, dark blue flowers
appearing from stem terminals to form
racemose inflorescences. Capsule ellipsoid,
slightly flat.

Properties and action: Has "han" cold
properties, slightly bitter to taste.
Clears fevers, detoxifies, and promotes
diuresis.

Conditions most used for: (1) Difficult
urination, ascites, gonorrhea; (2) colds,
malaria, laryngitis, conjunctivitis;
(3) snake and insect bites, boils and
abscesses.

Preparation: Whole plant is used medicinally, 1-2 liang of fresh product in
decoction; or suitable amount crushed
for external application.

366. Kuo-lou [Trichosanthes species]

Family: Cucurbitaceae

Scientific name: Trichosanthes kirilowii Maxim.

Synonyms: "Kua-wei" [withered melon], ch'uan-kuo-wei," "kua-wei p'i" [withered melon peel], "kua-wei jen" [withered melon seed], "t'ien-hua fen," "hua-fen," "shih-tung kua," "shih-kua-wei."

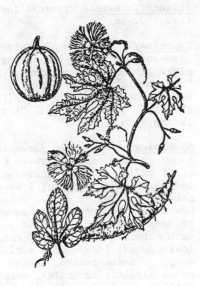

Morphology: Perennial herbaceous vine. Found growing wild along hillsides, in weed thickets, and along edges of woods. Stem tuber thick, cross-section white. Stem climbing, multibranching, surface shallowly grooved. Tendrils axillary, fine and long, 2-branching at ends. Leaves alternate, almost rounded, palmate 5-7, deeply cleft, margins sparsely serrated or notched, older leaves containing coarse spots on undersides. In summer-fall, axillary white flowers appearing. Fruit a gourd, ovate-rounded, orange-yellow when ripe. Seeds long-ellipsoid, dull yellow.

Properties and action: Has "han" cold properties, a pleasant, yet bitter taste. Clears fevers and detoxifies, promotes salivation and quenches thirst, aids pus drainage and reduces swelling.

Conditions most used for: (1) Parchness in high fever; (2) jaundice, difficult urination; (3) bronchitis, laryngitis, mumps, mastitis, and various boils and abscesses.

Preparation: Fruits, gourd, fruit peels, seeds, roots (t'ien-hua fen) are used medicinally, 2-4 ch'ien each time, in decoction. For external purposes, a suitable amount may be used.

367. Ku-sui-pu [Drynaria species]

Family: Polypodiaceae

Scientific name: Drynaria fortunei
(kze.) J. Sm.

Synonyms: "Mao-chiang" [hairy ginger],
"jou-sui-pu," "shih-pan chiang" [stony
plate ginger], "wang-chiang," "shih-chiang,"
"hou-chiang" [monkey ginger], "p'a shan
hu" [mountain-climbing tiger], "feng-
chiang," "pa-yen chiang," "hou-sheng
chiang," "hou chueh."

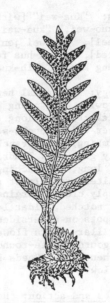

Morphology: Evergreen perennial herb.
Found growing on tree trunks or rocky
cliff walls. Rhizome creeping, fleshy
and thick, flat and long like ginger,
densely covered by golden yellow scales.
Leaves in two forms: leaves with no sori
rounded-ovate, non-petioled, overlapping
each other, greyish-brown, margins shallowly lobed; leaves with sori long oval,
deeply pinnate-parted, apexes acute,
bases slightly auricular, margins
notched, petioled, winged. Sori palm-brown,
growing on the underside of upper leaves,
with 1-3 sori arranged on both sides of
main rib.

Properties and action: Has warming properties, bitter to taste. Aids kidney function and helps knit bones, eliminates
flatulence and removes moisture.

Conditions most used for: (1) Rheumatoid
arthritis, pains and aches in back and legs;
(2) traumatic fractures; (3) neurasthenia;
(4) marasmus in infants and small children.

Preparation: Rhizomes are used medicinally,
5 ch'ien - 1 liang each time, in decoction.

368. Kuei-chien-yu (Wei-mao) [Winged spindle-tree]

Family: Celestraceae

Scientific name: Euonymus alata (Thunb.) Regel.

Synonyms: "P'i-chia shu," "lu-yueh-ling," "so-pi feng," "szu-mien feng" [four-sided wind], "szu-pa tao" [four knives], "chien-ku feng," "szu-fang feng."

Morphology: Deciduous shrub. Found growing wild on sunny slope shrub thickets. Stem height reaching 3 meters, with multiple branches, longitudinal furrows, with 2-4 brown woody wings (broad) growing out at an incline. Leaves opposite, oval or obovate, apexes short-acute or acuminate, bases sharp, margins finely serrated, main rib protruding on both surfaces. In summer, light yellowish-green small flowers appearing to form cymose inflorescences. Capsule ovoid, purple.

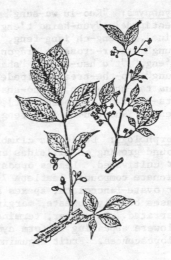

Properties and action: Has slightly warming properties, acrid and bitter to taste. Purges flatulence and dispels "han" cold, stimulates blood circulation and eliminates clots.

Conditions most used for: (1) "Cold" headache, general body aches, pruritus; (2) irregular menstruation, traumatic injuries, and other gynecological disorders.

Preparation: Stems and branches are used medicinally, 3 ch'ien - 1 liang each time, in decoction.

369. Liang-hsiao Hua [Chinese trumpet-flower]

Family: Bignoniaceae

Scientific name: Campsis chinensis Voss.

Synonyms: "Kuo-lu wu-sung" [transient centipede], "yun-hsiao t'eng" [cloud vine], "tseng-ch'iang-feng," "kuo-chiang lung" [river-crossing dragon], "ch'ing t'eng," "t'u hsu-tuan," "shang-shu wu-sung" [up-the-tree centipede], "huang-hua tao-shui-lien," "kuo-shan-lung," "ta-tou ken" [soybean root], "shou-ku-feng," "kuo-t'u-ch'iang-feng."

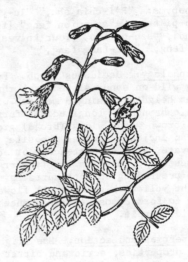

Morphology: Deciduous climbing vine. Found growing on hillsides and roadsides or cultivated. Leaves opposite, oddly pinnate compound, leaflets 7-9 ovate or ovate-lanceolate, apexes acute, bases broadly cuneate, margins sparsely serrated. In summer, terminal red flowers appearing to form cymose inflorescences. Fruit leguminous capsule.

Properties and action: Neutral, acrid and bitter to taste. Acts as a blood tonic, carminative, and diuretic.

Conditions most used for: (1) Amenorrhea, metrorrhagia, leukorrhea, and cramps in women; (2) Rheumatoid pains, traumatic injuries; (3) difficult urination; (4) pruritus and oozing dermaphytoses.

Preparation: Flowers or the whole plant is used medicinally, flowers 2-3 ch'ien, or the whole plant 3-5 ch'ien, each time, in decoction.

370. Sang Chih [Mulberry twigs]

Properties and action: Neutral, bitter to taste. Carminative and passage-clearing.

Conditions most used for: Rheumatic numbness and pain, blockage in meridians and associated pathways, spasms of hands and feet.

Preparation: For each dose, 3 ch'ien to 1 liang, in decoction.

371. Sang Shen-tzu [Mulberry achenes]

Properties and action: Slightly cooling, pleasant and tart to taste. Strengthens kidneys, aids vision, nourishes blood and yin element.

Conditions most used for: Agitation and insomnia, deafness and blurred vision, white patches in hair and beard, "hot" intestines and constipation, pain in back and knees, stiffness of muscle and joints.

Preparation: For each dose, 3-5 ch'ien, in decoction.

372. Sang Chi-sheng [Mulberry epiphyte (Ribes ambiguum?)]

Properties and action: Neutral, bitter to taste. Nourishes blood, and moisturizes sinews, eliminates flatus and clears passageways.

Conditions most used for: Backache, weakness of feet and knees, rheumatism numbness and pain, stiff joints, placenta previa [?], inadequate lactation.

Preparation: For each dose, 3-5 ch'ien, in decoction.

373. Sang P'iao hs'iao [Mantis cocoon found on mulberry trees]

Properties and action: Neutral, pleasant yet salty to taste. Strengthens kidneys and seminal control, relieves convulsions and calms nerves.

Conditions most used for: Impotency, seminal emission, premature ejaculation, enuresis, incontinence, apprehension, forgetfulness, excessive dreaming.

Preparation: For each dose, 1-3 ch'ien, in decoction.

374. Sang Hsieh [Mulberry leaves]

Properties and action: "Han" cooling, bitter yet pleasant to taste. Acts as carminative and antipyretic.

Conditions most used for: Fever from colds, headache, and bloodshot eyes, "hot" pulmonary coughing, sore throat, toothache.

Preparation: For each dose, 1.5-3 ch'ien, in decoction.

375. Sang Pai-p'i [Root bark of Morus Bombycis, Koidz]

Properties and action: "Han" cold, acrid, yet pleasant to taste. Relieves lung congestion and promotes diuresis.

Conditions most used for: "Hot" pulmonary coughing, asthma, excessive sputum production, edematous face, difficult urination.

Preparation: For each dose, 1.5-3 ch'ien, in decoction.

376. Kao-li Shen [Korean ginseng]

Properties and action: Has warming properties, pleasant to taste. Strengthens primary energy.

Conditions most used for: Weak yang energy, deficient and cold spleen and kidneys, anemia and shortness of breath, palpitation, insomnia, much dreaming, deficiency-related asthma, self perspiration, convalescent weakness, chronic sores.

Preparation: For each dose, 1-3 ch'ien, in decoction or steamed, to be taken internally.

377. Ts'an-sha (Appendix: Silkworm cocoon) [Silkworm droppings]

Properties and action: Has warming properties, pleasant yet acrid to taste. Reduces flatulence and removes moisture.

Conditions most used for: Rheumatoid aches and numbness, vomiting and diarrhea in cholera, abdominal cramps etc.

Preparation: For each dose, 1-3 ch'ien, in decoction; or a suitable amount may be boiled in water for external bathing of affected parts.

Appendix: Silkworm cocoons

Has warming properties, pleasant to taste. The cooked juice, taken internally, can quench thirst and cure polyuria. The burnt ashes taken by mouth can stop bleeding and cure blood in stools and metrorrhagia.

378. Tang Shen [Roots of Campanumaea pilosula, Franch.]

Properties and action: Neutral, pleasant to taste. Strengthens the spleen and stomach, fortifies central energy, promotes salivation and quenches thirst.

Conditions most used for: Weak spleen/stomach, inadequate pulmonary energy [shortness of breath], exhaustion, poor appetite, thirstiness.

Preparation: For each dose, 3-4 ch'ien, in decoction.

379. Kuei Chih [Cinnamon sticks]

Properties and action: Has warming properties, acrid yet pleasant to taste. Relaxes muscles and promotes hidrosis, warms the meridians and clears associated "lo" passageways.

Conditions most used for: Wind-cold symptoms, aches and pains in joints and body extremities, amenorrhea and abdominal cramps in females.

Preparation: For each dose, 5 fen to 2 ch'ien, in decoction.

380. Li-chi-ho [Seed of Nephilium litchi, Camb.]

Properties and action: Has warming properties, pleasant to taste. Warms the body center and corrects energy [balance], dispels "han" cold and alleviates pain.

Conditions most used for: Abdominal and gastric pain, pain due to hernia, and a "pins-and-needle pain" experienced by anemic women.

Preparation: For each dose, 1.5-3 ch'ien, in decoction.

381. Tieh-lo [Iron rinse water (used during forging process)]

Properties and action: Neutral, pleasant yet acrid to taste. Neutralizes the liver and relieves convulsions.

Conditions most used for: Proneness to anger and mania, fright, epilepsy, and convulsive spasms in infants.

Preparation: For each dose, 5 ch'ien to 1 liang, in decoction.

382. Ch'iu-yin [Earthworms]

Properties and action: Has "han" cold properties, salty to taste. Clears fevers, calms spasms, promotes diuresis and detoxifies.

Conditions most used for: Fevers and associated restlessness and headache, coughing, shortness of breath, convulsive spasms, difficult urination, ascites, hemiplegia.

Preparation: For each dose, 2-4 ch'ien, in decoction. Also effective for external application (dissolve with granulated sugar) over erysipelas and chronic open sores.

383. I-chih [Zingiber nigrum, Garth (fruit of)]

Properties and action: Has warming properties, acrid to taste. Warms the spleen and stomach, steadies energy and controls seminal emissions and ejaculations.

Conditions most used for: Cold-types of abdominal pain, vomiting and diarrhea, drowsiness, seminal emissions, noctrunal polyuria, placenta previa bleeding.

Preparation: For each dose, 1-3 ch'ien, in decoction.

384. Hai Ko [Oyster]

Properties and action: Neutral, bitter and salty to taste. Clears the lungs, and resolves phlegm, lowers energy [rise] and relieves asthma, moisturizes and dispels congestion.

Conditions most used for: "Pulmonary-heat" hemoptysis, dyspnea, tumors, stomach-ache, pain in chest and sides.

Preparation: For each dose, 3-5 ch'ien, in decoction.

385. Hai Tsao [Seaweed]

Properties and action: Has "han" cold properties, bitter and salty to taste. Resolves phlegm and relieves congestion, clears fevers, and promotes diuresis.

Conditions most used for: Scrophula, tumors, cysts, edema, congestion and hydrocele.

Preparation: For each dose, 1.5-3 ch'ien, in decoction.

386. Lien-tzu [Lotus seeds]

Properties and action: Neutral, pleasant yet acrid to taste. Strengthens spleen and cultivates the heart, controls peristalsis, and stabilizes sperm [seminal control?].

Conditions most used for: Spleen deficient diarrhea, excess dreaming and seminal emissions, metrorrhagia and leukorrhea.

Preparation: For each dose, 2-5 ch'ien, in decoction, or as food after cooking.

387. Lien-tzu Hsin [Fruit of Nelumbo nucifera]

Properties and action: Has "han" cold properties, bitter to taste. Calms the heart and reduces fever.

Conditions most used for: Agitation and hematemesis.

Preparation: For each dose, 5 fen to 1 ch'ien, in decoction.

388. Lien-fang [Floral receptacle of Nelumbo nucifera]

Properties and action: Has warming properties, bitter and acrid to taste. Resolves clots and stops bleeding.

Conditions most used for: Abdominal cramps (associated with blood clots), post-partum non-expulsion of amniotic sac, metrorrhagia, bloody discharge.

Preparation: For each dose, 1.5-3 ch'ien, in decoction.

- 863 -

389. Ch'uan-shan-chia [Crocodile]

Properties and action: Has slightly "han" chill properties, salty to taste.
Stimulates blood circulation, reduces swelling, aids pus drainage, and
promotes lactation.

Conditions most used for: Rheumatism-related numbness and pain, muscular
spasms, amenorrhea, ulcers and abscesses, scrophula, non-lactation.

Preparation: For each dose, 1.5-3 ch'ien, in decoction.

390. Yuan-tan [Massicot]

Properties and action: Has slightly "han" cold properties, acrid tasting.
Stops vomiting and calms nerves.

Conditions most used for: Vomiting and convulsions, convulsive spasms,
external sores, body odor.

Preparation: For each dose, 2-3 fen, in decoction. A suitable amount may
be used for external pruposes.

391. Ch'in-chiu [Justicia gendarussa, L.]

Properties and action: Neutral, bitter and acrid to taste. Relieves
flatulence and dispels moisture, clears fevers and promotes diuresis,
energizes blood and relaxes muscles.

Conditions most used for: Rheumatoid aches and numbness, muscular spasms,
jaundice, bloody stools, bone pains, marasmus [or intestinal parasites?] in
small children.

Preparation: For each dose, 1-3 ch'ien, in decoction.

392. Ya-tan-tzu [Brucea javanica, (Linne) Merri (fruit)]

Properties and action: Has "han" cold properties, bitter to taste. "Dries"
[counteracts] moisture, and kills insects.

Conditions most used for: Chronic diarrhea and dysentery, malaria, hemorrhoids,
external treatment of wens.

Preparation: For each dose, 5 to 20, to be taken with dried fruit of
longana. For external purposes, a suitable amount may be used.

393. Ho Hsieh [Waterlily leaves]

Properties and action: Neutral, bitter to taste. Raises stomach energy,
loosens up clots and stops bleeding.

Conditions most used for: Summer moisture and diarrhea, hematemesis,
epistaxis, metrorrhagia, bloody stools, bloody vaginal discharge.

Preparation: For each dose, 1-3 ch'ien, in decoction.

394. Yeh Shan-cha [Hawthorn species]

Family: Rosaceae

Scientific name: Crataegus cuneata Sieb et Zucc.

Synonyms: "Shan-cha" [hawthorn], "shan-cha," "wu-t'ai-shan," "yeh se-li" [wild acrid pear].

Morphology: Deciduous shrub. Found growing on sunny spots of upland wilds. Height attaining 1.5 meters. Stem with multiple branches, stiff thorns sparsely found on branches. Leaves alternate, obovate or obovate-elliptical, apexes acute, bases cuneate, margins irregularly serrated or shallowly parted, stipules almost ovate. In summer, white flowers appearing at terminal branches to form corymb inflorescences. Fruit orange-colored, globose, edible, tart and sweet when ripe.

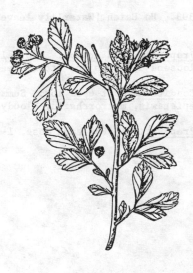

Properties and action: Has slightly warming properties, sour yet pleasant to taste. Aids digestion, stimulates blood circulation and stops diarrhea.

Conditions most used for: (1) Indigestion, infantile marasmus; (2) mentrual cramps, diarrhea and dysentery; (3) hernia.

Preparation: Roots and fruits are used medicinally, 2-4 ch'ien each time, in decoction.

395. Yeh Pai-ho [Rattlebox species]

<u>Family</u>: Leguminosae

<u>Scientific name</u>: Crotalaria sessiliflora
L.

<u>Synonyms</u>: "Hua ts'ao," "hua-ku ts'ao"
[bone-dissolving grass].

<u>Morphology</u>: Annual herb. Found growing
mostly in grass thickets on sunny hillsides. Stem cylindrical, height reaching
2 feet, with branches. Leaves alternate,
long elliptic-lanceolate, apexes acute,
bases cuneate, leaf surfaces dark green,
non-pubescent; leaf underside light
green, pubescent like the stem. In
summer-fall, dense cluster of disc-like
flowers appearing at terminal branches,
fresh purple, to form spike inflorescences.
Legume long-rounded, nonpubescent.

<u>Properties and action</u>: Neutral, pleasant
to taste. Serves as a detoxifier and a
softening agent.

<u>Conditions most used for</u>: (1) Bones
caught in throat; (2) intoxication
due to DDT, 666, arsenic, poisonous
mushrooms, and food poisoning; (3)
boils and sores.

<u>Preparation</u>: The whole plant is used
medicinally, 0.5-1.5 ch'ien each time,
pulverized and mixed with boiled
water for taking by mouth.

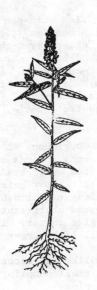

396. Yeh Nan-kua [Wild species of Spurge family]

Family: Euphorbiaceae

Scientific name: Glochidion puberum (L.) Hutch.

Synonyms: "Tieh chan-pan" [iron chop-block], "Tieh men-san" [iron gate], "man-t'ou kuo," "chi-p'i yen-shu," "hsueh-pao mu" [blood-bubble shrub], "tieh niu-tsao lan," "men-tzu shu" [door tree], "chi-pa shu," "suan-p'an tzu" [abacus], "tu-t'ung ta-yuan-shuai" [commander-in-chief], "mao-tzu t'o-t'o," "hung nan-kua shu."

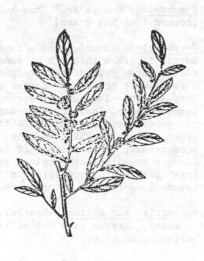

Morphology: Deciduous shrub. Found growing on sunny uplands or shrub thickets. Stem multi-branching, densely covered by soft brown hairs. Leaves alternate, long elliptic or oblong-rounded, apexes short-acute and somewhat obtuse, margins intact. In spring-summer, small light green flower appearing from leaf axils. Fruit a capsule, shape like an abacus bead, some-what like a small pumpkin, reddish purple when ripe.

Properties and action: Neutral, slightly bitter and acrid to taste. Clears fevers, detoxifies, dispels clots.

Conditions most used for: (1) Colds, influenza, malaria, laryngitis; (2) dysentery, enteritis; (3) sores and abscesses, poisonous snakebites; (4) traumatic injuries, amenorrhea, arteritis; (5) hernia (use fruit).

Preparation: Roots, stems, leaves or fruits are used medicinally, 2 ch'ien-2 liang each time, in decoction.

397. Yeh Hsiang-ju

Family: Labiatae

Scientific name: Orthodon fordu Maxim.

Synonym: "Hsi-hsieh ch'i-hsing-chien"
[small-leaf seven-starred sword].

Morphology: Annual herb. Found growing in virgin wilds, roadsides, also
cultivated. Whole plant highly fragrant. Stem height 30-60 cm, oblong,
multibranching, purplish-red. Leaves
opposite, linear-lanceolate, apexes
acuminate, bases narrowed, margins
serrated, with short petiole. In
fall, terminal or axillary small pink
flower appearing to form racemose inflorescences. Small nut growing
inside bell-shape calyx.

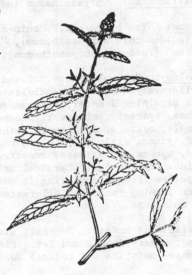

Properties and action: Has cooling
properties, acrid to taste, fragrant.
Breaks up clots and alleviates pain,
resolves gonorrheal [?] discharge and
neutralizes heat.

Conditions most used for: (1) Traumatic
bruises and pain; (2) poisonous snake
bites; (3) heatstroke fever; (4)
itching from oozing rash.

Preparation: The whole plant is used
medicinally, 3-5 ch'ien each time, in
decoction.

398. Yeh Chu-hua [Wild chrysanthemum]

Family: Compositae

Scientific name: Chrysanthemum indicum L.

Synonyms: "Yeh huang-chu," "chiñ-ch'ien chu" [golden coin chrysanthemum], "lu-pien chu" [roadside chrysanthemum].

Morphology: Perennial herb. Found growing wild everywhere. Stems clustered, height attaining 1 meter, with numerous branches, sparsely pubescent. Leaves alternate, ovate or long-ovate, pinnately parted, pinnae again shallowly pinnate-parted, apexes acute, bases cuneate, with stipules. In the fall, terminal and axillary yellow flowers appearing in corymb pattern forming racemose inflorescences. Fruit an achene.

Properties and action: Neutral, bitter-tasting, Clears fevers and detoxifies, eliminates moisture and reduces swelling.

Conditions most used for: (1) Swelling from boils and abscesses; (2) epidemic encephalomyelitis; (3) hypertension.

Preparation: The whole plant is used medicinally, 5 ch'ien- 1 liang in decoction each time. A suitable amount may be prepared for external use.

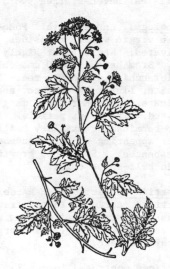

399. Huang Ching [Chaste tree species]

Family: Verbenaceae

Scientific name: Vitex negundo L.

Synonyms: "Chiang ts'ao" [sauce grass],
"huang-ching-t'iao," "t'u ch'ang-shan,"
"ma t'eng" [horse vine], "chiang-tzu hsieh"
[ginger leaf], "chiang ching-hsieh," "ching
ch'ai-shu," "ching-pa-ch'ai," "huang-chin
t'iao," "yang-chin t'iao."

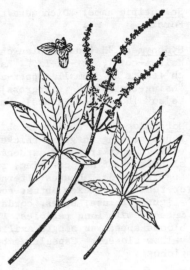

Morphology: Deciduous shrub. Found
growing wild in uplands and roadsides.
Stem branches oblong, greyish brown, densely pubescent. Leaves opposite, palmate
compound, with long petioles; leaflets
5, sometimes as few as 3, oval-lanceolate,
apexes long-acute, bases cuneate, margins
intact or shallowly and coarsely serrate,
leaf undersides greyish-white, densely
pubescent. In summer, terminal light
purple flowers appearing to form panicle
inflorescences. Drupe, brown globoid.

Properties and action: Neutral, acrid
and bitter to taste, fragrant. Clears
fevers, eliminates moisture, alleviates
diarrhea and dysentery.

Conditions most used for: (1) As a
malaria preventive, and for treatment
of colds, wheezing and coughing; (2)
acute bacterial dysentery, gastroenteritis.

Preparation: Fruit, leaves, and roots
are used medicinally: the dried and
pulverized fruits 2-3 ch'ien mixed with
boiled water each time for taking
internally, or roots and leaves 5 ch'ien
- 1 liang prepared in decoction.

400. Huang-tan Ts'ao [Dichondra species]

Family: Convolvulaceae

Scientific name: Dichondra repens, Forst.

Synonyms: "Hsiao pan-pien-ch'ien" [small half-a-coin], "ti-pu-la," "hsiao t'ung-ch'ien ts'ao" [small copper-cash grass], "hsing-tzu ts'ao" [stargrass], "ma-chiao ts'ao" [horse-hoof grass], "ma-t'i chin."

Morphology: Perennial climbing herb. Found growing in grass thickets along village outskirts and gardens. Stem slender and fine, creeping, roots growing from node. Leaves alternate, rounded or reniform, apexes obtuse-rounded and slightly retuse, bases, cordate, margins intact, with long petioles. In summer, blooms appear as single axillary small yellow flowers. Capsule membranous, globuse.

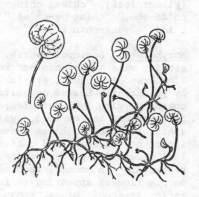

Properties and action: Has neutral properties, acrid to taste. Clears fevers, promotes diuresis, and stops bleeding.

Conditions most used for: (1) Jaundice; (2) dysentery; (3) mastitis; (4) hemoptysis.

Preparation: The whole plant is used medicinally, 5 ch'ien- 1 liang each time, in decoction.

401. Huang Tu [Yam species]

Family: Dioscoreaceae

Scientific name: Dioscorea bulbifera L.

Synonyms: "Huang-yao-tzu" [yellow kidney], "mao shen-tzu," "huang-yao," "ma-ch'iao-tan" [sparrow's egg], "t'ieh ch'en-t'o" [iron-scale weight], "mao-shih-erh," "yeh mien-shu," "yeh-chiao pan-shu."

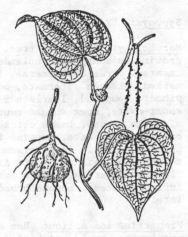

Morphology: Perennial herb. Found growing in shrub thickets in waste places, on hillsides, and along stream banks. Root tuber thick and large, fat globoid, with numerous fibrous roots. Stem climbing and entwining, length reaching 10 meters, smooth and non-pubescent. Leaves alternate, rounded or ovate-rounded, apexes sharply acute, bases broadly cordate, margins intact, leaf veins 7-9, very noticeable, all originating from base: bulbils in axils, brownish yellow and globose, with many nodules. In late summer, white purplish axillary flowers appearing to form panicle inflorescence. Capsule oblong-rounded, winged.

Properties and action: Has neutral properties, bitter to taste, slightly toxic. Clears fevers and detoxifies, reduces moisture and resolves phlegm.

Conditions most used for: (1) Hernia, goitre, food poisoning; (2) purulent inflammation.

Preparation: Root tubers and bulbils are used medicinally, 2-5 ch'ien each time, in decoction.

402. Huang T'an

Family: Leguminosae

Scientific name: Dalbergia hupeana
Hance.

Synonym: "T'an shu."

Morphology: Deciduous tree. Found
growing on sunny wild uplands or cultivated. Tree bark coarse, lenticels
marked. Leaves alternate, oddly
pinnate compound, leaflets 9-12,
short-ovate, apex obtuse-rounded or
slightly retuse, bases obtuse-rounded
or broadly cuneate, margins intact,
petioles short. In late summer,
terminal or axillary white disk like
flowers appearing to form panicle
inflorescences. Legume broad spatulate.

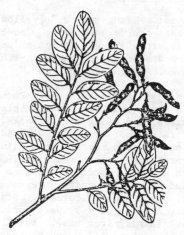

Properties and action: Has neutral
properties, acrid and bitter to taste,
slightly toxic. Used as an insecticide,
it also resolves bruises, breaks up
clots, and reduces swelling.

Conditions most used for: (1) Traumatic
injuries; (2) abscesses and boils.

Preparation: Leaves are used medicinally. To kill maggots, leaves are
crushed fine and thrown into the excreta.
For external use the leaves are crushed
and applied over affected parts; or
leaves may be crushed fine, then mixed with
water before application.

403. She-ch'uang [Cnidium species]

Family: Umbelliferae

Scientific name: Cnidium monnieri (L.) Cuss.

Synonyms: "Ch'ung ch'uang-tzu," "yeh hui-hsiang" [wild fennel].

Morphology: Perennial herb. Found growing alongside ditches and field edges. Young stem prostrate on ground like a snake, becoming erect with continuous growth, and showing longitudinal furrows and humps in midair. Leaves alternate, 2-3 times pinnately compound, final lobes linear-lanceolate, apexes acute non pubescent on both surfaces, leaf petioles expanded toward their stem attachment sections. Blooms in summer - fall, white flowers appearing to form compound umbellate inflorescences, terminal or lateral. Fruit broadly ovate.

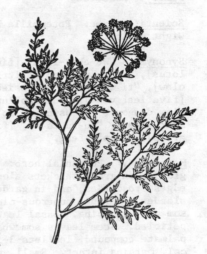

Properties and action: Has warming properties, acrid and bitter to taste, slightly toxic. Dispels "han" cold, eliminates flatulence and kills worms.

Conditions most used for: (1) Trichomonas vaginitis, leukorrhea; (2) uterine displacement; (3) weeping eczema of the skin and scrotum.

Preparation: Fruits or the whole plants are used medicinally, 1-3 ch'ien each time, in decoction. For external purposes, 5 ch'ien - 1 liang may be prepared in decoction and used for bathing affected parts.

404. She-han [Cinque-foil, five-finger]

Family: Rosaceae

Scientific name: Potentilla kleiniana
Wight et Arn.

Synonyms: "Wu-chao-lien" [five-claw
lotus], "hsiao wu-chao" [little five-
claw], "ti wu-chao," "wu-hsieh t'eng"
[five leaf vine], "wu-chao lung" [five-
claw dragon], "wu-hsing ts'ao" [five-
star grass], "wu-hu ts'ao" [five-tiger
grass], "wu-p'i feng."

Morphology: Perennial herb. Found
growing in grass thickets along field
edges, roadsides, and in gardens. Stem
slender and long, numerous-clustered,
somewhat creeping. Basal leaves long-
petioled. Stem leaves somewhat smaller,
palmate compound, leaflets 3-5, elliptical, margins intact. Small yellow flowers
appearing in summer, forming panicle-
like cymose inflorescences. Achene
wrinkled on surface.

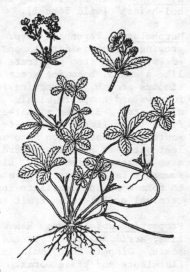

Properties and action: Has slightly "han"
cold properties, bitter to taste. Cools
fevers and detoxifies.

Conditions most used for: (1) Colds and
influenzea, sore throat; (2) traumatic
injuries; (3) poisonous snakebites.

Preparation: The whole plant is used
medicinally, 3-5 ch'ien each time in
decoction.

405. She Mei [Indian strawberry]

Family: Rosaceae

Scientific name: Duchesnea indica (Andr.) Focke.

Synonyms: "Ti-chin" [ground tapestry], "san-hsien ts'ao" [three-fairy grass], "wu-chao lung" [five-claw dragon], "tao-chun t'eng," "wu-lung ts'ao" [five-dragon grass], "wu-chao feng," "she-niao pao," "she-pao ts'ao" [snake bubble grass], "lung-han chu," "san-chia p'i," "san-chao feng," "feng-huang ts'ao" [phoenix grass], "san-ku feng," "sai-lung chu," "kuo-chiang lung" [river-crossing dragon], "san-chao ts'ao," "san-hsieh she-mei ts'ao" [three-leafed snake-berry grass], "wu-chih hu" [five-fingered tiger], "wu-p'i feng," "san-chao lung."

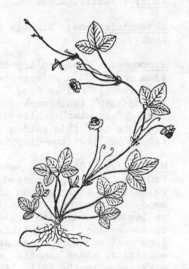

Morphology: Perennial herb. Found creeping in open woods, waste places, field edges, and roadsides. Whole plant covered by white hairs. Yellowish-white fibrous roots, slender stem noded, with adventitious roots growing from nodes; also branching from nodes. Palmate compound leaves 3-parted, the two lateral lobes somewhat smaller than central lobe, rhombic-ovate or obovate, margins serrated, basal margins intact. In late spring, single yellow flowers appearing from leaf axils. Red achenes growing in clusters similar to strawberry in shape.

Properties and action: Has cooling properties, slightly pleasant to taste, slightly toxic. Clears fevers and detoxifies, breaks up clots and reduces swelling.

Conditions most used for: (1) Boils and abscesses, weeping eczema, and ringworm; (2) stomatitis, laryngitis, acute tonsillitis; (3) snake and insect bites, traumatic injuries.

Preparation: The whole plant is used medicinally, 5 ch'ien - 1 liang, in decoction; or a suitable amount of the fresh plant may be crushed for external application or decocted for use to bathe affected parts.

406. Ch'ang-shan [Alum root]

Family: Saxifragaceae

Scientific name: Dichroa febrifuga
Lour.

Synonyms: "Huang ch'ang-shan" [yellow
alum root], "t'u ch'ang-shan" [native
alum root], "chi-ku feng," "chi-ku
ch'ang-shan" [chicken-bone alum root],
"pai ch'ang-shan" [white alum root],
"ta chin-tao" [big golden sword], "chi-
fen ts'ao" [chicken-droppings grass].

Morphology: Deciduous semi-shrub.
Found growing wild in open woods,
valleys and along stream edges. Root
woody and hard, cylindrical, surface
yellowish-brown, also yellowish on
cross-section. Single leaves opposite.
long oval or lanceolate. apexes
acuminate. bases cuneate. margins
serrated. In the fall. light blue
flowers appearing terminally or from
leaf axils to form umbellate inflorescences.
Berry blue and globose.

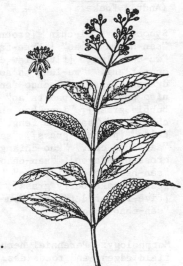

Properties and action: Has "han" cold
properties, bitter tasting, toxic. Used
as an antimalarial, expectorant and
sputum loosener, and as an emetic.

Conditions most used for: (1) Malaria;
(2) bronchitis.

Preparation: Roots and leaves are used
medicinally, 2-3 ch'ien, in decoction.

407. Ma-k'ou P'i-tzu Yao [Prickly ash species]

Family: Rutaceae

Scientific name: Zanthoxylum simulans var. podocarpum Huang.

Synonyms: "Tsung-kuan p'i," "men-shan hsiang" [fragrant mountain], "szu-p'i-ma," "tu chiao-tzu," "hsiao-shan-chiao" [small mountain pepper], "hung shan-chiao" [red mountain pepper], "yeh hua-chiao" [wild flowering pepper], "shan hu-chiao."

Morphology: Deciduous shrub. Found growing in virgin wilds, hillsides, or in open woods. Stem height 2-3 meters, greyish brown, thorns slender and long, tips sharply pointed, bases flat and broad. Leaves alternate, oddly pinnate-compound, leaflets 7-15, oval-lanceolate, apexes pointed, retuse, bases cuneate, margins finely dentate, almost non-petioled, leaf axils thorny. In summer, small light green flowers appearing from leaf axils to form racemose inflorescenses. Fruit a follicle, red.

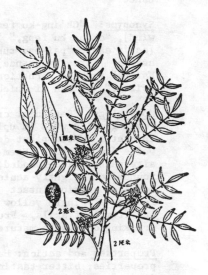

Properties and action: Has warming properties, acrid and biting to taste. Eliminates flatulence and stimulates the stomach, removes excess cold and alleviates pain, reduces swelling and kills worms.

Conditions most used for: (1) Rheumatism-related aching bones, traumatic injuries; (2) sore throats; (3) snakebites.

Preparation: Roots, stems, and bark are used medicinally, 1 ch'ien each time, in decoction, or chewed before swallowing.

408. Mien-mao Ma-tou-ling [Downy birthwort]

Family: Aristolochiaceae

Scientific name: Aristolochia mollissima
Hance.

Synonyms: "Ch'ing-ku feng" [bone-purifying
wind], "ch'un-ku feng," "mao-erh-t'o"
[cat's ear], "pai-mao tun," "mao-t'un
hsiang" [furry fragrance], "ti ting-
hsiang" [ground carnation], "huang mu-
hsiang," "ch'uan ti-chieh."

Morphology: Perennial crawling herb.
Found growing wild in uplands and bamboo
thickets. Whole plant densely pubescent,
white downy hairs. Stem climbing. Leaves
alternate, ovate-rounded, apexes obtuse-
rounded or slightly acute, bases deeply
cordate, margins intact, with petioles.
In summer, single yellow flowers appearing from leaf axils. Fruit a capsule,
cracking open when mature, seeds flat.

Properties and action: Has neutral
properties, bitter-tasting. Relieves
flatulence, moisturizes the body system,
opens up the meridians and activates
associated passageways, alleviates pain
and reduces swelling.

Conditions most used for: Rheumatoid aches
and pains.

Preparation: The whole plant is used
medicinally, 1 liang in decoction; or
plant may be steeped in wine before being
taken internally.

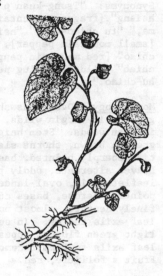

409. Mei-hsieh Tung-ch'ing [Holly species]

Family: Aquifoliaceae

Scientific name: Ilex asprolla Champ.

Synonyms: "Pai-chieh ch'a" [hundred-remedy tea], "ch'en-hsing shu," "ch'en-hsing-tzu ch'ai," [star wood], "pai-ch'ai," "ch'en-pai-ken" [weight-a-hundred roots], "kang mei" [mound plum], "pai-chieh ken" [hundred-remedy root], "huo-t'an mu," "tien-ch'en hsing," "ch'en-hsing mu," "t'u kan-ts'ao" [local lico-rice], "pai-tien ch'en" [white-spotted weighing scales].

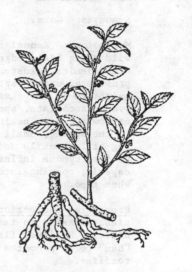

Morphology: Deciduous shrub. Found growing on hillsides, wild places, open woods or in shrub thickets. Subterranean root woody, yellowish white. Stem with numerous branches, bark bluish-green, with numerous scattered white lenticels, shaped like scale marks. Leaves alternate, ovate, obovate or elliptical, apexes acuminate or sharply acute, bases rounded, margins finely serrated. In spring-summer, yellowish white flowers appearing from leaf axils to form cymose inflorescences. Drupe globose, black when ripe.

Properties and action: Has "han" cold properties, bitter-tasting though slightly pleasant. Clears fevers and detoxifies, promotes salivation and quenches thirst, reduces swelling and resolves clots [bruises].

Conditions most used for: (1) High fever in colds, laryngitis, acute tonsillitis; (2) traumatic injuries, boils and abscesses.

Preparation: Roots are used medicinally, 5 ch'ien - 2 liang, in decoction. For external purposes a suitable amount may be used.

410. Chiao-she Ts'ao [Starwort species; Bird's tongue grass]

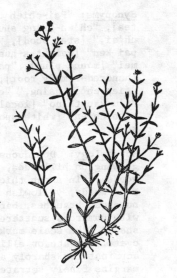

Family: Carophyllaceae

Scientific name: Stellaria alsine.

Synonyms: None.

Morphology: Annual herb. Found growing
wild along field edges and roadsides.
Stem slender, clustered, lower section
prostrate, upper part branching sparsely,
height 20-30 cm. Leaves small, opposite,
ovate-lanceolate, apexes acuminate, bases
narrowing, margins intact, non-petioled.
In the spring, small white flowers appearing at leaf axils and terminal branches
to form cymose inflorescences. Fruit a
capsule, opening into a 6-split crack
when ripe.

Properties and action: Has warming properties, pleasant to taste though slightly
bitter. Relieves flatulence and dispels
"han" cold, promotes hidrosis and detoxifies.

Conditions most used for: (1) Colds; (2)
traumatic injuries; (3) poisonous snakebites; (4) pimples.

Preparation: The whole plant is used
medicinally, 3-5 ch'ien each time in
decoction or in decoction mixed with
wine. For external purposes, the fresh
herb may be crushed for application
over affected parts.

411. Tan Chu-hsieh [Light bamboo leaf]

Family: Gramineae

Scientific name: Lophatherum gracile
Brongn.

Synonyms: "Chu-hsieh mai-tung" [bamboo
leafed lily turf], "chu-hsieh ts'ao"
[bamboo grass], "shui chu-hsieh" [aquatic
bamboo leaf].

Morphology: Perennial herb. Found growing along hillsides. Rhizomes almost woody,
fibrous roots expanded thick and fleshy like
spindles at tips or midsections. Stem
slender and long, rising in midair, yellow,
with longitudinal furrows. Leaves alternate,
lanceolate or broadly lanceolate, apexes
acuminate, bases sheathed and clasping
stem, ribs parallel, both surfaces pubescent,
white, noded at leaf ochrea. In summer,
small green terminal flowers appearing to
form panicle inflorescences. Caryopsis
dark brown.

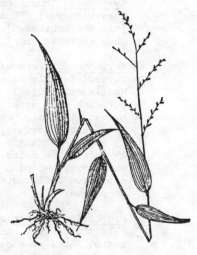

Properties and action: Has "han" cold
properties, bitter to taste. Clears
fevers, dispels feelings of agitation
and apprehension, promotes diuresis.

Conditions most used for: (1) Measles,
influenza, heatstroke; (2) restlessness
and insomnia in fevers, thirst, sore
throat, painful and difficult urination.

Preparation: Roots and leaves are used
medicinally, 1-3 ch'ien in decoction.

412.   Chu-hua [Chrysanthemum]

Family: Compositae

Scientific name: Chrysanthemum morifolium,
Ramat.

Synonyms: "Huang chu-hua" [yellow golden
chrysanthemum], "huang-kan-ch'u," "ch'a-ku"
[tea chrysanthemum], "Hang chu-hua" [Hang-
chow chrysanthemum].

Morphology: Perennial herb. Whole plant
covered densely by white downy hairs.
Mostly cultivated. Stem erect, slightly
purplish red, upper section multi-branching.
Leaves alternate, ovate-rounded to lanceolate, apexes obtuse, bases cuneate, pinnately lobed, margins serrated, undersides covered
by soft white hairs. Blooms in the fall,
white, yellow, pink flowers appearing in
capitulum inflorescences. Achene 4-angled,
no pappus.

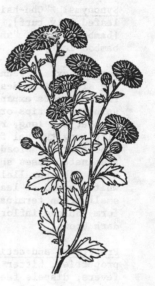

Properties and action: Has slightly "han"
cold properties, bitter yet pleasant to
taste. Acts as a carminative, antipyretic,
and detoxifying agent.

Conditions most used for: (1) Headache and
dizziness associated with wind-caused
fevers; (2) tinnitus, conjunctivitis; [or
trachoma] (3) boils and abscesses.

Preparation: Flowers are used medicinally,
2-4 ch'ien each time in decoction.

413. Chi Hua

Family: Hamamelidaceae

Scientific name: Loropetalum chinense,
Oliv.

Synonyms: "Chih-mu shu," "yang-yung shu,"
"t'u ch'iang- hua" [local wallflower], "t'u-
chiang shu" [local laquer tree?].

Morphology: Evergreen shrub or small tree.
Found growing along stream banks, hilly
slopes and roadsides. Back of stem and
branches deep brown. Leaves alternate,
ovate or oval, slightly inclined, margins
intact or finely serrated. In spring,
terminal white flowers appear. Fruit
a brown and globose capsule.

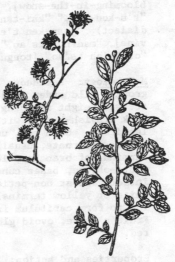

Properties and action: Has neutral
properties, acrid-tasting and slightly
bitter. Serves as a hemostatic, lung
purifier, and a detoxifying agent.

Conditions most used for: (1) Hematemesis
due to traumatic injuries, wound bleeding;
(2) coughing in tuberculosis; (3) dysenteries
and enteritis.

Preparation: The whole plant is used
medicinally, 3-5 ch'ien each time, in
decoction. For external purposes leaves
are crushed and pulverized for sprinkling
over wounds.

414. Hsueh-tung Hua (Jui-hsiang) [Mezereum]

Family: Thymelaceae

Scientific name: Daphne odora Thunb.

Synonyms: "Hsueh-li k'ai hua" [flowers
blooming-in-the-snow], "hsueh-hua p'i,"
"t'u-kou-p'i," "kai-tan-hsu" (Tung [minority]
dialect), "juan-ken t'eng" [sinew-softening
vine], "man-hua ts'ao," "shan-mien-p'i,"
"oh-hsieh ts'ao" [tongue-grass].

Morphology: Deciduous shrub. Found
growing wild under shade of upland
trees. Height reaching 2 meters. Tree
bark grayish-brown, with noticeable
lenticels. Stem red, usually fork-branched.
Leaves alternate, usually clustered at
terminal of branches, long oval, apexes
acute-obtuse, bases cuneate, margins
intact, almost non-petioled. In spring,
white or yellow terminal flowers appearing to form capitulum inflorescences.
Fruit a drupe, ovoid globose, bright
red.

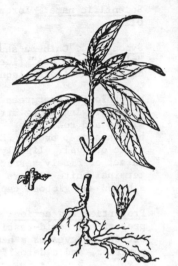

Properties and action: Neutral, acrid-
tasting. Relaxes muscles and connects
bones, reduces swelling and alleviates
pain, detoxifies and clears vision.

Conditions most used for: (1) Sciatica;
(2) traumatic injuries, backache; (3)
numbness of throat, skin diseases.

Preparation: Stem and flowers are used
medicinally, 3-5 ch'ien each time, in
decoction.

415. Man-t'o-lo

Family: Solanaceae

Scientific name: Datura metel L. f. alba.

Synonyms: "Nao-yang hua" [goat- 'provoking' flower], "shan ch'ieh-erh" [alpine eggplant], "la-pa hua" [trumpet flower], "feng ch'ieh-erh," "yang chin-hua," "tsui-hsien t'ao" [drunken-fairy peach].

Morphology: Erect and sturdy annual herb. Mostly found growing on hillsides, village outskirts, roadsides and river banks in sunny locations. Stem erect, cylindrical, young branches slightly purplish. Single leaves alternate, upper leaves frequently opposite, ovate-rounded, apexes acute, bases unequal on both sides, margins slightly undulate or irregularly shallow-parted. In summer, white trumpet-shaped flowers appearing singly at branch or leaf axils. Fruit a globose capsule, with coarse and short thorns.

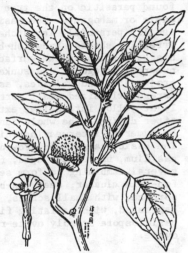

Properties and action: Has warming properties, bitter and acrid to taste, highly toxic. Anesthetizes, alleviates pain, stops coughing, and relieves asthma.

Conditions most used for: (1) Rheumatoid pains; (2) prolapse of rectum; (3) wheezing; (4) boils, ringworm, dermaphytosis; (5) rabies.

Preparation: Roots, leaves and flowers are used medicinally, 2-8 fen, in decoction or pulverized to be taken with water. For external purposes a suitable amount of fresh leaves may be used.

416. Chu Ling

Family: Polyparaceae

Scientific name: Grifola umbellata (Pers.)
Pilat.

Synonyms: "Yeh-chu fen" [wild boar dung],
"yeh-chu shih" [wild boar food].

Morphology: A basidiomycetic fungus. Mostly
found parasitic on the tree roots of oak,
maple or mahogany. The basidiocarp is
usually perennial, in patches or other
irregular shapes, brownish-black or
blackish-brown on the surface, with
numerous irregular and sunken tumor-like
projections and wrinkles, as well as many
irregularly sized small pores, white or
light yellow internally, extremely hard
after drying. The whole fungus formed
by numerous interweaving white hyphae.
The basidiocarp found growing from the
basidium, umbrella-shaped, frequently
several combining to form semi-circle
fan-like cluster, deep tea-brown on the
surface, with small scales, the center
depressed, with radiating fine lines. The
basidiospore broadly ovate-rounded to
ovate.

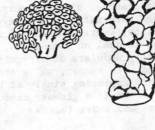

Properties and action: Has neutral
properties, pleasant to taste. Promotes
diuresis, and "leaks" moisture.

Conditions most used for: (1) Edema,
distension; (2) diarrhea; (3) leukorrhea,
and gonorrheal discharge.

Preparation: The basidiocarp is used
medicinally, 2-5 ch'ien each time, in
decoction.

417. Chu-sha Ken [Cinnabar root]

Family: Myrsinaceae

Scientific name: Ardisia crenata Sims.

Synonyms: "Shan-tou ken," "kuei-ta-san"
[devil's umbrella], "ti-chuang tzu,"
"tieh liang-san," "hsueh-li-k'ai-hua"
[flower-blooming-in-the-snow], "liang-
shan po," "liang-san-kai-chen-chu"
[parasol over pearls], "chin so-shih"
[golden key], "liang-shan-ken," "k'ai-hou
chien" [throat-splitting sword], "shang-
shan hu," "san t'iao ken," "hung-ch'en
hsiao" [red dust particles], "chin-chu-
lien," "tuan kang-ch'iao" [broken steel
bridge], "kao ch'a-feng," "ai-chiao niang-
tzu" [short-legged maiden], "san-liang chin,"
"huo-lung chu."

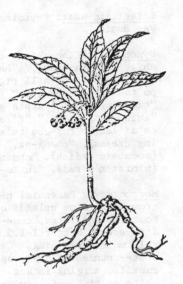

Morphology: Small evergreen shrub. Found
growing under forests or in shrub thickets.
Roots thick and solid, surface slightly
red. Stem erect, height about 1 meter.
Leaves alternate, oval-lanceolate, or
oblanceolate, apexes short-acute or
acuminate, bases cuneate, margins undulate. In summer-fall, white or pink axillary flowers appearing to form umbellate
inflorescences. Fruit a globose drupe.

Properties and action: Has cooling properties, bitter to taste. Clears fevers and
detoxifies, stimulates blood circulation
and alleviates pain.

Conditions most used for: (1) Diphtheria,
sore throat, toothache; (2) traumatic injuries, aches and pains in the back and
thighs; (3) poisonous snakebites, mad
dog bites.

Preparation: Roots are used medicinally,
5 ch'ien - 1 liang each time, in decoction.

418. Shang-lu [Pokeweed]

Family: Phytolaccaceae

Scientific name: Phytolacca esculenta
Van Houtt

Synonyms: "Niao-chi mu-tou," "pao mu-
chi," "niu ta-huang," "hsia-shan hu"
[descending-from-hill tiger], "ta lo-
po tou," "fei chu-t'ou" [fat hog's head],
"tzu yang-t'ou" [purple goat's head],
"chien-feng-hsiao," "t'ien ma," "hsien-
ts'ai lan," "fei-chu ts'ai" [hog-fatten-
ing greens], "chang-pa," "shan lo-po"
[mountain radish], "chuang-yuan hung"
[minister's red], "fu lo-po."

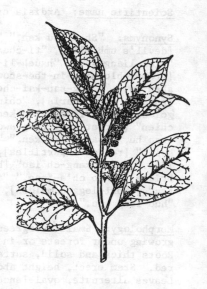

Morphology: Perennial herb. Found
growing wild on uplands or cultivated.
Root fat and large, cone-shaped, fleshy.
Stem erect, height 1-1.5 meters, cylindrical, multi-branching. Leaves alternate,
ovate-rounded to oval, apexes acute, bases
cuneate, margins intact. In summer, small
white or pink axillary and terminal flowers
appearing to form racemose inflorescences.
Berry globose, purplish back when ripe.

Properties and action: Has "han" cold
properties, bitter tasting, toxic. Promotes diuresis and reduces swelling.

Conditions most used for: (1) Edema,
abdominal distention; (2) numbness of
throat.

Preparation: Roots are used medicinally,
1-2 ch'ien each time, in decoction.

419. T'ou ku Ts'ao [Lopseed]

Family: Phrymaceae

Scientific name: Phryma leptastachya L.

Synonyms: "I-sao-kuan" [one-clean-sweep],
"ying-tu ts'ao" [fly-poison counteracting
grass].

Morphology: Perennial herb. Found growing on hillsides, forest edges and in grass
thickets in gullies. Stem erect, 4-angled,
densely pubescent, internodal distances
somewhat great, nodes enlarged, with longitudinal furrows on surface. Leaves opposite,
ovate, apexes acute or acuminate, bases
truncate to cuneate, margins coarsely
serrated. In summer, white purplish
flowers appear terminally or at leaf
axils to form spike-like racemose inflorescences. Fruit a capsule.

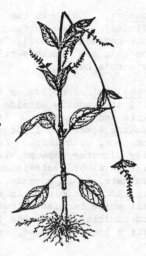

Properties and action: Has cooling
properties, biting to taste. Clears
fevers and detoxifies.

Conditions most used for: (1) "Huang-
shu" [muddy ? water] ulcers; (2) ringworms and scabies, etc.; (3) poisonous
insect bites; (4) as insecticide to
kill fly maggots.

Preparation: The whole plant is used
medicinally, mostly crushed and pulverized
for external application in suitable
amounts.

420. Chieh-ku Mu [Ground elder species]

Family: Caprifoliaceae

Scientific name: Sambucus racemosa L.

Synonyms: "Chieh-ku tan" [bone-knitting medicine], "chieh-ku feng," "hsu-ku mu" [bone-connecting wood], "mu shuo-t'iao," "shu-chin shu" [muscle-relaxing tree], "ch'a-ch'a huo."

Morphology: A deciduous shrub. Found cultivated mostly outside village out-skirts and in gardens. Stem height reaching 4 meters, light green, non-pubescent, pith thick. Leaves opposite, oddly pinnate-compound, leaflets 5-7 ovate, oval or ovate-lanceolate, apexes acuminate, bases cuneate, margins serrated, with short petioles. In early summer, small white terminal flowers appearing to form panicle-like cymose inflorescences. Fruit a berry, globose, bright red when ripe.

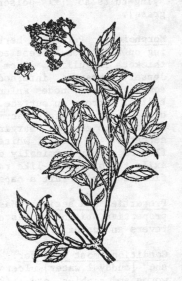

Properties and action: Has nuetral proper-ties, bitter tasting. Promotes callus formation and muscle and sinew healing, stimulates blood circulation and alleviates pain, dispels flatulence and moisturizes.

Conditions most used for: (1) Traumatic injuries, fractures; (2) rheumatoid arthralgia, gas pains: (3) acute and chronic nephritis.

Preparation: Leaves, stems and roots are used medicinally, 1-2 liang each time in decoction. Or decoction may be used for bathing affected parts.

421. Hsuan-fu Hua [Elecampane]

Family: Compositae

Scientific name: Inula japonica Thunb.

Synonym: "Fu-hua."

Morphology: Perennial herb. Found
growing on hillsides, roadsides, field
edges or damp lands. Stem height 30-80
cm, upper part multi-branching, with
horizontal angles. Leaves alternate,
oval or narrowly oval, upper leaves
somewhat smaller, apexes acute, bases
somewhat narrow, half clasping stem,
margins intact or finely serrated, densely
scabrous. Blooms in the fall, yellow
flowers appearing to form terminal
capitulum inflorescences in an umbellate arrangement. Fruit an achene,
long ellipsoid.

Properties and action: Has warming
properties, salty to taste. Lowers
excess, resolves phlegm and promotes
fluid elimination.

Conditions most used for: (1) Bronchitis,
coughing and shortness of breath; (2)
chest congestion and pain [pleurisy ?],
ascites.

Preparation: Flowers are used medicinally, 1-3 ch'ien each time in
decoction.

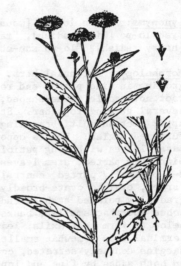

422. Hsu-tuan [Teasel]

Family: Dipsaceae

Scientific name: Dipsacus japonicus Miq.

Synonyms: "Shan lo-po" [mountain radish], "yeh lo-po [wild radish], "mao lo-po" [hairy radish], "lo-po san-ch'i."

Morphology: Perennial herb. Found growing in wild places and roadsides. Tap root noticeable, cone-shaped, frequently several growing together. Stem erect, upper section multi-branching, with furrowed angles. Leaves opposite; basal leaves with long petioles, pinnately parted; stem leaves mostly 3-5 pinnately parted, central part somewhat larger, oval to ovate-broadly oval, gradually pointed at both ends, lateral lobes somewhat smaller, bases extending below to form leaf axils; leaves at terminal stem somewhat smaller, 3-parted, margins coarsely serrated, covered densely on both sides by fine and long soft hairs. Blooms in the fall, reddish purple flowers appearing to form racemose inflorescences. Fruit an achene, wedge-shaped and oval.

Properties and action: Has slightly warming properties, bitter and acrid to taste. Strengthens the liver and kidneys, stimulates blood circulation.

Conditions most used for: (1) Rheumatoid anthralgia, traumatic injuries; (2) abortions[?], backache and weak knees, seminal emissions and polyuria.

Preparation: Roots are used medicinally, 2-4 ch'ien each time in decoction.

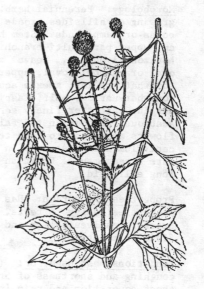

423. Yen So-shih [Silver key]

Family: Menispermaceae

Scientific name: Cyclea hypoglauca
(Schauer) Diels

Synonyms: "Fen-hsieh lun-huan t'eng"
[powdery leaf encircling vine], "pai-
chieh t'eng" [hundred-remedy vine],
"chin-hsien feng," "yu-mao-feng chi-
ma," "hei-p'i she" [black-skin snake],
"pai-chieh" [hundred remedies], "chia
shan-tou ken."

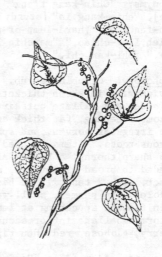

Morphology: Perennial herbaceous vine.
Found growing wild in open woods and
shrub thickets. Roots black, cross-
section showing radiating lines like
those of wheel spokes. Stem slender
with longitudinal furrows, covered by
long white hairs when young, vine and
leaves showing bubbly juice when crushed.
Leaves alternate, deltate-ovate to ovate,
peltate, apexes acute, bases rounded,
margins intact, with long petioles. In
summer, spike-like inflorescences appearing at leaf axils, consisting of
small light green flowers. Fruit similar to mung bean, red when ripe.

Properties and action: Has "han" cooling
properties, bitter to taste. Clears fevers
and detoxifies, eliminates flatulence and
alleviates pain, promotes diuresis.

Conditions most used for: (1) Sore throat,
toothache; (2) urinary tract infections,
rheumatoid arthralgia; (3) poisonous snake
bites.

Preparation: Roots are used medicinally,
5 ch'ien - 1 liang each time, in decoction.

424. Po-hsi [Chinaroot]

<u>Family</u>: Smilax family

<u>Scientific name</u>: Smilax china L.

<u>Synonyms</u>: "Chin-kang t'eng" [sturdy
vine], "chin-kang la" [sturdy thorn],
"yin-fan t'ou" [hard-lump-of-rice],
"t'ieh ling-chiao," "ma-chia le," "ma-
chia," "chi-kan chi."

<u>Morphology</u>: Climbing shrub. Found
growing wild in shrub thickets on
hillsides and village outskirts.
Rhizome creeping, fat thick and hard,
with irregular curves, and sparse,
fibrous roots. Stems rounded and hard,
with sharp thorns.   Leaves alternate,
rounded to broad-elliptical, margins
intact, with 2 tendrils at base of
petioles. In summer, small yellowish-
green flowers appearing at leaf axils
to form umbellate inflorescences. Fruit
a berry, globose, red when ripe.

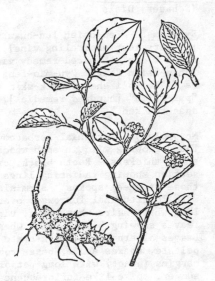

<u>Properties and action</u>: Has cooling
properties, pleasant and light to taste.
Eliminates flatulence and detoxifies,
removes [excess] moisture and promotes
diuresis.

<u>Conditions most used for</u>: (1) Boils
and abscesses; (2) rheumatoid arthritis;
(3) urinary tract infection; (4) enteritis
and diarrhea.

<u>Preparation</u>: Roots are used medicinally,
1-2 liang each time, in decoction.

425. Hsien-hou T'ao [Actinidia species]

Family: Actinidaceae

Scientific name: Actinidia chinensis
Plan ch.

Synonyms: "T'eng-li kuan," "t'eng-li
kuo," "yeh yang-t'ao" [wild carambola],
"chuan-ti feng," "t'eng-li shu," "yang-
t'ao t'eng" [carambola vine], "t'eng
li" [vine-pear].

Morphology: Climbing vine. Found growing in alpine forests. Stem reddish-
brown, pubescent. Leaves alternate,
broadly ovate or broadly oval, apexes
rounded-obtuse or slightly retuse,
bases rounded or cordate, margins with
fine serrations, undersides of leaves
grayish white, covered densely by downy
hairs. Blooms in summer, several yellowish white flowers clustered at leaf
axils. Fruit a berry, ovate-rounded,
covered by brownish black hairs, tart
and edible when ripe, with a banana
fragrance.

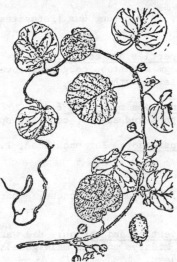

Properties and action: Has "han"
cold properties, tart and pleasant to
taste. Clears fevers and promotes diruesis,
relieves tension and quenches thirst,
counteracts cinnabar [mercury ?]

Conditions most used for: (1) Stones
in the urinary tract; (2) rheumatoid
arthralgia; (3) cancers of the liver and
esophagus.

Preparation: Fruits, stems and roots
are used medicinally, 5 ch'ien-1 liang
each time, in decoction.

426. Che Pei-mu [Fritillaria callicola]

Properties and action: Has "han" cold properties, bitter tasting. Clears fevers, moisturizes the lungs, resolves phlegm, and loosens up congestion.

Conditions most used for: Sputum productive "hot" coughs, lung abscess and throat numbness, scrophula and other boils and abscesses.

Preparation: For each dose, 1.5-3 ch'ien, in decoction.

427. K'uan-tung Hua [Petasites japonicus, Mig.]

Properties and action: Has warming properties, acrid tasting. Resolves phlegm and stops coughing, lowers the energy [slows the breathing?] and relieves asthma.

Conditions most used for: Chronic coughing and pulmonary "deficiency," dyspnea and asthma, constant sputum formation, pulmonary tuberculosis.

Preparation: For each dose, 1.5-3 ch'ien, in decoction.

428. So-yang [Orobanche, a parasitic herb]

Properties and action: Has warming properties, pleasant to taste. Strengthens the kidneys and the male gonads [potency and seminal control], moisturizes dryness.

Conditions most used for: Weak kidneys and impotency, weak back and knees, seminal emission, constipation.

Preparation: For each dose, 1.5-3 ch'ien, in decoction.

429. Hei Chih-ma [Black sesame seeds]

Properties and action: Neutral, pleasant to taste. Strengthens the liver and kidneys, moistens the five viscera (chuang).

Conditions most used for: Inadequate liver and kidney function, head-cold dizziness, numbness and paralysis, constipation.

Preparation: For each dose, 1-3 ch'ien, in decoction. Or, stir-fry for eating.

430. Huang Ching [Scutellaria baicalensis, Georg.]

Properties and action: Has "han" cold properties, bitter to taste. Removes moist heat, purges "solid" fire, and quiets the fetus.

Conditions most used for: Lungs-heated coughing, feverish restlessness, moist-heat diarrhea, jaundice, gonorrhea, red and swollen eyes [conjunctivitis and/or trachoma?], ulcers and boils, heat-caused nosebleed, restless fetus.

Preparation: For each dose, 1-3 ch'ien, in decoction.

431. Huang-lian [Coptis chinensis]

Properties and action: Has "han" cold properties, bitter to taste. Purges fire, detoxifies, and dries [excess] moisture.

Conditions most used for: Heat-dominating restlessness, abdominal fullness, emaciation, "fire-caused" diarrhea and abdominal cramps, hematemesis, epistaxis, "red" eyes, canker sores, skin sores and scabies.

Preparation: For each dose, 5 fen to 1 ch'ien, in decoction. For external purposes, a suitable amount may be used.

432. Huang-pai [Phellodendron]

Properties and action: Has "han" cold properties, bitter to taste. Purges [excess?] fire, removes moisture-heat.

Conditions most used for: Fever-associated dysentery, diarrhea, jaundice, gonorrhea, hemorrhoids, bloody stools, aching bones, conjunctivitis, tinnitus, canker sores, lameness, paralysis, boils, leukorrhea and bloody vaginal discharge.

Preparation: For each dose, 1.5-3 ch'ien, in decoction. For external purposes, a suitable amount may be used.

433. Huang-ch'i [locoweed, yellow vetch]

Properties and action: Has slightly warming properties, pleasant to taste.
Strengthens energy and maintains [body] resistance; transfers toxins and
aids tissue regeneration.

Conditions most used for: Low [body] resistance, self-perspiration, hidrosis,
anemia, spleen-deficient diarrhea, "non-ripening" of boils and non-healing
ulcers, and all illnesses due to inadequate prime energy.

Preparation: For each dose, 3 ch'ien to 1 liang, in decoction.

434. She-t'o [Snake exuviae (shed coat)]

Properties and action: Neutral, salty yet pleasant to taste, mildly toxic.
Relieves flatulence, retracts pterygium growth, kills insects.

Conditions most used for: Infantile convulsions, canker, abscesses, pterygiums,
hemorrhoids.

Preparation: For each dose, 1.5-3 ch'ien, in decoction, or pulverized and
mixed with water to be taken internally.

435. Mi-t'o-tseng [Lead oxide, a yellowish powder]

Properties and action: Neutral, acrid and salty to taste, toxic. "Dries"
dampness, kills insects, cleanses sores, resolves phlegm and quiets convulsions.

Conditions most used for: Moist sores and fungus infections, ulcers, treated
externally, excess phlegm-sputum and convulsions treated by drug taken internally.

Preparation: For external purposes, an appropriate amount is used. For
taking internally, 5 fen to 1.5 ch'ien, to be used with care.

436. Chu Sha [Cinnabar, vermillion]

Properties and action: Has slightly "han" cold properties, pleasant to taste. Settles nerves and controls convulsions. Also detoxifies.

Conditions most used for: Mania, apprehension, insomnia, nightmares; boils (treated externally).

Preparation: For each dose, 1-3 fen, used in pills. A suitable amount may be used for external purposes.

437. Tzu-shih [Fruit (nut) of lindera species]

Properties and action: Neutral, pleasant to taste. Diuretic and vermicidal.

Conditions most used for: Difficult urination, edema, abdominal distension; fungus infections and scabies treated externally.

Preparation: For each dose, 3-5 ch'ien, in decoction. For external application, a suitable amount may be used.

438. Fan Hsieh-hsieh [Senna leaves]

Properties and action: Has "han" cold properties, bitter to taste. Relieves "stoppage" distension and eliminates constipation.

Conditions most used for: Overeating and indigestion, abdominal fullness, constipation, ascites.

Preparation: For each dose, 5 fen to 1.5 ch'ien, in decoction.

439. Tzu-yuan [Aster tataricus L.]

Properties and action: Has slightly warming properties, acrid and bitter
to taste. Resolves phlegm and stops coughing.

Conditions most used for: Coughing and shortness of breath, difficulty
in loosening up phlegm, lung-deficient chronic cough, bloody sputum.

Preparation: For each dose, 8 fen to 3 ch'ien, in decoction.

440. Ma-huang [Ephedra]

Properties and action: Has warming properties, acrid to taste. Induces
perspiration and relieves asthma.

Conditions most used for: "Solid" fevers [that do not break up], fever and
chills with no perspiration, arthralgia, coughing [that drains energy], edema.

Preparation: For each dose, 5 fen to 2 ch'ien in decoction.

441. Liu-huang [Sulfur]

Properties and action: Has warming properties, acid to taste. Supplements
body fire and strengthens the male gonads, kills intestinal parasites.

Conditions most used for: Impotency, chronic dysentery, deficiency-cold
constipation in the aged; and sores, ringworms and scabies to be treated
externally.

Preparation: For each dose, 5 fen to 1 ch'ien, in decoction. A suitable
amount for external use.

442. T'ing-li-tzu [Seeds of Draba nemorosa subspecies]

Properties and action: Has "han" cold properties, acrid and bitter to taste. Loosens phlegm and promotes fluid elimination, slows respiration and re- lieves asthma.

Conditions most used for: Coughing and moist wheezes, obstruction in pulmonary energy [breathing], tightness in chest and sides, facial edema, difficult urination.

Preparation: For each dose, 1-3 ch'ien, in decoction.

443. Mi Meng-hua [Buddlea officinalis, Maxim.]

Properties and action: Neutral, with slightly "han" cold properties, pleasant to taste. Clears fevers and restores clarity of vision.

Conditions most used for: Edematous and painful red eyes, bleary eyes, photophobia, blinding cataracts.

Preparation: For each dose, 1-3 ch'ien, in decoction.

444. Pan-mao [Cantharis: Spanish fly]

Properties and action: Has "han" cold properties, acrid to taste, toxic. Lubricates to attach stoppage congestion, cauterizes tissues to control toxin spread.

Conditions most used for: Scabies, fungus infections, purulent boils and scrophula, rabid dog bites.

Preparation: One fly to be used each time, in decoction or pulverized for taking with boiled water. No set amount specified for external use.

445. Tzu chu [Purple bamboo]

Family: Graminea

Scientific name: Phyllostachys nigra
Munro.

Synonyms: "Hei chu" [black bamboo], "yu
chu" [oil bamboo].

Morphology: Evergreen bush. Found growing in fertile and moist places in remote
hill areas and alongside streams, also
cultivated. Height reaching 8 meters.
New stalks green, gradually changing to
black on attaining maturity. Stalks and
forking branches black, light black or
black spotted, cylindrical. Leaves growing terminally from small branches, 2-3,
lanceolate, apexes acute, bases obtuse,
with short petioles, parallel ribs, white
on dorsal surface, showing small tongues,
ochrea nonpubescent.

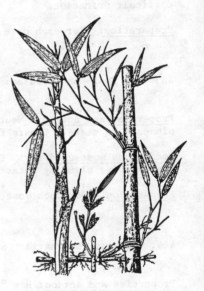

Properties and action: Has cooling
properties, bland to taste. Detoxifies
and promotes diuresis, clears fevers and
allays apprehension and restlessness.

Conditions most used for: (1) High
fevers; (2) nocturnal fretfulness in
infants; (3) rabies.

Preparation: The whip-like roots are
used medicinally, 5 ch'ien - 1 liang
each time in decoction.

446. Tzu Ssu [Perilla species]

Family: Labiatae

Scientific name: Perilla frutescens
(L) Brit. var. crispa Decne

Synonyms: "Yeh-ssu," "chi-ssu," "hung-
sha-yao," "ts'ao-t'ou tzu," "tsu-shih
ts'ao."

Morphology: Annual herb. Found growing in sunny and fertile locations,
cultivated in gardens. Stem oblong,
multi-branching, height about 1 meter,
purple or purplish-green. Leaves
opposite, broadly ovate or almost
rounded, apexes acuminate or aristate,
bases rounded, margins coarsely serrated,
both surfaces bluish-purple, or green
on the upper surface and purple on the
underside, slightly pubescent, long-
petioled. In summer, small purplish
axillary or terminal flowers appearing
to form racemose inflorescences. Nut
small, yellowish-brown.

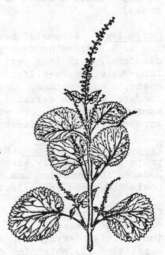

Properties and action: Has warming
properties, acrid to taste and aromatic.
Dispels "han"-cold and corrects energy
balance, relieves asthma, quiets restless fetus, and detoxifies.

Conditions most used for: (1) As a
preventive for epidemic influenza, colds,
and malaria; (2) vomiting, abdominal
distension and flatulence; (3) restless
fetus; (4) seafood (fish and crab)
poisoning.

Preparation: The whole plant is used
medicinally, 3-5 ch'ien each time, in
decoction.

447. Tzu-hua Ti-ting (Li-t'ou ts'ao) [Violet (plow-grass)]

Family: Violaceae

Scientific name: Viola japonica Langsd.

Synonyms: "Kuan-t'ou chien," "li-ts'iu ts'ao," "chien-t'ou ts'ao" [arrowhead grass].

Morphology: Perennial herb. Found growing on hillsides or damp places. Leaves clustered, with long petioles, leaves long-ovate, ovate-elliptical or deltoid-ovate, apexes obtuse, bases shallowly cordate, margins serrated. In spring-summer, purplish-red terminal flowers appear. Fruit an ellipsoid capsule.

Properties and action: Has "han" cold properties, slightly bitter to taste. Reduces inflammation and detoxifies, cools the blood and alleviates pain.

Conditions most used for: (1) Boils, ulcers and abscesses; (2) acute conjunctivitis, laryngitis, acute jaundice hepatitis; (3) poisoning due to "tuanch'ang ts'ao."

Preparation: The whole plant is used medicinally, 5 ch'ien - 1 liang each time, in decoction.

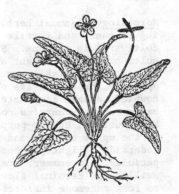

448. Tzu-Shen (Ts'ao-ho-che) [Buckwheat species]

Family: Polygonaceae

Scientific name: Polygonum bistorta L.

Synonyms: "Chung-lou," "tao-ken ts'ao,"
[inverted root grass], "tao-ch'iang yao"
[sword and gun drug].

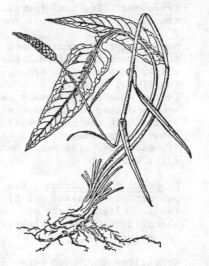

Morphology: Perennial herb. Found growing in alpine weed thickets. Rhizome
thick and fat, sturdy, crooked, in 1
piece, purplish-brown on the outside.
Single stem, erect, height 60-90 cm.
Basal leaves long-petioled, lanceolate,
apexes gradually narrowing, bases truncate
or gradually narrowing, extending below
to form narrow rings, leaf margins
frequently curled externally; stem leaves
alternate, linear-lanceolate to linear,
bases embracing stem, stipules sheath-
like. In summer-fall, light red or white
flower appearing to form spike inflorescences. Small nut 3-angled, blackish-
brown.

Properties and action: Has slightly "han"
cooling properties, bitter to taste.
Clears fevers and detoxifies, loosens
congestion and reduces swelling.

Conditions most used for: (1) Fever
convulsions, spasms of hand and feet,
tetanus; (2) cervical lymphadenopathy;
(3) swellings and scrophula, snake and
insect bites.

Preparation: Roots and stems are used,
1-2 ch'ien each time, in decoction.

Note: Another plant from the Labiatae, Salvia chinensis, Benth. is also
called "tzu shen," though it is commonly referred to as "shih-chien-ch'uan"
in the area around Shanghai.

449. Tzu Ts'ao [Borage species]

Family: Boraginaceae

Scientific name: Lithosperum erythrorhizon
Sieb et Zucc

Synonyms: "Tzu-ken" [purple root], "hung-
tzu ken" [reddish purple root].

Morphology: Perennial herb. Found growing on sunny hillsides. Roots large and
thick, purple. Stem erect, height reaching 60 cm, pubescent with white hairs.
Leaves alternate, broadly lanceolate,
apexes acute, bases cuneate, margins
intact. In the fall, white terminal
flowers appearing to form racemose inflorescences. The small nut ovoid,
light brown.

Properties and action: Has "han" cold
properties, pleasant yet biting to
taste. Clears fevers and cools the
blood, detoxifies and lubricates the
intestines.

Conditions most used for: (1) Measles
preventive; (2) burns, knife cuts and
bleeding; (3) oozing dermatitis,
abscesses; (4) constipation.

Preparation: The whole plant is used
medicinally, 3-5 ch'ien each time, in
decoction.

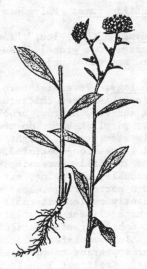

450. Tzu P'ing [Duckweed species]

Family: Lemnaceae

Scientific name: Spirodela polyrhizd (L.) Schleid.

Synonyms: "Shui p'ing" [pondweed], "hung p'ing" [red pondweed], "tzu-pei fou'p'ing" [purple-backed duckweed].

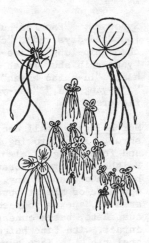

Morphology: Small herb floating on water. Found growing in rice paddies and swamps. Leaves somewhat flat, 1-5 clustered, obovate or rounded. Leaf surface stipule inverted inwardly, dark green, purple on the underside. Fibrous roots numerous. Blooms in summer, flowers growing from the notches found alongside margins of the leaf-life body, with 2 lipped spathes.

Properties and action: Has "han" cold properties, acrid to taste. Promotes perspiration and stimulates measles rash appearance, expels flatulence and promotes diuresis.

Conditions most used for: (1) Exposure-colds and fever, inadequate measles rash appearance; (2) acute nephritis; (3) hemorrhagic purpura; (4) urticaria.

Preparation: The whole plant is used medicinally, 1-3 ch'ien, in decoction.

451. Tzu Hui [Loosestrife species]

Family: Lythraceae

Scientific name: Lagerstroemia indica
L.

Synonyms: "Pao fan-hua," "pai-jih hung"
[hundred-days red], "ch'iung-hua," "wu-
chao chin-lung" [five-claw golden dragon],
"yang-shih shu" [goat dung tree], "ho-
hua," "lu-chiao hsieh" [deer antler leaves],
"p'a-yang shu," "ssu-yueh hua" [April
flowers].

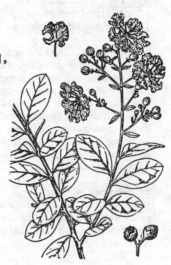

Morphology: Small deciduous tree or
shrub. Found growing along hillsides
and forest edges, also cultivated.
Height 2-7 meters, branches curved,
bark smooth and shiny, brown. Leaves
opposite or almost opposite, obovate
or oval, apexes rounded and slightly
cuspidate, bases cuneate, margins
intact, with fine hairs alongside central rib. In late summer, red, white
or purplish flowers appearing terminally
to form panicle inflorescences. Globoid
capsule somewhat ellipsoid.

Properties and action: Has neutral
properties, slightly bitter and biting
to taste. Detoxifies, breaks up and
purges clots [bruises], eliminates
[excess] moisture, promotes diuresis.

Conditions most used for: (1) Boils,
ulcers and abscesses, and "lei-kung
t'eng" (Tripterygium wilfordii)
poisoning; (2) jaundice, abdominal
distention, edema; (3) oozing dermatitis,
mucus dysentery; (4) post-partum abdominal
pain and dizziness.

Preparation: Roots are used medicinally,
3 liang - 8 liang (0.5 chin) each time,
in decoction.

452. Ching T'ien [Stonecrop]

Family: Crassulaceae

Scientific name: Sedum spectabile Boreau

Synonyms: "Kuan-yin shan" [Goddess-of-Mercy's fan], "ta-pu-ssu" [can-never-die], "ts'an-tou ch'i" [horsebean seven], "chiu-t'ou san-ch'i," "t'u san-ch'i," "hsiang-p'i ch'i," "chien-jo sheng."

Morphology: Perennial fleshy herb. Mostly cultivated; also found growing in valleys, rocky cliffs, and in damp places along woodlands. Height reaching 50 cm, stems cylindrical, erect. Leaves fleshy and thick, opposite or 3-leaf whorled, elliptical or obovate cuneate, apexes obtuse, bases narrowing, margins finely crenate, almost intact near base, with short petioles. In the fall, greenish-white axillary and terminal flowers appearing to form cymose inflorescences. Follicle red or pink.

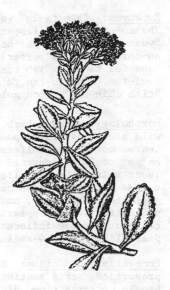

Properties and action: Has neutral properties, bitter tasting. Reduces inflammation and detoxifies, stops thirstiness and promotes salivation.

Conditions most used for: (1) Sore throat; (2) abscesses and erysipelas, (3) redness and swelling from traumatic injuries.

Preparation: The whole plant is used medicinally, 1-2 liang each time, in decoction; or fresh product may be crushed in suitable amounts for external application.

453. O-pu-sh'ih Ts'ao (Shih Hu-t'o) [Goose-will-not-eat herb (Stony coriander)]

Family: Compositae

Scientific name: Centipeda minima (L.)
A. Braun et Aschers

Synonyms: Chin ti-lo" [brocade carpet],
"hsiao-shih ts'ao" [appetite-curbing],
"yuan-tzu ts'ao," "hsi-hsi ts'ao," "ti
hu-chiao" [ground pepper], "ta-chiu chia,"
"sha-fei ts'ao," "yeh tung kao," "leng-
shui-tan," "ch'iu-tzu ts'ao" [ball-grass],
"tieh chin-hua" [iron golden flowers].

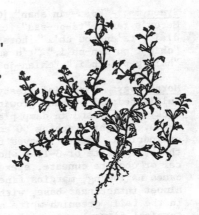

Morphology: Annual herb. Found growing
wild along roadsides, paddy field edges.
Leaves mostly stoloniferous, attaining
height of 20 cm, covered sparsely with
short hairs. Leaves alternate, obovate,
apexes serrated, bases cuneate, non-
petioled. In summer, small and light
yellowish flowers appearing from axilla
to form racemose inflorescences. The
pearl-like achene 4-angled.

Properties and action: Has warming
properties, acrid tasting and aromatic.
Breaks up congestion, dispels "han"
cold, stimulates blood circulation
[thereby removing clots], detoxifies.

Conditions most used for: (1) Rhinitis,
sinusitis, conjunctivitis, corneal
pterygium; (2) colds; (3) malaria.

Preparation: The whole plant is used
medicinally. For the dry product 1-3
ch'ien, or the fresh product 3-5 ch'ien,
each time in decoction; or the fresh
herb may be crushed and a suitable amount
is inserted into the nostrils.

454. T'u-ssu-tzu (Wu-ken t'eng) [Dodder (rootless vine)]

Family: Convovulaceae

Scientific name: Cuscuta japonica Choisy

Synonyms: "Wu-sung ma-huang" [centipede 'ephedra'] "huang-ssu t'eng" [yellow filament vine], "chin-ssu t'eng" [golden thread vine], "wu-ya t'eng," "men-ken t'eng."

Morphology: Annual parasitic herb. Found growing on the branches of shrubs located in sunny hill wilds, stream banks, and roadsides. Stem fine like silk, entwining other objects counterclockwise, yellow or purplish-red. Leaves small, forming scales, sparse, containing no chlorophyll. Blooms in the fall, orange-red bell-like flowers forming short spike inforescences. Capsule a flat globoid.

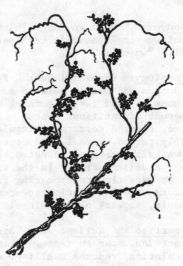

Properties and action: Has neutral properties, pleasant to taste. Strengthens the liver and kidney, builds up the blood, moisturizes the "dry," and strengthens sinews and bones.

Conditions most used for: (1) Enuresis, seminal emission, constipation; (2) backache and cold knees, rheumatoid paralysis.

Preparation: The fruit or the whole plant is used medicinally, 1-4 ch'ien each time, in decoction.

455. Lieh-hsieh Ch'iu-hai-t'ang [Split-leaf begonia]

Family: Begoniaceae

Scientific name: Begonia laciniata Roxb.

Synonyms: "Hsueh wu-sung" [bloody centipede], "shui wu-sung" [aquatic centipede], "wu-sung-ch'i," "wu-ch'i."

Morphology: Perennial herb. Found growing in damp shady places between mountains. Rhizome fat and large, forming nodes, with numerous adventitious roots. Leaves clustered, slanted cordate, irregularly 5-7 deeply parted, dorsal leaf covered by soft brown hairs, margins serrated, leaf petioles long, reddish-purple. In the summer, light red or pink flowers appearing from axilla to form umbellate inflorescences. Long capsule, showing narrow wings.

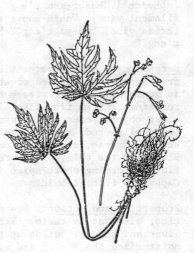

Properties and action: Has "han" cold properties, sour to taste. Stimulates blood circulation, reduces swelling, stops diarrhea.

Conditions most used for: (1) Hematemesis; (2) amenorrhea; (3) traumatic stagnant blood collection.

Preparation: The roots are used medicinally, 3-5 ch'ien each time, decocted in small amount of water.

456. Huo-hsieh Shih-ta Kung-lao [Broadleaf ten-great-awards]

Family: Berberidaceae

Scientific name: Mahonia bealei Carr.

Synonyms: T'u huang-pai [native phellodendron]

Morphology: Evergreen shrub. Found growing wild in uplands, or cultivated in gardens. Stem coarse and strong, height 2-4 meters, wood yellow. Leaves alternate, oddly pinnate-compound, petioles sheathlike at base enclosing stem. Leaflets 9-15 broadly ovate, apexes acute and sharply prickly, bases cuneate, margins curling back forming prickly dentate edges. In the fall, yellow flowers appearing in racemose inflorescences, terminally. Berry ovate-rounded, blackish-blue.

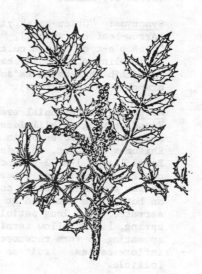

Properties and action: Has cooling properties, bitter to taste. Clears fevers, detoxifies, reduces inflammation.

Conditions most used for: (1) Pulmonary tuberculosis, recurring fever and cough in rundown body systems; (2) rheumatoid arthritis pains, backaches and weak knees; (3) dysentery, enteritis.

Preparation: Roots, stems are used medicinally, 5 ch'ien - 1 liang each time in decoction.

457. Yin Yang-huo [Barrenwort species]

Family: Berberidaceae

Scientific name: Epimedium sagittatum
(S. et Z.) Maxim.

Synonyms: "Chien-hsieh yin-yang-huo"
[Arrow-leaf barrenwort], "san-ch'a ku,"
"tieh p'a-t'ou" [iron cultivator],
"hsien-ling p'i," "pin-chang ts'ao,"
"san-chih chiu-hsieh ts'ao" [three-
branch nine-leaf grass].

Morphology: Perennial evergreen herb.
Found growing on hillsides, in damp
shady bamboo groves or in cliff crevices.
Rhizomes creeping, in nodular formation.
Basal leaves 1-3, 3-parted compound;
central leaflet oval to ovate-lanceolate,
apexes acuminate, bases cordate; leaflets
on both sides inclined at base, margins
serrated, with long petioles. In the
spring, light yellow terminal flowers
appearing to form racemose or panicle
inflorescences. Fruit an ovoid-rounded
follicle.

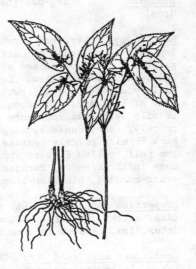

Properties and action: Has warming
properties, pleasant to taste. Warms the
kidneys and strengthens the yang element
[virility], removes excess moisture and
flatulence.

Conditions most used for: (1) Impotency,
weakness in back and knees; (2) neurasthenia;
(3) rheumatoid numbness and pain, in-
sensitivity.

Preparation: Leaves are used medicinally,
5 ch'ien each time, in decoction; can
also be steeped in white wine.

458. Hu-nan Lien-ch'iao [Hunan forsythia]

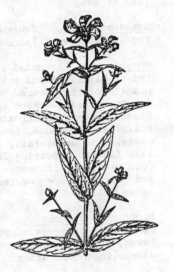

Family: Guttiferae

Scientific name: Hypericum ascyron L.

Synonyms: "Hung-ts'ao-lien"

Morphology: Perennial herb. Found growing on sunny hillsides and uplands. Height
reaching 1 meter. Stem erect, 4-angled.
Leaves opposite, broadly lanceolate, apexes
acute, bases clasping stem, margins intact.
In summer, golden yellow terminal flowers
appearing to form cymose inflorescences.
Capsule ovoid, containing several seeds.

Properties and action: Has slightly "han"
cold properties, bitter to taste. Clears
fevers and detoxifies, promotes pus drainage and tissue healing.

Conditions most used for: (1) Boils and
abscesses; (2) Stomachache and vomiting,
headache.

Preparation: The whole plant is used
medicinally, 3-5 ch'ien, in decoction.

459. Ko Ken [Kudzu vine?]

Family: Leguminosae

Scientific name: Pueraria pseudohirsuta
Tang et Wang.

Synonyms: "Ko," "fen-ko" [starchy arrow
root], "ko t'eng" [arrow-root vine].

Morphology: Perennial vine. Found growing on hillsides and roadsides. Whole
plant hirsute, covered by coarse yellowish-brown hairs. Root tuber thick and
fleshy. Leaves alternate, long-petioled,
trifoliate compound, leaflets broadly
ovate. In summer-fall, purplish-red disk-
like flowers appearing from leaf axils to
form racemose inflorescences. Legume long
and flat, surface covered by yellowish-
brown hairs.

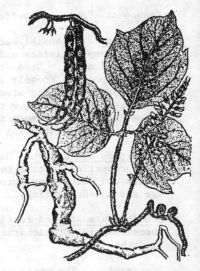

Properties and action: Neutral, pleasant
to taste. Relieves hunger and lowers
fever, stops diarrhea and counteracts
alcoholic intoxication.

Conditions most used for: (1) Exposure-
caused colds and fever, incomplete measles
rash breakout; (2) diarrhea, dysentery,
enteritis; (3) alcohol intoxication.

Preparation: Roots and flowers are used
medicinally: roots 1.5-3 ch'ien, or
flowers 1-2 ch'ien, in decoction.

460. P'i-ma [Castor bean]

Family: Euphorbiaceae

Scientific name: "Jen-ch'ang" [laxative],
"hung p'i" [red castor bean], "ta ma-tzu"
['cannabis'], "hung p'i-ma."

Morphology: Annual herb, similar to semi-
shrub. Cultivated or wild grown. Stem
hollow, cylindrical, covered on outside
by frosty bloom. Leaves alternate, large
and thin, 7-9 palmate cleft deeply, lobes
long-ovate or ovate-lanceolate, apexes
acute, margins serrated. Main venation
palmate, secondary venation pinnate. In
summer-fall, light yellow terminal flowers
appearing to form racemose inflorescences.
Capsule globoid, with prickly projections.

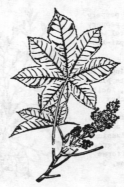

Properties and action: Neutral, pleasant
to taste, though slightly acrid and slightly
toxic. Draws out pus, stops pain, relieves
constipation, corrects prolapses.

Conditions most used for: (1) Gunshot
wounds, boils and abscesses, enlarged
lymph nodes; (2) joint pains, strabismus
and facial palsy; (3) constipation, anal
prolapse, prolapse of uterus.

Preparation: Seeds, roots and leaves are
used medicinally: seeds, a suitable amount
crushed and applied externally; or roots
and leaves 5 ch'ien - 1 liang, in decoction.

461. Po-lo-hui [Plume poppy]

Family: Papaveraceae

Scientific name: Macleaya cordata (Willd)
R. Br.

Synonyms: "Hao-t'ung keng," "t'ung-ta-
hai" [to-the-sea], "pao-t'ung-chu," "pien-
t'ien kao" [heaven's edge artemesia], "t'ung-
t'ien ta-huang."

Morphology: Large perennial herb, semi-
shrublike. Growing wild on plains, waste
places, and small hillsides. Rhizome
thick and large, yellowish-brown. Stem
erect, cylindrical, suspended in midair,
secreting yellowish fluid when broken in
half, exterior powdery. Leaves alternate,
broad-ovate, apexes obtuse, margins irregularly palmate-compound, 5-9 shallow-
parted, surfaces glabrous, undersides
powdery white, long petioles, shallowly
grooved, dorsal surface semicircular.
In summer, white or reddish terminal flowers
appearing to form panicle inflorescences.
Capsule slender and long-oval, turning
red when ripe, surface powdery white.

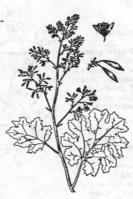

Properties and action: Has "han" cold properties, acrid to taste, slightly toxic.
Relieves flatulence and detoxifies, stimulates energy circulation and reduces edema;
kills insects and mosquito larvae.

Conditions most used for: (1) Hookworm
disease, constipation; (2) syphilitic
sores, skin diseases; (3) osteomyelitis,
arthralgia, abscesses, caries.

Preparation: Roots, stems and leaves
are used medicinally, 3-5 ch'ien each
time, in decoction. A suitable amount
may be used externally.

462. Pien-hsu [Knotgrass; goosegrass]

Family: Polygonaceae

Scientific name: Polygonum aviculare L.

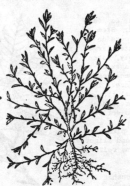

Synonyms: "Pai huo-la," [white peppery knotgrass], "pai la-liu" [white peppery willow], "tieh-hsien ts'ao" [steel wiregrass], "chieh-chieh ch'ing," "pai-lao-ya ts'ao," "tao-sheng ts'ao."

Morphology: Annual herb. Growing wild along roadsides, fields and waste places. Stem creeping or growing upward, inclined, height about 40 cm. Basal branches numerous, with pronounced nodes and longitudinal grooves. Leaves alternate, lanceolate to ovate-lanceolate, apexes obtuse, bases cuneate, ochrea clasping stem, margins intact. In summer, green flowers seen growing in cluster forms from leaf axils. Fruit an achene, 3-angled ovoid, blackish-brown.

Properties and action: Neutral, bitter to taste. Clears fevers, promotes diuresis, "dries" [excess] moisture, and kills worms and insects.

Conditions most used for: (1) pyelitis, stone formation in the urinary tract; (2) jaundice; (3) weeping eczema; (4) mucus and bloody vaginal discharge.

Preparation: The whole plant is used medicinally, 3-5 ch'ien each time, in decoction.

463. Tsa-chiang Ts'ao [Sorrel]

Family: Oxalidaceae

Scientific name: Oxalis Corniculata L.

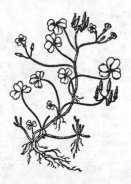

Synonyms: "Lao-ya ts'ao" [old crow grass], "huang-hua ts'ao" [yellow-flower grass], "lei-kung ch'ien" [thunder god's scissors], "san-hsieh suan" [three-leaf sour], "chiao-ling ts'ao," "szu-hsieh ts'ao" [four-leaf sorrel], "lao-ya suan-ts'ao" [old crow's sorrel], "yen-shih-hsiao," "lu-hsieh lien"

Morphology: Perennial herb. Found growing in damp and shady wild places. Stem creeping, slender and pubescent. Trifoliate compound leaves alternate, leaflets obcordate, apexes obtuse-rounded, with two shallow-parted lobes. In summer, small yellow flowers appearing to form umbellate inflorescences. Capsule cylindrical.

Properties and action: Has cooling properties, sour to taste. Clears fevers and detoxifies, resolves clots and bruises, reduces swelling.

Conditions most used for: (1) Influenza fever, urinary tract infections, enteritis, and diarrhea; (2) traumatic injuries and sprains, poisonous snakebites.

Preparation: Whole plant is used medicinally, 1-2 liang each time. Or a suitable amount of the fresh product may be crushed for external application.

464. Tsung-lu [Palm]

Family: Palmea

Scientific name: Trachycarpus excelsa
Wendl.

Synonyms: "Tsung-shu" [palm tree], "tsung
pa chiang," "ting-hai chen."

Morphology: Evergreen shrub. Found growing on sunny slopes, stream banks, or
cultivated. Height reaching 5 meters.
Stem erect, cylindrical, non-branching.
Leaves clustered at top, forming a spreading, umbrella-like crown. Fronds rounded
in fan-shape, digital-parted, highly fibrous,
bases covered by brown bractioles (sheaths).
In summer, small yellow terminal flowers
appearing to form spadix inflorescences.
Drupe globular.

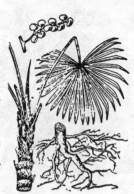

Properties and action: Neutral, bitter
and biting to taste. Hemostatic, astringent,
and contraceptive.

Conditions most used for: (1) Hemopytsis,
epistaxis, hematemesis, blood in stools,
metrorrhagia; (2) gonorrhea and other
venereal diseases.

Preparation: Coals ashes from silky hairs
of the palm are used medicinally, 3-5
ch'ien, mixed with boiling water in each
dose (to stop bleeding). Roots 3-5 liang,
or drupes 1-2 liang, in decoction (for
contraceptive effect).

465. Hsuan Ts'ao [Daylily; Miscanthus sinensis]

Properties and action: Cooling, pleasant to taste. Promotes diuresis,
cools the blood.

Conditions most used for: Edema, stones in the urinary tract, constipation,
jaundice, epistaxis, bloody stools, breast abscess.

Preparation: For each dose, 1.5-3 ch'ien, in decoction.

466. Hu-lu [Gourd]

Properties and action: Neutral, pleasant to taste. Promotes diuresis,
reduces swelling.

Conditions most used for: Edematous facies, ascites, berberi edema.

Preparation: For each dose, 5 ch'ien to 1 liang, in decoction.

467. Hsiung-huang [Realgar; spirits of sulfur]

Properties and action: Has warming properties, bitter and acrid to taste,
toxic. Exerts a cleansing and detoxifying action, "dries up" excess moisture,
and kills worms/insects.

Conditions most used for: Poisoning, abdominal pain, marasmus, malaria,
convulsions, scabies, fungus infections, snake and insect bites.

Preparation: For each dose, 1-4 fen, in decoction. A suitable amount may
be used for external application.

468. Hsi-chiao [Rhinoceros horns]

Properties and action: Has "han" cooling properties, bitter, sour, and
salty to taste. Clears fevers, cools the blood, detoxifies, and controls
convulsive spasms.

Conditions most used for: Low and high grade fevers, restlessness and
great thirst, cracked lips and parched tongue, delirium, epistaxis and
hematemesis, purpura, quinsy sore throat, fatigue, boils and abscesses.

Preparation: For each dose, 2-8 fen, in decoction.

469. Hu Mu [Chinese Ginseng]

Family: Araliaceae

Scientific name: Aralia chinensis L.

Synonyms: "La-lung-pao," "niao-pu-su"
[bird-will-not-sleep], "hai-t'ung-p'i,"
"t'ung-la," "huang-lung p'ao" [yellow
dragon robe], "mi-t'ou," "la ch'un-shu"
[prickly cedrela], "pai-hsin la" [white-
core thorn], "pai-niao pu-su" [hundred-
birds-will-not-sleep].

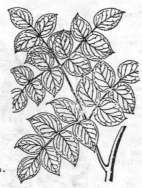

Morphology: Deciduous shrub or small
tree. Growing on uplands. Stem height
reaching 2 meters, branches and petioles
densely pilose and scabrous. Leaves
alternate, twice oddly pinnate-compound,
leaflets ovate-rounded, apexes acuminate,
bases rounded, margins dentate. In the
fall, small white flowers appearing terminally to form compound umbellate inflorescences.
Berry globose, black when ripe.

Properties and action: Has warming properties, acrid to taste. Relieves flatulence,
removes moisture, and alleviates pain.

Conditions most used for: (1) Rheumatoid
arthralgia, headache; (2) jaundice,
gastroenteritis.

Preparation: Roots and stems are used
medicinally, 1-2 liang each time, in
decoction.

470. P'u-kung-ying [Dandelion]

Family: Compositae

Scientific name: Taraxacum mongolicum
Hand-Mazt.

Synonyms: "Huang-hua ti-ting" [yellow-
flowered 'violets'], "ju-chi ts'ao"
[milky grass], "ai-chiao p'u-kung-ying"
[short-legged dandelion].

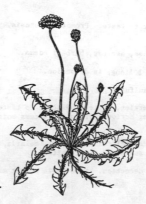

Morphology: Perennial herb. Found
growing along village outskirts, embankments, and damp roadsides. Height 25 cm,
whole stem containing white milky fluid.
Leaves covering the ground, clustered,
oblanceolate, apexes mucronate, bases
narrowing like petioles, margins irregularly serrated or shallow-parted. In
spring, flower styles emerging from leaf
cluster, with terminal yellow capitate
flowers. Fruit an achene, with slender
cylinder extending from apex, characterized by pappus at tip.

Properties and action: Has "han" cold
properties, bitter yet pleasant to taste.
Clears fevers and detoxifies, breaks up
congestion, strengthens the stomach and
stimulates milk flow.

Conditions most used for: (1) Mastitis,
boils and abscesses; (2) stomach-ache;
(3) inadequate milk supply.

Preparation: The whole plant is used
medicinally, 3-5 ch'ien each time, in
decoction

471. Lei-kung T'eng [Thunder God vine]

Family: Celastraceae

Scientific name: Tripterygium wilfordii
Hook. F.

Synonyms: "Huang-t'eng ken" [yellow-vine
root], "shui-mang ts'ao," "huang-yao,"
"tuan-ch'iang ts'ao" [intestines-breaking
grass], "shiu-nao-tzu ken," "huang-la
t'eng [yellow wax-vine], "sha-ch'ung
yao" [insect-killing drug], "nan-t'o ken,"
"La-hsin men" (Miao minority dialect),
"san-leng hua" [three- angled flower],
"tsao-ho hua" [early-rice flower].

Morphology: Deciduous shrublike vine.
Mostly found growing along field edges,
ditch edges, and stream banks. Small
branches angled, surface reddish-brown,
with small tubercle projections. Leaves
alternate, oval to broad-ovate, apexes
acute or acuminate, bases almost rounded
or slightly cuneate, margins finely serrate, with short petioles. In summer,
small white flowers appearing terminally
or axillary to form panicle inflorescences.
Fruit a samara, membranous, 3-angled.

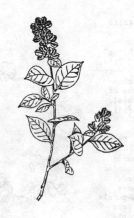

Properties and action: Bitter tasting,
highly toxic. Reduces inflammation,
detoxifies, kills maggots and larvae,
poisons rats and birds [by baiting], and
destroys oncomelania snails.

Conditions most used for: (1) Waistband
ulcers; (2) pruritus.

Preparation: Roots, leaves, flowers or
fruits are used medicinally for external
purposes in suitable amounts. Do not
take internally.

472. Wu-shui Ko [Misty 'arrowroot']

Family: Urticaceae

Scientific name: Pouzolzia zeylanica
(L.) Benn.

Synonyms: "Cho-nung kao" [pus-sucking
ointment], "kuan ts'ai."

Morphology: Perennial herb. Mostly
found growing in wild places, field edges,
and moist damp places in open woods. Root
fleshy, spindle-shaped, sticky and smooth
to feel when crushed. Stem multibranching,
curved or prostrate. Leaves alternate,
coarse and thin on both surfaces, ovate
to ovate-lanceolate, apexes cuspidate or
obtuse, bases rounded, margins intact.
In summer, light green or purple flowers
appearing from leaf axils. Achene ovoid,
black and lustrous.

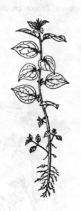

Properties and action: Has cooling properties, pleasant to taste. Draws out toxins
and promotes pus drainage, clears fevers
and hydrates.

Conditions most used for: (1) Urinary
tract infections; (2) dysentery, enteritis;
(3) boils, breast abscess, toothache.

Preparation: The whole plant is used
medicinally, 3 ch'ien to 1 liang, in
decoction.

473. Man-t'ien-hsing (T'ien Hu-t'o) [Sky-full-of-stars (heavenly coriander)]

Family: Umbelliferae

Scientific name: Hydrocotyle rotundifolia Roxb.

Synonyms: "I-tzu ts'ao," "p'ien-ti ch'ing" [green groundcover], "kuo-ting ts'ao," "p'o t'ung-ch'ien" [broken copper cash], "p'u-ti chin" [groundcover tapestry], "lo-ti chin-ch'ien" "szu-p'ien k'ung," [four-pieces of holes], "kuo-p'i ts'ao" [pot-scale grass], "tung-hsin mu," "hsi-p'i ts'ao" [tin-foil grass.]

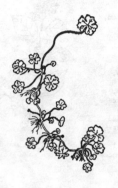

Morphology: Perennial slender herb. Found growing on shady and damp grasslands. Stem stoloniferous, adventitious roots growing from stem nodes. Leaves alternate, rounded or reniform, margins 5-7 shallow-parted, parted lobes with crenate margins, bases cordate. In summer, white or pinkish-purple flowers appearing from leaf axils to form umbellate inflorescences. Fruit a double cremocarp.

Properties and action: Cooling, pleasant to taste though slightly acrid. Clears fevers and detoxifies, hydrates, and re-solves mucus [formation].

Conditions most used for: (1) Colds and influenza, coughing and sore throat; (2) boils and abscesses; (3) jaundice and liver cirrhosis.

Preparation: The whole plant is used medicinally, 5 ch'ien to 2 liang each time, in decoction. Or a suitable amount of the fresh herb may be crushed and used for external application.

474. Lu-pien Ching (Lu-yueh Hsueh) [Roadside thorn (Snow in June)]

Family: Rubiaceae

Scientific name: Serissa foetida Comm.

Synonyms: "Tso-shan hu" [tiger-sitting-on-the-hill], "ch'ien-nien ai" [short-for-a-thousand years], "ch'ien-nien shu" [thousand-year tree], "pai-hua shu" [white-flower tree], "tieh-hsien shu" [wire tree], "lu-pien ts'ao" [roadside grass], "lu-pien chi" [roadside chicken], "huang-yang nao" [yellow goat brain].

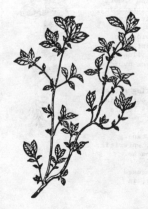

Morphology: Small semi-deciduous shrub. Found growing along fertile roadsides in wild places. Height reaching 1 meter, bark of stem grey, tender young branches sparsely downy. Leaves small, opposite, narrow oval, apexes acute or obtuse, bases gradually narrowing to form short petioles, margins intact, undersides covered by soft white hairs. Blooms in summer, several white flowers frequently clustered at branch terminals or leaf axils. Fruit a drupe, globose.

Properties and action: Neutral, acid to
taste. Expels flatulence and relieves
superficial symptoms, clears fevers and
helps maintain fluid balance.

Conditions most used for: (1) Influenza,
headache, hemialgic headache [caused by
malevolent excesses reaching one side
of the head via meridian passageways],
infantile convulsions, difficult eruption
of measles rash; (2) acute and chronic
hepatitis; (3) enteritis and diarrhea.

Preparation: The whole plant is used
medicinally, 3-5 ch'ien each time, in
decoction.

475. Ai fi-ch'a (Tz'u-chin niu) [Ardisia species (Myrsine)]

Family: Myrsinaceae

Scientific name: Ardisia japonica Bl.

Synonyms: "P'ing-ti mu" [level-land tree],
"ai ch'a-feng" [short tea-wind], "liang-
san kai chen-chu" [parasol-over-a-pearl],
"ch'ien-nien ai" [thousand years short],
"lao-pu-ta" [becoming-older-but-not-bigger].

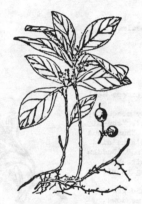

Morphology: Small evergreen shrub. Found
growing wild beneath woodland shade or in
shrub thickets. Whole plant somewhat short
and small. Subterranean stem stoloniferous,
dull red. Above-ground stem erect. Leaves
alternate, clustered at stem terminal, oval,
apexes acute, bases cuneate, margins finely
serrated. In summer, small white or pink
flowers appearing terminally or at leaf
axils. Fruit a globose drupe, red when
ripe.

Properties and action: Neutral, bitter
to taste. Stimulates blood circulation,
detoxifies, and resolves phlegm.

Conditions most used for: (1) Traumatic
injuries, tuberculous hemoptysis; (2)
swollen and painful eyes [? conjunctivitis];
(3) pulmonary tuberculosis, pneumonia, and
various respiratory tract infections.

Preparation: The whole plant is used
medicinally, 5 ch'ien - 1 liang each
time, in decoction.

476. Lan-ho Lien [Andrographis species]

Family: Acanthaceae

Scientific name: Andrographis paniculata
Nees.

Synonyms: "I-chien-hsi" [happiness-at-
first-sight], "ch'uan-hsin lien" [through-
the-heart lotus], "jih-hsing ch'ien-li"
[thousand-li traveled in a day], "chan-
she chien" [snake-chopping sword], "szu-
fang lien," "Yin-tu ts'ao" [Indian grass].

Morphology: Annual herb. Transplanted and cultivated. Height reaching 1 meter. Stem oblong and angled, multibranching, somewhat enlarged at nodes. Leaves opposite, ovate-oval, apexes acuminate, bases cuneate, margins intact, short-petioled, shaped like a pepper leaf. In summer-fall, small white terminal and axillary flowers appearing to form cymose inflorescences. Fruit a capsule, long ellipsoid.

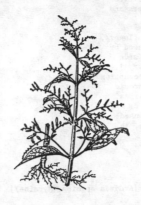

Properties and action: Has "han" cold properties, bitter to taste. Clears fever and detoxifies, reduces swelling and alleviates pain.

Conditions most used for: (1) Bacterial dysentery, gastroenteritis; (2) tonsillitis, pneumonia; (3) pyelonephritis; (4) abscesses; (5) poisonous snakebites.

Preparation: The whole plant is used medicinally, 2-5 ch'ien each time, in decoction. For external use, a tincture extract is applied over affected parts.

477. Shu-ch'u Ts'ao [Cudweed species]

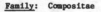

Family: Compositae

Scientific name: Gnaphalium multiceps Wall

Synonyms: "Shui wen-tzu" [swampy mosquito], "shu-erh ts'ao" [rat's ear grass], "shu-mi ai," "shui kao" [aquatic sedge], "huang-hua ts'ao" [yellow-flower grass], "p'a ts'ai" [cultivator greens], "Fu-erh ts'ao" [Buddha's ear grass], "pai-t'ou ts'ao" [white-head grass], "shui-ch'u," "ch'ing-ming ts'ai."

Morphology: Biennial herb. Found growing on hillsides, on arid lands and meadows. Stem erect, frequently branching from base and clustered, height 10-40 cm, covered densely by soft white hairs. Leaves alternate, basal leaves spatulate, upper-section leaves spatulate to linear-oblanceolate, apexes rounded-obtuse or slightly acute, bases gradually narrowing, margins undulate. In late spring, yellow flowers appearing from stem cluster to form umbellate-racemose inflorescences. Achenes small, pappi present.

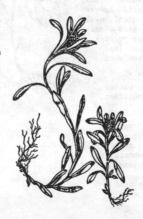

Properties and action: Has slightly warming properties, acrid to taste. Warms the lungs and eases breathing, resolves phlegm and stops coughing.

Conditions most used for: (1) Influenza, sore throat, productive coughing (with much mucus); (2) rheumatoid arthralgia, traumatic injuries; (3) leukorrhea, seminal emission; (4) hives, weeping pruritus of the skin.

Preparation: The whole plant is used medicinally, 5 ch'ien to 1 liang each time, in decoction.

478. La-liao Ts'ao [Shui Liao] [Common smartweed (Water smartweed)]

Family: Polygonaceae

Scientific name: Polygonum hydropiper Linn.

Synonyms: "Hung la-liao" [red smartweed], "han liao" [aridity resistant smartweed], "ping-yao ts'ao."

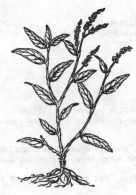

Morphology: Annual herb. Found growing mostly in shady and damp places along the water's edge. Height reaching 90 cm, the whole plant covered by glandular dots and downy fuzz. Stem erect, usually light reddish-purple, few branches, nodes enlarged. Leaves alternate, broadly lanceolate, apexes acuminate, bases cuneate, margins intact, surfaces covered by ∧-shaped black spots, ochrea thin and membranaceous, margins scabrous. In summer, flower style emerging from branch terminal and presenting small pink flowers in spike inflorescences. Achene 3-angled, envelope retained in calyx.

Properties and action: Has warming properties, acrid and bitter to taste. Removes moisture and resolves indigestion, strengthens the stomach and stops diarrhea.

Conditions most used for: (1) Bacterial dysentery, enteritis; (2) heat stroke, rheumatoid arthralgia.

Preparation: The whole plant is used medicinally, 1 liang each time, in decoction.

479. Chi-li [Caltrop]

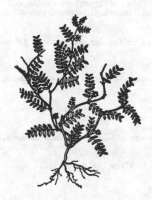

Family: Zygophyllaceae

Scientific name: Tribulis terrestris L.

Synonyms: "Tzu," "pai chi-li" [white caltrop], "la-chi-li" [prickly caltrop].

Morphology: Annual herb. Found growing wild along roadsides and stream embankments. Whole plant covered by white downy hairs. Steam creeping, multibranching, as long as 1 meter, superficially grooved. Leaves opposite, evenly pinnate-

compound, leaflets 5-7 pairs, long-oval,
leaflets at both ends somewhat smaller than
those in central portion, apexes acute,
bases varying, margins intact. Blooms in
summer, yellow flowers. Schizocarp consisting of 4-5 segments, each segment
resembling a triangular hatchet, with
many short and hard prickly spines,
yellowish-green, covering thick and tough.

Properties and action: Has warming
properties, bitter to taste. Neutralizes
the liver and dispels flatulence, clears
the lungs and overcomes moisture, stimulates blood circulation.

Preparation: Fruits are used medicinally,
3-5 ch'ien each time, in decoction.

480. Ch'un [Cedrela chinensis Juss.

Properties and action: Has "han" cooling properties, bitter and biting to
taste. Clears fever, "dries" moisture, cleanses the intestines, and arrests
bleeding.

Conditions most used for: Diarrhea, chronic dysentery, flatulence, bloody
stools, seminal emission, leukorrhea, metrorrhea, metrorrhagia, gonorrhea.

Preparation: Bark is used medicinally. For each dose, 2-3 ch'ien, in
decoction.

481. Huai [Sophora japonica]

Properties and action: Slightly "han" cold, bitter to taste. Cools blood
and stops bleeding, clears fevers and "moisturizes."

Conditions most used for: Hematemesis, epistaxis, bloody stools, hemorrhoids,
bloody dysentery, metrorrhagia, wind-caused fever, "red" eyes [conjunctivitis ?]
nervous agitation and apprehension, dizziness, moist pruritus of genitals.

Preparation: For each dose, 1.5 to 4 ch'ien, in decoction. (Buds, flowers,
and legumes of the sophora can all be used medicinally.)

482. Hua-shih [Talc]

Properties and action: Has "han" cold properties, pleasant to taste. Clears
fevers and promotes diuresis, relieves summer heat and releases moisture.

Conditions most used for: Restlessness and thirst due to summer heat, "moisture-heat" jaundice, bloody discharge, hematuria and painful penis, dysen-
tery-related edema, weeping dermatitis.

Preparation: For each dose, 2-5 ch'ien in decoction.

483. Suan [Leek]

Properties and action: Warming and acrid to taste. Warms the central [organs],
and opens up stoppages, cleanses intestines and kills worms.

Conditions most used for: Diarrhea and dysentery, colds and stopped-up noses,
tuberculosis-associated coughing, ascariasis-caused abdominal pain, ringworm,
boils and abscesses.

Preparation: For each dose, 1-3 ch'ien, or 1-3 onions, in decoction or chewed
and swallowed.

484. Lei-yuan [Omphalia lapidecens, a parasitic fungus found growing on
roots of the bamboo]

Properties and action: Has "han" cold properties, bitter-tasting, slightly
toxic. Kills worms and eliminates marasmus.

Conditions most used for: Hookworm disease, tapeworm disease, roundworm
disease, and marasmus.

Preparation: For each dose, 1-3 ch'ien, in decoction.

485. Shu-fu Ch'ung [Sow bug commonly found under bottom of crocks and in dirt; literally, a louse found on rats; also called ground louse.]

Properties and action: Has warming properties, sour to taste. Resolves blood clots and bruises, eliminates disease symptoms, and aids diuresis.

Conditions most used for: Amenorrhea symptoms, abdominal cramps, chronic malaria, difficult urination, edema.

Preparation: For each dose, 3 fen to 1 ch'ien, in decoction, or pulverized and mixed with boiled water.

486. Peng-sha [Borax]

Properties and action: Cooling, pleasant yet salty to taste. Clears fevers, resolves phlegm, detoxifies.

Conditions most used for: Sore throat, dental abscess and/or pyorrhea, canker sores, fever blisters, eye ailments, ulcerations etc.

Preparation: Mostly for external use. (Care should be taken when taken internally for relief of hiccups and as expectorant to bring up sputum, in amounts of 0.5-1 ch'ien for each dose.)

487. Feng-fang [Beehive]

Properties and action: Neutral, pleasant to taste, toxic. Relieves flatulence, counteracts toxicity, and kills worms.

Conditions most used for: Convulsions, epilepsy, hidden rashes and pruritus; and for external treatment of discharging scrophula, bleeding hemorrhoids, toothache, bee stings and insect bites.

Preparation: For internal use, 0.8 to 1.5 ch'ien in decoction, for each dose. For external purposes, use an appropriate amount.

488. Fu-shui Ts'ao [Ascites grass]

Family: Scrophulariaceae

Scientific name: Botryopleuron axillare Hemsl.

Synonyms: "Tiao-kan-feng," "tiao-ju t'eng" [fishing vine], "tiao-ju kan" [fishing pole], "hsien-jen ta-ch'iao" [fairies-building-a-bridge], "mei-hsieh shen-chin" [plum-leaves-extending-muscles], "chin-chi wei" [golden chicken tail], "tiao-ch'ien ts'ao" [charm-hanging grass], "tao-kua feng," "p'a-yen hung," "lao-chun tan," "tiao-kan wei," "tiao-kan ts'ao" [pole-hanging grass], "san-ch'ien tan," "hsiao tiao-kan ts'ao," "tiao-hsien feng."

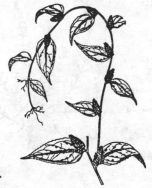

Morphology: Perennial herb. Found growing on hillsides and gulley edges. Stem slender and long, upper part vine-like, the upper section rooting wherever it touches the ground. Leaves alternate, long-oval or long-ovate, margins serrated. In fall, reddish-purple flowers appearing from leaf axils to form spike inflorescences. Capsule ovate-rounded.

Properties and action: Has warming properties, bitter and acrid to taste. Expels gas and detoxifies, stimulates blood circulation and reduces swelling, removes necrotic debri and promotes tissue regeneration, knits bones.

Conditions most used for: (1) Epidemic mumps, infected boils; (2) ascites; (3) rheumatoid arthralgia, traumatic injuries.

Preparation: The whole plant is used medicinally, 3-5 ch'ien each time, in decoction. For external purposes, a suitable amount is used.

489. Man Chu [?]-ma [Nettle species]

Family: Urticaceae

Scientific name: Momorialis hirta
Wedd.

Synonyms: "No-mi t'eng" [glutinous
rice vine], "no-fan t'eng."

Morphology: Perennial herb. Mostly
found growing along sunny stream banks,
in valleys and weed patches alongside
woodlands. Stem prostrate at base,
vinelike in its upper section, young
branches purplish. Leaves opposite,
long-ovate to ovate-lanceolate, apexes
acuminate, bases rounded, margins
intact, with 3 basal ribs. Blooms in
fall, small yellowish-white flowers
clustered around leaf axils. Achene
deltate-ovoid, black.

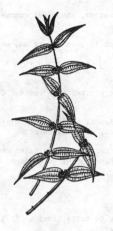

Properties and action: Has "han" cold
properties, sour and acrid to taste.
Clears fevers and detoxifies.

Conditions most used for: (1) Boils and
abscesses; (2) abdominal cramps in
females, leukorrhea.

Preparation: Roots, leaves or the whole
plant is used medicinally, 3 ch'ien to
1 liang each time, in decoction.

490. Ch'i-ku Ts'ao [Chickweed species]

Family: Carophyllaceae

Scientific name: Sagina maxima
A. Gray

Synonyms: "She-ya ts'ao" [snake-fang
grass], "ya-ch'ih tê'ao" [teeth grass],
"sha-tzu ts'ao" [sand grass], "pai-jih
ts'ao" [hundred-days grass].

Morphology: Biennial herb. Found
growing in gardens, along roadsides,
hilly slopes, and damp places along
stream banks. Stems clustered, multi-
branching at base, lower sections
prostrate, upper sections erect.
Leaves opposite, linear, apexes mucronate,
bases membranous, joining to form
short sheaths, margins intact. Blooms in
summer, terminal or axillary white
flowers. Capsule broadly ovate.

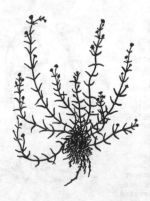

Properties and action: Has cooling
properties, sour yet pleasant to taste.
Reduces fevers and stimulates blood
circulation.

Conditions most used for: (1) "Angry"
boils, "lacquer" sores [allergic
dermatitis [?]; (2) dental caries; (3)
snakebites; (4) traumatic injuries;
(5) pterygiums.

Preparation: The whole plant is used
medicinally, 3 ch'ien to 1 liang in
decoction.

491. Hsi Ch'ien [Siegesbekia species]

Family: Compositae

Scientific name: Siegesbeckia orientalis
Linn var. pubescens Makino

Synonyms: "Chu-kuan ma-hsieh" [hog's-
head-hemp-leaves], "chu-mu-niang" [sow's
greens], "szu-ling ma" [4-angled sesame
seed ?], "ta-chieh-ku" [big bone-con-
nector], "nien-nien ts'ai" [sticky greens].

Morphology: Annual herb. Found growing
mostly on hilly roadsides. Stem erect,
height reaching 1.5 meters, with striped
furrows, covered densely by long greyish
white pilose or glandular hairs. Leaves
opposite, ovate-oval, apexes acuminate,
bases cuneate, extending below to form
wings. In the fall, terminal yellow
flowers in racemose inflorescences arranged in panicle pattern, outer row of
bracteal leaves covered by glandular hairs,
easily attached to clothing. Achene 4-
angled.

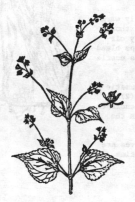

Properties and action: Has "han" cold
properties, bitter to taste, slightly
toxic. Dispels gas and opens up "lo"
passageways, stimulates blood circulation and alleviates pain, resolves
"moisture" heat.

Conditions most used for: Rheumatoid arthritis,
pains and aches in sides and legs, hemiplegia;
(2) hypertension, sciatica; (3) weeping
dermatitis, mastitis.

Preparation: The whole plant is used
medicinally, 3-5 ch'ien each time, in
decoction. Or, the plant may be mixed with
wine and "sun-dried evaporated" for further
refinement into pills which are taken 3
for a dose.

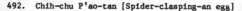

492. Chih-chu P'ao-tan [Spider-clasping-an egg]

Family: Liliaceae

Scientific name: Aspidistra elatior
Blume.

Synonyms: "Kan-shan pien" [rushing-over-
the-mountain whip], "niu-mao shen ken,"
"pein-tan shen-ken," "chiu-lung p'an"
[nine dragon disks], "liao-hsieh shen-ken"
[smartweed leaves extending sinews], "ta
shen-ken," "yao-pien chu," "lung-ku
ts'ao" [dragon-bone grass], "chu-chieh·
shen-ken," "tieh ma-pien" [iron horsewhip],
"kan-hsin wu-sung" [contented centipede],
"chu-ken ch'i," "ti wu-sung" [ground centi-
pede], "chiu-chieh lung" [nine-section
dragon], "wu-sung ts'ao" [centipede grass],
"I-ts'un shih-pa chieh."

Morphology: Perennial herb. Found mostly growing along roadsides, along ditches, and under trees. Underground stem creeping, ochreae clasping stem between nodes. Leaves coriaceous, oval-lanceolate or lanceolate, apexes acute, bases narrowing, parallel ribs 8-12, petioled. Blooms in summer, purple solitary flowers growing from leaf axils closer to the ground. Berry globose.

Properties and action: Has slightly warming properties, pleasant to taste, though slightly biting. Stimulates energy circulation, steps up blood flow, stops bleeding, reduces fever, and strengthens muscle and bones.

Conditions most used for: (1) Traumatic injuries, sore muscles and bones; (2) diarrhea, abdominal cramps; (3) amenorrhea and abdominal cramps; (4) stones in the urinary tract.

Preparation: Roots, stems, or leaves are used medicinally, 3-5 ch'ien each time, in decoction.

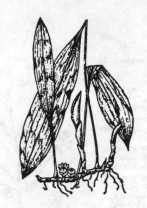

493. Suan Chiang [Winter-cherry]

Family: Solanaceae

Scientific name: Physalis alkekengi L.

Synonyms: "Hung-t'ien p'ao-tzu" [sky-red bubbles], "t'ien p'ao tzu" [heavenly bubbles], "t'ien p'ao ts'ao" [heavenly bubble grass], "hung ku-niang" [little red maid], "teng-lung kuo" [lantern fruit], "kua-chin-teng" [hanging golden lamp].

Morphology: Perennial herb. Mostly found growing on field edges, along roadsides, and in wild places. Subterranean stem creeping, stem erect, longitudinally angled, leaves alternate, broadly ovate, apexes apiculate, margins irregularly notched and coarsely dentate, bases broadly cuneate, extending below to form petioles. Blooms in summer, solitary white flowers growing from leaf axils. Berry globose, blood-red when ripe, enclosed within expanded and drooping lantern-like calyx.

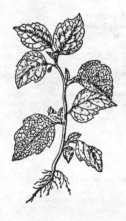

Properties and action: Has "han" cold properties, pleasant and sour to taste. Clears fevers, promotes diuresis, and resolves phlegm.

Conditions most used for: (1) Pemphigus, boils and abscesses; (2) diabetes, jaundice; (3) gas pains; (4) swollen sore throat, pertussis, dysentery.

Preparation: Roots, leaves, and fruits are used medicinally. For external use, a suitable amount. Or, for internal use, 1-3 ch'ien prepared in decoction. The whole plant has a purging effect. Overdose easily precipitates abortion.

494. Ch'iang-wei mei [Bramble species]

Family: Rosaceae

Scientific name: Rubus roseafolius
Smith.

Synonyms: "K'ung-hsin t'eng" [hollow
vine], "mao-tzu p'ao" [headgear bubble],
"huo-shang p'ao" [burn-injury bubble],
"szu-yueh p'ao" [April bubble].

Morphology: Deciduous prickly shrub.
Found growing on hillsides, in gulleys,
rock seams, and base of walls. Stem
erect or inclined, branches fragile
and weak, covered at random by short
thorns. Leaves alternate, oddly pinnate-compound, leaflets 5-11, ovate-

495. Fei-tzu [Torreya nucifera]

Properties and action: Neutral, pleasant to taste, yet biting. Kills
worms, eliminates stoppages [marasmuc caused], exerts laxative action.

Conditions most used for: Abdominal pain due to intestinal worms, constipation associated with hemorrhoids.

Preparation: For each dose, 3-5 ch'ien, or 10-20 seeds, in decoction.

496. Tzu-shih [Loadstone; magnetite]

Properties and action: Has "han" cold properties, acrid to taste. Relieves
convulsions and calms nerves, subdues the yang and restores energy.

Conditions most used for: Tinnitus and deafness associated with gonad
deficiency, dizziness and blurred vision, epilepsy, palpitation and insomnia,
anemia, senile shortness of breath.

Preparation: For each dose, 3 ch'ien to 1 liang, in decoction.

497. Ch'an T'ui [Cicada molting, the exuviae or outer shell shed by the
insect when it grows a new coat]

Properties and action: Has "han" cold properties, salty yet pleasant to
taste. Reduces fevers, clears the lungs, and relieves spasms.

Conditions most used for: Fever in influenza, coughing and hoarseness, sore
throat, hives and measles, infantile nocturnal fretfulness, spasms, tetanus.

Preparation: For each dose, 1-2 ch'ien, in decoction.

498. Suan Tsoa-jen [Seeds of Zizyphus vulgaris, Lamm var. spinosa Bunge]

Properties and action: Neutral, sour to taste. Calms nerves, soothes.

Conditions most used for: Nervous exhaustion and insomnia, apprehension and
forgetfulness, dizziness, chamminess.

Preparation: For each dose, 2-4 ch'ien, in decoction.

lanceolate, apexes acuminate, bases rounded;
lower venations, leaf axis, and petioles
all covered at random by prickly thorns
and glandular hairs. Blooms in summer-
fall, terminal white flowers. Drupe
ovate-globoid, bright red when ripe.

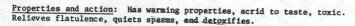

Properties and action: Neutral and sour-
tasting. Reduces inflammation, detoxifies, and alleviates pain.

Conditions most used for: (1) Infantile convulsions; (2) scalding burns;
(3) broken [amputated] fingers.

Preparation: Roots and leaves are
used medicinally, 3-5 ch'ien each
time, in decoction. For external
purposes, a suitable amount is used.

499. Wu-sung [Centipede]

Properties and action: Has warming properties, acrid to taste, toxic.
Relieves flatulence, quiets spasms, and detoxifies.

Conditions most used for: Infantile convulsions, spasms and cramps, lockjaw,
incoordination, erysipelas and scrophula, traumatic infections, "angry"
boils and snakebites.

Preparation: For each dose, 1-3 centipedes or 3 fen to 1 ch'ien, in decoction.

500. Pin-lang [Betelnut Areca catechu Linne]

Properties and action: Has warming properties, bitter, acrid, and biting to
taste. Kills worms and relieves stoppages, loosens energy stagnation for
smooth elimination of stools, aids diuresis and conversion of moisture.

Conditions most used for: Indigestion and fullness, abdominal pain due to
worms, energy stagnation in chest and abdomen, diarrhea and dysentery [con-
tinuous urge "to go"], beriberi edema, malaria.

Preparation: For each dose, 1.5-3 ch'ien, in decoction.

501. Chiang-lang ch'ugn [Dung beetle]

Properties and action: Has "han" cold properties, salty to taste, and toxic.
Quiets convulsions, dissipates clots and bruises, counteracts toxicity.

Conditions most used for: Convulsions and mania, hemorrhoidal bleeding, boils
and abscesses.

Preparation: For each dose, 3-8 fen, in decoction. For external purposes,
use an appropriate amount.

502. Chang [Camphor tree]

Family: Lauraceae

Scientific name: Cinnamonum camphora
(L.) Neeset Eberm.

Synonyms: "Hsiang chang" [fragrant
camphor], "niao chang," "pen chang,"
"fang chang" [aromatic camphor], "yu
chang" [oil camphor], "hou chang-mu."

503. Chieh Ts'ao [Valerian species, garden heliotrope]

Family: Valerianaceae

Scientific name: Valeriana officinalis
L.

Synonyms: "Ou chieh-ts'ao" [Europian
valerian], "shan she."

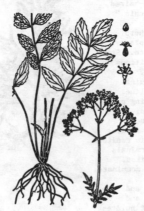

Morphology: Perennial herb. Found growing on sunny mountain locations. Root
emitting a characteristic odor. Stem
erect. Height 80-100 cm, with purple
keeled lines. Stem leaves opposite,
merging with short and broad ochreae,
leaves oddly pinnate-compound, divided
into numerous (4 to 10 pairs) segments;
upper segments curved-lanceolate, lower
segments ovate-rounded, both edges deeply
serrated; basal leaves with long petioles.
Blooms in fall, terminal compound cymose
inflorescences presenting small pink
flowers. Achene with pappus.

Properties and action: Has warming
properties, bitter and acrid to taste,
emitting characteristic odor. Carminative,
antispasmodic, and antipyretic.

Conditions most used for: (1) Influenza,
rheumatism; (2) neurasthenia, apprehension and insomnia; (3) traumatic injuries.

Preparation: Roots are used medicinally,
3-5 ch'ien in decoction each time. Or
crushed pulverized root 1-2 ch'ien, mixed
in boiled water to be taken by mouth.

504. Ch'u [Tree of Heaven]
Family: Simarubaceae

Scientific name: Ailanthus altissima
Swingle.

Synonyms: "Ch'ou-ch'un" [stinky quassia],
"hung-ch'un" [red cedrela], "mu-lung shu"
[wooden-mill tree].

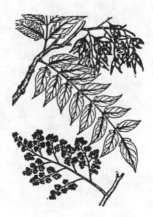

Morphology: Large deciduous tree. Growing wild in uplands. Height over 20
meters. Tree bark grey, with straight
cracked lines. Leaves alternate, oddly
pinnate compound, leaflets 13-25, ovate-
lanceolate, apexes acuminate, bases
broadly cuneate, margins intact or slightly
undulate. Blooms in summer, small greenish-white terminal flowers forming panicle
inflorescences. Samara long ellipsoid.

Properties and action: Has "han" cold
properties, bitter and biting to taste.
Clears fevers and converts moisture,
cleanses, and stabilizes peristaltic
action.

Conditions most used for: (1) Chronic
dysentery, gassy and bloody stools;
(2) Metrorrhagia and leukorrhea, "wet
dreams" and seminal emission.

Preparation: Roots and bark are used
medicinally, 2-3 ch'ien each time, in
decoction.

505. P'u-ti Wu-sung [Ground-covering centipede; Clubmoss species]
Family: Lycopodiaceae

Scientific name: Lycopodium cernuum L.

Synonyms: "Shen-chin ts'ao" [sinew extending herb], "ho-chin ts'ao" [alloy herb], "lu-mao shen-chin" [green-haired sinew-extender], "feng-wei shen chin."

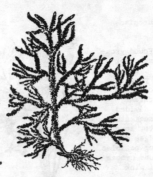

Morphology: Perennial evergree herb. Found growing on waste mountain places and meadows. Root yellowish-white. Stem prostrate on ground, with adventitious roots growing, numerous branches, stoloniferous at first, with terminal sections rising gradually on incline, as high as 60 cm, in fork-branching pattern. Leaves small, in spiralling arrangement, linear, pointed cone shape, apexes acuminate, margins showing numerous ciliate hairs. Sporangia reniform, sori attached to small branch terminals forming cylindrical sporangia spikes, sporangia leaves deltoid, apexes acuminate.

Properties and action: Neutral, and light and bland to taste. Expels gas and hydrates, relaxes muscles, and stimulates the "lo" passageways.

Conditions most used for: (1) Muscular spasms, leg cramps; (2) rheumatism aches and pains in muscles and bone, numbness of the four extremities; (3) traumatic falls, abscesses.

Preparation: The whole plant is used medicinally, 1-2 liang each time, decocted with water or sweet wine. For external use, a suitable amount is crushed and applied over affected parts.

506. Che-shih [Hematite]

Properties and action: Has "han" cold properties, bitter to taste. Impedes "retrograding" disease symptoms, cools the blood.

Conditions most used for: Vomiting, gagging, hiccups, asthma, hematemesis, epistaxis, flatulence, hemorrhoidal bleeding, metrorrhagia.

Preparation: For each dose, 3 ch'ien to 1 liang, in decoction.

507. Lou-ku [Mole cricket]

Properties and action: Has "han" cold properties, salty to taste. Promotes diuresis, eliminates edema.

Conditions most used for: Edema and difficult urination.

Preparation: For each dose, 1-2 crickets, roasted and pulverized, then mixed with boiled water before taken by mouth.

508. P'i-li [Fig species]

Family: Moraceae

Scientific name: Ficus pumila L.

Synonyms: "Mu-lien" [wood lotus], "t'ang man-t'ou" [sweet bun], "lo-shih t'eng," "man-t'ou kuo," "p'a-pi t'eng" [wall-climbing vine], "pang-pang tzu," "liang fen tzu," "kuei man-t'ou," "mu-kua [papaya], "shih-pi t'eng" [stone-wall vine], "pu-hsueh wang" [king of blood-building tonics], "chui-ku feng," "p'a-yen feng" [cliff-climbing wind], "kuo-ch'iang feng" [over-the-wall-wind].

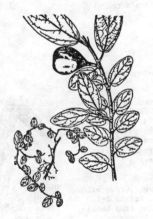

Morphology: Evergreen climbing vine. Found growing on uplands, rocks, trees, or walls. Stem prostrate or climbing, aerial roots growing frequently from nodes to support its growth while climbing on other objects. Leaves alternate, size covering a broad range, ovate or obovate, apexes obtuse-rounded, bases rounded or cordate, margins intact. Blooms in summer, flowers usually attached within floral receptacle, hypanthodium inflorescence pear-shaped, larger than a fig. Fruit a small nut.

Properties and action: Has "han" cold properties, bitter tasting. Clears fevers and detoxifies, counteracts moisture and promotes diuresis, allays thirst.

Conditions most used for: (1) Tuberculosis of the testicles, hernia, gonorrhea; (2) diarrhea, "heat"-caused dysentery; (3) backache, cancer.

Preparation: Stem or fruit peel is used medicinally, 5 ch'ien to 1 liang each time, in decoction.

509. I-I [Pearl barley; Job's tears]

Family: Graminea

Scientific name: Coix lachryma jobi L.

Synonyms: "Niao-tuan-tzu," "niao-chu-tzu" [urine pearl], "hui-hui mi" [every-time rice], "su chu ken," "he-yen-tzu shu" [blind man's tree], "t'u I-jen" [native barley], "ts'ui-sheng tzu" [labor-inducer], "shan I-mi" [mountain barley], "kuei-chu shu" [pearl barley], "pien-po chu," "liao ch'a-tzu," "ch'uan-hua-tzu."

Morphology: Perennial herb. Grows wild or cultivated. Stem erect, height 1-1.5 meters, aerial roots growing from basal nodes. Leaves alternate, linear to lanceolate, apexes acuminate, bases clasping stem, margins coarse and scabrous. Blooms in the fall, axillary spike inflorescences, staminate spikelets on top, in layered arrangement at each joint on the rachis; pistillate spikelets below, enclosed within the involucre, involucre ovoid or globoid, greyish-white when ripe. Fruit a caryopsis.

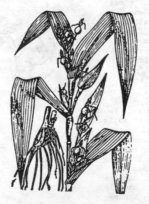

Properties and action: Has slightly "han" cold properties, pleasant and bland to taste. Strengthens the spleen, converts moisture, and promotes diuresis.

Conditions most used for: (1) Lung abscess, lobar pneumonia, appendicitis; (2) rheumatoid arthritis, beriberi; (3) diarrhea, edema, difficult urination.

Preparation: Seeds are used medicinally, 3-5 ch'ien each time, in decoction.

510. Po-ho [Mint species] Bo� ㅓㄷ

<u>Family</u>: Labiatae

<u>Scientific name</u>: Mentha arvensis L.

<u>Synonyms</u>: "Lung-nao po-ho" [camphor-mint],
"fan ho-ts'ai."

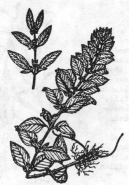

<u>Morphology</u>: Perennial herb. Mostly cul-
tivated. Whole plant emitting strong aroma.
Stem oblong, multibranching. Leaves
opposite, ovate-rounded to oblong-rounded
ovate, apexes acute, bases broadly cuneate,
margins serrated. Blooms in fall, purple,
pink, or white axillary flowers forming
verticillate inflorescences. Small nuts, 4.

<u>Properties and action</u>: Has cooling
properties, acrid to taste, aromatic.
Expels flatulence, clears fevers, promotes
perspiration and measles rash appearance,
reduces swelling and relieves itching.

<u>Conditions most used for</u>: (1) Influenza,
headache, cough; (2) incomplete measles
eruption, pharyngitis, conjunctivitis;
beriberi edema; (3) pruritus.

<u>Preparation</u>: The whole plant is used
medicinally, 5 fen to 3 ch'ien each time,
in decoction. For external use, the
fresh herb may be decocted, and fluid
used for bathing affected parts.

511. Chiao-ch'uang [Water-willow species]

<u>Family</u>: Acanthaceae

<u>Scientific name</u>: Justicia procumbens L.

Synonyms: "Chuang-yuan ts'ao" [highest
Hanlin scholar grass], "kan-chi ts'ao"
[marasmus grass], "chi-ku hsiang" [fragrant-
chicken bones], "chieh-chieh hung," "la-
tzu ts'ao" [pepper herb].

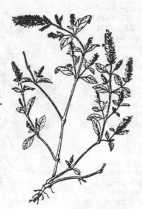

<u>Morphology</u>: Annual creeping herb. Found
growing in wild places, meadows, and damp
shady roadside spots. Whole plant pubescent.
Stem slightly oblong, 4-6 angled, nodes
expanded like knee-joints, mostly branching. Leaves opposite, ovate long-oval,
apexes acute or obtuse, bases obtuse,
margins intact. In the fall, axillary or
terminal inflorescences presenting with
small pink or purplish-red flowers. Linear
capsule, hairy.

<u>Properties and action</u>: Has "han" cold
properties, salty to taste. Reduces
fever, stimulates energy circulation,
relieves distention, clears the blood-
stream, removes moisture, and dissipates
swelling.

<u>Conditions most used for</u>: (1) Marasmus
in small children; (2) muscular and joint
pains, backache; (3) sore throat, canker
sores; (4) pressure sores, boils.

<u>Preparation</u>: The whole plant is used
medicinally, 3 ch'ien to 1 liang, in
decoction.

512. Ch'u-mai [Pink or carnation species]

Family: Carophyllaceae

Scientific name: Dianthus superbus Linn.

Synonyms: "Yeh-mai" [wild oats].

Morphology: Perennial herb. Found growing on hillsides, edges of open woods,
and weed patches along stream banks.
Stem clustered, height 30-60 cm, joints
protruding. Leaves opposite, linear-
lanceolate, apexes acute, bases clasping
stem, 3-5 ribbed. Blooms in the fall,
terminal pink flowers forming racemose
inflorescences. Capsule cylindrical.

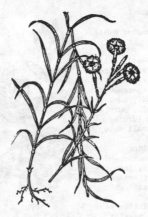

Properties and action: Has "han" cold
properties, bitter to taste. Clears
fever and promotes diuresis, stimulates
blood circulation and opens up meridian
passageways.

Conditions most used for: (1) Edema
and gonorrhea; (2) Irregular menstruation.

Preparation: The whole plant is used
medicinally, 3-5 ch'ien each time in
decoction.

513. Fan-pai Ts'ao [Cinquefoil species]

Family: Rosaceae

Scientific name: Potentilla discolor
Bunge.

Synonyms: "Yeh-chi pa," "t'u yang-shen"
[local ginseng], "t'u-ts'ai" [local herb],
"fu-ling ts'ao" [smilax herb], "lan-ch'i
pai-t'ou weng" [across-the-stream anemone],
"huang-hua ti-ting," [yellow-flowered
violet], "ti-ting," "ch'ien-ch'ui-ta"
[a thousand-hammerings], "chi-pa ch'ui,"
"chi-chao hsien."

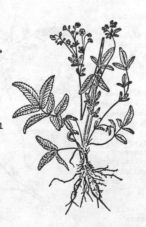

Morphology: Perennial herb. Found growing in virgin wilds, mountain slopes, and
uplands. Height reaching 30 cm. Perennial
roots thick and strong, spindle-shaped,
dull brown on surface. Basal leaves
clustered, prostrate, oddly pinnate-
compound, leaflets 5-9; Stem leaves
trifoliate compound, leaflets long oval,
margins serrated, dorsal surface covered
densely by soft white hairs, with long
petioles. Blooms in summer, terminal
yellow flowers in cymes. Small achene,
ovate or slightly reniform.

Properties and action: Cooling, pleasant
yet bitter to taste. Cools the blood and
detoxifies, stops bleeding and strengthens
the spleen.

Conditions most used for: (1) Hematemesis,
bloody stools, metrorrhagia; (2) enteritis,
dysentery.

Preparation: Roots are used medicinally,
1-2 liang each time, in decoction.

514. Huo-hsiang [Giant hyssop species]

Family: Labiatae

Scientific name: Agastache rugosa O. Kuntze.

Synonyms: "Hsing-jen hua" [almond blossoms].

Morphology: Annual herb. Growing wild on hillsides, stream banks, or cultivated in gardens. Height 1-1.5 meters. Whole plant emitting characteristic aroma. Stem erect, oblong. Leaves opposite, ovate or deltate, apexes acuminate, bases rounded or somewhat cordate, margins coarsely serrate, with long petioles. Blooms in summer-fall, small light purple flowers in racemose closely grouped like spikes. Nut long-oblong, yellow.

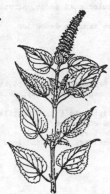

Properties and action: Has warming properties, pleasant yet acrid to taste. Clears fevers, resolves moisture, strengthens the stomach and stops vomiting.

Conditions most used for: (1) Wound injuries and summer moisture; (2) vomiting and diarrhea; (3) angina pains.

Preparation: Stems and leaves are used medicinally, 2-3 ch'ien each time, mixed with boiled water or in decoction.

515. Ou-chieh [Knotted separations in the nalumbo rootstock]

Properties and action: Neutral, pleasant yet biting to taste. Absorbs clots and bruises, stops bleeding.

Conditions most used for: Hematemesis, epistaxis, hemoptysis, bloody discharge, hematuria, bloody stools, bloody dysentery, metrorrhagia.

Preparation: For each dose, 1.5-3 ch'ien, in decoction.

516. Kao-pen [Nothosmyrnium japonicum Miq.]

Properties and action: Has warming properties, acrid to taste. Dispels excesses of wind [flatulence], "han" cold and moisture.

Conditions most used for: Wind-"han" cold headaches, "han" damp hernias, abdominal cramps and diarrhea. Used externally to treat ringworm and other fungus infections.

Preparation: For each dose, 8 fen to 2 ch'ien, in decoction. Use an appropriate amount for external application.

517. Chiang Ts'an [Dead silkworms]

Properties and action: Neutral, acrid and salty to taste. Relieves flatulence, resolves phlegm, loosens congestion, and stimulates meridian activity.

Conditions most used for: Apoplectic aphasia, convulsions, fever with phlegm present [bronchitis, pneumonia ?], headache, toothache, sore throat, numbness and spasms, eryispelas, tubercular cold sores, scrophula.

Preparation: For each dose, 1.5 to 3 ch'ien, in decoction.

518. Chang-lang [Mantis ?]

Properties and action: Has "han" cold properties, salty to taste, toxic. Resolves bruises and clots, reduces stoppages (marasmus), detoxifies.

Conditions most used for: Gonorrhea, diptheris [?], infantile marasmus, snake and insect bites, dysmenorrhea and abscesses.

Preparation: For each dose, use 3-5 mantises, heads and legs removed, then fried before eating.

519. Hsi-so [Cricket]

Properties and action: Has warming properties, acrid and salty to taste, toxic. Promotes diuresis.

Conditions most used for: Edema, difficult urination.

Preparation: For each dose, 5-6 crickets, toasted and crushed, mixed with boiled water, for taking by mouth.

520. Meng-shih [A mica type of mineral]

Properties and action: Neutral, pleasant and salty to taste. Expectorates sputum and lowers excess energy.

Conditions most used for: Raspy wheezing, convulsive spasms, resistant collection of phlegm in chest.

Preparation: For each dose, 3-5 ch'ien, in decoction.

521. Kuei-chia [Tortoise shell]

Properties and action: Neutral, salty to taste. Nourishes the yin and reduces fever, balances liver action and controls the yang, softens the hard and loosens up congestion.

Conditions most used for: Feverishness and aching bones, yin deficiency and flatulence, chronic fevers, malaria, stiffness of sides, movable "mass" in abdomen, amenorrhea, infantile convulsions.

Preparation: For each dose, 3-5 ch'ien, in decoction.

522. No-tao Ken [Roots of glutinous rice plant]

Properties and action: Has slightly warming properties, pleasant to taste. Counteracts perspiration and kills worms.

Conditions most used for: Drenching sweats, spontaneous hidrosis, filariasis.

Preparation: For each dose, 5 ch'ien to 1 chin, in decoction.

INDEX

A

Abdominal pain, 252, 80
Abscesses, 80
Acupuncture points, 98-125
Acupuncture therapy, 90-138
    ear acupuncture therapy, 127
    fluid puncture, 131
    incision therapy, 136
    "prick-open" therapy, 135
    suture implantation and ligation, 137-138
Adrenal glands, 11
Alkaline therapy, 139
Allergy tests, 143
Amebic dysentery, 310
Anemia, 401
Anesthetic agents, 150
Anesthesia, local infiltration, 149
Ankylostomiasis (hookworm), 343
Appendicitis, 439
Appendix, 22
Arthritis, 80, 81
    rheumatic, 383
    rheumatoid, 385, 139
Artificial respiration, 160
Ascarias (roundworm), 345
    in children, treatment by incision therapy, 136
    bile duct ascariasis, 444
Ascites (abdominal distension), 260, 22

B

Backache, 270, 81
Backstrain, 426
Bacterial dysentery, 307
Bandaging, 186
Bedbug elimination, 46
Beriberi, 409
Bile ducts, 22
Bile duct ascariasis, 444
Birth control, 173
Bleeding control, 182
    by pressure points, 184
    by pressure bandaging, 185
    by tourniquet, 185
Blood cells, 19
Blood circulation, 17
Blood-forming organs, 18
Blood letting, 80
Blood pressure, to check, 141
Blood vessels, 16

Boils, 428
Bone structure and function, 12
Bones stuck in throat, 217
Brain & cranial nerves, 9
Bronchial asthma, treatment by incision therapy, 136
Bronchitis, acute, 351
Bronchitis, chronic, 353
    treatment by incision therapy, 136
Bruises, 80
Bruise resorption, 76
Burns, 195-199

C

Calmette Guerin vaccine, 167
Calyces, 23
Cancer, 477-480
Carbon monoxide poisoning, 211
Carbuncles, 431
Cardiac massage, 162
Cardiac orifice, 21
Catarrhal headaches, 79
Cecum, 22
Cellulitis, 434
Chapping, 458
Chest pain, 238
Chicken pox, 291
Child delivery, 176
Children, characteristics of different systems, 26
Chills & fever, diagnosis of, 52
Chills, massaging acupuncture points, 86
Cholicystitis, acute (gallstones), 441
Circulatory system, 15
Cirrhosis of liver, 367
Colds, massaging acupuncture points, 86
Colic, 80, 521
Colon, 22
Conjunctivitis, acute (redeye), 539
Constipation, 249
    treatment by massaging acupuncture points, 86
Contraception, 173
    use of Chinese herbs, 173
    use of condoms, 174
    use of oral contraceptives, 174
    use of sterilization, 175
Convulsions, massaging acupuncture points, 86
    in children, treatment by moxibustion, 89
Corns & calluses, 460
Cortex, renal, 23
Coughing, 230
    types of, 230
    diagnosis of, 231
    treatment, 232

943

945

Trichiasis (eye pain), 545
Triple-warmer, 72
Tuberculosis, 300, 74
Tuberculosis of cervical nodes, 437
Tumors, 477-480
Tympanic distension, 73
Typhoid, 312

U

Ulcers, 364, 88, 136
Upper respiratory tract infections, 351
Urethra, 24
Ureters, 23
Urinary diseases, 372
    calculi in urinary system, 379
    glomerulonephritis, 372
    pyelonephritis, 377
    retention of urine, 380
Urinary system, 23
Urine, bloody, 282
Urine, diagnosis of, 53
Uterine bleeding, 494
Uterus, 24
    prolapse of, 497

V

Vagina, 24
Vaginal bleeding, 89
Vasectomy, 121
Visceral peritoneum, 22
Vomit-inducing method, 78
Vomiting, during pregnancy, 499
Vomiting, 242, 80, 87

W

Water sanitation, 35
Whooping cough, 292
Wound debridement, 153

Y

Yang deficiency, 75
Yang depletion, 74
Yang illness, 69
Yin deficiency, 75
Yin depletion, 74
Yin illness, 69